Pediatric and Adolescent Gynecology

Pediatric and Adolescent Gynecology

Editors

Sue Ellen Koehler Carpenter, M.D.

Assistant Professor, Department of
Gynecology and Obstetrics
Head, Section of Pediatric and Adolescent Gynecology
The Johns Hopkins University School of Medicine
Baltimore, Maryland

John A. Rock, M.D.

Professor, Departments of
Gynecology and Obstetrics, and Pediatrics
The Johns Hopkins University School of Medicine
and
Chairman, Department of Obstetrics and Gynecology
The Union Memorial Hospital
Baltimore, Maryland

Lippincott - Raven
PUBLISHERS
Philadelphia • New York

**Lippincott–Raven Publishers, 227 East Washington Square,
Philadelphia, Pennsylvania 19106**

Printed in the United States of America

9 8 7 6 5 4 3

Library of Congress Cataloging-in-Publication Data

Pediatric and adolescent gynecology/editors, Sue Ellen Koehler
Carpenter, John A. Rock.
p. cm.
Includes bibliographical references and index.
ISBN 0-88167-839-2
1. Pediatric gynecology. I. Carpenter, Sue Ellen Koehler.
II. Rock, John A.
[DNLM: 1. Adolescent Medicine. 2. Genital Diseases, Female—in adolescence. 3. Genital Diseases, Female—in infancy & childhood.
4. Pediatrics. WS 360 P3705]
RJ47P43 1991
618.92′098—dc20
DNLM/DLC
for library of Congress 91-33821

To our families

Contents

Contributors

Robert A. Ambros, M.D.
Assistant Professor
Department of Pathology
The Albany Medical College
Albany, New York 12208

Jean Anderson, M.D.
Assistant Professor
Department of Gynecology and Obstetrics
The Johns Hopkins University School of Medicine
600 North Wolfe Street
Baltimore, Maryland 21205

Ricardo Azziz, M.D.
Assistant Professor
Department of Obstetrics and Gynecology
Division of Reproductive Biology and Endocrinology
University of Alabama
619 South 19th Street
Birmingham, Alabama 35294

G. William Bates, M.D.
Vice President
Medical Education and Research
Greenville Memorial Hospital
701 Grove Road
Greenville, South Carolina 29605

Gary D. Berkovitz, M.D.
Assistant Professor
Department of Pediatrics
The Johns Hopkins University School of Medicine
600 North Wolfe Street
Baltimore, Maryland 21205

Sue Ellen Koehler Carpenter, M.D.
Assistant Professor
Department of Gynecology and Obstetrics
Head, Section of Pediatric and Adolescent Gynecology
Division of Reproductive Endocrinology
The Johns Hopkins University School of Medicine
600 North Wolfe Street
Baltimore, Maryland 21205

Sandra Ann Carson, M.D.
Assistant Professor
Department of Obstetrics and Gynecology
Chief, In Vitro Fertilization and Embryo Transfer
Division of Reproductive Endocrinology and Infertility
The University of Tennessee College of Medicine
956 Court Avenue
Memphis, Tennessee 38103

Andrew S. Cook, M.D.
Instructor, Department of Gynecology and Obstetrics
Division of Reproductive Endocrinology
The Johns Hopkins University School of Medicine
600 North Wolfe Street
Baltimore, Maryland 21205

Vanessa E. Cullins, M.D., MPH
Department of Obstetrics and Gynecology,
The Francis Scott Key Medical Center
and
Instructor, Department of Gynecology and Obstetrics
The Johns Hopkins University School of Medicine
4940 Eastern Avenue
Baltimore, Maryland 21224

Jeffrey L. Deaton, M.D.
Assistant Professor
Department of Obstetrics and Gynecology
Section on Reproductive Endocrinology
Bowman Gray School of Medicine
Winston-Salem, North Carolina 27157

David L. Dudgeon, M.D.
Professor of Surgery and Pediatrics
The Johns Hopkins University School of Medicine
600 North Wolfe Street
Baltimore, Maryland 21205

Michelle R. Dudzinski, M.D.
Assistant Professor
Department of Gynecology and Obstetrics
Division of Gynecologic Oncology
The Johns Hopkins University School of Medicine
600 North Wolfe Street
Baltimore, Maryland 21205

Peter J. Fagan, Ph.D.
Assistant Professor
Department of Psychiatry
Division of Medical Psychology
and
Director, Sexual Behaviors Consultation Unit
The Johns Hopkins University School of Medicine
550 North Broadway
Baltimore, Maryland 21205

John P. Gearhart, M.D.
Associate Professor
Department of Urology and Chief, Pediatric Urology
James Buchanan Brady Urological Institute
The Johns Hopkins University School of Medicine
600 North Wolfe Street
Baltimore, Maryland 21205

John S. Hesla, M.D.
Assistant Professor
Department of Gynecology and Obstetrics
Division of Reproductive Endocrinology
The Johns Hopkins University School of Medicine
600 North Wolfe Street
Baltimore, Maryland 21205

Ira R. Horowitz, M.D.
Assistant Professor
Departments of Gynecology and Obstetrics and Oncology
The Johns Hopkins University School of Medicine, and
Director, Division of Gynecologic Oncology
Department of Gynecology and Obstetrics
The Union Memorial Hospital
Baltimore, Maryland 21218

George R. Huggins, M.D.
Chairman
Department of Obstetrics and Gynecology
The Francis Scott Key Medical Center
Associate Professor, Department of Gynecology and Obstetrics
The Johns Hopkins University School of Medicine
4940 Eastern Avenue
Baltimore, Maryland 21224

Eugene Katz, M.D.
Assistant Professor
Department of Obstetrics and Gynecology
Division of Reproductive Endocrinology
The University of Maryland
405 West Redwood Street
Baltimore, Maryland 21201

William R. Keye, Jr., M.D.
The Beaumont Hospital Fertility Center
2662 Luckey John Drive
Royal Oak, Michigan 81432

Joel S. Krasnow, M.D.
Assistant Professor
Department of Obstetrics and Gynecology
Women's Endocrine Division
University of Wisconsin
Madison, Wisconsin 53792

Robert J. Kurman, M.D.
The Richard W. TeLinde Professor of Gynecologic Pathology
Professor
Departments of Gynecology and Obstetrics and Pathology
The Johns Hopkins University School of Medicine
600 North Wolfe Street
Baltimore, Maryland 21205

Claude J. Migeon, M.D.
Professor
Department of Pediatrics
Director, Division of Endocrinology
The Johns Hopkins University School of Medicine
600 North Wolfe Street
Baltimore, Maryland 21205

John Money, Ph.D.
Professor Emeritus
Department of Psychiatry
Division of Medical Psychology
The Johns Hopkins University School of Medicine
1235 East Monument Street
Baltimore, Maryland 21202

John E. Niederhuber, M.D.
Chairman
Department of Surgery
Stanford University School of Medicine
MSOB X-228, MC 5408
Stanford University Medical Center
Stanford, California 94305

Charles Paidas, M.D.
Assistant Professor
Department of Pediatric Surgery
The Johns Hopkins School of Medicine
600 North Wolfe Street
Baltimore, Maryland 21205

Donald E. Pittaway, M.D., Ph.D.
Associate Professor
Department of Obstetrics and Gynecology
Section on Reproductive Endocrinology
Bowman-Gray School of Medicine
Winston-Salem, North Carolina 27103

Leslie Plotnick, M.D.
Associate Professor
Department of Pediatrics
The Johns Hopkins University School of Medicine
600 North Wolfe Street
Baltimore, Maryland 21205

Janet S. Rader, M.D.
Assistant Professor
Department of Obstetrics and Gynecology
Division of Gynecologic Oncology
Washington University School of Medicine
St. Louis, Missouri 63110

John A. Rock, M.D.
Chairman
Department of Gynecology and Obstetrics
The Union Memorial Hospital
Professor
Department of Gynecology and Obstetrics
The Johns Hopkins University School of Medicine
600 North Wolfe Street
Baltimore, Maryland 21205

Ricardo Sainz de la Cuesta
Chief Resident
The Union Memorial Hospital
Baltimore, Maryland 21218

Sander S. Shapiro, M.D.
Professor
Department of Obstetrics and Gynecology
Director
Women's Endocrine Division
University of Wisconsin
1300 University Avenue
Madison, Wisconsin 53706

Joe Leigh Simpson, M.D.
Faculty Professor and Chairman
Department of Obstetrics and Gynecology
University of Tennessee College of Medicine
853 Jefferson Avenue
Memphis, Tennessee 38163

Melinda B. Stein, Ph.D.
Instructor
Department of Psychiatry
The Johns Hopkins University School of Medicine
Division of Medical Psychology
Francis Scott Key Medical Center
4940 Eastern Avenue
Baltimore, Maryland 21224

Sergio C. Stone, M.D.
Professor
Department of Obstetrics and Gynecology
Division of Reproductive Endocrinology and Infertility
University of California Irvine Medical Center
College of Medicine
100 The City Drive South
Orange, California 92668

Bruce L. Tjaden, M.D.
Instructor
Department of Obstetrics and Gynecology
Division of Reproductive Endocrinology
The Johns Hopkins University School of Medicine
600 North Wolfe Street
Baltimore, Maryland 21205

Eric A. Wiebke, M.D.
Indiana University
Department of Surgery
Indiana University Medical Center
545 Barnhill Drive
Indianapolis, Indiana 46202-5124

Carol A. Wilson, Ph.D.
Assistant Professor
School of Health, Physical Education, and Recreation
University of Nevada, Las Vegas
Las Vegas, Nevada 89154

Michele D. Wilson, M.D.
Assistant Professor
Department of Pediatrics
The Johns Hopkins University School of Medicine
600 North Wolfe Street
Baltimore, Maryland 21205

Lawrence S. Wissow, M.D., MPH
Assistant Professor
Department of Pediatrics
Director, Child Advocacy
The Johns Hopkins University School of Medicine
600 North Wolfe Street
Baltimore, Maryland 21205

J. Donald Woodruff, M.D.
Professor Emeritus
Department of Gynecology and Obstetrics
Johns Hopkins University School of Medicine
600 North Wolfe Street
Baltimore, Maryland 21205

Preface

This book brings a multidisciplinary approach to the gynecologic care of infants, children, and adolescents. The editors are truly fortunate to have outstanding contributors from the fields of pediatrics, urology, psychology, surgery, and gynecology discuss the recognition and treatment of medical illness in these specific age groups. The pathophysiology of disease is stressed. Knowledgeable handling of pediatric patients requires a background in genetics and developmental biology. Genital examination requires forethought and gentleness, particularly in children, so variations from a standard examination are discussed. Ultrasonography and laparoscopy have enhanced our ability to diagnosis routine gynecologic complaints of children and adolescents, but new norms for their use must be established.

Pediatric and adolescent gynecology is an emerging specialty. Since the broadest definition of adolescence includes the psychologic, mental, and social growth, as well as physical maturation, that begins with the appearance of secondary sexual characteristics and terminates with the cessation of somatic growth. Thus, this subspecialty has appealed to family practitioners, pediatricians, urologists, and reproductive endocrinologists.

The fertility potential and gynecologic and psychosexual health of our youngest patients must be protected, there is a great need to provide quality care for a wide variety of complaints. We hope this book will assist these providing quality care for gynecologic complaints in infants, children, and adolescents.

Sue Ellen Koehler Carpenter, M.D.
John A. Rock, M.D.

Acknowledgments

We would like to acknowledge the assistance of Ann Terry, Janice Scott, and Donna Knoll in preparation of this manuscript. We are especially grateful to the many fine contributors whose experience and research is represented in this book.

Pediatric and Adolescent Gynecology

Pediatric and Adolescent Gynecology,
edited by S. E. Carpenter and J. A. Rock.
Raven Press, Ltd., New York © 1992.

1

Genetics of Sexual Differentiation

Joe Leigh Simpson

Department of Obstetrics and Gynecology, University of Tennessee at Memphis, Memphis, Tennessee 38163

Abnormalities in sexual differentiation may involve gonads, genital ducts, or external genitalia. These abnormalities are usually manifested either at birth or at the expected time of puberty. The pediatric and adolescent gynecologist is usually called upon to help diagnose and manage affected individuals. In this chapter, we will emphasize the genetic basis of sexual differentiation, as delineated and illustrated through clinical perturbations. Clinical management is discussed in greater detail elsewhere, including other chapters of this volume.

This chapter inevitably reflects the author's other recent reviews on the subject (1,2).

REPRODUCTIVE EMBRYOLOGY

In the early embryo, the gonads are indistinguishable (indifferent). External genitalia are undifferentiated (female-like). Both Müllerian and Wolffian ducts exist side by side. If the embryo is 46,XY, the indifferent gonad differentiates into a testis, becoming identifiable about 6–7 weeks embryonic development (8–9 weeks gestation). If the embryo is not a normal 46,XY embryo, the indifferent gonad differentiates into an ovary. Ovarian differentiation is manifested slightly later than testicular differentiation.

Genital and Ductal Development

Although the precise nature of gonadal determinants on the X and Y are uncertain, genital and ductal differentiation proceed predictably once gonadal development is established. Genetic factors govern these steps.

Sertoli cells are the first cell to become evident in testicular differentiation, in fact organizing surrounding cells into tubules. Both Leydig cells (3) and Sertoli cells (4) function in dissociation from testicular morphogenesis, consistent with their earlier having directed gonadal development. These

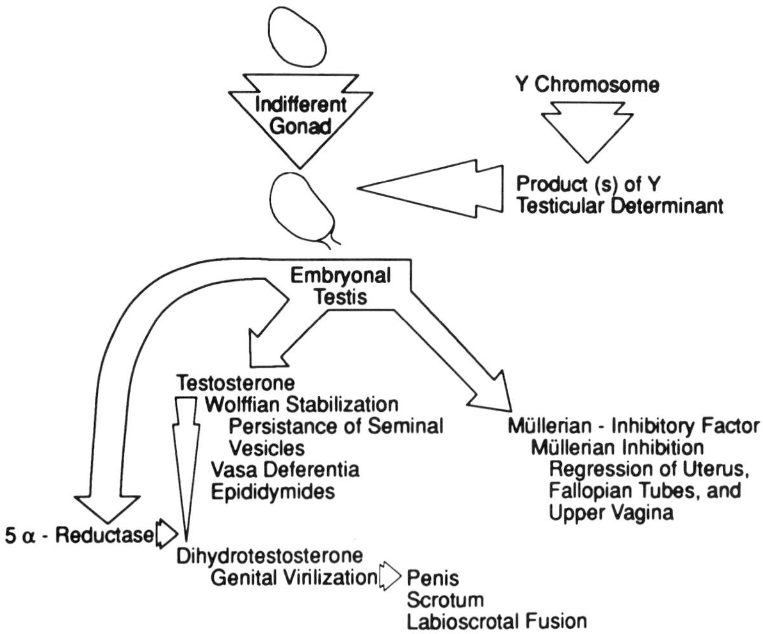

FIG. 1. Schematic diagram of normal male differentiation.

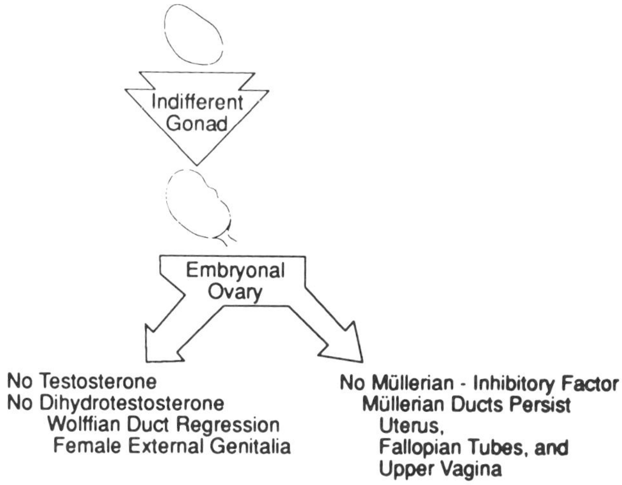

FIG. 2. Schematic diagram of normal female differentiation.

two cells secrete hormones that direct subsequent male differentiation (Fig. 1).

Fetal Leydig cells produce an androgen, probably testosterone, that stabilizes wolffian ducts and permits differentiation of vasa deferentia, epididymides and seminal vesicles. After conversion by 5α-reductase to dihydrotestosterone, the external genitalia are virilized. These actions can be mimicked by the administration of testosterone to female or castrated male embryos, as demonstrated clinically by existence of teratogenic forms of female pseudohermaphroditism (5). Fetal Sertoli cells produce a different hormone. This glycoprotein is believed to diffuse locally to cause regression of Müllerian derivatives (uterus and Fallopian tubes). The gene for anti-Müllerian hormone (AMH) has been isolated and localized to chromosome No. 19 (6). Although the above embryology is traditionally accepted, the situation may be more complex. The probability exists that the gene has other functions as well, as demonstrated by experiments in transgenic mice. When AMH is chronically expressed in XX mice, oocytes fail to persist and tubule-like structures develop in gonads (7).

In the absence of AMH and testosterone, internal genitalia develop along female lines (Fig. 2). Müllerian ducts develop into uterus and Fallopian tubes; Wolffian ducts regress. External genitalia also develop along female lines. First shown decades ago in rabbits (8), these changes also occur in 46,XX and in castrated 46,XY human embryos.

GENETIC CONTROL OF GONADAL DIFFERENTIATION

Localization of the Testis Determining Factor to the Y Short Arm

That 46,X,i(Yq) individuals were female in appearance led, over 20 years ago, to the assumption that the major testicular determinants [now called testis determining factor (TDF)] were localized to the Y short arm (Yp) (9). Later, the most distal portion of the Y short arm was excluded because nonmosaic ring Y individuals proved to be male (10). Such observations were consistent with the existence of an obligatory pairing region between Xp and Yp, presumed for decades but proved only recently (11). Because the X-Y pairing region is presumed to be pseudoautosomal, one would not expect it to contain sex determining genes. Later studies indicated that TDF was not located immediately near the centro-

TABLE 1. *An early study illustrating the principle of localizing TDF by analysis of presence or absence of selected cloned DNA sequences in XX males and XY males*[a]

Diagnosis	n	DNA sequences (probe) DXYS5 (47)	DXYS7 (13d)	DYS8 (118)	DXYS1 (DP34)	Interval (Vergnaud)
XX male	7	−	−	−	−	
XX male	1	+	−	−	−	1
XX male	6	+	+	−	−	2
XY male	5	+	+	+	−	3
XY male	5	+	+	+	+	4

[a]Interval 3 is never present without interval 2, nor is 2 present without 1. Thus, TDF lies closer to interval 1 than to other intervals. However, none of these clones correspond to TDF because some XX males lack all clones tested. Data of Vergnaud (14). Later TDF was localized to a small portion of interval 1 (36).
+, Present; −, absent.

mere. An individual with a distal Yp deletion proved female (12). XX males, which usually result from X-Y interchange during paternal meiosis, rarely showed heteromorphic X chromosomes (13); thus, the X-Y interchange causing sex-reversal must involve only a small portion of Yp.

Localizing TDF further required molecular technology. Investigations utilizing cloned Y-DNA sequences initially allowed TDF to be localized to a relatively distal portion of Yp11.2, specifically near sequence DXYS5 (14). This strategy is illustrated in Table 1 and the result in Fig. 3. In this initial study DXYS5 merely was that sequence most integrally related to presence of testes and, hence, presumably nearest to TDF. DXYS5 did not correspond to TDF, but strategies for "walking the chromosome" could next be applied to localize TDF.

TDF and Zinc Finger Y

In 1987, Page et al. (15) claimed to localize TDF to a 140-kb sequence near the pseudoautosomal region. This sequence was present in about 80% of 46,XX males, yet absent in some 46,XY females. The 140-kb region was purported to contain TDF codes for zinc finger proteins (16). Thus, the locus was termed ZFY (zinc finger Y). The amino terminal portion is acidic, 25% of its residues being glutamic or aspartic acid. The carboxy-terminal protein contains 13 zinc finger domains. If ZFY were truly TDF, TDF could be deduced to be a DNA binding protein because of its nucleotide sequence. A reasonable hypothesis would be that the protein binds to nucleic acids, perhaps in sequence-specific fashion. TDF might thus act by regulating transcription.

On the other hand, cogent reasons have arisen to suspect that ZFY is not truly

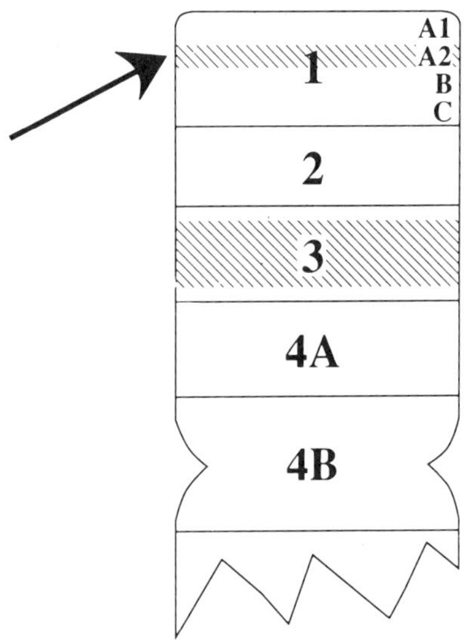

FIG. 3. Location of TDF and other loci on the Y chromosome. The region of Yp containing TDF is Interval 1, as originally defined by DNA sequence DXYS5 (14). Page et al. (15) further subdivided region 1 into subintervals, one of which is believed to contain TDF (1A2).

TDF. Actually one frequently one raised argument—that not all XX males contain ZFY—is not insurmountable because undetected mosaicism (46,XX/46,XY) can easily be postulated in this not uncommon condition. More puzzling is that sequences homologous to human ZFY are autosomal in marsupials (17). It can be argued that since many genes located on the human X are autosomal in marsupials (18), ZFX could be autosomal in marsupials, thus accounting for autosomal hybridization with human ZFY. In turn, it is postulated that the marsupial TDF has diverged from the human TDF and in doing so lost certain ZFY sequences homologous to those retained by the humans. This explanation is possible, but in my opinion tenuous. Claims that sex determining mechanisms in mammals and etherian species differ likewise seem nearly disingenuous.

Also unclear is why ZFY transcripts can be recovered not only from human testes but also from somatic tissues (19). The transcript recovered by Lau et al. (19) encoded an 801 amino acid protein of molecular weight 90.6 kD. ZFY was transcribed as a 3-kb mRNA transcript in testes and a 5.7-kb transcript in somatic cells. No transcript was recovered in ovarian cells. Differing-sized transcripts between gonadal and somatic tissues have been observed in oncogenes, raising the possibility that ZFY, like oncogenes, has a ubiquitous growth-promoting effect. If so, the hypothesis that ZFY is synonymous with TDF as traditionally imagined would be cast in doubt.

Even more convincing, a mouse mutant with testes failed to show ZFY (20), and XX males with genital ambiguity did likewise (21). Finally, ZFY is not detected in XX true hermaphrodites. In aggregate, we can conclude that ZFY is not TDF.

Sex-Determining Region Y

The latest candidate for TDF is called the sex-determining region Y (SRY), another finger protein located even nearer to the pseudoautosomal region than ZFY (22). Like ZFY, SRY is evolutionarily conserved. It was found within a 35-kb region distal to ZFY. Within this region was found a 2.1-kb subclone (Y53.3) that was present in two related sex-reversed individuals, an XX male and an XX true hermaphrodite (Fig. 4). Neither had ZFY. Point mutations within SRY have been found in XY gonadal dysgenesis cases (22a,22b). Moreover, XY mice lacking SRY (23) are female. More recently, the crucial transgenic experiments proving that SRY is in fact TDF have been performed (194).

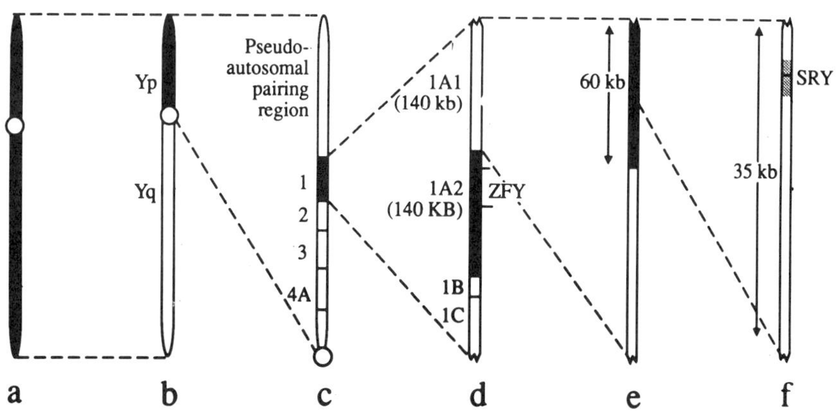

FIG. 4. The latest candidate for TDF is SRY (sex-determining region Y), contained within 2.1 kb clone encoding an 80 amino acid motif. (From ref. 193, with permission.)

H-Y Antigen

An earlier candidate for TDF was H-Y antigen (HYA), a topic still worth recounting given the great publicity engendered. The topic remains confusing because of uncertain number of types of H-Y antigen (serologic, transplantation, or both). Circumstantial data implicating H-Y as pivotal for testicular differentiation were well referenced by Wachtel (24), namely the apparent invariable correlation between presence of testes and H-Y antigen. XX males and XX true hermaphrodites were both H-Y positive. Antibodies against H-Y antigen also prevented reaggregation of disrupted testicular cells, which were then directed into follicular-like rather than tubular-like structures (25). On the other hand, Simpson (26) recovered H-Y positive female mice carrying Sxr (Sex-reversal) (X/XSxr), and McLaren et al. (27), observed testicular differentiation in X/XSxr mice lacking H-Y. Those groups believe that H-Y is necessary for spermatogenesis (28), but not testicular differentiation.

That H-Y was not synonymous with TDF further became clear when DNA sequence DXYS5 proved absent in 46,XY phenotypic females showing H-Y antigen (29,30). If governed by the Y, the locus for H-Y antigen must then exist in a region other than that localized to interval 1A (Fig. 3). In fact, H-Y is believed located on the Y long arm.

Lau et al. (19) suggested that the long arm for the Y chromosome codes for the H-Y transplantation antigen, whereas the short arm codes for H-Y serologic antigen. This is relevant because of prior observations by Wachtel (24) that almost all XX males contain H-Y serologic antigen.

Although no longer considered a candidate for TDF, HYA could still prove prognostically useful in predicting predisposition to neoplasia in XY gonadal dysgenesis. We shall see later that XY gonadal dysgenesis patients having H-Y antigen are more likely to develop neoplasia than similar patients lacking H-Y antigen.

Genes on the Y Long Arm

In addition to a locus integral for H-Y, the Y long arm (Yq) may contain several other genes that affect morbid anatomy. These include (a) a region that if deleted protects against neoplasia; (b) a region essential for spermatogenesis (designated AZO, or SP3); (c) a region exerting a positive effect on stature (cell growth) (CGY); and (d) a region exerting a positive effect on tooth size (TSY). Whether all these loci truly exist is uncertain, as is their relationship to one another.

The best candidate for a locus on Yq controlling morbid anatomical traits is one relating to growth. Yq has plausibly been said to contain factors exerting a positive effect on height (cell growth Y chromosome of CGY) (31) and tooth size (TSY) (32). These loci have been proposed on the basis of comparisons between normal and abnormal individuals, specifically XY males with androgen insensitivity. That a single locus (region) is responsible for both traits (CGY and TSY) also seems plausible (33).

A locus on Yq that if disrupted causes azoospermia [azoospermia (AZO) or so-called spermatogenesis Factor 3 (SP3)] has been postulated on the basis of the following observations: (a) infertile males may show deletions of Yq; and (b) infertile males showing nonfluorescent Y chromosomes may be deficient for Yq (34). However, potential pitfalls preclude readily accepting such a hypothesis. First, male infertility and azoospermia are both uncommon; thus, detecting a sex chromosomal abnormality in an azoospermic man may merely be coincidental. Second, alternative cytogenetic interpretations are often possible. In particular, nonfluorescent Y chromosomes are usually dicentric, an aberration invariably accompanied by monosomic lines because of the inherent instability of dicentric chromosomes (breakage-fusion-bridge cycle).

Loss of fluorescent Yq (and presumably at least a small contiguous nonfluorescent unique sequence region) was said by Lukusa et al. (35) to exert a protective effect against germ cell neoplasia. Page (36) refers to this locus as GBY (gonadoblastoma Y) and postulated that its wild-type function concerns spermatogenesis.

The various Yq loci postulated to influence somatic traits are certainly not necessarily mutually exclusive. Simpson (33) speculated that CGY, TSY, and GBY could all be synonymous.

X-Y Homologies, X-Inactivation, and Genetic Control of Testicular Development

Of relevance at this point in our discussion are more specific comments concerning possible homologies between gonadal determinants on the X and the Y. Such homologies would be in addition to the long established pseudoautosomal regions (Xp and Yp). In fact, homologies have been demonstrated between Yp and Xq, Yq and Xq, and Yq and Xp.

Chandra (37) first proposed X-inactivation as a mechanism for sex determination, based upon a variety of observations in invertebrates and lower mammals. In 1984, region Xq13-24 was shown to be highly (98%) homologous to a region on Yp (38). Not only was this considered the basis for presuming the human Y evolved from duplication and transposition of Xq to Yp, but it rekindled interest by several investigators (33,39–42) in Chandra's (37) hypothesis that sex determination is governed by X-inactivation. Moreover, in both the nematode *Caenorhabditis elegans* (43) and in *Drosophila melanogaster* (44), there is solid evidence that gene inactivation is pivotal for sex determination. One wonders whether ovarian and testicular determinants might be identical, with gonadal determinants governed by gene inactivation (33,39). Males might have twice the gonadal gene product as females because Y-loci are not inactivated. If this thesis or a modification thereof were correct, unique sequence TDF will never be recovered. Instead, structural genes for testicular differentiation might be autosomal. Conversely, if SRY truly is the elusive testicular determinant (TDF), X-inactivation is not the crucial mechanism in gonadal differentiation.

Autosomal Factors in Testicular Differentiation

Certain disorders affecting ovarian and testicular differentiation are caused by autosomal genes. Thus, one can deduce that not only sex chromosomes, but also autosomes are necessary for development of the normal ovary or testis.

In addition to familial aggregates of various human disorders (discussed below), animal studies point to autosomes as pivotal to gonadal differentiation. In mice, Eicher et al. (45) crossed C57BL females to Mus posciavinus males. The F1 males were then back-crossed to C57 females, placing the Mus posciavinus Y on a predominantly C57 autosomal background. The Y sometimes proved incapable of directing testicular differentiation, demonstrating capacity of autosomes to affect male differentiation. The autosomal region responsible for this perturbation appeared localized to mouse chromosome 17 (46). In humans, some have postulated chromosome 11p as an analogous region given localization to that region of the gene for Wilms' tumor. [Sometimes Wilms' tumor is associated with male pseudohermaphroditism and aniridia (47).] Consistent with autosomal localization for testis-determining factors are two other groups of disorders that we shall discuss below. There include several forms of male pseudohermaphroditism in which XY individuals manifest sex reversal, and the occurrence of abnormalities of autosomal genes capable of affecting germ cell development in both sexes, presumably due to autosomal genes acting at a site common to early germ cell development.

That autosomal factors affect testicular

differentiation is perhaps most strongly supported by reports of familial aggregates. Sibships with XX true hermaphroditism are shown in Fig. 5 (48–51). In addition, genetic factors are presumably responsible for the coexistence of 46,XX males and 46,XX true hermaphrodites in the same kindred (52–55). In two families, the disorder was present in more than one generation.

Given the existence of autosomal genes causing sex-reversal in mice (45,46), it is tempting to postulate that perturbation of an ordinarily dormant autosomal gene induces inappropriate sex reversal in XX true hermaphroditism. Moreover, human familial true hermaphroditism is more likely to be characterized by bilateral ovotestes than is a nonfamilial case (56). This is consistent with a central control mechanism, disturbance of which would exert a bilateral ef-

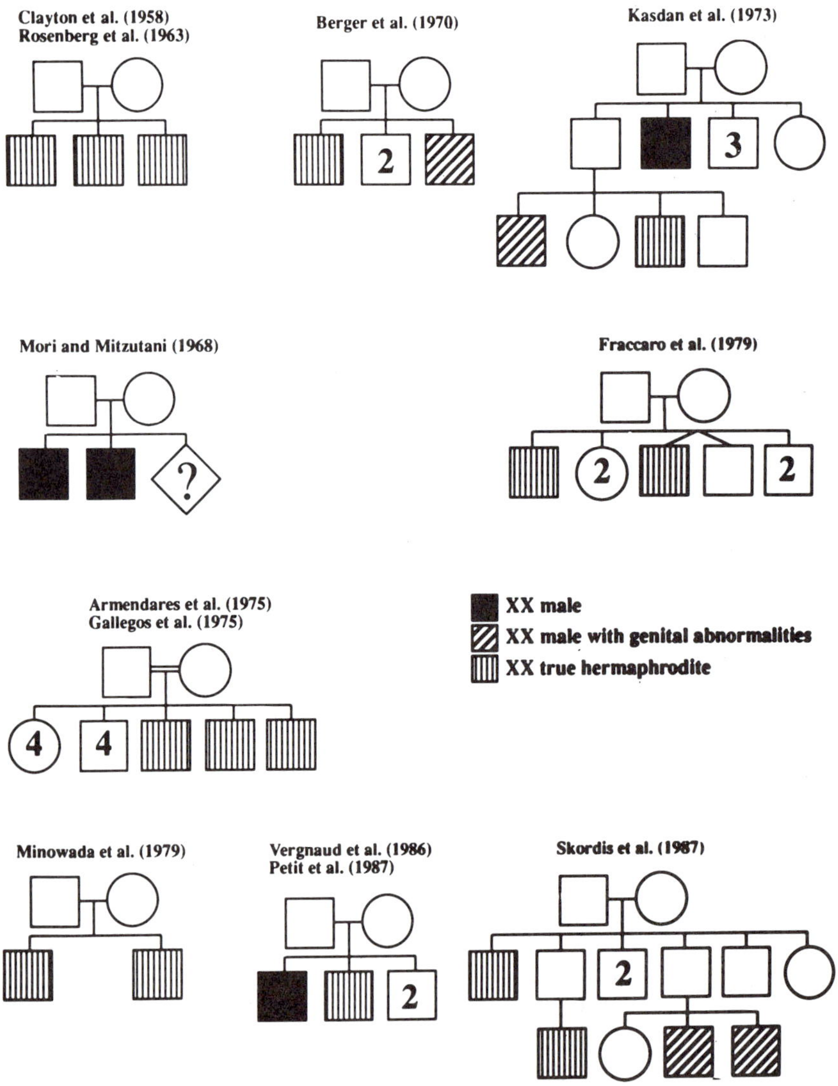

FIG. 5. Abbreviated pedigrees of families in which multiple family members are either 46,XX true hermaphrodites or 46,XX sex-reversed males. Simplified pedigrees of families with more than one XX male or XX true hermaphrodite (48–55,170).

fect. The mechanism could resemble that postulated for inducing certain neoplasias. A gene normally suppressed in females could, if induced, be responsible for directing testicular development in 46,XX males. Alternatively, the gene might be one whose wild type function involves a "switch" mechanism capable of directing an indifferent gonad in either testicular or ovarian direction. Indeed, such mechanisms may exist in *C. elegans* (43) and *D. melanogaster* (44).

Ovarian Differentiation

In the absence of a Y chromosome, the indifferent gonad develops into an ovary. Germ cells exist in 45,X human fetuses (57). In fact, monosomy X in mice (58) and in most other mammals confers little reproductive disadvantage; thus, the pathogenesis of germ cell failure involves increased germ cell attrition, not failure of germ cell formation. If two intact X chromosomes are not present, 45,X ovarian follicles usually degenerate by birth. The second X chromosome is therefore responsible for ovarian maintenance, rather than ovarian differentiation, further supporting constitutive ovarian differentiation and observations that oocyte development occurs in infants with XY gonadal dysgenesis (59) and genitopalatocardiac syndrome (60). Oocyte development in the presence of a Y chromosome is also well documented in mice.

For years efforts have been directed toward localizing those regions of the X chromosome important for ovarian maintenance. Reviewed and updated on several occasions by this author (1,33,39,61), ovarian maintenance determinants can be deduced on the basis of phenotypic-karyotypic correlations to exist on both the X short arm and the X long arm. Each arm probably has at least two regions of importance for ovarian development.

With respect to the X short arm, a locus in regions Xp11.2→11.4 clearly seems important for ovarian maintenance (Fig. 6). More telomeric terminal deletions [del(X)(p21)] can be deduced to be less important because all reported women with deletions have menstruated. However, half of these del(X)(p21) women are infertile, manifesting secondary amenorrhea. Thus, a second region on Xp may be important for ovarian maintenance, albeit less integral than region Xp11.2→11.4.

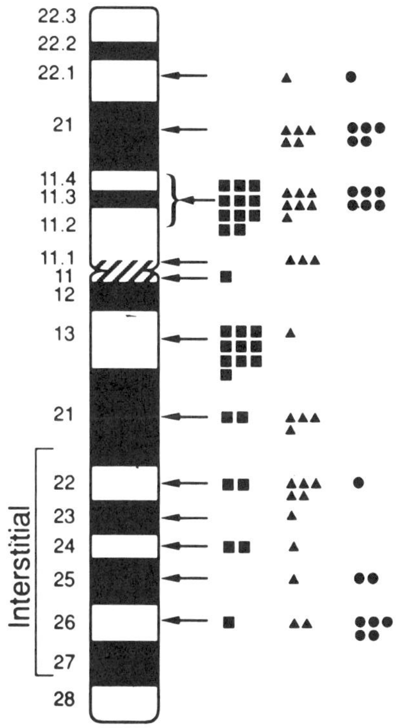

FIG. 6. Schematic diagram of X chromosome, showing ovarian function as function of terminal deletion. The bracketed area to the left connotes the interstitial deletion reported by Krauss (62). Key: ■, 1° Amenorrhea; ▲, 2° Amenorrhea oligomenorrhea; ● Fertility or regular menses. (Adapted from ref. 62.)

Similar topography appears to exist on the X long arm (Xq). Deletions involving Xq11.3 or proximal Xq 21 are usually associated with complete ovarian failure. However, region Xq25 or Xq26 also seems necessary. An interstitial deletion involving this region resulted in secondary amenorrhea in a mother and her daughters (62). Familial terminal deletions at Xq25 (33) and Xq26 (63) yielded similar phenotypes. Thus, two or more regions on Xq must play roles in ovarian maintenance, with the region nearer the centromere of greatest importance.

That multiple genes (regions) on the X are necessary for ovarian maintenance is not dissimilar from the well documented systems in nematodes *(Caenorhabditis elegans)* (43) and fruit flies *(Drosophila)* (44). The temptation to postulate evolutionary conservation is almost irresistible, although human genes and those in lower animals need not necessarily be homologous.

In addition to determinants on the X, the autosomal recessive disorders of XX gonadal dysgenesis (see below) make it clear that autosomal genes must remain intact for normal ovarian maintenance. Finally, in other kindreds, unexplained premature ovarian failure is ostensibly transmitted in autosomal dominant fashion (64).

OVARIAN DYSGENESIS

Individuals with ovarian dysgenesis have deficient numbers of oocytes, often resulting in so-called streak gonads. Many different chromosomal complements have been associated with gonadal dysgenesis, only a few of which we shall discuss here. There also exist forms associated with normal chromosomal complement (XX and XY gonadal dysgenesis).

The term most frequently applied to individuals with gonadal dysgenesis is "Turner syndrome," a term that unfortunately connotes different features to different investigators. Here we apply the term "gonadal dysgenesis" to any individual with streak gonads, restricting the term "Turner stigmata" for those with short stature and certain other somatic anomalies. By itself, the term "Turner stigmata" would not imply the presence of streak gonads.

Monosomy X (45,X)

Gonads

In most 45,X adults with gonadal dysgenesis, the normal gonad is replaced by a white fibrous streak, 2–3 cm long and about 0.5 cm wide, located in the position ordinarily occupied by the ovary (Fig. 7). A streak gonad is characterized histologically by interlacing waves of dense fibrous stroma, indistinguishable from normal ovarian stroma (Fig. 8). Oocytes are usually completely absent in 45,X adults, but germ cells are present in 45,X embryos (57). Thus, the pathogenesis of germ cell failure is increased atresia, not failure of germ cell formation. That adult 45,X individuals showing ovarian failure could involve (a) key loci on the normal heterochromatic (inactive) X not being inactivated in humans, (b) key loci being inactivated but become reactivated in oocytes, or (c) inactivation never occurring in oocytes (65).

Although streak gonads are usually present in 45,X individuals, about 3% of adult cases menstruate spontaneously at least twice and 5% show breast minimal development. Fertile patients have even been reported. Undetected 46,XX cells should be suspected in menstruating 45,X patients; however, it is plausible that a few 45,X individuals could be fertile, inasmuch as germ cells are present in 45,X embryos. The rare offspring of 45,X women are probably not at increased risk for chromosomal abnormalities (66,67), despite some authors holding contrary opinions (68,69). The above comments notwithstanding, menstruation and fertility occur so rarely that 45,X patients should be counseled to anticipate primary amenorrhea and sterility. However, hormone therapy (estrogen and cyclic progestogens) can produce normal uterine size, allowing 45,X women to carry pregnancies obtained through donor oocytes [*in vitro* fertilization or gamete intrafallopian transfer (GIFT)].

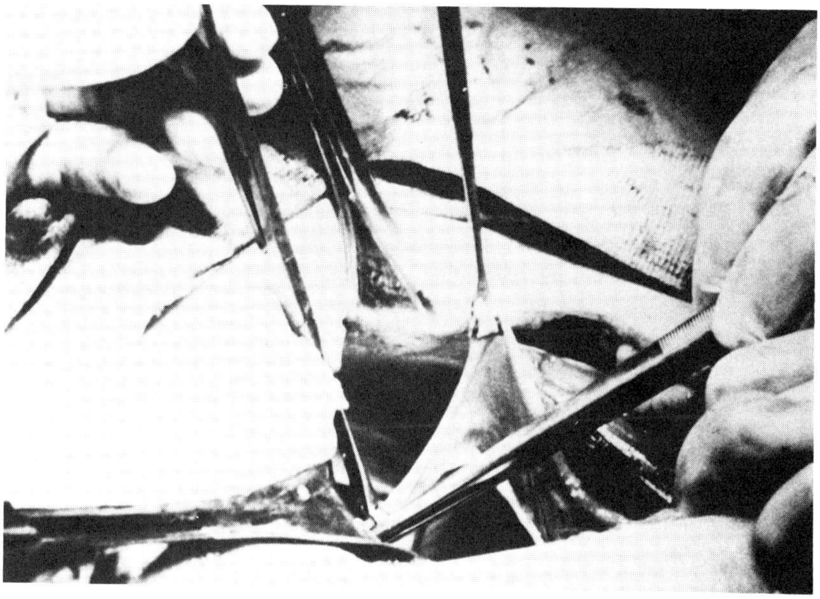

FIG. 7. A streak gonad. (From ref. 114, with permission.)

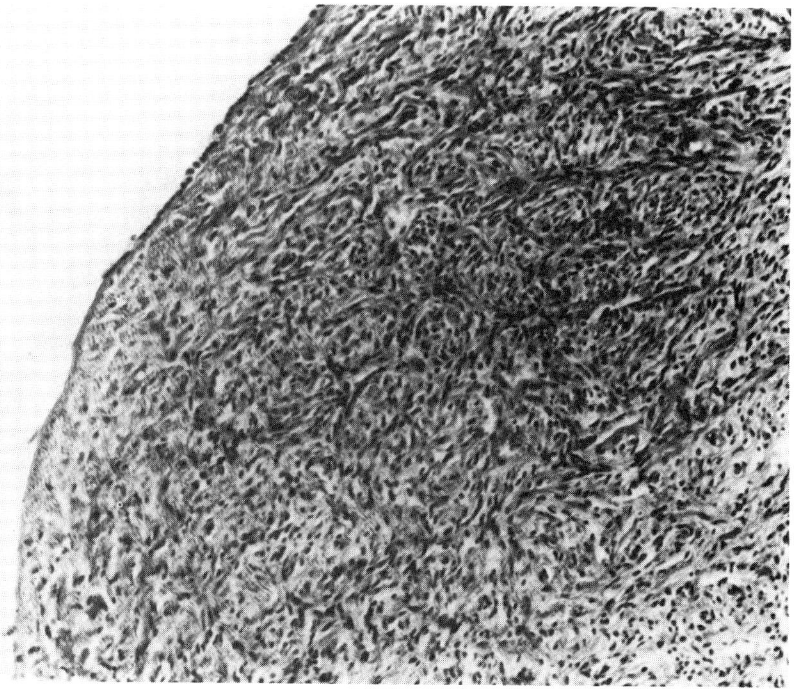

FIG. 8. Histologic appearance of streak gonad showing lack of oocytes. (From ref. 114, with permission.)

In untreated women, lack of normal ovarian development predictably leads to deficient secretion of sex steroids. Estrogen and androgen levels are decreased; follicle-stimulating hormone (FSH) and luteinizing hormone (LH) levels are increased. Estrogen-dependent processes show effects predictable for hormonal deficiency. At puberty, pubic and axillary hair fail to develop in normal quantity (Fig. 9). Breasts contain little parenchymal tissue, and the areolar tissue is only slightly darker than the surrounding skin; the well-differentiated external genitalia, vagina and mullerian derivatives remain small.

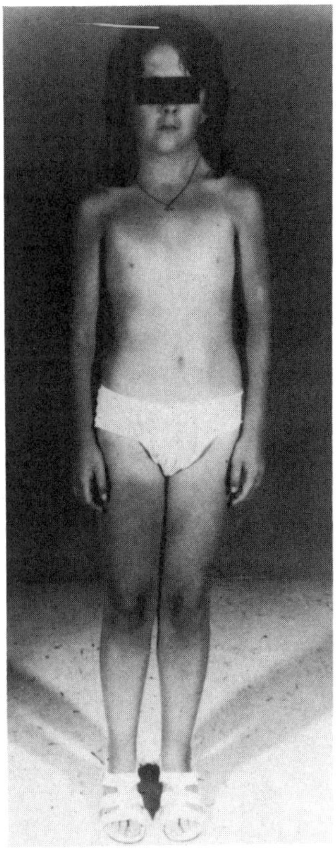

FIG. 9. Seventeen-year-old 45,X individual showing sexual infantilism, webbing of the neck, low nuchal hair line, and pigmented nevi. Patient of the author. (From ref. 114, with permission.)

Somatic Anomalies

The 45,X individuals not only are short (<4 feet 10 inches) but often exhibit many features of Turner stigmata (Table 2). None of these features is pathognomonic, but in aggregate a characteristic spectrum of anomalies is observed that is more likely to exist in individuals with a 45,X complement than in individuals with most other sex chromosomal abnormalities. Verifying normal renal, vertebral, cardiac and auditory function is therefore obligatory.

Growth

Individuals with a 45,X karyotype have decreased birthweight (68). Total body length at birth is sometimes less than normal, but often is close to 50th percentile. However, height velocity before puberty generally lies in the 10th to 15th percentile (69) and the mean height of 45,X adults ($\geq$16 years old) approximates 141 to 146 cm (70,71).

Various treatments for short stature in 45,X patients have been proposed: growth hormone, anabolic steroids and low dose estrogen. Growth hormone abnormalities have long been proposed; however, their existence is still contentious, and perturbations could be only secondary to lack of gonadal activity (72). Irrespective, various treatment regimens involving growth hormone, anabolic steroids or low dose estrogens show ostensible benefit, especially in the first few years of therapy. The consensus is that final height is increased by approximately 6–8 cm (73). Most pediatric endocrinologists appear to favor use of human recombinant-DNA derived methionyl human growth hormone (Genentech).

One reason to doubt efficacy of growth hormone or other treatment is that epiphyses in patients with a 45,X complement are structurally abnormal. Not only are

TABLE 2. *Somatic features associated with 45,X chromosomal complement*

Feature
Growth
Decreased birth weight
Decreased adult height (141–146 cm)
Intellectual function
Verbal IQ > performance IQ
Cognitive deficits (space-form-blindness)
Immature personality, probably secondary to short stature
Cranofacial
Premature fusion sphenoccipital and other sutures, producing brachycephaly
Abnormal pinnae
Retruded mandible
Epicanthal folds (25%)
High-arched palate (36%)
Abnormal dentition
Visual anomalies, usually strabismus (22%)
Auditory deficits: sensorineural or secondary to middle ear infections
Neck
Pterygium coli (46%)
Short broad neck (74%)
Low nuchal hair (71%)
Chest
Rectangular contour (shield chest) (53%)
Apparent widely spaced nipples
Tapered lateral ends of clavicle
Cardiovascular
Coarctation of aorta or ventricular septal defect (10–16%)
Renal (38%)
Horseshoe kidneys
Unilateral renal aplasia
Duplication ureters
Gastrointestinal
Telangiectasias
Skin and lymphatics
Pigmented nevi (63%)
Lymphadema (38%) due to hypoplasia superficial vessels
Nails
Hypoplasia and malformation (66%)
Skeletal
Cubitus valgus (54%)
Radial tilt of articular surface of trochlear
Clinodactyly V
Short metacarpals, usually IV (48%)
Decreased carpal arch (mean angle 117°)
Deformities of medial tibial condyle
Dermatoglyphics
Increased total digital ridge count
Increased distance between palmar triradii a and b
Distal axial triradius in position t′

Percentages refer to number of 45,X individuals with a given feature.
From ref. 114.

long bones abnormal but also teeth (74) and skull (75). Thus, individuals with a 45,X karyotype might be said to have a skeletal dysplasia.

Intelligence

Most 45,X patients have normal intelligence, but any given 45,X patient has a slightly higher probability of being retarded than a 46,XX individual (70). Performance IQ is lower than verbal IQ, the latter being similar to 46,XX matched controls (76). 45,X individuals also have a cognitive defect characterized by poor spatial processing skills (space-form blindness) (76–78). Predictable psychosocial deficits occur, primarily involving immaturity and social relationships.

45,X/46,XX and 45,X/47,XXX Mosaicism

Individuals with a 45,X/46,XX complement show fewer anomalies than do 45,X individuals. Twelve percent of 45,X/46,XX individuals menstruate, compared with only 3% of 45,X individuals (70). Of 45,X/46,XX individuals, 18% undergo breast development compared with 5% of 45,X individuals. Mean adult height is greater in 45,X/46,XX than in 45,X; more mosaic (25%) than nonmosaic (5%) patients reach adult heights of >152 cm (68). Somatic anomalies are less likely to exist in 45,X/46,XX than in 45,X.

Individuals with 45,X/47,XXX are rarer but phenotypically similar to 45,X/46,XX individuals.

The 45,X/46,XY individuals may also show bilateral streak gonads; however, they often show a unilateral streak gonad and a contralateral dysgenetic testis (mixed gonadal dysgenesis). For this reason, discussion is deferred until our consideration of male pseudohermaphroditism.

Deletions of the X Short Arm

As already discussed, the most common breakpoint for a terminal deletion of the X short arm is band Xp11 (Fig. 6). The breakpoint may also occur at Xp21 or Xp22, and interstitial deletions have been reported. Of 24 reported del(X)(p11.2→11.4) individuals, 13 individuals (54.2%) menstruated spontaneously; however, menstruation was rarely normal (66,78). Functioning ovarian tissue thus persists more often in these del(Xp) individuals than in 45,X individuals. In fact, individuals with more distal deletions [del(X)(p21)] usually menstruate spontaneously, although approximately half are infertile (secondary amenorrhea). Thus, the terminal portion of Xp[X(pter→p21)] plays some role in ovarian development, in contrast to previous beliefs that it was unimportant (79).

Figure 10 shows heights of women with short arm deletions. Statural determinant(s) can be localized to Xp2→Xpter because del(X)(p21) women are short even if they display normal ovarian function (39,79). Thus, regions on Xp responsible for ovarian and statural determinants must be distinct (33,39,61,79). Page et al. (80) presented evidence that the Y pseudoautosomal region and the X long arm contain a sequence that is not subject to inactivation and that if deleted may produce short stature and the Turner stigmata.

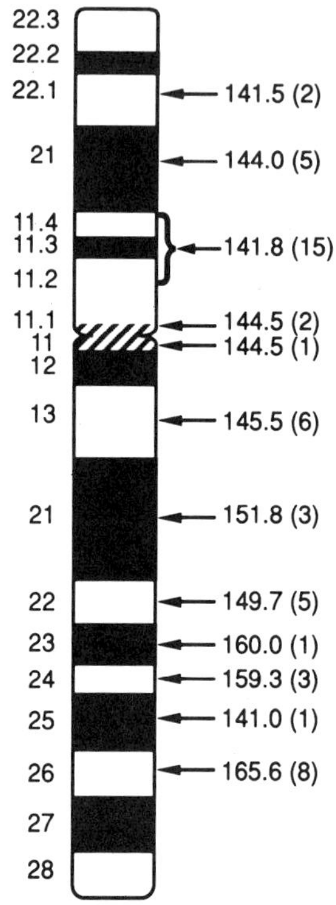

FIG. 10. Heights in adults reported to have terminal deletions at various regions of the X. Samples restricted to adult cases (older than 15 years of age) in which mosaicism was excluded. (From ref. 73, with permission.)

Isochromosome for the X Long Arm

Division of the centromere in the transverse rather than in the longitudinal plane results in an isochromosome, a metacentric chromosome consisting of isologous arms. Both arms are structurally identical and contain the same genes. An isochromosome for the X long arm [i(Xq)] differs from a terminal deletion of Xp in that not just the terminal portion but all of the Xp is deleted. An isochromosome for the X long arm is the most common X-structural abnormality, but coexisting 45,X lines (mosaicism) are common.

Almost all reported 46,X,i(Xq) patients show streak gonads. Short stature and Turner stigmata are common as well (70). Occasional 46,X,i(Xq) individuals have menstruated, but surveys support that of this author (70) in showing rarity of menstruation. The almost complete lack of gonadal development in 46,X,i(Xq) individuals contrasts to that in 46,X,del(Xp11) individuals, about half of whom menstruate or develop breasts. This difference could be explained if gonadal determinants exist at several different locations on Xp. If so, one locus on Xp might be deficient in i(Xq) yet retained in del(X)(p11).

The mean height of nonmosaic 46,X, i(Xq) patients is 136 cm (70). Somatic anomalies of the Turner stigmata occur about as frequently in 46,X,i(Xq) as in 45,X, and the spectrum of anomalies associated with the two complements is similar.

Deletions of the X Long Arm

In non-mosaic deletions of the X long arm (39), many different break points have been reported (39). However, region Xq13 or Xq21 is probably the single most important region for ovarian maintenance deletions. Deletions originating at Xq13 are usually (Fig. 6) associated with primary amenorrhea, lack of breast development, and complete ovarian failure (33,39,61). Deletions involving region Xq25→27 are less deleterious, affected individuals usually showing only premature ovarian failure (33,39,61,81).

Figure 10 suggests that the effect of distal Xq deletions on height may also be less deleterious than the effect of more proximal deletions.

Isochromosome of X Short Arm

Of particular note are those individuals claimed years ago to have a 46,X,i(Xp) complement. Such women showed primary amenorrhea, and were usually normal in stature. None have been restudied with molecular techniques, but the consensus now appears to be that i(Xp) probably does not exist or is very rare. Rather, the karyotype in previously suspected individuals is now presumed to be del(X) (q22 or q24).

Other X Abnormalities

Many other X abnormalities have been reported. Centric fragments, dicentric and ring X chromosome are mitotically unstable rearrangements, frequently associated with monosomic lines. The latter may be responsible for gonadal dysgenesis rather than the structurally abnormal X. Irrespective, it is not the rearrangement per se but rather the deficient loci that are responsible for associated abnormalities. Translocations between an autosome and an X chromosome may be associated with ovarian dysgenesis. Those involving the X long arm are especially likely to cause ovarian failure. X/autosome translocations may lead to familial gonadal dysgenesis (79,82).

Abnormalities of the Y Chromosome

The initial step in localizing the TDF occurred over 20 years ago when 46,X,i(Yq) individuals were observed to be female in appearance (9). Because 46,X,i(Yq) individuals lacked Yp, TDF could be localized to the Y short arm. Thus, interstitial Yp deletion, terminal Yp deletion, or isochromosome for Yq may all lead to gonadal failure.

XX Gonadal Dysgenesis

Gonadal dysgenesis histologically similar to that detected in individuals with an abnormal sex chromosomal complement has been observed repeatedly in 46,XX individuals in whom mosaicism is reasonably excluded. The term XX gonadal dysgenesis is applied to affected individuals (83–86).

External genitalia and streak gonads of affected individuals are indistinguishable from those of individuals who have gonadal dysgenesis due to an abnormal chromosomal complement. Likewise, both endocrine findings (elevated FSH and LH) and lack of secondary sexual development are similar to those of other individuals with streak gonads. Most individuals with XX gonadal dysgenesis are normal in stature (mean height, 165 cm) (84). Somatic features of the Turner stigmata are usually absent.

XX gonadal dysgenesis is inherited in autosomal recessive fashion. Of gynecologic interest are families in which affected sibs showed different phenotypes: one with streak gonads, the other with primary amenorrhea and extreme ovarian hypoplasia (i.e., presence of a few oocytes) (84, 87,88). Such families suggest that the mutant gene responsible for XX gonadal dysgenesis does not necessarily always cause complete ovarian failure. It follows that a similar mutation may also be responsible for sporadic cases of premature ovarian failure.

XX gonadal dysgenesis may occur alone or it may coexist with patterns of somatic anomalies. The combination of XX gonadal dysgenesis and neurosensory deafness (Perrault syndrome) is accepted as a separate entity (85,86,89–91). Other possible syndromes include XX gonadal dysgenesis and myopathy (92); XX gonadal dysgenesis and cerebellar ataxia (93); and XX gonadal dysgenesis, microcephaly, and arachnodactyly (94).

Gonadal dysgenesis in 46,XX individuals may also result from nongenetic causes (phenocopies). Plausible mechanisms include infections (e.g., mumps), infarctions, infiltrative processes (e.g., tuberculosis, neoplasia), and autoimmune phenomena (95). Sometimes familial aggregates are observed, illustrating that familial and genetic are not synonymous (96).

XY Gonadal Dysgenesis

Gonadal dysgenesis may occur in individuals with apparently normal male (46, XY) chromosomal complements. In at least some cases, the gonads of these individuals appeared to have been ovaries during embryologic development (59). Irrespective, the pathogenesis could be explained by loss of testicular tissue before 7–8 weeks embryogenesis. This would produce a female phenotype, as shown in castration experiments performed decades ago by Jost (8,97).

Individuals with XY gonadal dysgenesis show female external genitalia, a uterus and Fallopian tubes. At puberty, secondary sexual development fails to occur. Height is normal and somatic anomalies usually absent. However, a relationship between XY gonadal dysgenesis and renal failure exists (98,99).

Approximately 20–30% of XY gonadal dysgenesis patients develop a dysgerminoma or gonadoblastoma. Often the neoplasia arises in the first or second decade. About two-thirds of XY gonadal dysgenesis individuals are H-Y antigen positive, and such individuals are far more likely to develop neoplasia than H-Y antigen negative individuals (24). Because of the relatively high probability of undergoing neoplastic transformation, gonads should at present be extirpated from all individuals with XY gonadal dysgenesis. The uterus and Fallopian tubes should not be removed, even though it is technically easier to remove all these organs than solely to extirpate the streaks. Retention of the uterus allows pregnancy through donor oocytes or donor embryos.

Genetic heterogeneity exists with respect to XY gonadal dysgenesis (100). At least one form segregates in the fashion expected of an X-linked recessive (66,85). Neoplasia and H-Y positivity has been observed in some X-linked kindreds (101). An autosomal recessive form of XY gonadal dysgenesis may or may not also exist (66), and it is clear that clinically indistinguishable cases can result from deletion of TDF from Yp (29,36,102). Specifically, deletion or point mutations within SRY may occur (22,22a,22b). However, relatively few cases result from deletions of Yp.

At least three syndromes have XY gonadal dysgenesis as one of their components: (a) XY gonadal dysgenesis and campomelic dwarfism (103,104), (b) XY gonadal dysgenesis and ectodermal anomalies (105), and (c) genitopalatocardiac (Gardner-Silengo-Wachtel) syndrome (60,106).

Germ Cell Failure in Both Sexes

In each of five sibships, male and female sibs have each shown germinal cell failure.

Affected females showed streak gonads, whereas affected males showed germ cell aplasia (Sertoli-cell only syndrome or del Castillo phenotype) (see below). In two families, parents were consanguineous, and in each no somatic anomalies coexisted (107,108). In three other families, seemingly unique patterns of somatic anomalies suggested existence of distinct entities. Hamet et al. (109) reported germ cell failure, hypertension and deafness; Al-Awadi et al. (110) reported germ cell failure and alopecia; Mikati et al. (111) reported germ cell failure, microcephaly, short stature, and minor anomalies.

Although clinically rare, these families are biologically important in demonstrating that several different autosomal genes are capable of affecting germ cell development in both sexes. Presumably they act at a site common to early germ cell development.

FEMALE PSEUDOHERMAPHRODITISM

Female pseudohermaphrodites are 46,XX individuals whose external genitalia fail to develop as expected for normal females. Affected individuals may result from either genetic or teratogenic causes. Usually anomalies are limited to the external genitalia, but in a few cases abnormalities of embryonic hindgut, cloacal membrane, or urogenital membrane coexist.

Congenital Adrenal Hyperplasia

General Considerations

The most common cause of genital ambiguity, syndromes of adrenal hyperplasia result from deficiencies of the various enzymes required for steroid biosynthesis (Fig. 11). Deficiencies of 21-hydroxylase, 11-hydroxylase, and 3β-ol-dehydrogenase produce female pseudohermaphroditism. In these disorders, the common pathogenesis involves decreased production of adrenal cortisol. Cortisol regulates secretion of ACTH through negative feedback inhibition mechanism. If cortisol production is decreased, ACTH secretion is not inhibited. Elevated ACTH leads to increased quantities of steroid precursors, from which androgens can be synthesized (Fig. 11). Because the fetal adrenal begins to function during the third month of embryogenesis, excessive production of adrenal androgens will virilize external genitalia. Müllerian and gonadal development remain unaffected because neither is androgen-dependent.

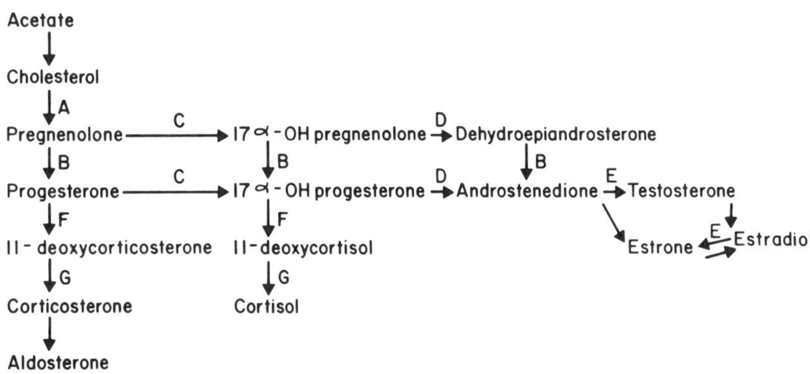

FIG. 11. Important adrenal and gonadal biosynthetic pathways. *Letters* designate enzymes required for the appropriate conversions: A, 20 α-hydroxylase, 22 hydroxylase, and 20,22 desmolase; B, 3β-ol-dehydrogenase; C, 17α-hydroxylase; D, 17,20-desmolase; E, 17-ketosteroid reductase; F, 21-hydroxylase; G, 11-hydroxylase. (From ref. 114, with permission.)

The syndromes of adrenal hyperplasia represent the most common causes of genital ambiguity. They must be excluded immediately when assessing an individual with genital ambiguity because cortisol and corticosterone deficiencies result in sodium wasting.

Cortisol administration should be begun immediately following birth in order to maximize height. If cortisol is not administered, affected individuals initially experience increased growth during early childhood; however, premature epiphyseal closure leads to a final adult height below the third percentile.

Deficiency of 21-Hydroxylase without Sodium Wasting

The gene for 21-hydroxylase is coded by a gene on chromosome number 6. If the enzyme is deficient, 17α-hydroxyprogesterone cannot be converted to 11-desoxycortisol (Fig. 11). In this most common cause of genital ambiguity, cortisol and deoxycortisol levels are decreased unless a compensatory increase in ACTH secretion occurs. Irrespective, 17α-hydroxyprogesterone, androstenedione, estrone, and testosterone increase; the latter causes genital masculinization. Increased 17α-OHP serves as the basis for diagnosis, both in serum (affected neonate) and amniotic fluid (affected fetus).

Females deficient for 21- or 11β-hydroxylase show clitoral hypertrophy, labioscrotal fusion, and displacement of the urethral orifice to a location more nearly approximating that of a normal male. Extent of virilization may vary among individuals with the same type of enzyme deficiency. Wolffian derivatives (vasa deferentia, seminal vesicles, epididymides) are rarely present, probably because fetal adrenal function begins too late in embryogenesis to stabilize the Wolffian ducts. Müllerian derivatives develop normally, as expected in the absence of the nonandrogenic hormone AMH. Ovaries likewise develop normally. Genital (scrotal) and areolar hyperpigmentation may occur, presumably because ACTH has melanocyte-stimulating properties. In fact, presence of hyperpigmentation suggests the diagnosis of 21- or 11β-hydroxylase deficiencies in males, whose genitalia are normal at birth. If not ascertained at birth, males usually pass undetected until approximately 2 years of age, when pubic hair develops and increased statural growth is noted. If the sex of rearing is established by 18 months and genital reconstruction accomplished at 2–4 years of age, the child should be unequivocally female in psychosexual development.

In 21-hydroxylase deficiency, sodium wasting may or may not occur. In the form of 21-hydroxylase deficiency not associated with sodium wasting, it is assumed that increased secretion of ACTH results in levels of aldosterone and cortisol sufficient to prevent sodium wasting.

In the neonatal period attention must be given to administration of cortisol, correction of hyperkalemia, and restoration of fluid-electrolyte balance. If untreated, these deficiencies can lead to hyponatremia, hyperkalemia, dehydration, and death due to renal insufficiency. Salt-retaining hormones (e.g., fluorinated hydrocortisone) are necessary, if salt wastage occurs. Cortisol administration must be continued into adulthood, although requirements per unit weight may diminish. Mineralocorticoids may not be necessary after 5 years of age.

The 21-hydroxylase deficiency is an autosomal recessive trait, closely linked to HLA and located on the short arm of chromosome 6. HLA linkage facilitates heterozygote identification and antenatal diagnosis.

Deficiency of 11β-Hydroxylase

Less common than 21-hydroxylase deficiency, 11β-hydroxylase deficiency is inherited in autosomal recessive fashion. Deficiency of 11β-hydroxylase results in decreased conversion of 11-deoxycortisol to cortisol. Desoxycortisol, desoxycorticosterone, and testosterone are increased.

Tetrahydrocortisol, the major metabolite of 11-deoxycortisol, is increased.

Because desoxycortisol and desoxycorticosterone are potent salt-retaining hormones, increased levels may lead to hypervolemia and, hence, hypertension. Patients with 11β-hydroxylase deficiency thus not only manifest the genital virilization characteristic of 21-hydroxylase deficiency, but also hypertension. Salt-wasting does not occur. Deficiency for the 11β-hydroxylase gene located on chromosome number 8 is inherited in autosomal recessive fashion.

Deficiency of 3β-ol-Dehydrogenase

If 3β-ol-dehydrogenase (Fig. 11) is deficient, the only androgen synthesized is dehydroepiandrosterone (DHEA). This relatively weak androgen cannot be converted to androstenedione and testosterone. Females with 3β-ol-dehydrogenase deficiency are thus less virilized than females with 21- or 11β-hydroxylase deficiencies. On the other hand, DHEA is such a weak androgen that males with 3β-ol-dehydrogenase deficiency fail to masculinize completely (male pseudohermaphroditism). 3β-ol-Dehydrogenase deficiency is therefore the only form of adrenal hyperplasia in which both males and females show genital ambiguity. 3β-ol-Dehydrogenase activity is believed to reach its maximum capacity earlier in embryonic testes (third month) than in embryonic adrenals and ovaries (fourth month). Otherwise, one might expect the external genitalia to be identical in affected males and affected females.

Complete deficiency of 3β-ol-dehydrogenase results in severe salt wasting because of deficiency of salt-retaining hormones. Sodium wasting is often so pronounced that affected infants die precipitously. However, less severe deficiencies are compatible with long-term survival, increasing numbers of cases now being detected in older infants (112). The trait is inherited in autosomal recessive fashion, and is best diagnosed on the basis of elevated urinary pregnenetriol.

Deficiency of 17α-hydroxylase

If 17α-hydroxylase is deficient, pregnenolone cannot be converted to 17α-hydroxypregnenolone. Cortisol, androstenedione, testosterone, and estrogens cannot be synthesized if the defect is complete; however, 11-desoxycorticosterone and corticosterone can be synthesized. As ACTH secretion compensatorily increases, 11-desoxycorticosterone and corticosterone increase. This results in hypernatremia, hypokalemia, hypervolemia, and hypertension. Aldosterone is decreased, presumably because hypervolemia suppresses the renin-angiotensin system.

Females with 17α-hydroxylase deficiency have normal external genitalia, but at puberty they fail to undergo normal secondary sexual development (primary amenorrhea). Their oocytes appear incapable of reaching diameter of >2.5 mm (113). Affected males usually have genital ambiguity (male pseudohermaphroditism). 17α-Hydroxylase deficiency is assumed to be an autosomal recessive trait.

Cloacal Anemalies

Genital abnormalities may also result from maldevelopment of the genital tubercle, cloacal membrane, urogenital membrane, or the entire hind end of the embryo (caudal regression syndrome). In some of these malformations the external genitalia may be so abnormal that the sex of rearing is in doubt. Discussed elsewhere in detail (114), these rare disorders include exstrophy of the bladder, exstrophy of cloaca, and sirenomelia. Gearhart and Rock (115) also reported some unusual forms of female pseudohermaphroditism.

Teratogenic Female Pseudohermaphroditism

Female pseudohermaphroditism can result from administration of androgens or certain progestins during pregnancy. These forms of female pseudohermaphroditism are now rare, but still important because they are preventable. Administration of testosterone and other androgens to pregnant women may masculinize their female offspring: phallic enlargement, labioscrotal fusion, displacement of the urogenital sinus invagination, and Wolffian duct development. Again, excessive androgen production does not affect Müllerian differentiation or ovarian differentiation.

The phenomenon of androgen-induced female pseudohermaphroditism in humans was clinically important several decades ago, when women were routinely treated during pregnancy with high doses of synthetic progestins. Virilized female offspring often resulted (116). Administration of progestins during pregnancy is now rarely indicated.

Not every female fetus exposed to a given progestin is masculinized. Teratogenesis depends upon the specific agent, the dosage, the time during gestation when the agent is administered, and genotype of mother and fetus. All this would be predicted in accordance with known principles of teratogenicity. Some hormones are more likely to produce female pseudohermaphroditism than others (5). Testosterone, ethinyl testosterone, norethindrone acetate, and norethindrone are proved teratogens. Norethynodrel, medroxyprogesterone and 17α-OH-progesterone caproate have rarely been implicated. In order to interfere with genital differentiation, a teratogen must also be present during organogenesis. Prior to that time organ-specific structural abnormalities do not arise. In humans, the genital tubercle first becomes evident at about 5 weeks of embryogenesis (seven weeks gestation). By 10–12 weeks, male and female embryos are anatomically distinguishable. Labioscrotal fusion thus occurs only if a teratogen is administered prior to 12 weeks. After 12 weeks, an androgenic teratogen may cause clitoral enlargement, but not labioscrotal fusion.

Often cited as a cause for masculinizing female fetuses, androgen-secreting tumors in pregnant women are actually an extraordinarily rare cause of female pseudohermaphroditism. Fetal masculinization has been reported in pregnancies associated with arrhenoblastoma, Leydig cell tumor, luteoma of pregnancy, and certain adenocarcinomas metastatic to the ovary (Krukenberg tumor). However, patients with pre-existing androgen-secreting tumors rarely become pregnant. In 1973 Verhoeven (117) could collect only 45 reports in which virilizing tumors were associated with pregnancy. Among the offspring were 18 females whose external genitalia were described; nine had clitoral or labial hypertrophy, but only one had labioscrotal fusion.

Other Forms of Female Pseudohermaphroditism

Jones and Park (118) and Park et al. (119) described two sibs with clitoral hypertrophy, a single perineal orifice leading anteriorly to a urethra and posteriorly to a vagina, and numerous skeletal anomalies (hypoplasia of the mandible and maxilla, brachycephaly, narrow vertebral bodies, relatively long slender bones, dislocation or fusion of the radial heads leading to abnormal-appearing elbows, coxa valga, and phalangeal fusion of several toes). Müllerian derivatives and ovaries were normal. Both sibs developed breasts and pubic hair, but failed to menstruate. Their parents were consanguineous; thus, autosomal recessive inheritance seemed probable.

Female pseudohermaphroditism of unknown etiology can also be associated with one or more of the following anomalies: absence or duplication of the uterus; absence, duplication, or hydronephrosis of the kidneys; and imperforate anus (120). Short stature, mental retardation, deafness, ear and nose malformation, and blindly ending colon are less often associated; ovaries are usually normal.

Occasionally clitoral hypertrophy seems idiopathic. Recent evidence that placental aromatase perturbation can be associated with female pseudohermaphroditism (120a)

may help explain otherwise perplexing cases.

MALE PSEUDOHERMAPHRODITISM

Male pseudohermaphrodites are individuals with a Y chromosome whose external genitalia fail to develop as expected for normal males. Some authors apply the appellation only to those whose external genitalia are ambiguous enough to confuse the sex of rearing; however, applying the term more liberally seems more useful clinically. Cytogenetic forms of male pseudohermaphroditism (45,X/46,XY and variants) are also discussed here in order to contrast their phenotype with those of genetic male pseudohermaphroditism.

Cytogenetic Forms

The 45,X/46,XY individuals have both a 45,X cell line and at least one cell line containing a Y chromosome. They may manifest a variety of phenotypes, ranging from almost normal males with cryptorchidism or penile hypospadias to females indistinguishable from those with the 45,X Turner syndrome (114,121). Different phenotypes presumably reflect different tissue distributions of the various cell lines. Not infrequently a structurally abnormal Y chromosome is present.

The 45,X/46,XY individuals may be grouped clinically into one of three categories, specifically individuals with (a) unambiguous female external genitalia, (b) ambiguous external genitalia, i.e., the sex of rearing is in doubt, or (c) nearly normal male external genitalia.

Female External Genitalia

These 45,X/46,XY individuals may have the Turner stigmata (Table 2) and thus be clinically indistinguishable from 45,X individuals. Usually, such individuals are normal in stature and show no somatic anomalies. Like other types of gonadal dysgenesis, the external genitalia, vagina, and Müllerian derivatives remain unstimulated because of the lack of sex steroids. Breasts fail to develop. If breast development occurs in a 45,X/46,XY individual, one should suspect an estrogen-secreting tumor like a gonadoblastoma or dysgerminoma (122). Occasionally virilization is claimed to result from gonadotropin stimulation of streak gonads (123).

Although the streak gonads of 45,X/46,XY individuals are usually histologically indistinguishable from the streak gonads of individuals with 45,X gonadal dysgenesis, gonadoblastomas or dysgerminomas develop in about 15–20% of 45,X/46,XY individuals. Neoplasia may develop in the first or second decade. Despite the possibility that loss of a region (locus) on Yq has been claimed to confer a protective effect with respect to neoplasia (35), we recommend gonadal extirpation for all 45,X/46,XY individuals having female external genitalia. The uterus should not be removed, in deference to prospects of pregnancy through donor oocytes or donor embryos.

Ambiguous Genitalia

The term asymmetric or mixed gonadal dysgenesis is applied to individuals with one streak gonad and one dysgenetic testis. Such individuals usually have ambiguous external genitalia and a 45,X/46,XY complement. Occasionally only 45,X or only 46,XY cells are demonstrable. Many investigators believe that the phenotype is invariably associated with 45,X/46,XY mosaicism, ostensibly nonmosaic cases merely reflecting inability to sample appropriate tissues.

An important clinical observation is that 45,X/46,XY individuals with ambiguous external genitalia usually have Müllerian derivatives (e.g., a uterus). Presence of a uterus is diagnostically helpful because that organ is absent in almost all genetic (Mendelian) forms of male pseudohermaphroditism (discussed elsewhere in this section). If an individual has ambiguous external genitalia, bilateral testes, and a uterus, it is therefore reasonable to infer that such an individual has 45,X/46,XY mosaicism, regardless of whether both lines can be demonstrated cytogenetically. Occasionally the uterus is rudimentary, or a Fallopian tube may fail to develop ipsilateral to a testis.

Almost Normal Male Genitalia

The 45,X/46,XY mosaicism may be detected in individuals with almost normal male external genitalia. In fact, this phenotype may be the single most common form, based on 45,X/46,XY fetus ascertained at amniocentesis usually (90%) having a normal male phenotype (124). That neonates with genital ambiguity seem the more common reflects biases of selection. 45,X/46,XY individuals having almost normal male external genitalia do not seem to develop neoplasia as often as 45,X/46,XY individuals with female or frankly ambiguous genitalia. Gonadal extirpation is thus probably not necessary if a male sex-of-rearing is chosen, provided gonads can be assessed periodically within the scrotum.

Disorders with Multiple Malformation Patterns

Genital ambiguity may be part of multiple malformation patterns caused by mutant genes. Long recognized is the coexistence of genital ambiguity with the Meckel syndrome, the Smith-Lemli-Opitz (type I) syndrome, the brachioskeletal-genital syndrome (125) and the esophageal-facial-genital syndrome (126). These disorders are inherited in autosomal recessive or X-linked recessive fashion. Descriptions are provided in standard text books of dysmorphia (127,128).

Several recently recognized disorders are of special interest to gynecologists. "Drash syndrome" is the term now applied to individuals with Wilms' tumor, aniridia, and male pseudohermaphroditism (47,129). Because Wilms' tumor is associated with deletion of chromosome 11p13, its association with the Drash syndrome could be interpreted as localizing an autosomal region integral for male development. Smith-Lemli-Opitz syndrome, type II, is an autosomal recessive condition in which 46,XY individuals not only show genital abnormalities but also female external genitalia (sex-reversal) (130). In the genitopalatal-cardiac (Gardner-Silengo-Wachtel) syndrome, 46,XY individuals show phenotypic variability not only in external genitalia but also in gonads (60); complete sex-reversal can even occur, 46,XY individuals showing ovaries (60). Implications of these syndromes for sex determining mechanisms are discussed in detail elsewhere (106).

Deficiencies in Testosterone Biosynthesis

Male pseudohermaphroditism may result from deficiencies of 17-α-hydroxylase, 3β-ol-dehydrogenase, 17-ketosteroid reductase, 17-20 desmolase, or one of the enzymes required to convert cholesterol to pregnenolone (congenital adrenal lipoid hyperplasia) (Fig. 11). Deficiencies of 21- or 11β-hydroxylase, the most common causes of female pseudohermaphroditism, do not cause male pseudohermaphroditism.

An enzyme deficiency should be suspected if testosterone or its metabolites is decreased. Although diagnosis of the conditions to be discussed below is not difficult in older children, detection may be difficult during infancy because neonatal testosterone levels are normally low. Provocative tests (hCG) are usually recommended to facilitate diagnosis.

Congenital Adrenal Lipoid Hyperplasia

In this condition male pseudohermaphrodites show ambiguous or female-like external genitalia, severe salt wasting and adrenals characterized by foamy-appearing cells filled with cholesterol. Approximately 30 cases have been described (131,132). Accumulation of cholesterol has long indicated that this compound cannot be converted to pregnenolone (Fig. 11). The enzyme responsible for this defect is that causing side chain cleavage (scc). This enzyme is required to convert cholesterol to pregnenolone: 20α-hydroxylase, 20,22-desmolase, 22α-hydroxylase. Inheritance is presumed to be autosomal recessive on the basis of increased parental consanguinity.

3βol-Dehydrogenase Deficiency

Deficiency of 3β-ol-dehydrogenase, also an autosomal recessive disorder, results in decreased synthesis of both androgens and estrogens (Fig. 11). By 1985, Perrone et al. (133) had collected 27 cases in males. The major androgen produced is DHEA, which as a weaker androgen than testosterone cannot produce adequate virilization. Diagnosis is usually made on the basis of elevated urinary 16-hydroxypregnenolone. In addition to genital abnormalities, 3β-ol-dehydrogenase deficiency is often associated with severe salt wasting because aldosterone and cortisol are decreased.

The incompletely developed external genitalia in 3β-ol-dehydrogenase deficiency are clinically similar to the external genitalia of most other male pseudohermaphrodites: small phallus, urethral opening proximal on the penis, incomplete labioscrotal fusion. Testes and Wolffian ducts differentiate normally. Given that affected females (46,XX) also show genital ambiguity, 3β-ol-dehydrogenase is the only enzyme that when deficient produces male pseudohermaphroditism in males and female pseudohermaphroditism in females.

17α-Hydroxylase Deficiency

Males deficient of 17α-hydroxylase usually show ambiguous external genitalia; however, Wolffian duct development and testicular development are normal. Severely affected males may even show female external genitalia (134). Males deficient for 17α-hydroxylase usually display normal blood pressure, although females (46,XX) show hypertension. Inheritance is autosomal recessive.

17,20-Desmolase Deficiency

Zachmann et al. (135) reported a family in which two maternal cousins had genital ambiguity, bilateral testes, and no Müllerian derivatives. A maternal "aunt" was said to have abnormal external genitalia and bilateral testes. The deficient enzyme was deduced to be 17,20-desmolase deficiency on the basis of both cousins showing low plasma testosterone and DHEA despite normal urinary excretion of pregnanediol, pregnanetriol, and 17-hydroxycorticoids. In testicular tissue testosterone could be synthesized from androstenedione or dehydroepiandrosterone, excluding 17-ketosteroid reductase deficiency (see below) but suggesting 17,20-desmolase deficiency. Later, however, 17,20 demolase and 17α-hydroxylase enzymes were shown to be closely related, if not identical, given that a single enzyme is capable of both steroid interconversions (136). It remains unclear whether this disorder is autosomal recessive or X-linked recessive.

Deficiency of 17-Ketosteroid Reductase

Inability of testes to convert dehydroepiandrosterone to testosterone is the result of deficiency of 17-ketosteroid reductase (Fig. 11). Approximately 25 cases are reported (137). Plasma testosterone is usually decreased; androstenedione and dehydroepiandrosterone are increased. Affected males show ambiguous external genitalia, bilateral testes, and no Müllerian derivatives. Breast development may or may not be present, apparently depending upon the estrogen/testosterone ratio (138). Pubertal virilization is greater than in some other enzyme deficiencies, gynecomastia sometimes not even being evident (139). In one remarkable case, the sex of rearing of an affected individual was changed from female to male after puberty (138). The disorder could be either autosomal recessive or X-linked recessive.

Complete Androgen Insensitivity

In complete androgen insensitivity (complete testicular feminization), 46,XY individuals have bilateral testes, female external genitalia, blindly-ending vagina, and no Müllerian derivatives. Affected individuals undergo breast development and pubertal feminization (Fig. 12).

Despite pubertal feminization, some individuals with androgen insensitivity show clitoral enlargement and labioscrotal fusion; the term incomplete (partial) androgen insensitivity (incomplete testicular feminization) is applied to these patients. Both complete and incomplete (partial) androgen insensitivity are inherited in X-linked recessive fashion. Not only are the two disorders genetically distinct, but heterogeneity exists for each. The gene for complete androgen insensitivity has been localized to the X long arm and cloned.

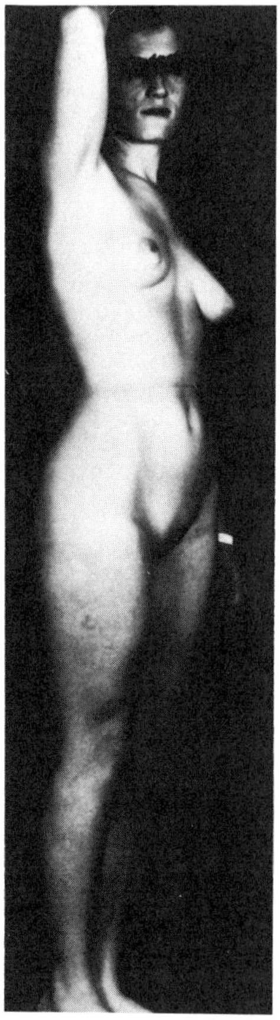

FIG. 12. Photograph of individual with complete androgen insensitivity. (From ref. 114, with permission.)

Clinical features of complete androgen sensitivity are well-known to clinicians. Some affected individuals may be quite attractive and show excellent breast development, but most are similar in appearance to unaffected females in the general population. Breasts contain normal ductal and glandular tissue, but areolae are often pale and underdeveloped. Pubic and axillary hair are usually sparse, but scalp hair is normal. The vagina terminates blindly. Sometimes vaginal length is shorter than usual, presumably because Müllerian ducts fail to contribute to formation of the vagina. Occasionally, the vagina is only 1–2 cm long or represented merely by a dimple. Surgery may then be necessary to create a neovagina.

Neither a uterus nor Fallopian tubes are ordinarily present. Occasionally one detects fibromuscular remnants, rudimentary Fallopian tubes or even a uterus (140). Absence of Müllerian derivatives is not unexpected because the AMH secreted by the fetal Sertoli cells is not an androgen; therefore, Müllerian regression would be expected to occur in males with androgen sensitivity, just as in normal males. The only other condition in which a uterus is absent in a phenotypic female is Müllerian aplasia, readily distinguishable on the basis of pubic hair and a 46,XX complement.

Testes are usually normal in size. They may be located in the abdomen, inguinal canal, or labia, i.e., anywhere along the path of embryonic testicular descent. If located in the inguinal canal, testes may produce inguinal hernias. One-half of all individuals with testicular feminization develop inguinal hernias. It is, therefore, worthwhile to determine cytogenetic status of prepubertal girls with inguinal hernias; however, most will prove 46,XX. Height is slightly increased compared to normal women, but unremarkable compared to 46,XY males.

Frequency of gonadal neoplasia is increased, but the exact magnitude is uncertain. Once considered relatively high (141), the actual risk is probably no greater than 5% (14,122). Risk of neoplasia is certainly relatively low before 25–30 years of age, thereafter increasing. Benign tubular adenomas (Pick adenomas) are especially common in postpubertal patients, probably as result of increased secretion of LH. Although orchiectomy is eventually necessary, it is acceptable to leave the testes in situ until after pubertal feminization. Most surgeons would, however, perform orchiectomies if herniorrophies prove necessary before puberty. There may also be psychologic benefit in prepubertal orchiectomies.

Pathogenesis of complete androgen insensitivity clearly involves end-organ insensitivity to androgens. This has long been deduced on the basis of baseline plasma testosterone being normal, yet patients neither virilizing nor retaining nitrogen after administration of androgen (testosterone or dehydrotestosterone). In addition, hyperplastic Leydig cells and elevated LH levels suggest an abnormal gonadal-hypothalamic axis.

Genetic heterogeneity exists. In 60–70% of cases, androgen receptors are not present (receptor negative). In 30–40%, receptors are present (receptor positive). In the latter, a defect at a more distal step in androgen action must be postulated. Receptor positive and receptor negative cases are clinically indistinguishable. Enormous recent progress has been made by applying molecular genetic technology to receptor negative androgen insensitivity. A number of different mutations have been uncovered. All mutations are in the androgen binding domain (exons 5, 6, and 7) (Fig. 13). No particular exon is preferentially involved, nor any particular codon (142).

Incomplete or Partial Androgen Sensitivity and the Reifenstein Syndrome

At puberty we have already noted that certain 46,XY individuals feminize (show

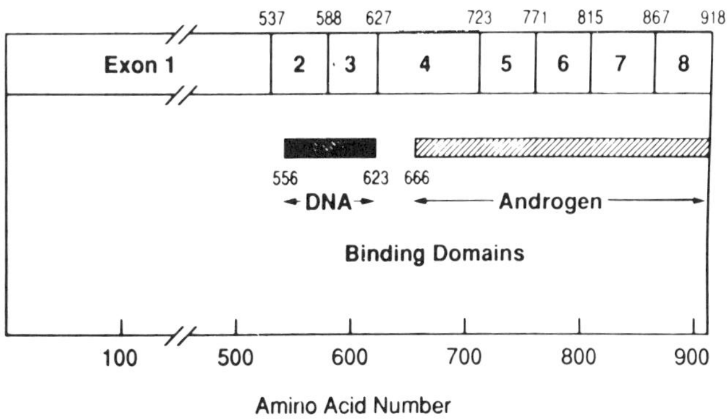

FIG. 13. Schematic diagram showing androgen receptor gene whose mutations cause complete and partial androgen insensitivity. (From ref. 142, with permission.)

breast development) despite having external genitalia characterized by phallic enlargement and partial labioscrotal fusion. Such individuals are said to have incomplete or partial androgen insensitivity (incomplete testicular feminization). Both incomplete and complete androgen insensitivity share the following features: bilateral testes with similar histologic findings, no Müllerian derivatives, pubertal breast development, lack of pubertal virilization, normal (male) plasma testosterone and failure to respond to androgen (85,114,143). The pathogenesis of partial androgen insensitivity probably involves decreased numbers or qualitative defects of androgen receptors (2,144–146). As noted above, molecular analysis detected several different mutations in the androgen binding domains (exons 5, 6, and 7). There is as of yet no correlation between the region involved and phenotype.

Irrespective, incomplete (partial) androgen insensitivity is an X-linked recessive condition that encompasses several entities once considered separate: Lubs syndrome, Gilbert-Dreyfus syndrome, Reifenstein syndrome.

In 1974, Wilson et al. (147) demonstrated occurrence in a single kindred of both the Reifenstein phenotype and incomplete androgen insensitivity phenotype as traditionally defined, and in 1984 the same group confirmed partial androgen receptor deficiency in two individuals with the Lubs syndrome phenotype (148). Thus, the traditional separation between Reifenstein syndrome, Lubs syndrome and incomplete androgen insensitivity as defined above was not valid. All these disorders merely represent different spectrums of a single X-linked recessive disorder, here called incomplete (partial) androgen insensitivity. Incidentally, this author believes that individuals characterized by female external genitalia yet failure of posterior labioscrotal fusion also fit into this spectrum, disagreeing with those who apply a separate appellation. Genetic heterogeneity still exists, but the basis is molecular and for now should not be considered to exist solely on the basis of differences in clinical appearance.

Of course, the clinical significance of incomplete (partial) androgen insensitivity is that this disorder must be excluded before a male sex of rearing is assigned. Presence of androgen receptors and demonstration of a response to exogenous androgen excludes the condition.

5α-Reductase Deficiency

For over 20 years, it has been recognized that some genetic males show ambiguous external genitalia at birth, yet at puberty virilize like normal males. They undergo phallic enlargement, increased facial hair, muscular hypertrophy, voice deepening, and no breast development. Their external genitalia consist of a phallus that resembles a clitoris more than a penis, a perineal urethral orifice, and usually a separate blindly ending perineal orifice that resembles a vagina (pseudovagina) (Fig. 14). Testes of relatively normal size secrete testosterone in normal amounts.

By 1971–1972, this trait, then called pseudovaginal perineoscrotal hypospadias (PPSH), was shown to be inherited in autosomal recessive fashion (149,150). The disorder was later shown to result from deficiency of the enzyme 5α-reductase (151–153). This enzyme converts testosterone to dihydrotestosterone. That intracellular 5α-reductase deficiency results in the PPSH phenotype is consistent with observations that virilization of the external genitalia during embryogenesis requires dihydrotestosterone; Wolffian differentiation requires only testosterone. Pubertal virilization also can be accomplished by testosterone alone.

The 5α-reductase deficiency is autosomal recessive (151). Diagnosis is most easily made on the basis of an elevated testosterone (T)/dihydrotestosterone (DHT) ratio after administering hCG or testosterone propionate (154). The ratio of the respective

urinary metabolites of T and DHT (i.e., etiocholanolone/androsterone) is also elevated. In infants, baseline levels of testosterone and dihydrotestosterone are so low that distinguishing normal from affected individuals may be difficult. Imperato-McGinley et al. (155) suggest elevated urinary tetrahydrocortisol/5α-tetrahydrocortisol ratio as the basis for diagnosis, utilizing gas chromatography/mass spectrometry.

Agonadia

In agonadia gonads are absent, external genitalia abnormal, and all but rudimentary Müllerian or Wolffian derivatives absent. External genitalia usually consist of a phallus about the size of a clitoris, underdeveloped labia majora, and nearly complete fusion of labioscrotal folds. A persistent urogenital sinus is often present. By definition, gonads are undetectable. Neither normal Müllerian derivatives nor normal Wolffian derivatives are ordinarily present; however, rudimentary structures may be present along the lateral pelvic wall. Somatic anomalies (craniofacial, vertebral, mental retardation) may coexist (156).

Pathogenesis of agonadia must take into account not only absence of gonads, but also abnormal external genitalia and absence of internal ducts. Two explanations seem plausible: (a) Fetal testes functioned sufficiently long to inhibit Müllerian development, yet not sufficiently long to complete male differentiation (hence the appellation testicular regression syndrome, preferred by some). (b) Alternatively, gonadal, ductal, and genital systems could have all developed abnormally as result of either defective anlage, defective connective tissue, or teratogenic action. The frequent coexistence of somatic anomalies is most consistent with the latter hypothesis.

Among the approximately 30 reported cases are several sibships of affected males (157). Autosomal recessive inheritance seems likely, but X-linked recessive inheritance cannot be excluded.

Leydig Cell Agenesis

46,XY patients showing complete absence of Leydig cells (158,159) have female external genitalia, no uterus, and bilateral testes devoid of Leydig cells. Epididymides and vasa deferentia are present. LH is elevated. Affected sibs have been reported (160,161), and parental consanguinity observed (161,162).

TRUE HERMAPHRODITISM

True hermaphrodites display both ovarian and testicular tissue. They may have a separate ovary and a separate testis, or, more often, one or more ovotestes. Most (60%) true hermaphrodites have a 46,XX chromosomal complement; however, others have 46, XX/46,XY, 46,XY,46,XX/47,XXY, or other complements (56). Although there are suggestions that phenotype depends upon karyotype (56,163), it is preferable here to generalize about the phenotype of all true hermaphrodites.

Phenotype

About two-thirds of true hermaphrodites are raised as males, although their external genitalia may be frankly ambiguous or predominantly female. Irrespective, breast development usually occurs at puberty even with predominantly male external genitalia.

Gonadal tissue may be located in the ovarian, inguinal, or labioscrotal regions. A testis or an ovotestis is more likely to be present on the right than the left. Spermatozoa are rarely present (164); however, apparently normal oocytes are often present, surprisingly in ovotestes. Five 46,XX true hermaphrodites have become pregnant (165,166), usually but not always after removal of testicular tissue.

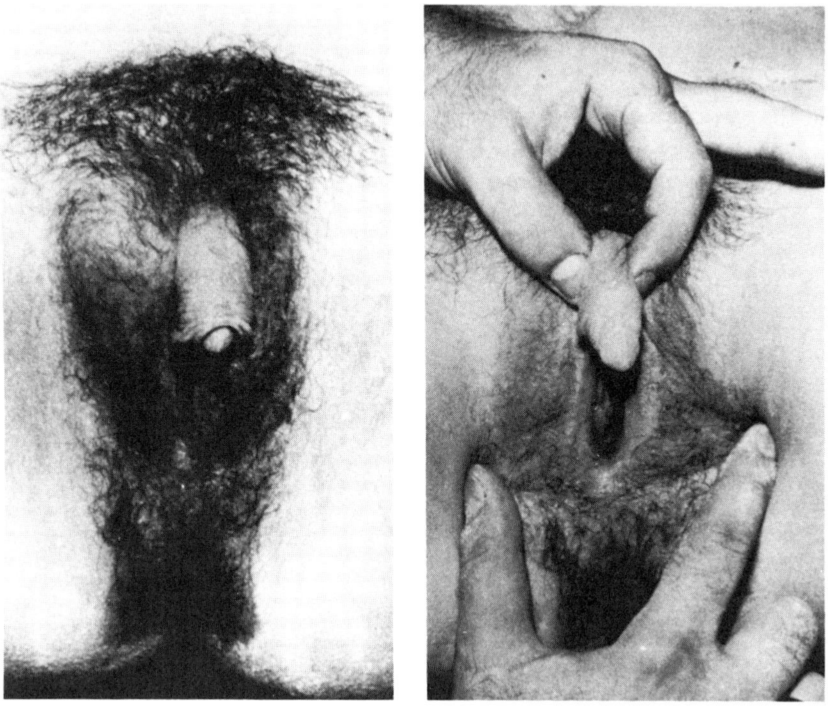

FIG. 14. Photographs of the external genitalia of an individual with pseudovaginal perineoscrotal hypospadias. At puberty, phallic enlargement occurred and breast development did not. Some individuals with this phenotype have a 5α-reductase deficiency. (From ref. 150, with permission.)

The greater the proportion of testicular tissue in an ovotestis, the greater the likelihood of gonadal descent. In 80% of ovotestes, testicular and ovarian components are juxtaposed end-to-end (167). An ovotestis can thus be detected by inspection or by palpation because testicular tissue is softer and darker than ovarian tissue. Ultrasound evaluation may also be useful. Accurate identification is particularly necessary if one wishes to extirpate the inappropriate portion of an ovotestis.

A uterus is usually present, albeit sometimes bicornuate or unicornuate. Absence of a uterine horn usually indicates an ipsilateral testis or ovotestis. The fimbriated end of the Fallopian tube may be occluded ipsilateral to an ovotestis, and squamous metaplasia of the endocervix may occur (167). Menstruation is not uncommon, occasionally manifested as cyclic hematuria (168).

Diagnosis is usually made only after excluding male and female pseudohermaphroditism. If a female sex-of-rearing is chosen, extensive surgery may or may not be necessary. genital reconstruction and selective gonadal extirpation is invariably indicated. Both gonadal neoplasia as well as breast carcinoma have been reported (56,122).

Etiology

The etiology of true hermaphroditism is heterogenous and doubtless reflective of chromosomal complement. 46,XX/46,XY true hermaphroditism is caused by chimerism. Chimerism is the presence in a single individual of two or more cell lines, each derived from different zygotes, in a single individual. Simpson (56) believes that most 46,XY cases are unrecognized chimeras.

Although a few 46,XX true hermaphro-

Expression of H-Y antigen by female mice carrying SXR. *Transplantation* 1984;37:1721–3.
27. McLaren A, Simpson E, Tomonari K, et al. Male sex differentiation in mice lacking H-Y antigen. *Nature* 1984;312:552–5.
28. Burgoyne PS, Levy ER, McLaren A. Spermatogenic failure in male mice lacking H-Y antigen. *Nature* 1986;320:170–2.
29. Page DC. Sex reversal: deletion mapping the male determining function of the Y chromosome. *Cold Spring Harbor Symp Quant Biol* 1986;51:229–35.
30. Simpson E, Chandler P, Goulmy E, et al. Separation of the genetic loci for the H-Y antigen and for testis determination on human Y chromosome. *Nature* 1987;326:876–8.
31. Smith DW, Marokus R, Graham JM Jr. Tentative evidence of Y-linked statural gene(s). Growth in the testicular feminization syndrome. *Clin Pediatr* 1985;24:189–92.
32. Alvesalo L, de la Chapelle A. Tooth size in two males with deletion of the long arm of the Y chromosome. *Ann Hum Genet* 1981;54:49–54.
33. Simpson JL. Genetic control of sexual development. In: Ratnam SS, Teoh E, Anandakumar C, eds. *Advances in fertility and sterility: releasing hormones and genetics and immunology in human reproduction, vol 3. Proceedings of the 12th World Congress on Fertility and Sterility (Singapore 1986).* Lancaster: United Kingdom Parthenon Press. 1987:165–73.
34. Tiepolo L, Zuffardi O. Localization of factors controlling spermatogenesis in the non-fluorescent portion of the human Y chromosome long arm. *Hum Genet* 1976;34:119–24.
35. Lukusa T, Fryns JP, Van den Berge H. Gonadoblastoma and Y-chromosome fluorescence. *Clin Genet* 1986;29:311–6.
36. Page DC. Hypothesis: a Y-chromosome gene causes gonadoblastoma in poorly dysgenetic gonads. *Development* 1987;101:151–5.
37. Chandra HS. Is human X chromosome inactivation a sex determining device?: *Proc Natl Acad Sci USA* 1985;82:6947–9.
38. Geldwerth D, Bishop CE, Guaellaen G, et al. Extensive DNA sequence homologies between the human Y and the long arm of the X chromosome. *EMRO J* 1985;4:1739–43.
39. Simpson JL. Phenotypic-karyotypic correlations of gonadal determinants: Current status and relationship to molecular studies. In: Sperling K, Vogel F, eds. *Human genetics. Proceedings of the 7th International Congress Human Genetics (Berlin, 1986).* Heidelberg: Springer-Verlag, 1987:224–32.
40. de la Chapelle A. The Y-chromosomal and autosomal testis-determining genes. *Development* 1987;101:33–8.
41. de la Chapelle A. The complicated issue of human sex differentiation. *Am J Hum Genet* 1988;43:1–3.
42. German J. Gonadal dimorphism explained as a dosage effect of a locus on the sex chromosomes, the Gonad-Differentiation Locus (GDL). *Am J Hum Genet* 1988;42:414–21.
43. Hodgkin J. Primary sex determination in the nematode C. elegans. *Development* 1987;101: 5–16.
44. Nothiger R, Steinman-Zwicky M. Genetics of sex determination: what can we learn from Drosophila? *Development* 1987;101:17–24.
45. Eicher EM, Washburn LL, Whitney JB III, et al. Mus posciavinus Y chromosome in C57BL/65 murine genome causes sex reversal. *Science* 1982;217:535–7.
46. Washburn LL, Eicher ME. Sex reversal in XY mice caused by dominant mutation on Chromosome 17. *Nature* 1983;303:338–40.
47. Habib R, Loirat C, Gubler MC, et al. The nephropathy associated with male pseudohermaphroditism and Wilms' tumor (Drash syndrome): a distinctive glomerular lesion—report of 10 cases. *Clin Nephrol* 1985;24:269–36.
48. Clayton GW, Smith JD, Rosenberg HS. Familial true hermaphroditism in pre- and postpuberal genetic females. Hormonal and morphologic studies. *J Clin Endocrinol Metab* 1958; 18:1349–58.
49. Rosenberg HS, Clayton GW, Hsu TC. Familial true hermaphroditism. *J Clin Endocrinol Metab* 1983;23:203–6.
50. Armendares S, Salamanca F, Canty SD, et al. Familial true hermaphroditism in three siblings. *Humangenetik* 1975;29:99–109.
51. Fraccaro M, Tiepolo L, Zuffardio-Chiumello G, et al. Familial XX true hermaphroditism and H-Y antigen. *Hum Genet* 1979;48:45–51.
52. Berger R, Abonyi D, Nodot A, et al. Hermaphroditism vrai et "garcon XX" dans une fratrie. *Revue Europeenne de Etudes Clinique Biologie* 1970;15:330–33.
53. Kasdan R, Nankin HP, Troen P, et al. Paternal transmission of maleness in XX human beings. *N Engl J Med* 1973;288:539–45.
54. Petit C, de la Chapelle A, Levilliers J, et al. An abnormal terminal X-Y interchange accounts for most but not all cases of human XX maleness. *Cell* 1987;49:595–602.
55. Skordis NA, Stetka DG, MacGillivray MH, et al. Familial 46,XX coexisting with familial 46,XX true hermaphrodites in same pedigree. *J Pediatr* 1987;110:244–8.
56. Simpson JL. True hermaphroditism. Etiology and phenotypic considerations. *Birth Defects* 1978;14(6):9–35.
57. Jirasek J. Principles of reproductive embroyology. In: Simpson JL, ed. *Disorders of sexual differentiation.* New York: Academic Press, 1976:51–111.
58. Burgoyne PS, Baker TG. Perinatal oocyte loss in XO mice and its implication for the etiology of gonadal dysgenesis in XO women. *J Reprod Fertil* 1987;75:633–45.
59. Cussen LK, McMahon R. Germ cells and ova in dysgenetic gonads of a 46,XY female dizygote twin. *Arch Dis Child* 1979;133:373–5.
60. Greenberg F, Gresik MW, Carpenter RJ, et al. The Gardner-Silengo-Wachtel or Genito-Palato-Cardiac syndrome: male pseudohermaphroditism with micrognathia, cleft palate, and conotruncal cardiac defects. *Am J Med Genet* 1987;26:59–64.

126. Opitz JM, Howe JJ. The Meckel syndrome (dysencephalic splanchnocystica, the Gruber syndrome). *Birth Defects* 1969;5:167.
127. Jones KL. *Smith's recognizable patterns of human malformation*. 4th ed. Philadelphia: W.B. Saunders, 1988.
128. Buyse ML. *Birth defects encyclopedia*. Edinburgh: Blackwell Scientific Publishers, 1990.
129. Eddy AA, Mauer M. Pseudohermaphroditism, glomerulopathy and Wilms tumor (Drash syndrome): frequency in end-stage renal failure. *J Pediatr* 1985;106:584–7.
130. Curry CRJ, Carey JC, Holland JS, et al. Smith-Lemli-Opitz syndrome-type II: multiple congenital anomalies with male pseudohermaphroditism and frequent early lethality. *Am J Med Genet* 1987;26:45–57.
131. Degenhart HJ. Prader's syndrome (congenital lipoid adrenal hyperplasia). In: Laron Z, ed. *Pediatric adolescence endocrinology, Vol 13*. Basel: Karger, 1984:125–44.
132. Frydman M, Kauschansky A, Zamir R, et al. Familial lipoid adrenal hyperplasia: genetic marker data and an approach to prenatal diagnosis. *Am J Med Genet* 1986;25:319–25.
133. Perrone, Criscuolo T, Sinisi AA. Male pseudohermaphroditism due to 3β-hydroxysteroid dehydrogenase-isomerase deficiency associated with atrial septal defect. *Acta Endocrinol* 1985;110:532–9.
134. Heremans GFP, Moolenaar AJ, Van Geldere HM. Female phenotype in a male child due to 17α-hydroxylase deficiency. *Arch Dis Child* 1976;51:721–3.
135. Zachmann M, Vollmin JA, Hamilton W, et al. Steroid 17,20-desmolase deficiency: a new cause of male pseudohermaphroditism. *Clin Endocrinol* 1972;1:369–85.
136. Zachmann M. Male pseudohermaphroditism. In: Wachtel SS, Simpson JL, eds. *Molecular genetics of sex discrimination*. Oxford: Blackwell Scientific Publications (in press).
137. Balducci R, Toscano V, Wright F, et al. Familial male pseudohermaphroditism with gynaecomastia due to 17β-hydroxysteroid dehydrogenase deficiency. A report of 3 cases. *Clin Endocrinol* 1985;23:439–44.
138. Imperato-McGinley J, Peterson RE, Stoller R, et al. Male pseudohermaphroditism secondary to a 17α-hydroxysteroid dehydrogenase deficiency: gender role with puberty. *J Clin Endocrinol Metab* 1979;49:391–5.
139. Caufriez A. Male pseudohermaphroditism due to 17-ketoreductase deficiency: report of a case without gynecomastia and without vaginal pouch. *Am J Obstet Gynecol* 1986;154:148–9.
140. Ulloa-Aguirre A, Mendez PJ, Chavez A, et al. Incomplete regression of Mullerian ducts in the androgen insensitivity syndrome. *Fertil Steril* 1990;53:1024–8.
141. Morris JM, Mahesh VB. Further observations on the syndrome "testicular feminization." *Am J Obstet Gynecol* 1963;87:731–48.
142. Pinsky L, Trifiro M, Prior L, et al. The molecular genetics of androgen insensitivity syndromes in man. In: Wachtel SS, Simpson JL, eds. *Molecular genetics of sex determination*. Oxford: Blackwell Scientific Publications (in press).
143. Simpson JL, Rebar RW. Normal and abnormal sexual differentiation and development. In: Becker LK, ed. *Principles and practice of endocrinology and metabolism*. Philadelphia: JB Lippincott, 1990:710–39.
144. Pinksy L, Kaufman M. Genetics of steroid receptors and their disorders. *Adv Hum Genet* 1985;16:299–472.
145. Griffin JE, Punyashthiki K, Wilson JD. Dihydrotestosterone binding by culture human fibroblasts. Comparison of cells from control subjects and from patients with hereditary pseudohermaphroditism due to androgen resistance. *J Clin Invest* 1976;57:1342–51.
146. Pinsky L, Kaufman M, Levitzsky LL. Partial androgen resistance due to a distinctive qualitative defect of the androgen receptor. *Am J Med Genet* 1987;27:459–66.
147. Wilson JD, Harrod MJ, Goldstein JL, et al. Familial incomplete male pseudohermaphroditism, type 1: evidence for androgen resistance and variable clinical manifestations in a family with the Reifenstein syndrome. *N Engl J Med* 1974;290:1097–103.
148. Wilson JD, Carlson BR, Weaver D, et al. Endocrine and genetic characterization of cousins with male pseudohermaphroditism: evidence that the Lubs phenotype can result from a mutation that alters the structure of the androgen receptor. *Clin Genet* 1984;26:363–70.
149. Simpson JL, New M, Peterson RE, et al. Pseudovaginal perineoscrotal hypospadias (PPSH) in sibs. *Birth Defects* 1971;7(6):140–4.
150. Opitz JM, Simpson JL, Sarto GE, et al. Pseudovaginal perineoscrotal hypospadias. *Clin Genet* 1972;3:1–36.
151. Imperato-McGinley J, Guerrero L, Gauiter T, et al. Steroid 5δ-reductase deficiency: an inherited form of male pseudohermaphroditism. *Science* 1974;186:1213–5.
152. Walsh C, Madden JD, Harrod MJ, et al. Familial incomplete male pseudohermaphroditism, type 2. *N Engl J Med* 1974;291:944–9.
153. Peterson RE, Imperato-McGinley J, Gautier T, et al. Male pseudohermaphroditism due to steroid 5δ-reductase deficiency. *Am J Med* 1977; 62:170–91.
154. Green S, Zachmann M, Mannella B. Comparison of two tests to recognize or exclude 5 alpha-reductase deficiency in prepubertal children. *Acta Endocrinol (Copenh)* 1987;114: 113–7.
155. Imperato-McGinley J, Gautier T, Pichardo M, et al. The diagnosis of 5 alpha-reductase in infancy. *J Clin Endo Metab* 1986;63:1313–8.
156. Sarto GE, Opitz JM. The XY gonadal agenesis syndrome. *J Med Genet* 1973;10:288–93.
157. de Grouchy J, Gompel A, Salmon-Bernard Y. Embryonic testicular regression syndrome and severe mental retardation in sibs. *Ann Genet* 1985;28:154–60.

158. Brown M, Markland C, Dehner LP. Leydig cell hypoplasia: a case of male pseudohermaphroditism. *J Clin Endocrinol Metab* 1976;46:1–7.
159. Lee PA, Rock JA, Brown TR, et al. Leydig cell hypofunction resulting in male pseudohermaphroditism. *Fertil Steril* 1981;37:675–9.
160. Perez-Palacios G, Scaglia HE, Kofman-Afaro S. Inherited male pseudohermaphroditism due to gonadotropin unresponsiveness. *Acta Endocrinol* 1982;98:148–55.
161. Saldanha PH, Arnhold I JP, Mendonca BB, et al. A clinico-genetic investigation of Leydig cell hypoplasia. *Am J Med Genet* 1987;26:337–44.
162. Schwartz M, Imperato-McGinley J, Peterson RE, et al. Male pseudohermaphroditism secondary to an abnormality in Leydig cell differentiation. *J Clin Endocrinol Metab* 1981;53:123–7.
163. Van Niekerk WA, Retief AE. The gonads of human true hermaphrodities. *Hum Genet* 1981;58:117–22.
164. Aaronsen I. True hermaphroditism. A review of 41 cases with observations on testicular histology and function. *Br J Urol* 1985;57:775–9.
165. Tegenkamp TR, Brazzell JW, Tegenkamp I, et al. Pregnancy without benefit of reconstructive surgery in a bisexually active true hermaphrodite. *Am J Obstet Gynecol* 1979;135:427–8.
166. Minowada S, Fukutani K, Hara M, et al. Childbirth in a true hermaphrodite. *Eur Urol* 1984;10:414.
167. Van Neikerk WA. *True hermaphroditism*. New York: Harper and Row, 1974.
168. Raspa RW, Subramanian AP, Romas NA. True hermaphroditism presents as intermittent hemitura and groin pain. *Urology* 1986;28:133–41.
169. Ramsay M, Bernstein R, Zwane E, et al. XX true hermaphroditism in South African Blacks: an enigma of primary sexual differentiation. *Am J Hum Genet* 1988;43:4–13.
170. Mori V, Mitzutani S. Familial hermaphroditism in genetic families. *Jpn J Urol* 1968;59:857–63.
171. LeMarguand HS. Congenital hypogonadotropic hypogonadism in 5 members of a family, 3 brothers and 2 sisters. *Proc R Soc Med* 1954;47:442–6.
172. Betend B, Lebacq E Jr, David L, et al. Familial idiopathic hypogonadotrophic hypogonadism. *Acta Endocrinol (Copenh)* 1977;84:246–53.
173. Toledo SP. Leydig cell hypoplasia determining familial hypergonadotrophic hypogonadism. *Prog Clin Biol Res* 1983;200:311–4.
174. Carson SA. Hypogonadotropic hypogonadism. In: Buyse ML, ed. *Birth defects encyclopedia*. 1990:805.
175. Santen RJ, Paulsen CA. Hypogonadotrophic eunuchoidism. I. Clinical study of the mode of inheritance. *J Clin Endocrinol Metab* 1973;36:47–54.
176. Rabin D, Spitz I, Bercovici B, et al. Isolated deficiency of follicle-stimulating hormone clinical and laboratory features. *N Engl J Med* 1972;287:1313–7.
177. Bell J, Benveniste R, Spitz I, et al. Isolated deficiency of follicle-stimulating hormone. Further studies. *J Clin Endocrinol Metab* 1975;40:790–4.
178. McKusick VA, Weilbaecher RG, Gregg CW. Recessive inheritance of a congenital malformation syndrome. *JAMA* 1968;204:113–8.
179. Carson SA, Simpson JL, Malinak LR, et al. Heritable aspects of uterine anomalies II. Genetic analysis of Mullerian aplasia. *Fertil Steril* 1983;34:86–90.
180. Opitz JM. Vaginal atresia (von Mayer-Rokitansky-Kuster or MRK anomaly) in hereditary renal adysplasia (HRP). *Am J Med Genet* 1987;26:873–6.
181. Shokeir MHK. Aplasia of the Mullerian system: evidence for probable sex-limited autosomal dominant inheritance. *Birth Defects* 1978;14(6):147–65.
182. Cramer DW, Ravnikar VA, Craighill M, et al. Mullerian aplasia associated with maternal deficiency of galactose-1-phosphate uridyl transferase. *Fertil Steril* 1987;47:930–4.
183. Kaufman F, Kogut MD, Donnell GN, et al. Ovarian failure in galactosemia. *Lancet* 1979;2:737–8.
184. Hoefnagel D, Wurster-Hill DY, Dupree WB, et al. Campomelic dwarfism associated with XY gonadal dysgenesis and chromosome anomalies. *Clin Genet* 1978;13:489–99.
185. Simpson JL. Gynecologic disorders. In: King RA, Rotter JI, Motulsky AG, eds. *The genetic basis of common disease*. Oxford: Oxford Press, in press.
186. Elias S, Simpson JL, Carson SA, et al. Genetic studies in incomplete Mullerian fusion. *Obstet Gynecol* 1984;63:276–9.
187. Verp ML, Simpson JL, Elias S, et al. Heritable aspects of uterine anomalies. I. Three familial aggregates with Mullerian fusion anomalies. *Fertil Steril* 1983;34:80–5.
188. Weiss EB, Kiefer JH, Rowlatt UF, et al. Persistent Müllerian duct syndrome in male identical twins. *Pediatrics* 1978;61:797–800.
189. Sheenan SJ, Fobbia IN, Ismail MA, et al. Persistent Müllerian duct syndrome: review and report of 3 cases. *Br J Urol* 1985;57:548–51.
190. Sloan WR, Walsh PC. Familial persistent Müllerian duct syndrome. *J Urol* 1976;115:459–61.
191. Naguib KK, Teebi AS, Farag TI, et al. Familial uterine hernia syndrome: report of an Arab family of four affected males. *Am J Med Genet* 1989;33:180–1.
192. Harbison MD, Magid ML, Josso N, et al. Antimullerian hormone in three intersex conditions. *Annales de Genetique* (in press).
193. McLaren A. What makes a man a man? *Nature* 1990;346:216–7.
194. Koopman P, Gubbay J, Vivian N, et al. Male development of chromosomally female mice transgenic for SRY. *Nature* 1991;351:117–121.

Pediatric and Adolescent Gynecology,
edited by S. E. Carpenter and J. A. Rock.
Raven Press, Ltd., New York © 1992.

2

Normal Growth and Development of the Genitalia in Infancy and Childhood

Andrew S. Cook

Department of Gynecology and Obstetrics, Division of Reproductive Endocrinology, Johns Hopkins University School of Medicine, Baltimore, Maryland 21205

OVERVIEW

Changes that occur in the prepubertal female genitalia are a reflection of both the changes in the hormonal environment and the physical growth of the child. The genitalia of the newborn and child is hormonally responsive. At birth, the newborn is under the influence of estrogen via passive transmission across the placenta from the mother. The effects of this hormonal stimulation usually resolve within the first 6–8 weeks of life. The most common hormonally related changes include vulvar edema, vaginal discharge, vaginal bleeding, and breast enlargement. The external genitalia of the newborn are swollen and edematous. The hymen is usually thickened and prominent, protruding at the introitus. The hymen can remain thick and redundant as a result of maternal hormonal stimulation for up to 2 years after birth (1).

The vaginal epithelium of the newborn is thickened with glycogen rich cells in response to estrogen stimulation. The estrogen response is also reflected in the increased number of superficial cells present on the maturation index (2). The newborn physiologic vaginal discharge is the same as that seen in women in the reproductive age group. About 10% of female infants will experience withdrawal vaginal bleeding in the newborn period (3). A significant number of newborn infants experience some enlargement of the breast tissue by the fifth or sixth day. Approximately two-thirds of these infants will secrete a colostrum-like fluid followed by small amounts of milk (4). Secretion has been reported to persist up to 1 year.

The above findings are much less pronounced in the premature infant. The most prominent feature of the female genitalia in the premature infant is the relatively large clitoris. This is a normal finding, but a potential cause for concern to the unsuspecting parent or physician.

Once out of the neonatal period, the child enters a time of relative quiescence until puberty approaches. This time period is influenced primarily by the physical growth of the patient. The uterus undergoes regression from its hormonally influenced size at birth. The initial size of the uterus is not regained until the patient is 5 years old.

PHYSICAL EXAMINATION OF THE PREPUBERTAL FEMALE GENITALIA

The physical examination of the prepubertal female genitalia is unique. Success of the physical examination is highly dependent upon the rapport and interaction established with the patient. The physician should be sensitive to the child's emotions and fears, displaying gentleness, patience, and time. A lack of empathy towards the pediatric patient may, at minimum, adversely affect the ability to obtain adequate information from the physical examination and may at worst increase the potential risk of inadvertent nosocomial sexual abuse (5).

The office evaluation of the female prepubertal genitalia also requires both an understanding of the range of normal findings in a given age group and the advantages and disadvantages of the various examination techniques.

Examination Techniques in Evaluation of Prepubertal Female Genitalia

Explanation to both the mother and child of the examination process and the instruments (if any) used, is an important precursor to the genital examination. The perception that the virginal introitus is completely covered by the hymen is not uncommon. Reassurance that the exam will not alter the hymen should help to alleviate potential fears and increase the cooperation of both the patient and her mother. A great deal of information can be gained during the office examination of the female genitalia. The goal of the exam is to obtain the necessary information without causing long term emotional sequelae. In many cases the necessary information can be obtained in the office without instrumentation. Occasionally the use of general anesthesia will be necessary to perform an adequate examination. If vaginal instrumentation is necessary, the preferred type of instrument is dependent upon the age of the patient. The Cameron-Miller vaginoscope is both financially economical and efficient (Fig. 1).

An initial evaluation of hormonally sensitive tissue will provide a guide of the patient's endocrine status. Stage of breast development, vaginal mucosal maturation index, pattern of hair growth, and apocrine gland activity will provide information as to sex steroid production. In the child, an ovarian cyst or mass will present as an abdominal rather than pelvic mass, underscoring the importance of a good abdominal exam. The inguinal areas should be examined for the presence of an inguinal hernia or gonad. An inguinal gonad may represent the undescended testes of an undiagnosed male pseudohermaphrodite (6).

A prepubertal gynecologic examination

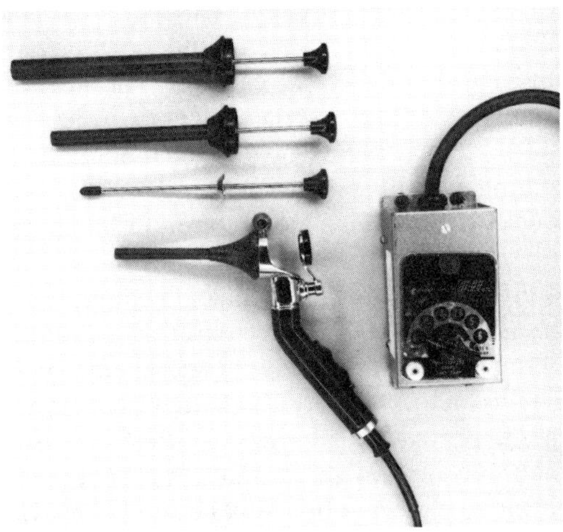

FIG. 1. Cameron-Miller vaginoscope.

should include evaluation of the external genitalia, including the clitoris, labia, perineal body and hymen, the vagina, and the cervix. The presence and size of the uterus may be determined by a rectoabdominal examination. The normal values and findings of prepubertal female genitalia will be detailed subsequently.

Three different methods used in examination of prepubertal female genitalia have been compared. Initially 172 children were each examined colposcopically using all three techniques (7). The exam techniques included (a) the supine position with labial separation, (b) the supine position with labial traction, and (c) the knee-chest position. Each technique was evaluated for the ability to open the vaginal introitus.

For examination in the supine position, the child is placed in a frog leg position, with her legs abducted and the soles of her feet together. The supine separation method involves the examiner separation of the labia with the fingertips in a lateral and downward direction until the introitus opens. The lower aspect of the labia majora are grasped between the thumb and index fingers and with gentle traction pulled, outward and slightly upward with the supine traction technique. The knee-chest examination technique employs the knee-chest position with the child's chest on the table and knees separated by 6–8 inches. The introitus is opened by placing the examiner's thumbs on the gluteus maximus at the level of the introitus and lifting, moving the perineal body and posterior fourchette dorsally.

The ability of the three examination techniques to open the introitus was compared. The knee-chest and supine traction techniques (98% and 96%) were superior to the supine separation technique (86%) in the overall ability to open the vaginal introitus. The difference in the ability to open the introitus was especially marked in the younger children. The separation technique opened the introitus in only 29% of infants and 76% of preschoolers (Table 1). The knee-chest examination method is most successful in opening the vaginal orifice and providing visualization of the cervix but requires an increased level of cooperation from the child. The vertical transhymenal diameters obtained with the knee-chest technique were consistently greater than with the other two techniques.

Normal Appearance and Values in the Examination of the Prepubertal Female Genitalia

A recent study by McCann et al. (1) details the normal values and appearance of the prepubertal female genitalia. Ninety-three nonabused girls from the ages of 10 months to 10 years old were examined using the three examination techniques described above. Examination of the prepubertal external female genitalia in the supine position (both traction and separation) yielded a greater incidence of positive findings than did examination in the knee-chest position. Labial adhesions, posterior fourchette raphe, and midline avascularity of

TABLE 1. *Ability of methods to open the vaginal introitus*

Group	Age (years)	Numbers opened with separation method	Numbers opened with traction method	Numbers opened with knee-chest method
Infant	Birth–1 11/12	2/7 (29)	7/7 (100)	7/7 (100)
Preschool	2–4 11/12	51/67 (76)	61/67 (91)	63/67 (94)
Early school age	5–7 11/12	53/55 (96)	54/55 (98)	55/55 (100)
Preadolescent	8–11 4/12	42/43 (98)	43/43 (100)	43/43 (100)

(From ref. 7, with permission.)

the posterior fourchette are common findings, whereas isolated vascularity and friability of the posterior fourchette are uncommon. Vestibular erythema, periurethral bands, and follicles are seen in a significant portion of patients. The majority of the labial adhesions were <2 mm in length. The authors felt that these small adhesions accounted for the midline avascularity with traction (supine or knee-chest) and bleeding with further traction.

Labial adhesions, which are probably related to the hypoestrogenic state of the prepubertal female, are usually asymptomatic and do not require treatment. Most labial adhesions will resolve spontaneously with puberty. The patient may present to the physician as a result of maternal concern that her daughter has vaginal agenesis. Treatment is required if the labial adhesions impede urination or drainage of vaginal secretions. Application of an estrogen cream b.i.d. to the adhesion line should be performed by a parent for 2 weeks, then once a day at bedtime for another week or two, until there is complete resolution of the labial adhesions. Gentle traction on the adhesion line at the time of estrogen application is required. Subsequent application of an ointment (e.g., vaseline) for a couple of weeks or months may help to prevent adhesion reformation.

All patients in the study by McCann et al. (1) had a hymen present. A crescent shaped hymen was the most commonly observed hymenal shape followed by the concentric hymen. The septate, cribriform, and imperforate shaped hymens were rarely seen. Redundancy of the hymenal membrane was reduced and, as a result, visualization of the hymen was increased with the supine traction and knee-chest examination techniques.

The colposcopic transhymenal diameters were measured using the three different examination techniques in preschoolers (2–4 11/12 years), early school age (5–7 11/12 years), and preadolescent (8 years to Tanner II) (Table 2). On average, the transhymenal diameters increased with the age of the child. The greatest vertical transhymenal diameters were measured with the

TABLE 2. *Colposcopic transhymenal diameter means and ranges by age group and examination method*[a]

Age group	Method	Plane	n	Mean ± SD (mm)	Range (mm)
II: Preschool (2–4 11/12 years)	Separation	Vertical	21	5.5 ± 2.2	2.5–10.0
		Horizontal	21	3.9 ± 1.4	1.0–5.5
	Traction	Vertical	24	5.5 ± 1.7	3.0–8.5
		Horizontal	24	5.2 ± 1.4	2.0–8.0
	Knee-chest	Vertical	29	6.3 ± 1.7	3.0 – 10.0
		Horizontal	29	4.6 ± 1.3	2.5–7.5
III: Early school age (5–7 11/12 years)	Separation	Vertical	39	5.6 ± 2.3	1.0–11.0
		Horizontal	39	4.2 ± 1.7	1.0–8.0
	Traction	Vertical	43	6.1 ± 2.1	1.0–10.0
		Horizontal	43	5.6 ± 1.8	1.0–9.0
	Knee-chest	Vertical	41	7.0 ± 2.0	3.0–11.5
		Horizontal	41	5.6 ± 1.5	2.5–8.5
IV: Preadolescent (8 to Tanner II)	Separation	Vertical	19	8.4 ± 2.2	5.0–13.5
		Horizontal	19	5.7 ± 1.6	3.0–8.5
	Traction	Vertical	20	8.3 ± 2.8	2.0–15.0
		Horizontal	20	6.9 ± 2.0	2.5–10.5
	Knee-chest	Vertical	21	8.7 ± 2.6	5.0–15.0
		Horizontal	21	7.3 ± 1.7	4.0–11.0

[a]n = 72. Infant age group not included because of small n.
(From ref. 1, with permission.)

supine traction technique while the largest horizontal diameters were seen with the knee-chest method.

The primary advantage of using the colposcope in examination of the prepubertal genitalia, is the capability for photographic documentation of the genital findings. An increased sensitivity, in comparison with gross visual examination, in diagnosis of genital findings or measurement of the vaginal introitus has not been documented.

The percentage of the introitus that was covered by the hymen varied over a wide range and was dependent upon the examination technique. Eighty-four patients were examined using the three examination techniques described above. The ability to visualize the cervix was highly dependent upon the examination technique used. The cervix was seen in 58 patients (69%) with the knee-chest examination technique, but was seen in none of the patients using the supine traction or separation techniques (1).

NORMAL OVARIAN DEVELOPMENT AND FINDINGS

At birth, the infant has high levels of circulating sex steroids as a result of passive placental transfer. Gonadotropins begin to rise after birth as the infant clears the placental steroids. Gonadotropin levels reach a peak in the first couple of months of life, with a slow return to low levels as the "gonadostat" is reset. This period of gonadotropin activity in the first year of life results in normal follicular activity and occasionally the formation of functional ovarian cysts. With suppression of the gonadotropins, follicular activity is reduced, but the ovary does not become quiescent. Continuous follicular growth and atresia occurs in both infancy and childhood (8). In contrast to the menstruating female who has cyclic follicular maturation and ovulation, the premenarcheal child rarely develops a dominant follicle or functional ovarian cyst.

Ovarian Morphology

Follicular growth in infancy and childhood has been documented by both morphologic and sonographic studies. An interesting study by Peters et al. (8) histologically evaluated 52 ovaries at autopsy of children who died in an accident or after an acute illness. The children ranged in ages from 2 months to 11 years. Ovarian growth was classified as (a) quiescent—small, resting follicles, with no growth; (b) early growth—preantral follicles present but not larger than 0.5 mm in diameter; and (c) actively growing—with antral follicles larger than 0.5 mm and evidence of degeneration and "scars." None of the ovaries were quiescent; three were in early growth and 49/52 were actively growing. Antral follicles measuring 3, 4, and 5 mm were commonly seen at all ages. The authors subjectively felt that both the number and size of antral follicles increased after the age of 6 years.

The ovarian architecture of infants and premenarcheal children has been evaluated sonographically. Ovaries can be classified as homogeneous, microcystic or macrocystic. The homogeneous ovary is void of cystic structures, the microcystic ovary has cysts of <9 mm, and the macrocystic ovary has at least one cyst of >9 mm (9). Follicular activity is noted from early childhood, with an increasing percentage of children demonstrating microcystic ovaries with increasing age (Fig. 2). Macrocystic ovaries were not observed before 12 years of age (9–11). Stanhope et al. (12) defined a megalocystic ovary as containing more than six follicles of >4 mm. They noted a progressive increase in the proportion of megalocystic ovaries in normal premenarcheal girls over the age of 8.5 years. Ovarian cysts are considered abnormal in girls <12 years of age if they are >9 mm in diameter. Ovarian cysts of >9 mm are seen in 12- and 13-year-old girls, even if they are premenarcheal (10). Most ovarian cysts up to the age of 2 years are functional cysts (13). Be-

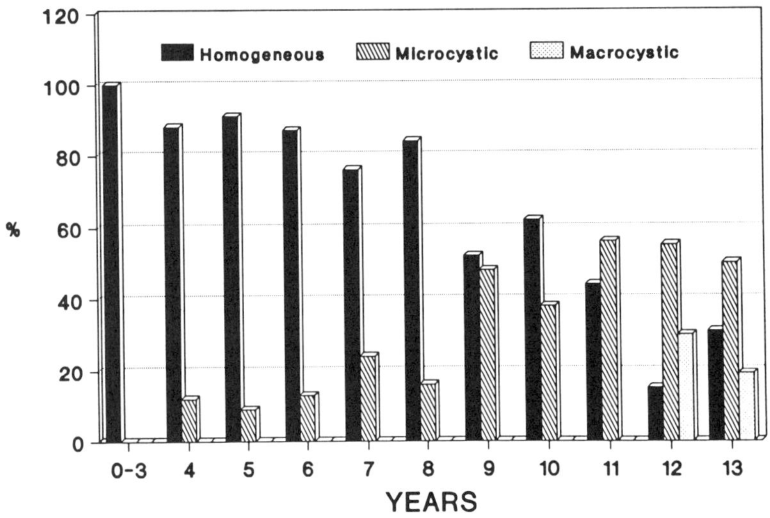

FIG. 2. Frequency of types of ovarian morphology. Classification of ovarian morphology defined in text. (Modified from data of ref. 9 and ref. 11.)

tween the ages of 5 and 15, most ovarian masses are teratomas, 30% of which are malignant.

Ovarian Size

Ovarian size has been evaluated sonographically in premenarcheal, menstruating, and postmenopausal women. These studies agree that the normal ovarian size is different in each group, however, the actual value is subject to controversy. The ovarian volume of menstruating women has been most widely studied and is the standard against which the premenarcheal and postmenopausal ovarian size is compared. Classically, the ovary of a menstruating woman was described as measuring $1 \times 2 \times 3$ cm (14). Using the mathematical formula to estimate the volume of an prolate ellipse (height $\times$ width $\times$ length $\times$ 0.523), this represents an ovarian volume of approximately 3 cm^3. An ovarian volume, in menstruating women, of 6 cm^3 has been also quoted as normal. This corresponds to dimensions of $2 \times 2 \times 3$ cm^3. A range in ovarian volume from 4.4 cm^3 to 9.8 cm^3 has been documented by sonographic evaluation (14).

Sonographic estimates of premenarcheal ovarian size have also varied. Difficulty in sonographic visualization of the ovaries in young girls was experienced initially (15). Recent reports have visualized the majority of premenarcheal ovaries, including those in infants. Ivarsson et al. (15) demonstrated an average ovarian volume of 0.7 cm^3 by sonographic evaluation. The authors also used Simkins (16) histologic data to calculate the ovarian volume using the prolate ellipsoid formula. Patients 6 months to 2 years had an average ovarian volume of 0.41 cm^3 and patients 7–9 years had an average ovarian volume of 0.74 cm^3. Stanhope et al. (12) sonographically evaluated 40 premenarcheal girls age 6 months to 14 years. At 2 years of age, the average volume was 1 cm^3 and at 12 years a volume of 2 cm^3.

Cohen et al. (14) studied ovarian volume of 725 consecutive patients (1157 ovaries) by ultrasound. The average volume of menstruating women in this study was 9.8 cm^3, which is on the upper end of normal values reported in the literature. The age range of premenarcheal patients was 3–15 years,

TABLE 3. *Ovarian volume*[a]

Age (years)	Number of patients	Ovarian volume (cm³) By chronologic age	By bone age
2	5	0.75 ± 0.41	0.78 ± 0.38
3	6	0.66 ± 0.17	0.64 ± 0.18
4	14	0.82 ± 0.36	1.00 ± 0.45
5	4	0.86 ± 0.02	0.95 ± 0.52
6	9	1.19 ± 0.36	1.05 ± 0.65
7	8	1.26 ± 0.59	1.23 ± 0.47
8	10	1.05 ± 0.50	1.29 ± 0.33
9	11	1.98 ± 0.76	1.35 ± 0.71
10	12	2.22 ± 0.69	1.47 ± 0.56
11	12	2.52 ± 1.30	2.45 ± 0.86
12	6	3.80 ± 1.40	3.10 ± 1.29
13	4	4.18 ± 2.30	4.38 ± 2.74

[a]As determined by ultrasonography in 101 girls from age 2 to 13.
(From ref. 9, with permission.)

with an average of 9.5 years. The average volume of 32 premenarcheal ovaries was 3.0 cm³. The mean volume of patients in the first decade of life (19 ovaries) was 1.7 cm³. Salardi et al. (10) measured the ovaries sonographically on 101 premenarcheal girls. The mean ovarian volume was determined for each year, from age 2 to 13 years (Table 3). Ovarian size is stable until about 5 years, when age-related growth begins.

Management of Premenarcheal Ovarian Cysts

Thind et al. (17) performed a retrospective study of 64 girls who were diagnosed with an ovarian cyst or tumor. Twenty-eight of these patients were managed surgically, of which 27 were benign and half were functional cysts. Fifty of the patients presented with pain or a palpable abdominal mass. The majority of these cysts were managed conservatively and resolved over a 6–8-week period. Management of ovarian cysts in premenarcheal girls is virtually the same as management of ovarian cysts in the adult female. Sonographic findings that are suggestive of a malignancy or a cyst which does not begin to resolve in 6–8 weeks

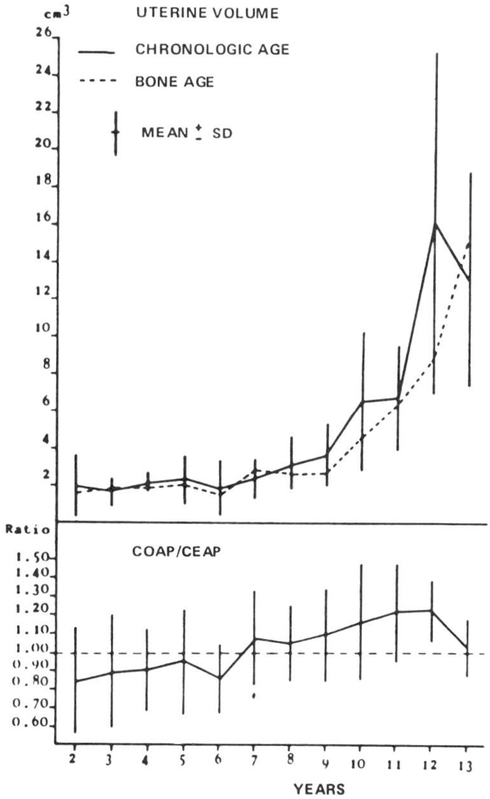

FIG. 3. Normal age-related sonographic values of uterine volume and ratio of anteroposterior diameter of the corpus (COAP) and the cervix (CEAP). (From ref. 9, with permission.)

TABLE 4. *Uterine diameters and volume*[a]

Age (years)	Numbers of patients	Uterine diameters (mm) TUL	COAP	CEAP	COAP/CEAP	Uterine volume (cm^3) By chronologic age	By bone age
2	7	33.1 ± 4.4	7.0 ± 3.4	8.3 ± 2.0	0.84 ± 0.29	1.98 ± 1.58	1.76 ± 0.72
3	8	32.4 ± 4.3	6.4 ± 1.3	7.6 ± 2.2	0.89 ± 0.29	1.63 ± 0.81	1.80 ± 0.74
4	15	32.9 ± 3.3	7.6 ± 1.8	8.6 ± 1.8	0.90 ± 0.22	2.10 ± 0.57	1.97 ± 0.74
5	7	33.1 ± 5.5	8.0 ± 2.8	8.4 ± 1.6	0.95 ± 0.28	2.36 ± 1.39	2.19 ± 1.16
6	9	33.2 ± 4.1	6.7 ± 2.9	7.5 ± 1.8	0.86 ± 0.18	1.80 ± 1.57	1.65 ± 0.93
7	9	32.3 ± 3.9	8.0 ± 2.2	7.7 ± 2.5	1.08 ± 0.26	2.32 ± 1.07	2.81 ± 1.44
8	11	35.8 ± 7.3	9.0 ± 2.8	8.4 ± 1.7	1.05 ± 0.20	3.12 ± 1.52	2.70 ± 1.43
9	11	37.1 ± 4.4	9.7 ± 3.0	8.8 ± 2.0	1.10 ± 0.24	3.70 ± 1.62	2.69 ± 1.83
10	13	40.3 ± 6.4	12.8 ± 5.3	10.7 ± 2.6	1.17 ± 0.31	6.54 ± 3.78	4.66 ± 3.03
11	13	42.2 ± 5.1	12.8 ± 3.1	10.7 ± 2.6	1.22 ± 0.26	6.66 ± 2.87	6.24 ± 3.07
12	6	54.3 ± 8.4	17.3 ± 5.3	14.3 ± 5.2	1.23 ± 0.16	16.18 ± 9.15	8.88 ± 3.65
13	5	53.8 ± 11.4	15.8 ± 4.5	15.0 ± 2.4	1.03 ± 0.15	13.18 ± 5.64	15.55 ± 5.98

[a]As determined by ultrasonography in 114 girls from age 2 to 13. Mean ± SD.
TUL, total uterine length; *COAP,* anteroposterior diameter of the corpus; *CEAP,* anteroposterior diameter of the cervix.
(From ref. 9, with permission.)

should be explored surgically. In addition, one must be aware that in the pediatric population an ovarian cyst more commonly results in torsion than in the adult or may cause ureteric compression with resulting hydronephrosis and persistent pyrexia may represent an undiagnosed appendicial abscess.

NORMAL UTERINE DEVELOPMENT AND SIZE

The fetal uterus enlarges in response to maternal hormonal stimulation. The infant experiences postnatal regression of uterine size. The size of the uterus remains stable until about 7 years of age. The cervix is larger than the corpus in the young child, resulting in an inverted pear shape of the uterus. The predominance of the cervix over the corpus persists until uterine growth begins at about age 7. Both the total uterine volume and the ratio of the corpus to the cervix begins to significantly increase between 6 and 8 years (Fig. 3) (9,10). The normal age related values of the uterine dimensions, as determined by sonographic evaluation of 114 normal premenarcheal girls, are presented in Table 4 (9).

REFERENCES

1. McCann J, Wells R, Simon, and Voris J. Genital findings in prepubertal girls selected for nonabuse: a descriptive study. *Pediatrics* 1990;86:428.
2. Cowell CA. The gynecologic examination of infants, children, and young adolescents. *Pediatr Clin North Am* 1981;28:247.
3. Edmonds DK. Patterns of childhood and adolescent gynaecology. In: *Dewhurst's practical paediatric and adolescent gynaecology.* 2nd ed. London: Butterworth & Co., 1989:1.
4. Bronstein IP, Cassorla E. Breast enlargement in pediatric practice. *Med Clin North Am* 1946;30:121.
5. Money J, Lamacz M. Genital examination and exposure experienced as nosocomial sexual abuse in childhood. *J Nerv Mental Dis* 1987;175:713.
6. Emans SJH, Goldstein DP. *Pediatric and adolescent gynecology.* 2nd ed. Boston: Little, Brown, 1982:1.
7. McCann J, Voris J, Simon M, Wells R. Comparison of genital examination techniques in prepubertal girls. *Pediatrics* 1990;85:182.
8. Peters H, Himelstein-Braw R, Faber M. The normal development of the ovary in childhood. *Acta Endocrinol* 1976;82:617.
9. Orsini LF, Salardi S, Pilu G, Bovicelli L, Cacciari E. Pelvic organs in premenarcheal girls: real-time ultrasonography. *Radiology* 1984;153:113.
10. Salardi S, Orsini LF, Cacciari E, Bovicelli L, Tassone P, Reggiani A. Pelvic ultrasonography in premenarcheal girls: relation to puberty and sex hormone concentrations. *Arch Dis Child* 1985;60:120.
11. Salardi S, Orsini LF, Cacciari E, Partesotti S,

Brondelli L, Cicognani A, Frejaville E, Pluchinotta V, Tonioli S, Bovicelli L. Pelvic ultrasonography in girls with precocious puberty, congenital adrenal hyperplasia, obesity, or hirsutism. *J Pediatr* 1988;112:880.

12. Stanhope R, Jacobs HS, Brook CGD. Ovarian ultrasound assessment in normal children, idiopathic precocious puberty, and during low dose pulsatile gonadotropin releasing hormone treatment of hypogonadotrophic hypogonadism. *Arch Dis Child* 1985;60:116.
13. Fleischer AC, Shawker TH. The role of sonography in pediatric gynecology. *Clin Obstet Gynecol* 1987;30:735.
14. Cohen HL, Tice HM, Mandel FS. Ovarian volumes measured by US: bigger than we think. *Radiology* 1990;177:189.
15. Ivarsson SA, Nilsson KO, Persson PH. Ultrasonography of the pelvic organs in prepubertal and postpubertal girls. *Arch Dis Child* 1983; 58:352.
16. Simkins CS. Development of the human ovary from birth to sexual maturity. *Am J Anat* 1932;51:465.
17. Thind CR, Carty HML, Pilling DW. The role of ultrasound in the management of ovarian masses in children. *Clin Radiol* 1989;40:180.

Pediatric and Adolescent Gynecology,
edited by S. E. Carpenter and J. A. Rock.
Raven Press, Ltd., New York © 1992.

3

Normal Pubertal Development

Joel S. Krasnow and Sander S. Shapiro

*Department of Obstetrics and Gynecology, Women's Endocrine Division,
University of Wisconsin, Madison, Wisconsin 53792*

Puberty refers to the developmental processes initiated in late childhood that culminate in adult reproductive competence. It involves a group of qualitative changes which depart from the generalized somatic growth processes that are dominant throughout childhood. Attainment of puberty is associated with profound hormonal alterations, the acquisition of secondary sexual characteristics, a short-lived increase in longitudinal growth rate, and numerous psychosocial changes (1). None of these changes, however, either alone or in concert, absolutely signify that an individual has established a reproductive capacity. Thus, puberty is a rather general term that connotes the transition period between childhood and adulthood.

The age at which the somatic changes associated with puberty occur is highly variable. A majority of North American females initiate pubertal alterations between 8 and 13 years of age. Their male counterparts initiate analogous pubertal development at 9–14 years of age (2). Between 1 and 2% of the population will start their transition outside of this range and thereby invite evaluation for either precocious or delayed puberty (3).

The first somatic change that occurs in females is either the beginning of breast (thelarche) or pubic hair (pubarche) development. The onset of both thelarche and pubarche are variable, with a mean of 10.9 and 11.2 years, respectively, for North American females. Tanner has described five stages of breast and pubic hair development as outlined in Figs. 1 and 2. An even earlier, but seldom documented change, is the onset of the "adolescent growth spurt." This change in growth velocity has a mean onset of 9.6 years (4). The peak height velocity (PHV) occurs almost 2.5 years later and precedes the onset of menses (mean age, 12.7 years). The interval between the onset of breast development and menarche is 2.3 ± 1.0 years and is independent of the age at which thelarche occurs. However, a wider temporal range exists for the onset, duration and completion of these transforming events. Within the spectrum of normal pubertal development, it is possible to see physical changes as much as 5 years prior to menarche. It is

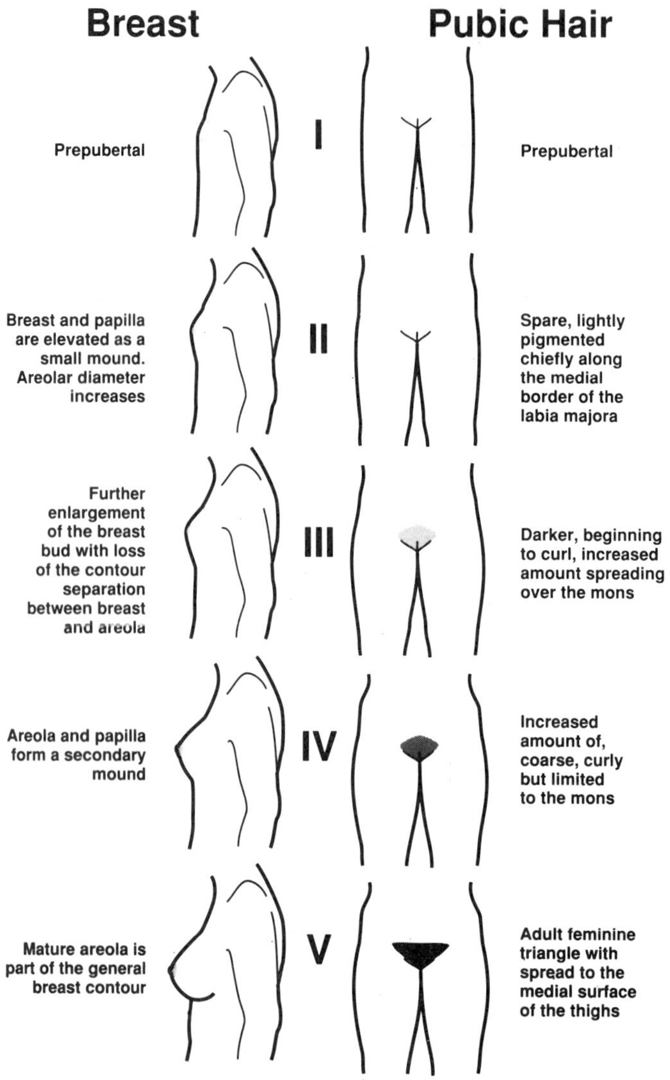

FIG. 1. Stages of female breast and pubic hair development during puberty as described by Marshall and Tanner. (From ref. 48, with permission.)

also possible for the sequence of physical changes to vary considerably from the order discussed above. Such variability can lead to expressions of concern on the part of the adolescent and their parents. Therefore, it is helpful for medical practitioners to have a firm sense of the wide temporal range of pubertal events and an understanding of when to initiate an evaluation for those who present outside popularly perceived norms.

The average age of pubertal onset, as well as the age of first menses (menarche), has declined steadily over the last century in this country and throughout the industrialized world. Currently, the average age of menarche is 12.7 years (5). This has been attributed to improved nutritional and general health conditions, as well as to altered lifestyles. In isolated nomadic tribes, where living conditions and socialization practices have not changed significantly during re-

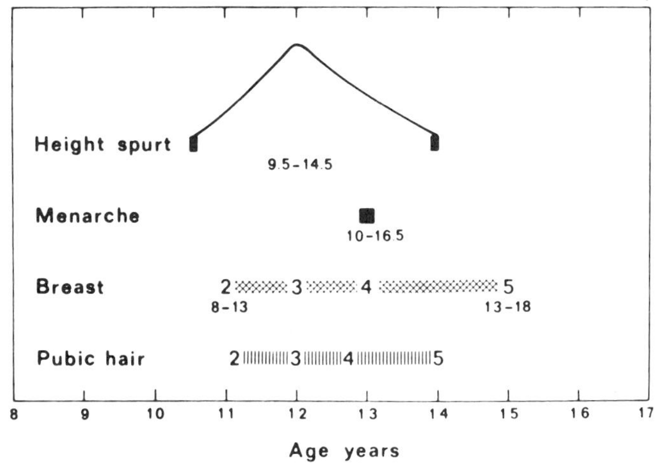

FIG. 2. Relationship of breast and pubic hair development to the adolescent growth spurt and menarche. Ranges are given for the changes illustrated. (From ref. 48, with permission.)

cent times, the trend towards earlier menarche is not found. In addition, strenuous physical activity, decreased body fat content, chronic disease and malnutrition are all associated with delayed puberty. Conversely, females with moderately increased fat content tend to experience menarche at an earlier age. Thus, geographic, nutritional and sociologically determined factors may affect the time at which puberty begins and its rate of progression. Furthermore, daughters frequently experience menarche at an age that is close to their mother's menarchical age, suggesting that genetic factors may also contribute to the timing of pubertal events.

ETIOLOGY OF PUBERTY

The principle factors involved in the initiation of puberty are contained within the hypothalamic-pituitary-gonadal (HPG) axis as represented in Fig. 3. The arcuate nucleus which is located in the medial basal hypothalamus contains a group of cells that have the ability to secrete gonadotropin hormone releasing hormone (GnRH). GnRH is released into the hypothalamic-portal circulation in a pulsatile manner, achieving a high concentration in the pituitary gland. This results in the secretion of follicle stimulating hormone (FSH) and luteinizing hormone (LH). These gonadotropins (FSH and LH) stimulate the production of sex steroids by the gonads. Circulating androgens, estrogens and the gonadal peptide inhibin have inhibitory actions at the level of the pituitary and hypothalamus, which also serve to maintain homeostasis.

Two major systems are known to modulate hypothalamic GnRH secretion. The central nervous system (CNS) exerts its influence through synaptic connections terminating in the region of the medial basal hypothalamus. The summation of all neural inputs usually results in an inhibitory effect, referred to as the "intrinsic CNS inhibitory mechanism." The second modulating system involves the negative feedback of sex steroids at the level of the hypothalamus. Thus, the relative sensitivity of the GnRH neurons in the hypothalamus to (a) the negative feedback effects of circulating sex steroids and (b) the neural inputs from the CNS, determine the activity of the entire HPG axis (Fig. 3). Puberty represents the disinhibition of these cells from the

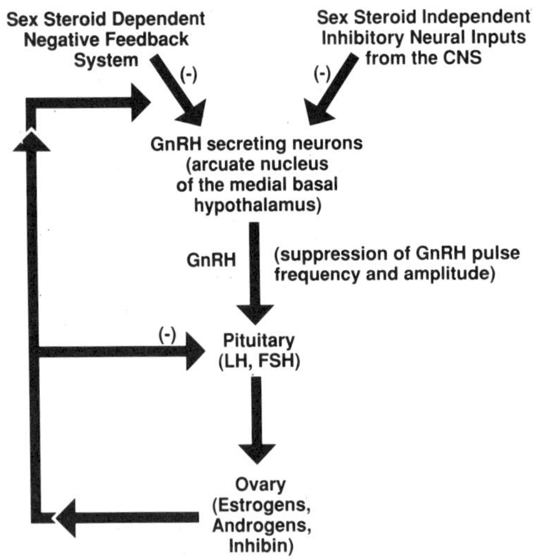

FIG. 3. Model of the major factors influencing the GnRH secreting neurons in the region of the medial basal hypothalamus. Prior to puberty, both the sex steroid dependent and independent systems exert primarily inhibitory influence on GnRH secretion. Pulsatile GnRH secretion causes the pituitary to release LH and FSH. The gonadotropins, in turn, stimulated ovarian activity. Ovarian secretion of sex steroids and inhibin maintain homeostasis by exerting feedback inhibition at the pituitary and hypothalamus.

aforementioned influences and result in regular, pulsatile GnRH secretion.

DEVELOPMENT AND MATURATION OF THE HYPOTHALAMIC-PITUITARY-GONADAL AXIS

During the fourth week of embryonic development, the germ cells, which have their origin in the yolk sac endoderm of the early fetus, migrate to the genital ridge and form an undifferentiated gonad. Organization of mesenchyme at this site progresses rapidly so that by the seventh week of gestation primordial testes are distinguishable. Expression of the testis determining factor (TDF) gene, which is located on the short arm of the Y chromosome, induces this differentiation (6). Absence of TDF gene expression leaves the gonad to differentiate into an ovary. Ovarian differentiation can be positively identified by ten weeks of gestation. The germ cells then undergo multiple mitotic divisions with meiosis being initiated at about 20 weeks (7). When oocytes enter the diplotene stage of prophase, they are surrounded by a single layer of granulosa cells forming a primordial follicle. The number of oocytes reaches a maximum of approximately 7 million during the fifth month of gestation; from that point it declines to about 2 million at term (8). After approximately the fifth month of gestation, the ovaries became responsive to gonadotropin stimulation resulting in follicular growth and estrogen production. Follicular development in utero usually proceeds to the early antral stage (1–2 mm in diameter) and is then followed by atresia. The maintenance of a normal complement of primary oocytes depends upon the presence of two normal X-chromosomes. This supposition is supported by the finding that fetuses with a 45 XO karyotype have a normal complement of oocytes at midgestation but a reduced number of follicles at birth. Follicular atresia continues after birth so that few of these X chromosome deficient girls experience menarche. On the other hand, children with 46 XX/45 XO karyotypes often have sufficient follicular development to experience menstruation and even conception. They, however, usually experience ovarian failure long before the time for normal menopause.

The hypothalamic-pituitary-gonadal (HPG) axis is established early in fetal development. In the human fetus, GnRH is present in the hypothalamus by 8 weeks of gestation (9) and the hypothalamic-portal system is functional by 11.5 gestational weeks. Detection of LH and FSH in the fetal pituitary is demonstrable by 12 gestational weeks. Fetal pituitary cells respond to GnRH with the synthesis and secretion of LH and FSH (9). The production of gonadotropins by the fetal pituitary appears to be necessary for normal ovarian development. Hypophysectomy of Rhesus monkey fetuses decreases the number of germ cells found in their ovaries (10). Similar changes are noted in anencephalic human fetuses. Female fetuses experience a significantly higher concentration of FSH in their serum and their pituitaries than do males (11). In the male, placental human chorionic gonadotropin (hCG) stimulates fetal Leydig cell differentiation and the secretion of testosterone (T). Fetal testosterone levels rise, peaking at 15–18 weeks (12). The elevated level of testosterone in males is thought to account for the sex difference in FSH through a negative feedback effect on the male hypothalamus and pituitary. The presence of such an inhibitory effect further suggests that a functional hypothalamic-pituitary-gonadal endocrine system exists in utero. Since this sex difference persists postnatally, a direct effect of testosterone on differentiation of the hypothalamic-pituitary unit has been postulated (13).

In utero, the fetoplacental unit is the primary estrogen secreting organ. Thus, at delivery, FSH and LH are low in cord blood due to the suppressive effect brought on by high levels of circulating estrogens. Estrogen levels fall abruptly following birth. This decreases the inhibitory influence on the GnRH pulse generator causing serum LH and FSH concentrations to rise gradually. As a result, gonadotropin levels remain low for the first 3 days postpartum and then increase to a peak during the third month of life (14–16). The sexual dimorphism in FSH secretion seen at midgestation is again observed following the third postpartum day. In females, plasma FSH levels rise earlier, and attain higher peak values as compared to males. Moreover, males experience a rapid decline in plasma FSH levels by 6 months, whereas slightly higher FSH levels may persist in the female until 4 years of age (16). FSH release following exogenous stimulation by GnRH is also greater in females than in males during this period (17). In females ovarian production of estradiol rises in response to increasing levels of FSH during the early part of infancy (18).

In males, postpartum testosterone levels fall immediately after birth as a consequence of the loss of testicular stimulation by placental hCG. The secondary rise in testosterone that occurs several days after birth is coincident with the rise in pituitary gonadotropins. After the third postnatal month, decreasing pituitary gonadotropin secretion results in a decline in serum testosterone levels. The role of gonadotropins in testosterone secretion can be inferred from the observation that infants with panhypopituitarism do not exhibit this secondary rise. In contrast to FSH levels, the rise in plasma LH occurs earlier in males than in females during the first 2 months postpartum. In both sexes, LH levels peak in the third to fourth months and then decline, reaching low levels by one year of age.

As illustrated in Fig. 3, GnRH secretion is dependent on both sex steroid dependent and sex steroid independent systems. From the third trimester of pregnancy through the first few months of life, fluctuations in LH and FSH can be explained largely by the negative feedback effects of circulating sex steroids. The sex steroid independent system represents the sum of all neural inputs to the GnRH secreting neurons. These inputs are primarily inhibitory. With continued growth and differentiation of the CNS, additional maturational changes occur resulting in increased inhibitory input to the GnRH secreting neurons. Evidence for the role of the "intrinsic CNS inhibitory mechanism" comes from neuroendocrine studies of the human neonate. When infants born prematurely are compared to infants born at term, both groups being of similar postnatal age and having similar sex steroid levels, the premature infants are found to have significantly higher serum LH and FSH levels. Presumably this is due to the relative immaturity of the intrinsic CNS inhibitory system (19). Similarly, premature male infants have a normal pattern of fall in their serum testosterone levels at birth due to withdrawal of hCG. Yet, they have a higher and more sustained secondary rise in T levels, reflecting decreased inhibition of GnRH and consequently LH secretion (19).

Agonadal patients provide a unique model for investigating the activity of the intrinsic CNS inhibitory system. These individuals secrete no gonadal steroids; therefore, the contribution of the sex steroid dependent feedback mechanism is minimal and solely dependent on intrinsic CNS factors. Following birth, gonadotropin levels rise to menopausal levels, peaking between 1 and 2 years of age (Fig. 4) (20).

The subsequent decline in gonadotropins to their nadir between 6 and 8 years of age suggests that an intrinsic CNS inhibitory mechanism is responsible for restraining the GnRH pulse generator during this period. In midchildhood, LH and FSH begin to rise again, demonstrating the reversibility of the intrinsic CNS inhibitory mechanism. This results in an increased secretion of sex steroids by the gonad which is referred to as "gonadarche." Dickerman was the first to postulate the role of increased GnRH pulse frequency in the initiation of puberty (21). He demonstrated that administering a bolus of GnRH resulted in the release of pituitary FSH and LH in prepubertal children. Subsequently, Knobil (22) eloquently demonstrated the central role of

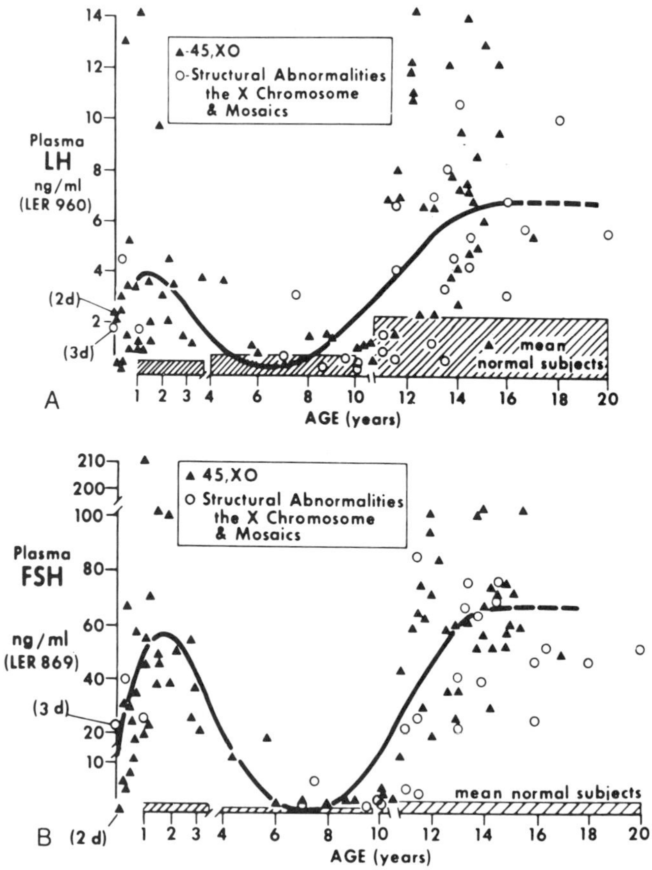

FIG. 4. Plasma LH (**A**) and FSH (**B**) levels in patients with gonadal dysgenesis compared to normal subjects. The *curved line* represents the mean of values from females with gonadal dysgenesis; the *hatched area* represents the mean for normal females. (From ref. 20, with permission.)

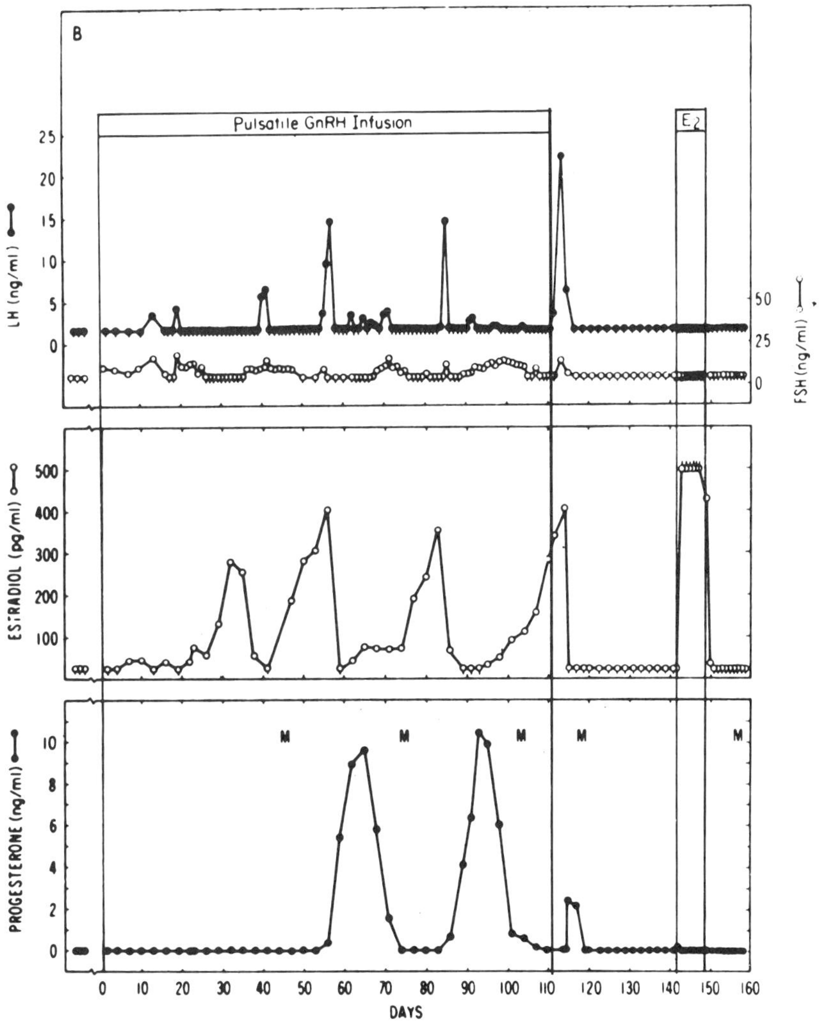

FIG. 5. The effect of an unvarying hourly pulsatile dose of GnRH in a prepubertal rhesus monkey. Gonadotropin and estradiol levels were undetectable prior to initiating stimulation with GnRH. At time 0, pulsatile GnRH was begun. This was followed by small, yet physiologically significant increases in gonadotropins. This resulted in elevated estradiol levels reflecting advancing ovarian folliculogenesis. The first rise in estradiol was ineffective in elicitating a gonadotropin surge. Nevertheless, menstruation (M) occurred as a consequence of estrogen withdrawal. The next rise in estradiol elicited an LH surge resulting in ovulation and progesterone secretion by the corpus luteum. Continued GnRH stimulation resulted in another ovulatory cycle 28 days later. Two days following discontinuation of the GnRH infusion, a gonadotropin surge occurred in response to rising estradiol levels. Progesterone secretion was only transient due to the absence of continued hypophysiotropic stimulation. The area labelled E_2 indicates implantation of estradiol containing silastic capsules. In the absence of hypophysiotropic stimulation, rising estradiol levels failed to induce a gonadotropin surge. (From ref. 22, with permission.)

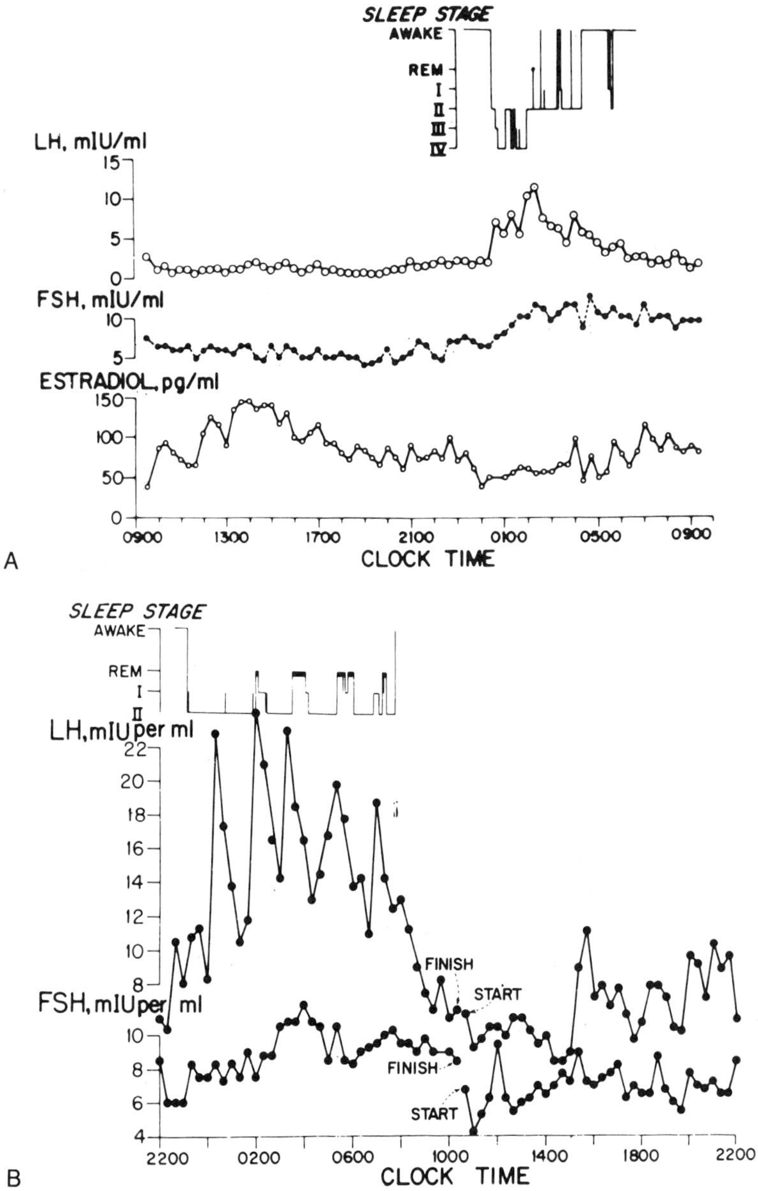

FIG. 6. The relationship between the onset of sleep and gonadotropin secretion in early (**A**) and mid puberty (**B**). Gonadotropins are released in association with the onset of sleep. A sleep histogram indicating the subject's sleep stage is superimposed. The sleep stages are REM (rapid eye movement), sleep, and stages I–IV. Advancing puberty (B) is associated with increased gonadotropin pulse frequency and amplitude. (From refs. 23 and 24, with permission.)

GnRH in pubertal development. He administered GnRH in a regular pulsatile manner to prepubertal rhesus monkeys (Fig. 5). Initially FSH and LH were not detectable. After 15 days of regular GnRH pulses, FSH rose to detectable levels. At 30 days, serum estradiol increased followed by an LH surge which was not great enough to induce ovulation. Subsequently, estrogen levels declined and menses occurred. Continued

GnRH administration resulted in a second rise of estradiol sufficient to produce an LH surge which resulted in ovulation. Adequate progesterone secretion demonstrated the presence of a functional corpus luteum. Continuation of GnRH administration produced regular 28-day menstrual cycles. When GnRH therapy was discontinued, the animals reverted to their prepubertal state. Subsequently, these animals experienced menarche at the expected age. Thus, Knobil's studies in the monkey support the hypothesis that reactivation of GnRH pulsatility leads to puberty.

The first identifiable endocrinologic sign of puberty is the release of GnRH only at night and coincident with onset of sleep (Fig. 6). Subsequently, LH pulses become more frequent but continue to occur primarily during sleep (23). With further maturation, LH pulses appear during the daytime and increase in amplitude. As menarche approaches, these pulses are detected at all hours and a diurnal variation in pulse frequency is no longer demonstrable (24). A similar change in secretory pattern is noted for FSH. Thus, puberty represents a limited disinhibition of the GnRH neurons, resulting in a progression of secretory activity which culminates in the adult form of regular pulsatile GnRH secretion. In concert with these maturational changes, LH levels rise and the serum ratio of LH to FSH, which had been less than one, reverses and ovulatory menstrual cycles occur (25).

Menarche, which is the most easily identified event during pubertal development, can be influenced by many factors. The factor(s) responsible for initiation of the hypothalamic pubertal changes described here are currently unknown. Frisch (26) has proposed that a critical body weight and body fat content are required for the initiation of menarche. Her theory is supported by the finding that in states of malnutrition and chronic disease there is a delay in menarche. Individuals who participate from an early age in highly competitive athletic training and consequently have low fat/lean muscle mass also experience menarche later than their nonathletic peers (27–29). Girls with anorexia nervosa exhibit a regression to the prepubertal pattern of gonadotropin secretion as body weight declines, and revert to normal secretory patterns as their weight increases (30). In order to test Frisch's hypothesis that increased body weight and fat content are required for the occurrence of menarche, urinary gonadotropin and anthropometric data have been obtained from healthy children. The changes in body composition in these children do not precede, but rather occur simultaneously with the rise in gonadotropin secretion (31). This suggests that changes in body composition are not a prerequisite to the initiation of puberty. Nevertheless, the regressive modifications in gonadotropin secretion associated with severe weight loss, noted by Boyars (30), point to the possibility that a strong link exists between nutritional status and the initiation of puberty. Presumably, that link operates at a CNS level exerting a direct influence upon hypothalamic activity.

INITIATION OF ADRENARCHE

Adrenarche refers to the process of adrenal gland maturation which results in increasing androgen secretion. At approximately 3 years of age, the zona reticularis begins to form. As that zone enlarges changes in its capacity for steroid production result in increased secretion of androgens, principally dehydroepiandrosterone (DHEA) and its sulfate (DHEAS) (32). A rise in plasma DHEAS is first detectable at about 7 years and reaches adult levels at about 15 years of age. During this period plasma DHEAS levels rise as much as 20-fold in both sexes (33). The increased production of adrenal androgens results in the development of pubic and axillary hair and contributes to the development of acne. Adrenal androgens also contribute to advancing bone age and linear growth. Individuals who experience premature adrenarche will have a diminished adult height since the effect of androgens upon bone maturation is considerably greater than upon skeletal growth (34).

The increase in androgen synthesis during adrenarche occurs in the absence of any detectable change in ACTH or cortisol secretion. A corticotropin androgen stimulating hormone (CASH) has been postulated as the agent responsible for adrenarche, but to date no such molecule has been positively identified. The onset of adrenarche typically precedes any rise in gonadotropins or change in growth rate. For this reason, the initiation of adrenal androgen production has been postulated as playing a role in the onset of puberty. Although the initiating factors in both adrenarche and gonadal puberty remain unknown, considerable experimental evidence supports a lack of association between the two processes. This evidence originates primarily from studies of patients with gonadal dysgenesis or isolated gonadotropin deficiency who almost universally experience normal adrenarche. Moreover, patients with true precocious puberty experience gonadal puberty prior to adrenarche. It has also been observed that children with chronic adrenal insufficiency, who consequently have deficient adrenal androgen secretion, will progress through puberty normally while receiving replacement doses of only glucocorticoids and mineralocorticoids.

INITIATION OF GONADARCHE

The alterations in physical characteristics that occur around puberty are largely dependent upon sex steroid production by the gonads. The process of ovarian follicular growth and atresia is a continuous process initiated in utero. Both ultrasound and autopsy studies have documented cystic changes in the ovaries from birth to puberty (35,36). It is not uncommon to note ovarian follicular cysts in utero or in the neonatal period which regress spontaneously following chorionic gonadotropin withdrawal. Throughout childhood, follicles continue to develop and undergo atresia resulting in a gradual increase in ovarian stromal tissue, but with only minimal estrogen secretion. The initiation of follicular development is thought to occur independent of pituitary gonadotropin stimulation. Sustained progression of follicular development to the antral stage with significant estrogen production does, however, require gonadotropins (37).

Following the reactivation of the HPG axis at puberty, multiple (>5) follicles develop to a size of ≥4 mm. With maturation of the neuroendocrine unit, gonadotropin pulse frequency increases and ovarian follicles develop to a progressively larger size. As follicular maturation progresses, steroidogenic competency develops. There is a direct relationship between follicular size and steroid synthesizing capacity (37). Follicular development to 16 mm in diameter may be expected to provide sufficient estrogen for endometrial proliferation. The earliest follicles to attain this degree of maturation usually fail to induce an LH surge and, therefore, undergo atresia without effecting ovulation. Thus, menarche follows and is usually the result of a non-ovulatory cycle. However, should ovulation take place during the initial cycle, pregnancy would be possible without the onset of a first menses.

Even after ovulatory competence has been achieved, abnormalities of the luteal phase (short luteal phase, inadequate luteal phase) commonly occur (38). These abnormalities are thought to be the result of inadequate follicular stimulation by the pituitary and provide evidence that the HPG axis has not achieved full maturity. With complete maturation of the HPG axis, a dominant follicle develops in each cycle, becomes fully mature and ovulates.

Both the onset and rate of progression through puberty correlate with the age of menarche and the age at which regular ovulatory menstrual cycles are established (39). Progression from Tanner Stage II breast and pubic hair to menarche occurred in 1.4 ± 0.1 years and 1.1 ± 0.2 years, respectively, in Finnish girls experiencing menarche prior to age 13. The majority of menstrual cycles were ovulatory within 18 months of menarche. In contrast, those girls experiencing menarche after age 13 progressed through these same developmental stages in 2.1 ± 0.2 years and 2.0 ± 0.2 years, respectively. In this group, only 50% of all menstrual cycles were ovulatory by the fifth year after menarche (40). This observation is thought to reflect the variable velocity at which integration of the HPG axis occurs (41).

PHYSICAL EVENTS OF PUBERTY

In utero, the fetus is exposed to high estrogen levels. Acute withdrawal of estrogen at birth can result in endometrial shedding which manifests clinically as vaginal bleeding. In infant girls between 1 and 6 months of age, the uterus decreases in size achieving an average length of 32 mm. The ratio of corpus-to-cervix in the prepubertal uterus is 1:2. When GnRH pulse frequency increases sufficiently to cause multiple follicular development and estradiol production, uterine growth begins. The first change is a lengthening of the corpus followed by an increase in the width and thickness of both corpus and cervix. This process is initiated between 7 and 9 years of age. A uterine cross sectional area of 4 × 2 cm is usually achieved by 12 years of age. Prior to initiation of puberty, the endometrium consists of a single layer of cuboidal cells. As estradiol levels increase, the endometrium begins to proliferate. A rapid increase in endometrial thickness immediately preceding menarche can be visualized by ultrasonic evaluation.

Like the uterus, the vagina is an estrogen responsive tissue. During puberty newly elevated estrogen levels stimulate overall growth as well as epithelial proliferation. Under the influence of estrogen, the vaginal epithelium increases in thickness, with cornification of the superficial cell layers. This change has been quantified and the karyopyknotic index used as a sign of estrogenic status. Multiple metabolic alterations of the epithelium also result from estrogen exposure. These effect a change in vaginal secretions and pH, providing greater resistance to local infection.

Both the labia minora and majora respond to estrogen by increasing in size and thickness. Concomitantly the hymen thickens and its orifice enlarges to about 1 cm in diameter. At the same time, the vestibular glands begin active secretion and the clitoris undergoes general enlargement. The relative contribution of estrogen and androgens to this latter change remain ill defined.

Breast development is often the first visible change of puberty, although it may follow pubarche by many months. Prior to thelarche, male and female breast tissue is histologically indistinguishable. Breast development at puberty requires the presence of multiple hormones including prolactin, glucocorticoids and insulin (42). However, it is gonadarche with its production of estrogens that induces thelarche. It is the direct estrogen stimulation of mammary epithelium which causes ductal proliferation and the site specific adipose deposition that accounts for the majority of female breast development. Males fail to produce significant breast mass, primarily because they lack optimal levels of circulating estrogen. The extent to which testosterone inhibits breast development remains uncertain. In complete testicular feminization, substantial breast tissue is usually present despite only minimal increases in estrogen as compared to the testosterone sensitive, normal male, suggesting the potential importance of androgens in limiting male breast development. Once thelarche begins, the duration of time at each Tanner stage is variable. Overall, breast development usually proceeds smoothly to maturity in about 3 years (4).

Temporally associated with the development of secondary sexual characteristics is a marked increase in growth which is referred to as the "adolescent growth spurt." This growth spurt, which is measured by a change in skeletal growth rate, actually represents a more global process involving an increase in muscle mass and growth of almost all internal organs. These processes are dependent upon both growth hormone and sex steroids. Adrenal, as well as gonadal hormones, are thought to contribute to this change in growth rate (43). In addition to their direct anabolic effects, sex steroids have been demonstrated to increase the secretion of growth hormone and consequently insulin-like growth factor (44). The rise in serum sex steroid levels initiates a change in growth velocity which often antedates pubarche and thelarche. A sudden increase in shoe size is frequently observed coincident with onset of the linear growth spurt. Peak growth velocity is usually attained midway in the course of pubertal maturation in females which is two years earlier than in males. Prior to the adolescent growth spurt, growth velocity averages 3–6 cm/year. Peak height velocity (PHV) in males averages 8.8 cm with a standard deviation of 1.05 cm/year. In females, PHV is 8.13 cm, with a standard deviation of 0.78 cm/year. By the time PHV is reached, approximately 90% of the final adult height has been achieved. Upon completion of the adolescent growth spurt, very little additional height is gained. The average increase in height from the onset of the growth spurt to the cessation of growth is 25 cm in females and 28 cm in males. Thus, the greater final height achieved in males is a function of both the delay in onset of the growth spurt and a greater gain in height during the growth spurt. Children who progress through puberty earlier tend to attain a greater PHV but ultimately have a shorter final adult height than their peers.

There are several common variations in normal pubertal development. For example, one breast may begin to develop up to 6 months before the other. This may lead to an asymmetry which persists into adult life. Premature development of the breast bud is referred to as premature thelarche. When this occurs in early infancy, it usually represents a delay in establishing the negative feedback effects of sex steroids on the hypothalamus. In the older child, it may be an attenuated form of sexual precocity. In both instances, endocrinologic findings may reveal increased gonadotropins or increased gonadotropin response to GnRH. Total or free estradiol may be elevated in plasma. Radiologic evaluation usually reveals some ovarian follicular activity. Follow up is necessary to distinguish premature thelarche from true precocious puberty. In premature thelarche, breast development ceases and may even regress, bone age is not advanced, and there are no further signs of pubertal development (45). In contrast, during premature puberty bone age will advance significantly and other signs of continued pubertal development such as the appearance of pubic hair will occur.

Premature development of sexual hair is referred to as premature pubarche. The majority of children with premature pubarche have early activation of adrenal androgen secretion. ACTH stimulation of these individuals will reveal responses in between those of adults and prepubertal children (46). Levels of DHEAS are usually elevated. Since puberty and adrenarche are independent events, there are no other signs of sexual precocity and bone age is not significantly advanced in these children.

In assessing children for suspected disorders of growth and development, charts displaying normative data provide valuable information. North American children grow faster and are on the average taller than British children; therefore, appropriate standards for the population being studied should be employed. The onset of gonadarche is associated with increased growth velocity. Because the time of initiation of gonadarche is quite variable, the range of heights in pubertal aged children will be greater than the range of prepubertal children. Therefore, the use of cross-sectional population curves to follow the growth of an individual child, once puberty has begun, is invalid (47). The use of the growth curves for North American children published by Tanner in 1985 take into account the variability in pubertal progression (Figs. 7 and 8). For example, take two girls both destined for an adult height of 164 cm (50th percentile). At age 12, an "early maturer" (+2 SD) will have completed her growth spurt and measure 160 cm. The "late maturer" (−2 SD) will measure 144 cm. Since these curves are derived by averaging data

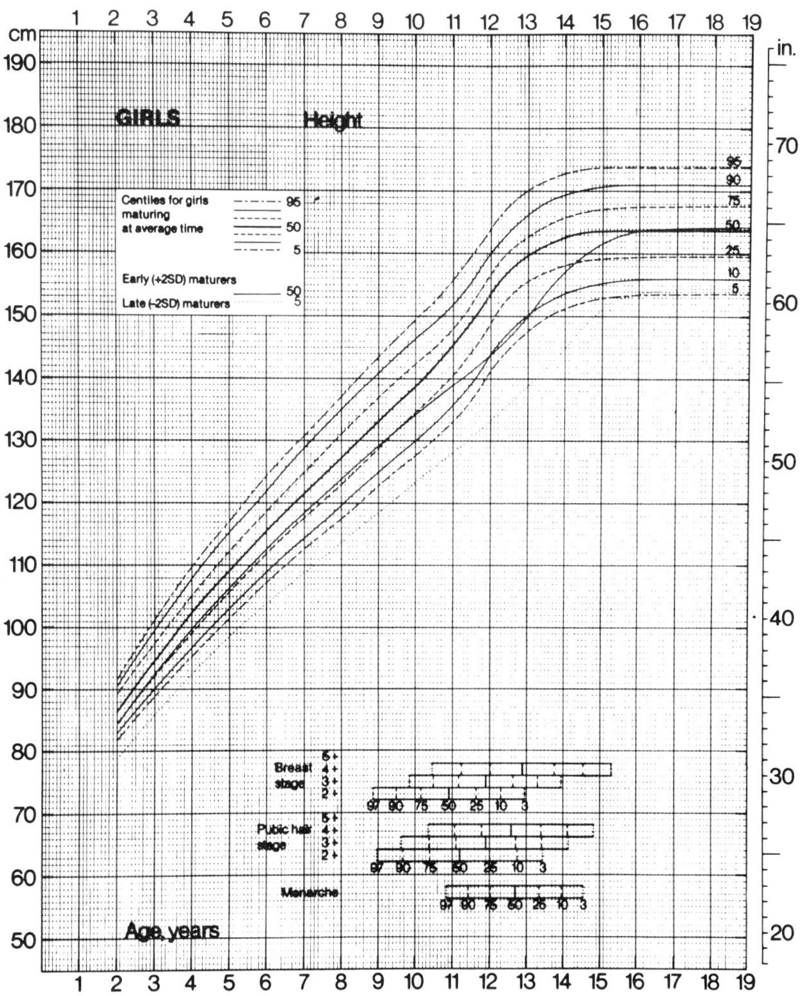

FIG. 7. Longitudinal growth curves for North American girls adjusted for the timing of pubertal development: the 50th and 95th centile for girls with accelerated maturation (*symbol*) and the 50th and 5th centile for girls with later maturation. Percentiles for Tanner stages and menarche are given for North American girls. (From ref. 2, with permission.)

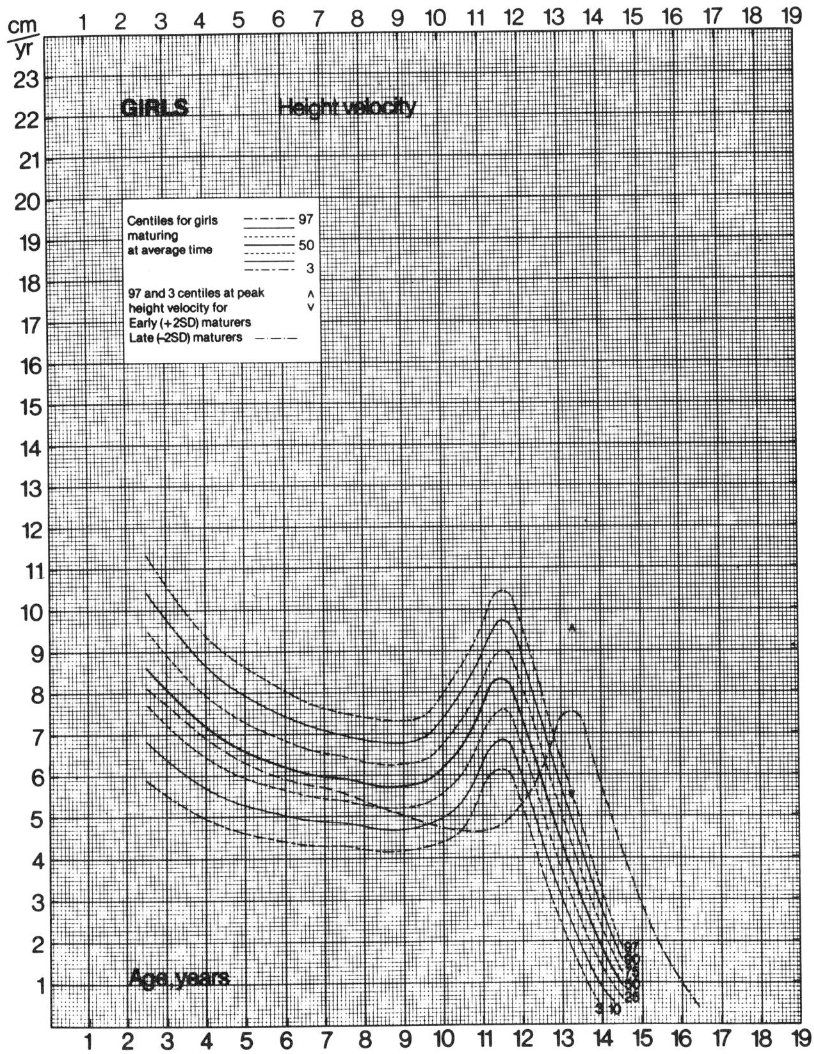

FIG. 8. Height velocity in North American girls adjusted for the timing of pubertal development. (From ref. 2, with permission.)

from a large population, no single individual should be expected to follow the curve precisely. These graphs are particularly useful in evaluating girls with primary amenorrhea. When height, breast and pubic hair development are all progressing in accordance with the norms and an intact reproductive tract is present, the patient can be assured that menarche is imminent.

A distinction must be made between the "late maturer" who makes slow but steady progress and the individual exhibiting an arrest of pubertal development. Individuals who have initiated breast and pubic hair growth will usually have also noticed an increase in the size of their hands and feet. As indicated above, increasing shoe size is an indicator of normal pubertal development. Arrest of pubertal development is relatively rare, but when detected may indicate hypothalamic, pituitary, gonadal, or systemic disease. Since the interval from thelarche to menarche is 2.3 ± 1.0 years (48), the absence of advancement in breast and pubic hair development and the absence of growth in the hands and feet over a 2–3-year period deserves further evaluation.

Girls who tend to initiate pubertal development late also tend to progress through puberty at a slower rate. Therefore, it would not be unusual for an individual initiating breast development at age 14 to not experience menarche until age 18. As a general rule, one should expect healthy girls of 14 years to have begun to demonstrate the physical changes of puberty. Those that have not require special attention. When a young woman does demonstrate substantial pubertal development yet has not experienced menarche by age 18, she too deserves thorough evaluation.

One of the more commonly seen variations from normal puberty is the failure to develop secondary sexual characteristics by age 14. These individuals are usually smaller than their peers due to the lack of initiation of a growth spurt. Commonly, their mothers also exhibited a delay in the onset of puberty. Bone age is useful in evaluating such patients since it is more closely correlated with pubertal events than chronologic age. Clinical signs of pubertal development are present in approximately 95% of individuals when the bone age reaches 12.5 years (49). Constitutional delay in growth and pubertal development occurs as a result of a delay in maturation of the HPG axis. Most cases of delayed development are constitutional, but other causes of delayed puberty, as discussed in the chapter by Plotnick need to be considered (50). In individuals with constitutional delay of pubertal development, endocrinologic evaluation should be consistent with the stage of development and may indicate impending onset of clinical signs (51).

In addition to changes in linear growth, the skeleton also undergoes a series of characteristic alterations in its osseous composition. These patterns define a bone age, which, during adolescence, more closely correlates with the individual's state of pubertal development than with their chronological age. A radiographically defined bone age of 11 years is usually associated with the onset of either pubarche, thelarche or both.

In conjunction with the physical changes described above, the appearance of acne, axillary hair growth, and phenotypical alterations in adipose distribution are part of the pubertal process. Each of these can be directly associated with the newly integrated hormonal changes that underpin puberty. On the other hand, there is little current evidence to support a direct relationship between adolescent patterns of social behavior and the chemical alterations that are an integral part of the pubertal process. This concept may change as a more thorough understanding of the effects that pubertal hormonal changes have on neurobiochemical processes evolves.

Growth and development throughout childhood usually progresses in an orderly fashion (52). Any deviation from the perceived norm usually results in the child being brought to medical attention. Precocious, delayed and aberrant development can cause alarm to parents, school officials, and medical personnel. Wide variation in the onset of developmental milestones evokes concern, as comparisons are usually made within children of similar chronological age. The physician faced with such concerns must thoroughly evaluate the child's current and past developmental status and utilize compilations of normative data including height, weight, skeletal age and time of onset of individual pubertal events to determine the presence or absence of pathological processes. For those children who deviate significantly from these established norms, a more thorough evaluation will be necessary. This can involve further radiologic as well as endocrinologic testing as described in the chapter by Plotnick.

REFERENCES

1. Sizonenko PC. Physiology of puberty. *J Endocrinol Invest* 1989;12(suppl 3):59–63.
2. Tanner JW, Davies PWS. Clinical longitudinal standards for height and height velocity for North American children. *J Pediatr* 1985;107: 317.
3. Grumbach MM, Kaplan SL. Recent advances in the diagnosis and management of sexual precocity. *Acta Paediatr Jpn* 1988;30(suppl):155–75.
4. Largo RH, Prader A. Pubertal development in girls. *Pediatrician* 1987;14:212–8.
5. Tanner JM. Trend toward earlier menarche in Long, Oslo, Copenhagen, the Netherlands and Hungary. *Nature* 1973;243:95.
6. Page DC. Sex reversal: deletion mapping the male-determining function of the human Y chromosome. *Cold Spring Harbor Symp Quant Biol* 1986;51:229.
7. Peters H. Migration of gonocytes in the mammalian gonad and their differentiation. *Philos Trans R Soc Lond [Biol]* 1970;259:91.
8. Baker TG. A quantitative and cytological study of germ cells in human ovaries. *Proc Roy Soc [Biol]* 1963;158:417.
9. Gluckman PD, Grumbach MM, Kaplan SL. The human fetal hypothalamus and pituitary gland; the maturation of neuroendocrine mechanisms controlling the secretion of fetal pituitary growth hormone, prolactin, gonadotropin, and adrenocorticotropin-related peptides. In: Tulchinsky D, Ryan KJ, eds. *Maternal-fetal endocrinology*. Philadelphia: WB Saunders, 1980:196–232.
10. Gulyas BJ, Hodgen GD, Tullner WW, et al. Effects of fetal or maternal hypophysextomy on endocrine organs and body weight in infant rhesus monkeys *(Macaca mulatta)*: with particular emphasis on oogenesis. *Biol Reprod* 1977;16: 216.
11. Kaplan SL, Grumbach MM. The ontogenesis of human foetal hormones. II. Luteinizing hormone (LH) and follicle stimulating hormone (FSH). *Acta Endocrinol* 1976;81:808–29.
12. Kaplan SL, Grumbach MM. Pituitary and placental gonadotropins and sex steroids in the human and subhuman primate fetus. *Clin Endocrinol Metab* 1978;7:487–511.
13. Gorski RA, Gordon JH, Shryne JE, et al. Evidence for a morphological sex difference within the medial preoptic area of the rat brain. *Brain Res* 1978;148:333.
14. Winter JSD, Hughes IA, Reyes FI, et al. Pituitary-gonadal relations in infancy: 2. Patterns of serum gonadal steroid concentrations in man from birth to two years of age. *J Clin Endocrinol Metab* 1976;42:679.
15. Winter JSD, Faiman C. Pituitary-gonadal relations in female children and adolescents. *Pediatr Res* 1973;7:948.
16. Winter JSD, Faiman C, Hobson WC, Prasad AV, Reyes FI. Pituitary-gonadal relations in infancy. I. Patterns of serum gonadotropin concentrations from birth to four years of age in man and chimpanzee. *J Clin Endocrinol Metab* 1975; 40:545.
17. Plauchu H, Claustart B, Betend B, David M, Francois R. Le test a l'hormone hypothalamique synthetique LHRH chez infant normal de la naissance a l'age adulte. *Pediatrie* 1980;35:119–31.
18. Bidlingmaier F, Knorr D. Oestrogens: physiological and clinical aspects. *Pediatr Adolesc Endocrinol* 1978;4:43.
19. Tapanainen J, Koivisto M, Vihko R, Huhtaniemi I. Enhanced activity of the pituitary-gonadal axis in premature human infants. *J Clin Endocrinol Metab* 1981;52:235–8.
20. Conte FA, Grumbach MM, Kaplan SS. A diphasic pattern in gonadotropin secretion in patients with the syndrome of gonadal dysgenesis. *J Clin Endocrinol Metab* 1975;40:670–5.
21. Dickerman Z, Prager-Lewin R, Laron Z. Response of plasma LH and FSH to synthetic LH-RH in children at various pubertal stages. *Am J Dis Child* 1974;130:634.
22. Wildt L, Marshall G, Knobil E. Experimental induction of puberty in the infantile rhesus monkey. *Science* 1980;207:1373–5.
23. Boyar R, Finkelstein J, Roffwarg H, et al. Synchronization of augmented luteinizing hormone secretion with sleep during puberty. *N Engl J Med* 1972;287:582.
24. Boyar RM, Wu RHK, Roffwarg H, et al. Human puberty: 24-hour estradiol patterns in pubertal girls. *J Clin Endocrinol Metab* 1976;43:1418.
25. Kulin HE, Reiter EO. Gonadotropins during children and adolescence: a review. *Pediatrics* 1973;51:260.
26. Frisch RE, Revelle R. Height and weight at menarche and a hypothesis of critical body weights and adolescent events. *Science* 1970;169:397.
27. Frisch RE, Wyshak G, Vincent L. Delayed menarche and amenorrhea in ballet dancers. *N Engl J Med* 1980;303:17.
28. Frisch RE, Gotz-Welbergen AV, McArthur JW, et al. Delayed menarche and amenorrhea of college athletes in relation to age of onset of training. *JAMA* 1981;246:1559.
29. Warren MP. The effects of exercise on pubertal progression and reproductive function in girls. *J Clin Endocrinol Metab* 1980;50:1150.
30. Boyar RM, Katz J, Finkelstein JW, et al. Anorexia nervosa. Immaturity of the 24-hour luteinizing hormone secretory pattern. *N Engl J Med* 1974;291:861–5.
31. Penny R, Goldstein IP, Frasier SD. Gonadotropin secretion and body composition. *Pediatrics* 1978;61:294.
32. Schiebinger RK, Albertson FG, Cassorla FG, et al. The developmental changes in plasma adrenal androgens during infancy and adrenarche are associated with changing activities of adrenal microsomal 17-hydroxylase and 17,20 desmolase. *J Clin Invest* 1981;67:1177.
33. Hopper BR, Yen SSC. Circulating concentrations of dehydroepiandrosterone and dehydroepiandrosterone sulfate during puberty. *J Clin Endocrinol Metab* 1975;40:458.

34. Sizonenko PE, Paunier L. Hormonal changes in puberty. III. Correlation of plasma dehydroepiandrosterone, testosterone, FSH, and LH with stages of puberty and bone age in normal boys and girls and in patients with Addison's disease or hypogonadism or with premature or late adrenarche. *J Clin Endocrinol Metab* 1975; 41:894.
35. Peters H, Byskov AG, Grinsted J. Follicular growth in fetal and prepubertal ovaries of humans and other primates. *Clin Endocrinol Metab* 1978;7:469.
36. Stanhope R, Adams J, Jacobs HS, Brook CGD. Ovarian ultrasound assessment in normal children, idiopathic precocious puberty, and during low dose pulsatile gonadotropin releasing hormone treatment of hypogonadotropic hypogonadism. *Arch Dis Child* 1985;60:116.
37. Ross GT. Gonadotropins and preantral follicular maturation in women. *Fertil Steril* 1974;25:522.
38. Knobil E. The neuroendocrine control of the menstrual cycle. *Recent Prog Horm Res* 1980; 36:53.
39. Apter D, Vihko R. Premenarcheal endocrine changes in relation to age at menarche. *Clin Endocrinol* 1985;22:753–60.
40. Apter D, Vihko R. Early menarche, a risk factor for breast cancer, indicates early onset of ovulatory cycles. *J Clin Endocrinol Metab* 1983; 57:82–6.
41. Vihko R, Apter D. Endocrine characteristics of adolescent menstrual cycles: impact of early menarche. *J Steroid Biochem* 1984;20:231–6.
42. Rosen JM, Paget P, Goodman H, Lee KE. Mechanisms by which prolactin and glucocorticoids regulate casein gene expression. *Biochem Soc Symp* 1989;55:115–23.
43. Wierman ME, Beardsworth DE, Crawford JD, et al. Adrenarche and skeletal maturation during luteinizing hormone releasing hormone analogue suppression of gonadarche. *J Clin Invest* 1986; 77:121–6.
44. Cara JF, Rosenfield RL, Furlanetto RW. A longitudinal study of the relationship of plasma somatomedin-C concentration to the pubertal growth spurt. *Am J Dis Child* 1987;41:562–4.
45. Pescovity OH, Hench KD, Barnes KM, Loriaux DL, Cutler GB Jr. Premature thelarche and central precocious puberty: the relationship between response of luteinizing hormone-releasing hormone. *J Clin Endocrinol Metab* 1988;67:474.
46. Rich BH, Rosenfield RL, Lucky AW, et al. Adrenarche: changing adrenal response to ACTH. *J Clin Endocrinol* 1981;52:1129.
47. Sorva R, Tolppanen E-M, Lankinen S, Perheentupa J. Growth evaluation: parent and child specific height standards. *Arch Dis Child* 1989; 64:1483–7.
48. Marshall WA, Tanner JM. Variations in pattern of pubertal changes in girls. *Arch Dis Child* 1969;44:291.
49. Rosenfeld RL. The ovary and female sexual maturation. In: Kaplan SA, ed. *Clinical pediatric endocrinology*. 2nd ed. Philadelphia: Saunders, 1989:259–323.
50. Rosenfield RL. Clinical review 6. Diagnosis and management of delayed puberty. *J Clin Endocrinol Metab* 1990;70:559–62.
51. Ehrmann DA, Rosenfield RL, Cuttler L, Burstein S, Cara JF, Levitsky LL. A new test of combined pituitary-testicular function using the gonadotropin-releasing hormone agonist nafarelin in the differentiation of gonadotropin deficiency from delayed puberty: pilot studies. *J Clin Endocrinol Metab* 1989;69:963–7.
52. Nottelmann ED, Susman EJ, Dorn LD, et al. Developmental processes in early adolescence. *J Adolesc Health Care* 1987;8:246–60.

surgery, hernias, and masses. Palpation of the liver edge, spleen, and kidney should be attempted; abdominal tenderness, rebound, or guarding noted. The presence of ascites should be ruled out.

Breast Examination

The breast exam should search for masses and elicit any nipple secretion present. Breast development should be staged according to the Tanner classification. However, the classification is a morphological classification and may not always reflect the glandular and ductal development of the breast during adolescence, which itself reflects a myriad of hormones and growth factors acting in concert. In a patient with precocious or delayed puberty, or patient with abnormal breast development, ultrasound examination of the breast seems more reproducible and documentable. In addition, serial ultrasound examinations over time probably will prove a more reliable reflection of pubertal progression and therapeutic efficacy than Tanner staging (16) (Fig. 1). This is an opportune time to instruct the adolescent in self-examination of her breasts. Although 93% of surveyed physicians thought this important, only 60% taught it (17).

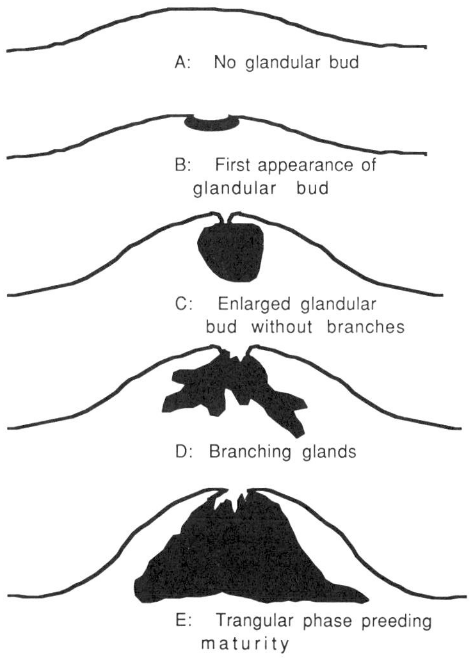

FIG. 1. Ultrasound stages of the breast are schematically depicted. (Adapted from ref. 16.)

Pelvic Examination

The best position for a pelvic examination in an adolescent patient depends on the comfort of the patient and maximal visualization for the physician. Although Huffman reported that the knee chest position frightens children (9), this position may be necessary to obtain full view of the vagina as well as demonstrate abnormalities of the hymen. In a questionnaire survey, adolescents at their first pelvic exam seemed more comfortable when examined in a semi-sitting position (18). One method is to begin the examination in the position most comfortable to the patient and then change it as necessary for visualization once she is more relaxed.

The patient must be informed of what is to happen prior to each step. "This is not going to hurt" is just as unwise as "This is going to hurt." Explaining each step prior to gently performing it and allowing the patient to decide how painful it is or is not paves the way for patient trust and better cooperation.

Vulva

The external genitalia should be staged according to the Tanner classification. The clitoris should be measured with a small ruler. The clitoris should not be larger than the average adult clitoris, 5.4 × 4.4 mm (9).

Hymen

The hymen should be examined for patency as well as caruncles. The normal hymen will change as the patient changes position. In the knee-chest position, gravity causes the lower edge to roll outward. Examining the hymen in this position allows confirmation of hymenal abnormalities and may also confirm suspect child abuse. In addition, labial traction will also allow gaping of the hymen and sizing of the hymeneal opening (19). An infected urethral meatus, at the superior aspect of the hymen, will often elicit tenderness or thickness upon palpation.

Vaginal Discharge

In early puberty, an adolescent may present with a thick, white, cloudy discharge that she or her parent may interpret as an infection. Usually, this is a physiologic leukorrhea resulting from the unopposed estrogen production which occurs prior to menarche and stimulates vaginal and cervical secretions. Microscopic examination reveals voluminous squamous cells without white blood cells or organisms. The patient should be reassured that no pathology is present and instructed in proper perineal hygiene. Indeed, improper perineal hygiene is the most common cause of adolescent vulvovaginitis resulting from *E. coli* colonization (9). Daily bathing, cotton panties, dresses, and panty hose with cotton crotches will help keep the perineum dry and prevent local pruritis, itching and odor. These instructions will be much more beneficial than attempting to change the patient's direction of tissue wiping after a bowel movement from "back to front" to "front to back." "Mini-pads" or "panty liners" may be recommended rather than messy, uncomfortable talcum powder to maintain dryness during the day.

Although usually physiologic, all discharge should also be examined for yeast, trichomonas, and *Gardnerella vaginalis*. Vulvovaginal infection is treated with the same medicines in the adolescent as in the adult except application is adjusted for the size of the vagina and inexperience of the patient (20).

Vagina and Cervix

Pelvic examination will rule out most congenital anomalies of the vagina. Visual examination of the vagina and cervix is best performed with a Huffman adolescent speculum (Fig. 2). The introitus of an adolescent who uses tampons or is having intercourse will easily admit the speculum. The speculum blades are 1.5 cm wide and 11 cm long. However, if the introitus is too narrow, a limited exam can be performed with a Peterson speculum or a pediatric vaginoscope (Fig. 3). Although the pediatric vaginoscope is useful for removal of a foreign body, it rarely allows enough visualization for an adequate cervical examination. In most cases, this instrument causes so much discomfort that the patient is less compliant for the succeeding bimanual examination; it is usually preferable to perform an examination under anesthesia in cases where cervical examination is mandated but the Huffman speculum is too large.

The speculum used should be *warm* and *lubricated*. If a cytologic smear is to be taken, then lubrication with warm water is substituted for jelly. The patient may be asked to perform a valsalva maneuver to relax the muscles of the pelvic diaphragm while inserting the speculum. The instrument should be inserted *slowly* with posterior pressure exerted on the perineal body to avoid the more tender urethra. Insertion should proceed with the blades close and pointed posteriorly toward the coccyx.

The cervix should be examined for lesions, infections or congenital abnormalities. Although it is unlikely that anyone born after 1970 will have been exposed *in utero* to diethylstilbesterol (DES), vaginal

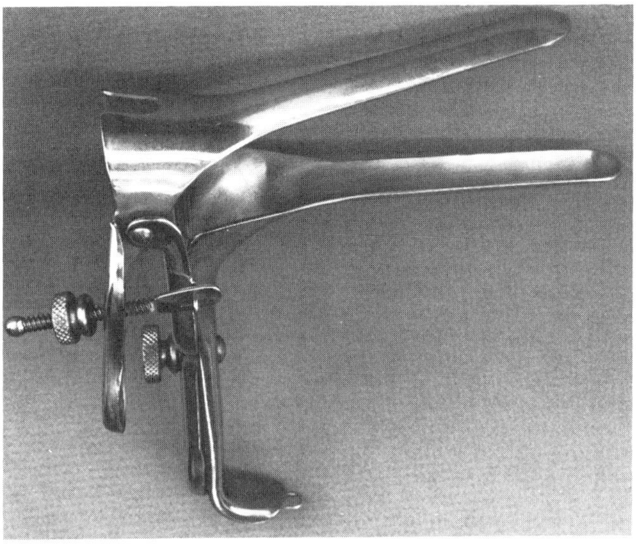

FIG. 2. The Huffman vaginal speculum is specially designed to fit the adolescent vagina. Its blades are 1.5 cm wide and 11 cm long. (From ref. 20, with permission.)

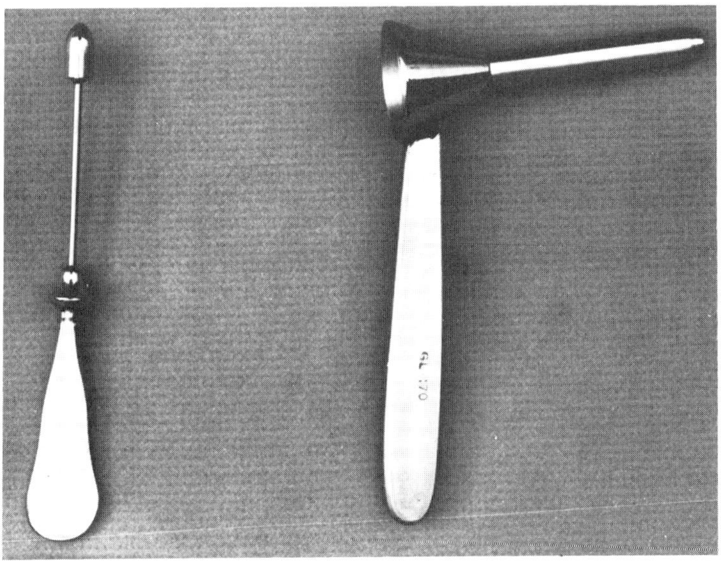

FIG. 3. A pediatric vaginoscope limits exposure and causes considerable discomfort, but may be useful for removal of a foreign body (From ref. 20, with permission.)

adenosis and clear cell carcinoma do occur *de novo*. The knee chest position will help position an eccentrically placed cervix into view.

An annual Pap smear is warranted in all sexually active adolescents. If adolescents have an easily identifiable cervix, a Pap smear may be obtained at the time of examination but, if normal, not repeated annually until she becomes sexually active.

Uterus

One lubricated finger can usually be inserted in the vagina for a bimanual examination. If the introitus is too small, the digital examination must be rectal. After entry, it is advisable to stop, allow the patient to regain composure and become accustomed to the finger in her vagina or rectum before proceeding with actual palpation. Ectopic gestation, endometriosis, and inflammation will often elicit cervical tenderness to palpation. The uterine fundus can be palpated and its position, size, shape and consistency noted (Table 1). During adolescence, the uterine length enlarges from approximately 3 cm at 7–8 years to almost 7 cm at 15–16 years (21). This increase in length is accompanied by a change in proportion of a relatively larger uterine fundus compared to cervix (21). Normal tubes cannot be palpated.

Ovaries

Normal ovaries can usually be palpated in thin patients. An ultrasound survey of 75 peripubertal girls with no ovarian pathology revealed a symmetric increase in ovarian size during puberty which parallels the increase in uterine length. Most girls had multiple, bilateral, 3–10-mm ovarian cysts. Occasionally, a 3–5-cm follicular cyst was found and resolved without incident (21) (Table 1). Thus, enlarged ovaries in the presence of an infantile uterus or a unilateral ovarian enlargement that does not resolve is suspect of neoplasia.

Rectovaginal Examination

A rectovaginal examination with one finger in each orifice is too painful for the adolescent. Thus, this exam should be avoided. A rectal exam alone will suffice.

INFORMATION AND THERAPY

Findings of the examination should be discussed with the patient immediately upon completion of the examination. A brief description while the patient is still on the examining table may be followed by a more detailed discussion after she is dressed. It is a nice gesture to ask her permission to explain the findings to her parent and have the more detailed discussion along with therapeutic plans in a consultation room with both patient and parent present. Patients should be reassured of normal findings repeatedly.

At some point in the discussion, the adolescent should be informed that intercourse does not feel the same as a pelvic exam. The physician should stress that fore-

TABLE 1. *Ovarian volume and uterine length increase during normal adolescence as viewed in 75 peripubertal girls undergoing ultrasonographic measurements*

Age	Mean uterine length (cm)	Corpus-to-cervix ratio	Mean ovarian volume (cm^3)
7–8 years	3.28 ± 1.3	1.1:1	1.91 ± 0.7
15–18 years	6.98 ± 1.0	1.3:1	3.52 ± 0.4
Commonly accepted adult values	8	3	12

From ref. 21.

play will increase vaginal compliance and lubrication allowing pleasurable lovemaking. This is, of course, a good time to inform the patient of her contraceptive choices.

Contraception

A teenager who consults a physician for contraception should be applauded, not given a lecture on being too young to have sex. Such lectures are not contraceptive and may result in teenage pregnancy. A physician willing to give contraception to a teenager only after she has demonstrated a previous pregnancy should not be taking care of adolescents. The adolescent who has decided to have intercourse will not change her mind if not given contraception. In fact, most of these young women have already had intercourse before seeking contraception (22).

Contraception does not increase adolescent promiscuity—it decreases adolescent pregnancy. Of course, it is difficult to make parents understand that withholding contraception will not decrease the sexual activity of their daughter or son. Nonetheless, sex education courses do reduce adolescent pregnancy rates (23). The laws governing prescription of contraceptives to minors vary from state to state even though the U.S. Supreme Court ruled that minors have a constitutional right to nonprescription contraceptives (24). The physician should take the time to describe the risks and benefit of each contraceptive method available (see the chapter by Huggins and Cullins) and allow the patient a choice. When afforded the opportunity, adolescents make surprisingly wise decisions for themselves. The physician should offer guidance and stress the importance of follow-up visits.

Prescribing for Minors

Individuals younger than 21 years of age are sometimes considered minors and require parental consent for surgery and treatment of nonvenereal disease, but most states have now lowered the age to 18 (25). In all 50 states, physicians can treat minors for venereal disease without parental consent. (25) An individual younger than 18 who is married, has parental consent, is self-supporting and living apart from her parents, has parents who have failed their legal responsibilities, or has a judicial decree deeming her of the majority, is an emancipated minor (25). Although emancipated minors may be a "legal" adult and therefore may give informed consent for medical and surgical therapy, they are not always emotionally and physically mature. Thus, the attitude and cautions that a physician displays to an emancipated minor should mimic that used in any adolescent examination. Prudent physicians are wise to consult their legal counsel regarding laws governing prescriptions for minors in their state.

Summary

Before dismissing the patient, it is wise to briefly summarize all findings and therapy plans. Asking the patient to repeat her understanding of the instructions may be the best way to confirm communication. In addition, giving the patient, and not her parent, a card with the physician's name and number along with instructions to call before prematurely stopping any medication or experiencing any side effect will identify the patient as the responsible person and codify the doctor-patient rather than doctor-parent relationship.

CONCLUSION

The care of the adolescent patient requires patience and time. Besides the initial visit, the adolescent also requires more vigilant attention to phone calls, as she may be frequently calling between classes or from a pay phone. Confidentiality may prevent return calls at a time more convenient for the physician.

REFERENCES

1. Millstein SG, Adler NE, Irwin CE Jr. Sources of anxiety about pelvic examinations among adolescent females. *J Adolesc Health Care* 1984; 5:105.
2. Muram D, Gold JJ. Physician dress style and the examination of young children. *Adolesc Pediatr Gynecol* 1990;3:158.
3. Dunn JJ, Lee TH, Percelay JM, et al. Patient and house officer attitudes on physician attire and etiquette. *JAMA* 1987;257:65.
4. Neinstein LS, Stewart D, Gordon N. Effect of physician dress style on patient-physician relationship. *J Adolesc Health Care* 1985;6:456.
5. Rapp CE Jr. The adolescent patient. *Ann Intern Med* 1983;99:52.
6. Dewhurst C, et al. The regularity of early menstrual cycles. *J Obstet Gynaecol Br Comm* 1971;78:1093.
7. Kantero R, Widholm O. Correlation of menstrual traits between adolescent girls and their mothers. *Acta Obstet Gynecol Scand [Suppl]* 1971;14:30.
8. Batrinos ML, Panitsa-Faflia C, Courcoutsakis N, Chatzipavlou V. Incidence, type and etiology of menstrual disorders in the age group 12–19 years. *Adolesc Pediatr Gynecol* 1990;3:149.
9. Huffman JW, Dewhurst CJ, Capraro VJ. *The gynecology of childhood and adolescence*. 2nd ed. Philadelphia: WB Saunders, 1981:85–87.
10. Apter D, Vihko R. Hormonal patterns of the first menstrual cycles. In: Flamigni C, Venturoli S, Givens JR, eds. *Adolescence in females*. Chicago: Year Book Medical Publishers, 1985.
11. Wilson L, Kurzrok R. Studies on the motility of the human uterus in vivo. A functional myometrial cycle. *Endocrinology* 1983;23:79.
12. Bichers W. Dysmenorrhea and menstrual disability. *Clin Obstet Gynecol* 1960;3:233.
13. Masters WH, Johnson VE. *Human sexual response*. Boston: Little Brown, 1966.
14. Buchta RM. Adolescent females' preferences regarding use of a chaperone during a pelvic examination. Observations from a private-practice setting. *J Adolesc Health Care* 1986;7:409.
15. Buchta RM. Use of chaperones during pelvic examinations of female adolescents. Results of a survey. *Am J Dis Child* 1987;141:666.
16. Bruni V, Dei M, Deligeoroglou E, et al. Breast development in adolescent girls. *Adolesc Pediatr Gynecol* 1990;3:201.
17. Nussbaum MP, Shenker IR, Feldman JG. Attitudes versus performance in providing gynecologic care to adolescents by pediatricians. *J Adolesc Health Care* 1989;10:203.
18. Seymore C, DuRant RH, Jay MS, et al. Influence of position during examination, and sex of examiner on patient anxiety during pelvic examination. *J Pediatr* 1986;108:312.
19. Bays J, Chewning M, Keltner L, Sewell R, Steinberg M, Thomas P. Changes in hymenal anatomy during examination of prepubertal girls for possible sexual abuse. *Adolesc Pediatr Gynecol* 1990;3:42.
20. Carson SA. Gynecologic problems of adolescence and puberty. In: Sciarra JJ, ed. *Gynecology and obstetrics, vol. 1*. Philadelphia: JJ Lippincott, 1986;1–10.
21. Winer-Muram HT, Emerson DE, Muram D, Boulden TS. The sonographic features of the peripubertal ovaries. *Adolesc Pediatr Gynecol* 1989;2:160.
22. Kanter JF, Zelnik M. Contraception and pregnancy: experience of young unmarried women in the United States. *Fam Plann Perspect* 1973;5:21.
23. Mecklenburg F. Pregnancy: an adolescent crisis. *Minn Med* 1973;56:101.
24. 431, US678, 1977 (United States Supreme Court Decision).
25. Annas GJ, Glantz LH, Katz BF. *Informed consent to human experimentation: the subject's dilemma*. Cambridge: Ballinger Publisher Company, 1977.

Pediatric and Adolescent Gynecology,
edited by S. E. Carpenter and J. A. Rock.
Raven Press, Ltd., New York © 1992.

5

Congenital Defects of the External Genitalia in the Newborn and Prepubertal Child

Claude J. Migeon and Gary D. Berkovitz

Department of Pediatrics, Division of Pediatric Endocrinology, Johns Hopkins University School of Medicine, Baltimore, Maryland 21205

In this section, we discuss mainly the problem of ambiguous genitalia observed at delivery, as this is usually the time at which the problem becomes apparent.

At every birth, two major events take place: the first cry of the baby at the perception of the harshness of the outside world, and the first glance by the world at the external genitalia of the baby. The first cry is, of course, vitally important. But the first glance at the baby is also significant as it establishes the sex of the individual for a lifetime. In the vast majority of cases, that casual glance is adequate in establishing sex. However, we strongly advise careful palpation of the scrotum to confirm the presence of testes before declaring the maleness of an infant.

The presence of ambiguous genitalia is always troubling to those witnessing the abnormality. At that point, it is of great importance to consult the pediatric endocrinologist, helped by the gynecologist, urologist, and psychologist experienced in problems of sex differentiation. In particular, the problem must be considered as an emergency. The first step to be taken is to explain to the parents that it is not possible to establish the sex of the infant by simple examination. Even the presence of palpable gonads does not necessarily indicate that one is dealing with testes (they can be ovotestes) or that they have a normal function. Furthermore, the parents must be told that various examinations will be needed before a decision can be made, that the laboratory tests may take a few days, and that the rest of the family and friends are to be told that the baby has a "congenital malformation of the external genitalia" and that it will take 1–2 weeks for doctors to determine the sex of the baby.

Ideally, the infant should be kept in the hospital until a decision is made about the sex of rearing. The mother, after her discharge, should be encouraged to stay with the baby in order to establish the appropriate bonding as well as breastfeeding and general care. Unfortunately, it is not always possible to do so.

The role of the pediatric endocrinologist will be important not only in determining the etiology of the ambiguous genitalia but also in guiding and advising the parents about the decision for the sex of rearing. The guiding of the family will include support and reassurance but also teaching about sexual differentiation. This will permit the physician to identify later the specific step responsible for the abnormality.

In the early stages of discussion with parents, physicians should keep an open mind about the sex of rearing of the infant. At that time, it is preferable to use neutral terms such as the baby (rather than girl or boy), the gonads (rather than testes or ovaries), and phallus (rather than penis or clitoris).

After the decision about gender has been made, then it is appropriate to emphasize the elected choice and to give a first name that is unambiguously male or female.

PHYSIOLOGY OF SEXUAL DIFFERENTIATION

The first step in sex differentiation is the determination of genetic sex (XX or XY) at the time of conception. Nonetheless, the external genitalia of the male and female fetus appear to be identical at 6 weeks of gestation. This neutral genitalia includes the genital tubercle, the labioscrotal folds, the urethral folds, and a urogenital sinus. Simultaneously, a variety of bipotential structures also develops (1). The first among these are the gonads, which become apparent as a genital ridge at about 5 weeks. These structures are populated by germ cells, which migrate from the wall of the yolk sac. The fate of these germ cells (whether they develop as oocytes or spermatozoa) will be under the control of the ovary or testis that will subsequently develop from the bipotential gonad. Two sets of ducts appear at about the sixth week of fetal life: the male, Wolffian ducts, and the female, Müllerian ducts. These structures will give rise later to the internal accessory sex organs.

Gonadal Differentiation

The primary event in specific male sex determination is the commitment of the bipotential gonad to testicular development at about the sixth week of gestation (1). The trigger for this process is a Y chromosomal gene, termed the "testis determining factor" (TDF). The locus of this gene has been mapped to the distal segment of the short arm of the Y chromosome near the pseudoautosomal boundary (2). A gene termed "sex-determining region of the Y chromosome" (SRY) was isolated from this region (3), and several lines of evidence suggest that SRY is indeed the testis-determining gene (Fig. 1) (4–6). However, other genes also appear to be necessary for testicular determination. In particular, a role for an X-linked gene (7–9) and for one or more autosomal genes (10–12) has been proposed in the cascade of events that starts with the action of TDF. The first histologic sign of testicular determination is the appearance of Sertoli cells, which then proliferate and aggregate about germs cells to form testicular tubules (13,14). Three weeks after the appearance of Sertoli cells, Leydig cells also appear within the developing testis (1).

In the absence of TDF, the bipotential gonad undergoes ovarian determination (15). The primordial cells, which gave rise to Sertoli cells in the testis, differentiate as

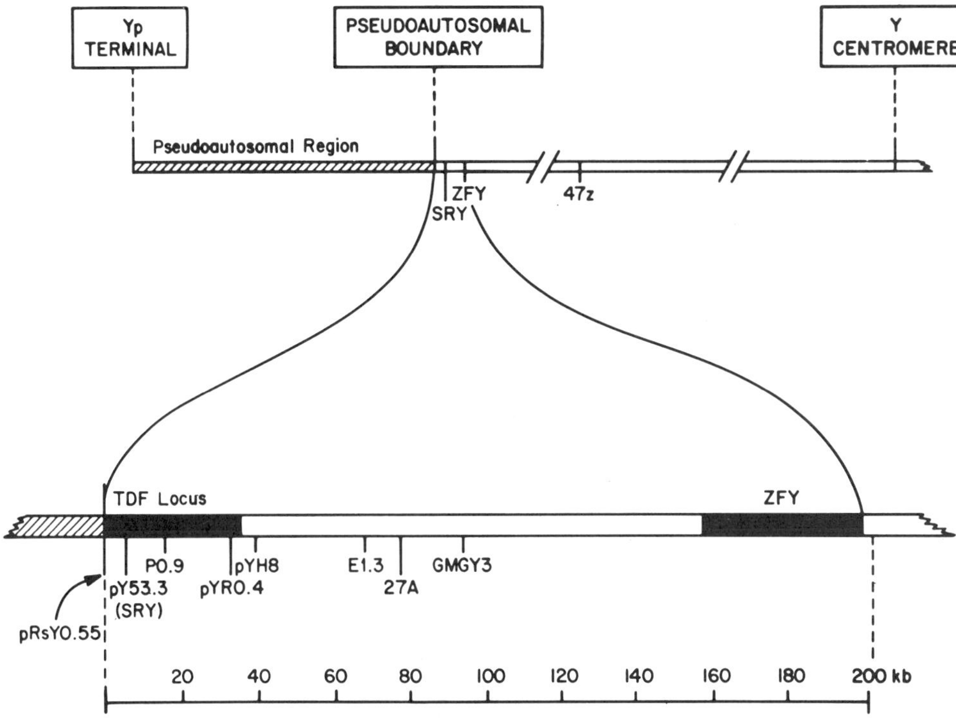

FIG. 1. Genetic map of the short arm of the human Y chromosome based on the work of Peter N. Goodfellow's laboratory (3).

granulosa cells in the developing ovary and surround germ cells to form primordial follicles.

Differentiation of Accessory Sex Organs

Differentiation of accessory sex organs (Wolffian ducts or Müllerian ducts) occurs between the eighth and 11th weeks of gestation. In the developing testis, Sertoli cells produce Müllerian inhibiting substance (MIS) which promotes the regression of female internal ducts (16). At about the same time, fetal Leydig cells begin to produce testosterone under the stimulus of maternal human chorionic gonadotropin. Biosynthesis of testosterone from cholesterol involves the action of four enzymes (17), including side chain cleavage, 3β-hydroxysteroid dehydrogenase, 17α-hydroxylase/17, 20-desmolase, and 17-ketoreductase (Fig. 2). In the presence of high local concentrations of testosterone, Wolffian ducts proliferate, giving rise to the epididymis, vas deferens, and seminal vesicles (10).

MIS is also produced in the female fetus, probably by the granulosa/theca cells, but it is not secreted until a later stage of development (18). The delay in MIS production beyond a critical commitment period permits the proliferation of Müllerian ducts and the formation of the fallopian tubes, uterus, and the upper two-thirds of the vagina. In the absence of fetal testosterone, Wolffian ducts in the female fetus regress (16).

Differentiation of External Genitalia

Masculinization of the external genitalia in the male fetus begins at around 8 weeks of gestation. This process begins with the

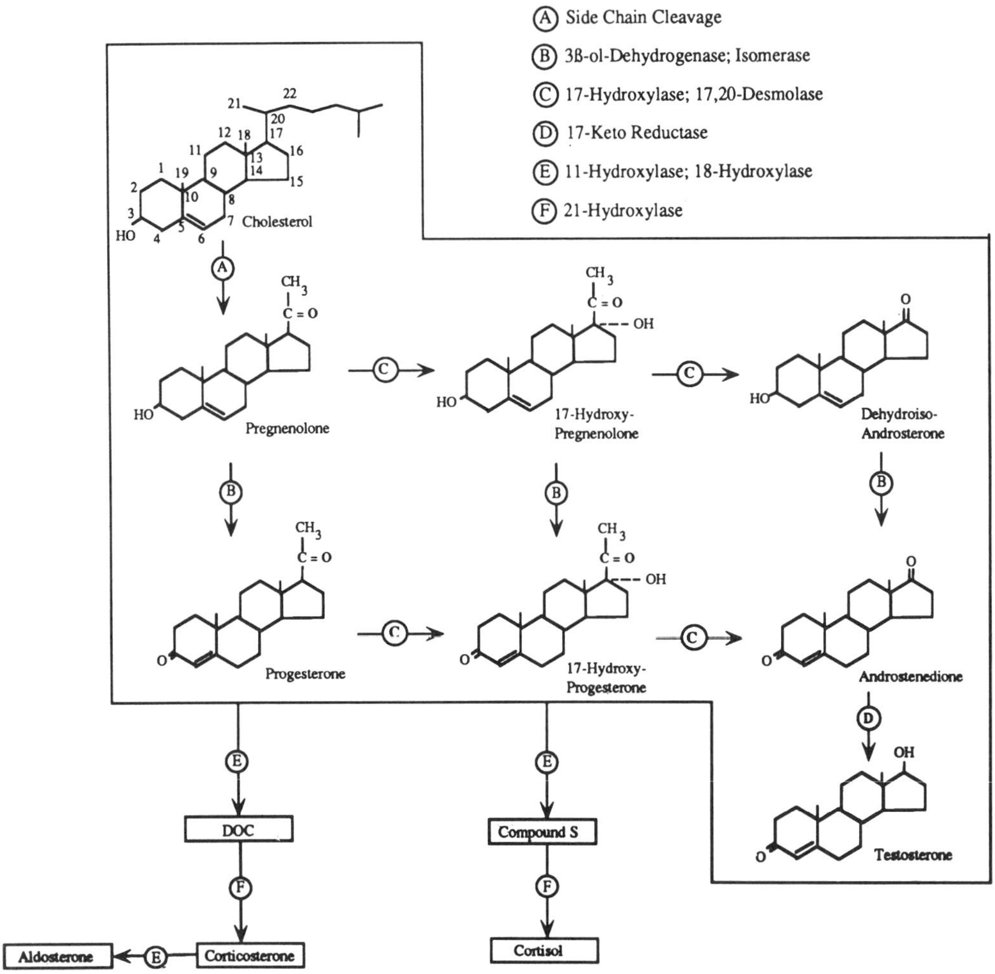

FIG. 2. Pathway for the biosynthesis of testosterone from cholesterol. Also shown is the pathway for the biosynthesis of glucocorticoids (cortisol, corticosterone) and mineralocorticoids (aldosterone, 11-deoxycorticosterone).

lengthening of the anogenital distance. It results in fusion of the labioscrotal folds to form the scrotum, growth of the genital tubercle to form the penis, and fusion of urethral folds to form the urethra and regression of the utriculovaginal pouch to form the prostatic utricle (1).

Development of male external genitalia requires the conversion of testosterone to the more biologically active metabolite dihydrotestosterone (19) by the 5α-reductase pathway. Dihydrotestosterone must then bind to specific protein receptors within target tissues to permit the expression of its androgenic effects (20). These androgen receptors are part of a family of steroid hormone receptors. They consist of three major structural and functional domains: a transcriptional activation domain, a DNA-binding domain, and a ligand-binding domain (21) (Fig. 3). The amount of androgen receptor protein is the same in the target tissue of men and women, the difference in androgenic effects being regulated principally by the amount of androgen available to the cells (22). The gene encoding the hu-

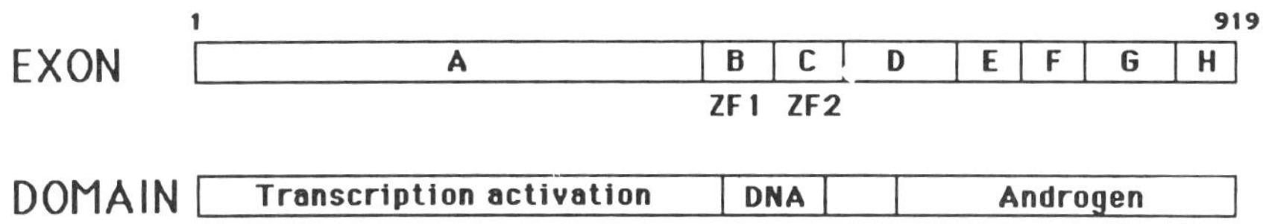

FIG. 3. Structural and functional domains of the human androgen receptor gene. This gene has been mapped to the long arm of the X chromosome (Xq12).

man androgen receptor has been mapped to the long arm of the X chromosome near the centromere (Xq12) (23). In addition, the complete human androgen receptor cDNA has been isolated recently facilitating a variety of studies of androgen receptors in health and disease (24,25).

In the absence of androgenic effects, the external genitalia develop along female lines. The labioscrotal folds become the labia majora, the urethral folds become the labia minora, the genital tubercle becomes the clitoris, and the urogenital sinus differentiates to form a separate urethral and vaginal opening (1).

WORK-UP OF NEWBORNS WITH AMBIGUOUS EXTERNAL GENITALIA

As already stated, it is an emergency to determine the etiology of the ambiguous genitalia because it will help in the decision making as far as the sex of rearing is concerned. It can also be a medical emergency as, in some cases, the mutation responsible for the abnormal genitalia results in life threatening symptoms. Following is an example of a schedule for tests which need to be ordered: day 1, karyotype (fluorescent Y chromosome); day 2, plasma testosterone, dihydrotestosterone, and androstenedione; day 3, plasma progesterone, 17-hydroxyprogesterone, 17-hydroxypregnenolone, and androstenedione; day 4, sonogram (gonads-uterus), genitogram with or without IVP; and day 6, repeat plasma 17-hydroxyprogesterone, 17-hydroxypregnenolone, and androstenedione.

At least once a day, it is necessary to check the levels of serum electrolytes and blood glucose (dextro-stick). The infant must also be weighed carefully every day.

The results of the tests listed above will help in arriving at the etiology of the ambiguous genitalia. The importance of the karyotype is self-evident. Although the search for a fluorescent Y chromosome is of interest, it is important to remember that the locus of the fluorescence is on the long arm of that chromosome, whereas the gene that initiates testicular formation (TDF) is located on the short arm. A buccal smear is not sufficient as a technique for determining the sex chromosome complement and should not be used.

The study of androgens (androstenedione, testosterone, and dihydrotestosterone) must be done on a single blood sample to permit the determination of the ratios of androstenedione/testosterone and of testosterone/dihydrotestosterone. Abnormally elevated ratios would be evidence of a deficiency in 17-ketosteroid reductase and 5α-steroid reductase, respectively. This investigation is timed for day 2 of life because testicular androgen levels tend to go down on days 3–8, prior to returning later to values of 150–250 ng/dl for testosterone (26).

The concentrations of 17-hydroxyprogesterone and progesterone are normally elevated in cord blood and shortly after birth (27). However, by day 3 of life they have reached levels that make possible the differentiation of normal values from those observed in patients with congenital adrenal hyperplasia due to 21-hydroxylase deficiency (28). This comment also applies to the levels of androstenedione. On occasion, it is appropriate to repeat the assays of various steroids if the original results are not conclusive.

Sonogram and genitogram permit the determination of the nature and localization of the internal ducts and their relationship to the urethra. In a markedly masculinized female, the vagina may open in the urethra via a narrow canal. In undermasculinized males, a utricular-vaginal pouch can be observed, opening in the urethra but ending blindly, without cervix or uterus.

Deficiency of some of the enzymes necessary for the biosynthesis of cortisol and aldosterone (21-hydroxylase, 3β-hydroxy steroid dehydrogenase-isomerase, side-chain cleavage) (Fig. 2) results also in abnormalities of the external genitalia. In such cases, an acute adrenal crisis with hyponatremic, hyperkalemic acidosis, and hypoglycemia can develop usually between day 2–6 of life. Hence, adequate monitoring of serum electrolytes and glucose are of great importance. Dehydration and marked weight loss are also symptoms of the adrenal crisis. A lack of adequate therapy may have catastrophic results (28).

WORK-UP OF PREPUBERTAL CHILDREN WITH AMBIGUOUS GENITALIA

The work up of ambiguous external genitalia that we described in the previous section was devised for newborn infants. Indeed, it is extremely important to establish early in life the etiology of the ambiguous genitalia and the preferred sex of rearing. Experience has shown that it is hazardous to make a change in sex after 1 or 2 years of age. In fact, the optimal time is in the first month of life.

On occasion, one is obliged to deal with a prepubertal child. Although the work-up of the prepubertal child with abnormal external genitalia is directed to ask the same questions as those raised in infancy, the gonadal physiology has changed in certain aspects. In particular, Leydig cell function that was quite active during the first 3–4 months of life remains quiescent throughout childhood and until puberty. In order to determine the potential of the gonads for androgen secretion, it is necessary to stimulate the Leydig cells by intramuscular administration of gonadotropins, usually human chorionic gonadotropin (hCG). The daily dose of hCG is adjusted for body size (3,000 IU per M^2 of body surface area). One injection is given every day for 5 consecutive days. A blood sample is obtained prior to the injections and on the morning of the sixth day (29).

The interpretation of the values of the various androgens is similar whether after hCG stimulation in childhood or without exogenous stimulation in infancy. An hCG stimulation test can also be helpful in the rare infants with ambiguous genitalia and suspected hypopituitarism.

In some children, the adequacy of penile response to androgen stimulation may be questioned. On such occasions, the hCG stimulation is prolonged to 6 weeks, giving two or three injections weekly. This sustained stimulation results normally in increased penile size. This diagnostic test is also used for therapeutic purposes in male children with small phallus.

DETERMINATION OF ETIOLOGY OF AMBIGUOUS GENITALIA

The first step in determining the etiology is the karyotype (Fig. 4). If it is 46,XY, one is dealing with an undermasculinized infant with a "male" karyotype. If testicular determination is normal, the condition is termed male pseudohermaphroditism, but if gonadal differentiation is abnormal, then it is a partial gonadal dysgenesis. On occasion, the abnormal gonadal differentiation can lead to true hermaphroditism, defined as the presence of well-characterized ovarian and testicular elements in the same in-

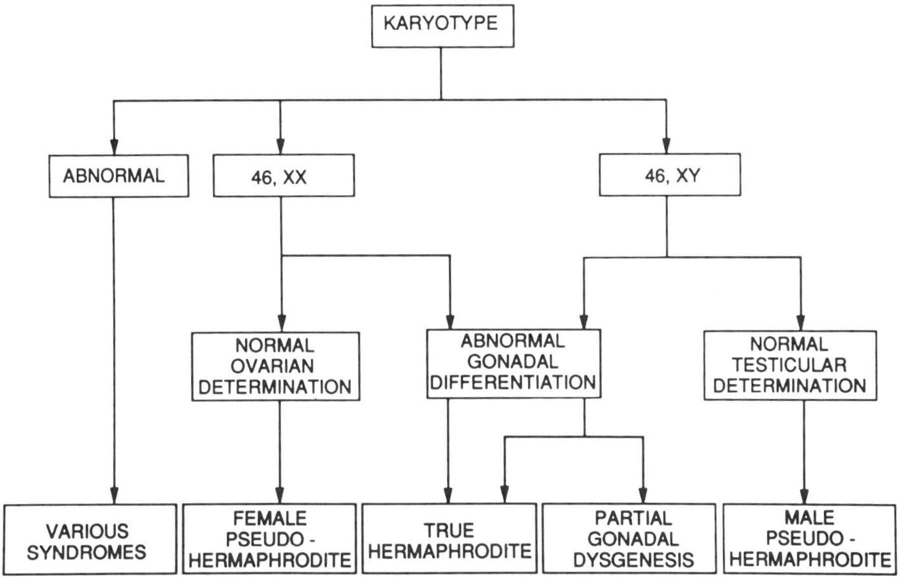

FIG. 4. Scheme for the determination of the pathology related to ambiguous genitalia based on the karyotype. In 46,XY infants with normal testicular formation, the condition is termed male pseudohermaphroditism. In 46,XX infants with normal ovarian formation, the condition is termed female pseudohermaphroditism. In 46,XX or 46,XY infants with abnormal gonadal differentiation, the condition may be true hermaphroditism or partial gonadal dysgenesis.

dividual. Often, the two tissues are combined to form an ovotestis.

If the karyotype is 46,XX and if the ovaries developed normally, the subject is a masculinized infant with a "female" karyotype and the condition is called female pseudohermaphroditism. A few subjects with XX sex chromosome complement will be true hermaphrodites.

Finally, in rare instances, an abnormality of sex chromosomes is found. This situation will be discussed separately, even though some cases may have an etiology similar to that of certain of the conditions mentioned above.

For etiologic classification, the determination of the karyotype permits the distinction of three groups of patients: 46,XY infants with ambiguous external genitalia, 46,XX infants with ambiguous genitalia, and infants with abnormal karyotype.

46,XY Infants with Ambiguous External Genitalia

The results of the study of the concentration of androgens will permit another practical and important consideration, namely to distinguish whether the function of the Leydig cells is normal or diminished; in other words, whether testosterone levels are normal or abnormally low (Fig. 5).

If testosterone is normal, a high testosterone/dihydrotesterone ratio (>12:1 in the newborn period) will be indicative of 5α-reductase deficiency (30). This syndrome is characterized by poor masculinization of the external genitalia but normal development of epididymis, vas deferens, and seminal vesicles (Table 1). This has permitted the conclusion that 5α-reduction of testosterone to dihydrotestosterone is necessary for masculinization of the external genitalia

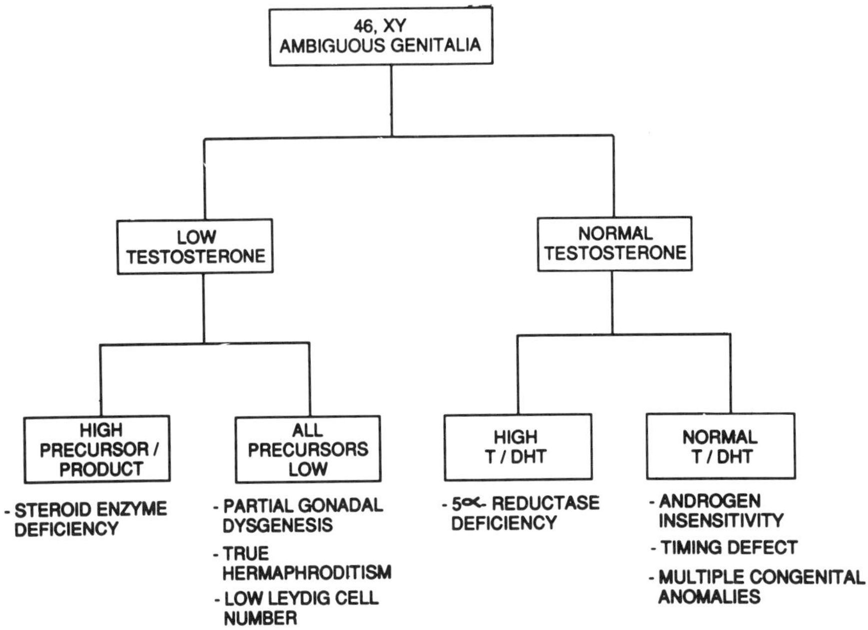

FIG. 5. Scheme for the determination of the pathophysiology related to ambiguous genitalia in 46,XY infants.

but not for proliferation of Wolffian structures. Individuals with 5α-reductase deficiency who are raised as males may have normal sperm production in adult life. There is virilization at puberty with improvement in phallic length, increased muscle mass, and deepening of the voice. However, there is usually poor development of facial and body hair, and little or no hairline recession (31,32).

TABLE 1. *Effects of various steroid enzyme deficiencies on the development of the external genitalia*

Enzyme deficiency	Genitalia in Males	Genitalia in Females	Other symptoms	Congenital adrenal hyperplasia
SCC				
Partial	Ambiguous	Female	—	+
Complete	Female	Female	Salt loss	+
3βol				
Partial	Ambiguous	Ambiguous	—	+
Complete	Female	Female	Salt loss	+
17OH				
Partial	Ambiguous	Female	Hypertension	+
Complete	Female	Female	Hypertension	+
11-Hydroxylase	Male	Ambiguous	Hypertension	+
21-OH				
Partial	Male	Ambiguous	—	+
Complete	Male	Ambiguous	Salt loss	+
17-Keto-reductase	Ambiguous	Female	—	0
5α-Reductase	Ambiguous	Female	—	0

SCG, Side-chain cleavage; 3β-ol, 3β-hydroxysteroid dehydrogenase; 17-OH, 17 hydroxylase; 21-OH, 21 hydroxylase.

A normal testosterone/dihydrotestosterone ratio will be characteristic of androgen insensitivity, a syndrome related to abnormal androgen receptor activity resulting in an inability to express androgen effects (33). In the complete form of androgen insensitivity, patients have normal female external genitalia but lack Müllerian as well as Wolffian structures (Fig. 6). Often, diagnosis is delayed until later in childhood when subjects present bilateral inguinal hernia, or at puberty when they present with primary amenorrhea despite normal breast development. Partial androgen insensitivity is characterized at birth by ambiguous genitalia and at puberty by poor development of secondary sexual characteristics, particularly with lack of growth of the phallus (Fig. 7). The diagnosis of androgen insensitivity can be made if there is an abnormality of androgen receptor binding in cultured genital skin fibroblasts and/or an X-linked family history of partial androgen insensitivity (33). The recent availability of cDNA clones for the androgen receptor make it possible now to evaluate androgen receptor defects at the molecular level (24,25).

A normal ratio is also found in the timing-defect syndrome: androgen secretion and expression of androgen effects are normal, but they started too late in embryonic life to permit complete masculinization of the external genitalia (34,35). Patients with the timing defect cannot be distinguished from those with partial androgen insensitivity on the basis of hormone profile alone. Furthermore, androgen receptor binding studies in cultured cells may sometimes be equivocal. Because patients with the timing defect develop normally at puberty whereas those with partial androgen insensitivity virilize poorly, it is important to dif-

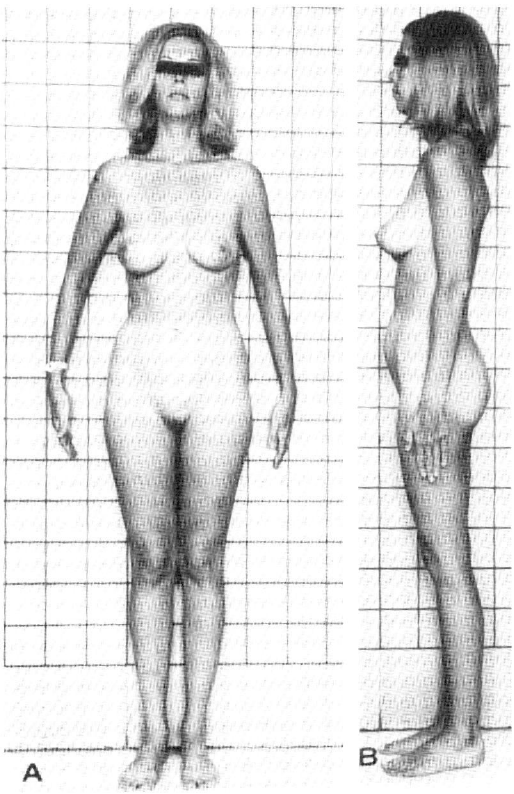

FIG. 6. Complete form of androgen insensitivity syndrome in a 46,XY adult subject. A mutation of the androgen receptor gene (deletion or point mutation) results in an inability to express androgen effects.

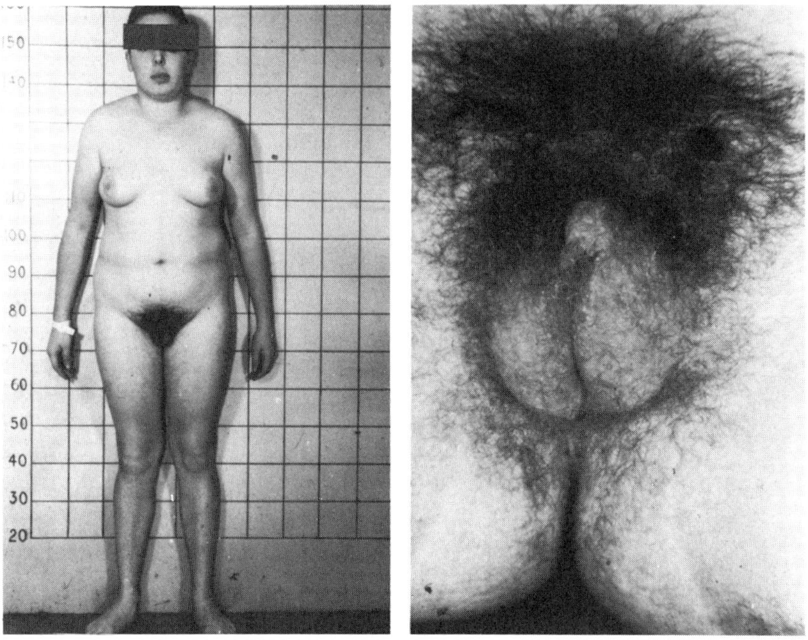

FIG. 7. Partial form of androgen insensitivity syndrome in a 46,XY young adult raised inappropriately as a male. The mutation of the androgen receptor gene results in a partial inability to express androgen effects.

ferentiate between the two at the time of gender assignment. It is now possible to use recently developed molecular techniques for the study of androgen receptors which permit us to detect mutations of the receptor gene in the newborn period (36,37).

A normal testosterone/dihydrotestosterone ratio can also be observed in infants with congenital malformations involving the genitourinary/gastrointestinal tracts. For example, a male infant with imperforate anus can also have an unusual external genitalia. This can also be seen in prune-belly syndrome (absence of abdominal wall) and in extrophy of the bladder.

When the testosterone concentrations are low, an increase in one of its precursors suggests an enzyme deficiency at the level of the abnormal precursor/product ratio. For example, an increase in androstenedione/testosterone ratio is indicative of a 17-ketosteroid reductase abnormality (38). The other enzymes (Table 1) involved in the formation of testosterone from cholesterol include: side chain cleavage enzyme (20-hydroxylase/22-hydroxylase/20,22-desmolase), 3β-hydroxysteroid dehydrogenase, and 17-hydroxylase/17,20-desmolase. A deficiency of either the side-chain cleavage enzyme (39) or 3β-hydroxysteroid dehydrogenase (40) is rare but results in a salt-losing form of congenital adrenal hyperplasia. These two conditions are often lethal in infancy. However, mild deficiencies without salt loss have been reported in children. By contrast, 17-hydroxylase deficiency results in an hypertensive form of congenital adrenal hyperplasia. It is associated with an absence of androgen secretion in the complete form, resulting in female-appearing genitalia in the affected infants. In the partial form, the genitalia are ambiguous (28).

If the levels of testosterone and its precursors are all low, then the problem might be related to 46,XY gonadal dysgenesis involving both tubules and Leydig cells. In the complete form of the disorder (pure gonadal dysgenesis), subjects develop bilateral streak gonads, normal Müllerian structures, and female external genitalia. Such subjects are usually diagnosed at 12–15 years of age when they present with hypergonadotrophic hypogonadism (41). The 46,XY partial gonadal dysgenesis is characterized by incomplete testicular differentiation. The gonads consist of poorly formed testicular tubules mixed with ovarian stroma. The external genitalia are ambiguous and there is frequently a mix of Müllerian and Wolffian structures. The degree of Leydig cell function determines the extent of the masculinization of the external genitalia (42,43). Early diagnosis of 46,XY partial gonadal dysgenesis is important as patients with this disorder are at increased risk for developing gonadal malignancy (44). The syndrome of 46XY true hermaphroditism might be considered to be a form of gonadal dysgenesis. Finally, in rare cases of diminished testosterone production, the tubules appear to have normal Sertoli cells and germ cells but the number of Leydig cells is decreased. This is sometimes referred to as Leydig cell hypoplasia.

46,XX Infants with Ambiguous External Genitalia

In female pseudohermaphroditism, the source of excessive androgen can be either the fetus or the mother (Table 2). Excessive production of fetal androgens is related to congenital adrenal hyperplasia (Table 1). Although there are several forms of this disorder, they all have a common etiology: a deficiency of one of the enzymes needed for the formation of cortisol from cholesterol (Fig. 2). In turn, the decreased cortisol secretion results in a compensatory increase in corticotropin releasing hormone/adrenocortitropic hormone (CRH/ACTH) output which produces adrenal hyperplasia and hypersecretion of adrenal androgens (except in side-chain cleavage enzyme deficiency).

TABLE 2. *Classification of female pseudohermaphroditism*

Excess fetal androgen
21-Hydroxylase deficiency
Partial (simple virilizing form)
More Complete (salt-losing form)
11-Hydroxylase deficiency (hypertensive form)
3β-Hydroxysteroid dehydrogenase deficiency
Excess maternal androgen
Iatrogenic
Virilizing tumor of ovary or adrenal
Congenital anormalities
Structural or teratogenic factors

The most frequent form is the 21-hydroxylase deficiency. The overproduced C_{19}-steroid is androstenedione, an androgen with little or no biological activity. However, 10% of it is metabolized to testosterone, which will masculinize the female fetus (Fig. 8). Two of the cortisol precursors that are also hypersecreted are 17-hydroxyprogesterone and progesterone. They produce a salt-losing tendency that is compensated by an increased aldosterone secretion in the partial form of 21-hydroxylase deficiency (simple virilizing form). In the more complete form, aldosterone secretion cannot be increased resulting in a salt-losing crisis (salt-losing form) with low Na, Cl, CO_2 and elevated K (28).

In the 11-hydroxylase deficiency (hypertensive form), the mechanism responsible for masculinization of the female fetus is similar to that of 21-hydroxylase deficiency. However, the hypersecreted precursors of cortisol are different. They are 11-deoxycortisol that has low glucocorticoid activity and 11-deoxy-corticosterone (DOC) that produces hypertension (28).

Deficiency in 3β-hydroxysteroid dehydrogenase/isomerase (28,40) is extremely rare, and so is that of cytochrome P450 side-chain cleavage enzyme (28,39), which permits 20-hydroxylation, 22-hydroxylation, and 20,22 desmolase. The complete deficiency of both of these enzymes result in a total lack of biologically active adrenal steroids. In such cases, there is salt loss and

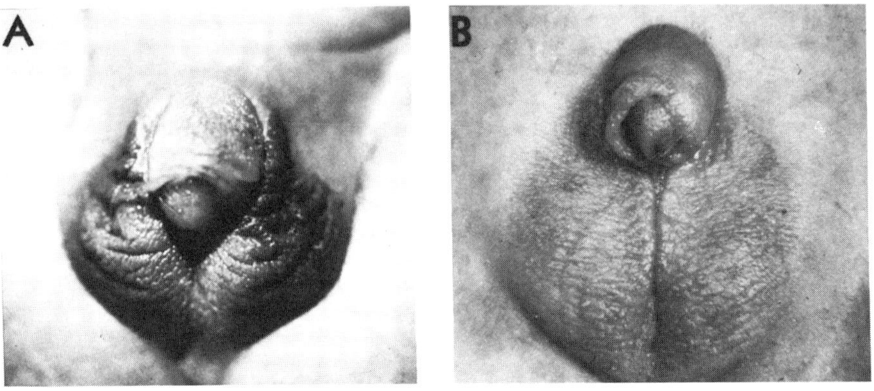

FIG. 8. Masculinization of the external genitalia of two 46,XX infants with congenital adrenal hyperplasia caused by 21-hydroxylase deficiency (salt-losing form). **A:** Typical abnormality including enlargement of the clitoris, scrotalization of the labia and urogenital sinus. **B:** Marked masculinization resulting in penile urethra.

a lack of androgen biosynthesis. Hence, female fetuses are not virilized and male fetuses present a female genitalia. When the deficiency of 3β-hydroxysteroid dehydrogenase is only partial, some androgens are secreted and there is a mild degree of masculinization in female fetuses and an almost complete feminization in male fetuses.

A deficiency of 17-hydroxylase, also rare, leads to feminization of the male fetus with no masculinization of female fetuses, if the deficiency is complete (45,46). In partial forms, both males and females present ambiguous genitalia.

On rare occasions, the source of androgens is the testicular component of the gonads of a subject with 46,XX true hermaphroditism.

Excessive androgens arising in the mother can cross the placenta and masculinize the external genitalia of a female fetus. The source of abnormal amounts of maternal androgens can be related to a virilizing tumor of the ovary (Hilar cell tumor, Adrenal-rest tumor, Krunkenberg tumor) or adrenal gland (47). Such tumors usually arise after fecondation as excess androgens prevent ovulation and therefore pregnancy. Some of the synthetic progestins have a mild androgenic activity. Given in large amounts shortly after the start of pregnancy (as done sometimes in habitual abortion), they can masculinize the female fetus (48).

Congenital abnormalities can, on occasion, mimic abnormalities of the external female genitalia. For example, moles or hemangioma located on the hood of the clitoris may suggest an hypertrophic phallus.

Abnormal Karyotype

As shown in Table 3, abnormal sex chromosome complements can result in various syndromes, some of them with unquestion-

TABLE 3. *Various syndromes with abnormal sex chromosome complement*

Ambiguous genitalia
X/XY
XX/XY
XX/XXY
Triploidy 69,XXY
Rare syndromes: Opitz, Opitz-Frias. Others: 47XXY, 47XYY.
Male genitalia
47,XXY and variants (Klinefelter syndrome)
47,XYY and variants (XYY syndrome)
46,XX Males
Female genitalia
45,X and variants (Turner syndrome)
47,XXX and variants (super female syndrome)
Pure gonadal dysgenesis (TDF gene deletion or mutation): 46,XY females; 46,X,i(Yq); 46,X,Yp-

ably male or female external genitalia, others with ambiguous genitalia.

In cases of triploidy (69 chromosomes), the XXY sex chromosome complement results in ambiguous genitalia in about 50% of subjects (49). However, triploidy is quite lethal: Most triploidy cases are detected in abortuses, and if pregnancy is carried to term the baby dies early in infancy.

Rare syndromes like those described by Opitz are often accompanied by various degrees of hypospadias (49). A few individuals with 47,XXY and 47,XYY may also present ambiguous genitalia (49).

In sex chromosome mosaicisms such as 45,X/46,XY or 46,XX/46,XY or 46,XX/47, XXY, the appearance of the external genitalia will vary in relation to the amount of testicular tissue present (50). The spectrum ranges from normal male genitalia with normal testes to normal female genitalia with ovaries (46,XX/46,XY) or streak gonads (45,X/46,XY) (Fig. 9). Ambiguous genitalia will be observed with abnormal gonadal differentiation of the partial gonadal dysgenesis type. Some of the patients with 45,X/46,XY present a streak gonad on one side and a dysgenetic testis on the other, whereas others are true hermaphrodites. The reason for the diversity of phenotypes seems to be related to the cloning of 45,X or 46,XX or 46,XY cells in the gonads.

GENDER ASSIGNMENT

Gender assignment is often a complex issue, and yet decisions need to be made as quickly as possible after the birth of a child. It is best handled by an experienced medical team including a pediatric endocrinologist/urologist/gynecologist and medical psychologist. The team should be organized as a standing committee with its own self-imposed rules. One rule is to use only the neutral terms in early discussions with the parents (e.g., phallus rather than penis or clitoris, gonad rather than testis or ovary).

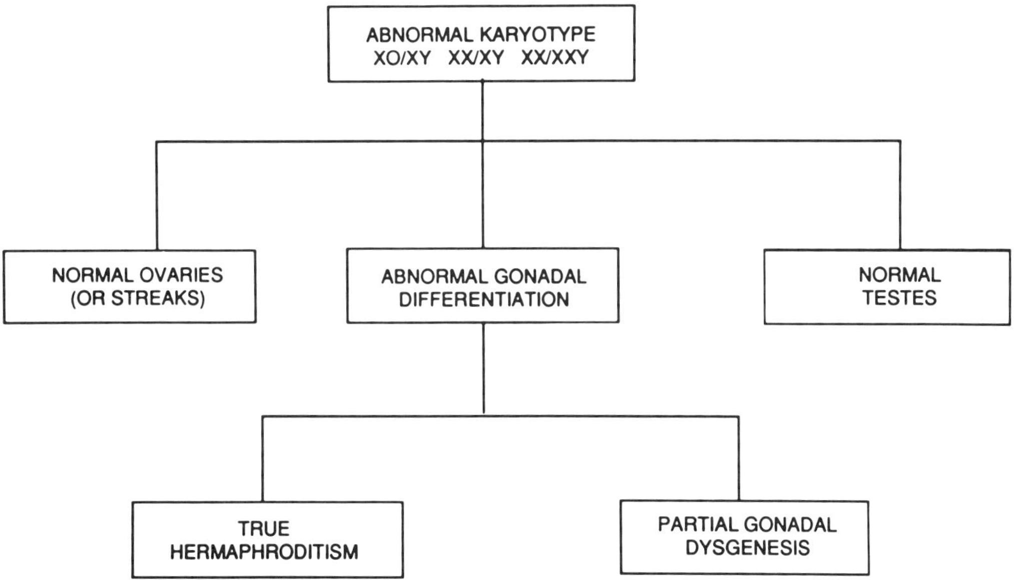

FIG. 9. Gonadal differentiation in subjects with karyotype showing sex chromosome mosaicism and including a Y chromosome.

This rule should also be imposed on all hospital personnel in contact with the family. One other important rule is that, following appropriate discussion, the members of the team should come up with a unanimous decision as to advice for gender to be presented to the parents. Although the team members would be expected to attempt to persuade the parents of the value of their advice, the parents should be made to understand that the final decision will be theirs. Furthermore, the team should make it clear, that whatever the parental decision, support will be given to the family in the future. In general, decisions about gender assignment depend on the results of studies performed as part of the etiologic evaluation of the child. In particular, informed decisions will require detailed information from the physical examination, karyotype, genitourethrogram and/or sonogram, studies of androgen production, including 5α-reductase activity, and, if possible, studies of androgen receptor function.

Decisions regarding gender assignment in infants with an XX karyotype tend to be easier. A 46,XX individual who has been virilized by the hyperandrogenism associated with adrenal hyperplasia, or by maternal androgens, has a normal uterus, fallopian tubes, and ovaries. Hence, the potential for normal reproductive function in these patients makes a female gender assignment the reasonable choice no matter how severe the masculinization.

Infants with an abnormal karyotype such as 45,X/46,XY present a somewhat special situation. Infertility, the potential for gonadal malignancy and the likelihood of short stature (50) suggest that female gender assignment is the better choice in the majority of these patients. The exception is in cases with well-masculinized external genitalia and with testes that are located or can be brought into the scrotum so the development of a gonadal tumor can be monitored.

Gender assignment in individuals with a 46,XY karyotype can be particularly complex. In making decisions, a variety of criteria regarding anatomy of the genitalia and the potential for future function need to be examined:

1. Phallic length should be determined by measuring the "stretched length" from the tip of the glans to the base of the phallus at the pubic symphysis. This can be easily accomplished in the newborn by applying slight pressure with the second and third finger at the base of the phallus to cause erection of phallic tissue. In considering the potential for normal function if the child is raised male, one needs to question whether the penile length will be adequate for the child to urinate standing up and whether it will be adequate for normal sexual function later in life. A phallic length of 1.9 cm is of 2.5 SD below the mean for a normal newborn male (51) and may be considered as a lower limit in assessing future function.

2. The position of the urethral meatus is important as it determines, in part, the number and complexity of the surgical procedures necessary to reconstruct the child as a male. In general, recent advances in surgical technique have greatly improved the outlook for repair of severe hypospadias.

3. The presence of a vaginal pouch may also strongly influence the decision regarding gender assignment. Removal of a large utriculovaginal pouch is often necessary if the child is raised as a male as it can otherwise become the site of urinary stasis and recurrent infection. However, removal of a utriculovaginal pouch in a male invariably damages the vas deferens and results in infertility. By contrast, the absence of a vaginal pouch may argue against a female gender assignment as construction of a vaginal pouch *de novo* may also be a difficult procedure.

4. The presence of normal Müllerian structures is important as their presence raises the possibility of menses or even a future pregnancy with a donor egg (52).

5. The adequacy of testosterone production can be assessed by determining blood levels in the first three months of life or following hCG stimulation. This information is useful in judging the potential for normal testosterone production at puberty and in adult life.

6. Evidence of androgen insensitivity in an infant with ambiguous genitalia creates a special case. As mentioned above, male subjects with partial androgen insensitivity virilize poorly at puberty despite high levels of androgens, usually develop gynecomastia and are invariably infertile (53). For these reasons, we recommend female gender assignment for infants with partial and of course, complete androgen insensitivity.

Advances in medical diagnosis and surgical technique have had a significant impact on our approach to gender assignment over the past twenty years. Longterm follow-up of patients born with ambiguous genitalia will ultimately provide information on the soundness of these decisions.

MANAGEMENT

One of the major steps in the management of infants and children with ambiguous genitalia is the decision on the sex rearing. This has been discussed in the previous section. The other steps will include consideration of the medical, surgical and psychological needs of the patient.

Medical Therapy

Adrenal Steroid Replacement Therapy

As shown in Table 1, deficiency of enzymes required for cortisol steroidogenesis may result in undermasculinized males (partial deficiency of side-chain cleavage enzymes, 3β-hydroxysteroid dehydrogenase, 17-hydroxylase) or overmasculinized females (partial or complete deficiency of 21-hydroxylase; 11-hydroxylase or 3β-dehydrogenase). Concomittently, there is adrenal hyperplasia. If the abnormality is quite marked, there can be hypertension in 11-hydroxylase deficiency or salt loss in the others.

Classically, the treatment includes replacement cortisol therapy (cortisol, cortisone, prednisone, dexamethasone), along with aldosterone replacement therapy (9α-Fluoro-cortisol) if there is salt loss. Such treatment is required in both male and female patients, and must be continued for a lifetime (28).

A deficiency of 17-ketosteroid reductase or 5α-reductase does not affect adrenocortical function (Table 1) and results in incomplete masculinization of male fetuses.

Sex Steroid Replacement Therapy at Puberty

Sex steroid therapy is usually not needed until pubertal age. Then, male patients with ambiguous genitalia and steroid enzyme deficiencies will often require supplemental androgen administration (testosterone enanthate, 200–300 mg intramuscularly, once a month). Female patients with deficiency of side-chain cleavage enzyme, 3β-hydroxysteroid dehydrogenase, and 17-hydroxylase require estrogen administration at puberty (Premarin, 0.3–0.6 mg po, daily for 1 year, then a contraceptive pill, the first 21 days of each month).

Patients raised as male and presenting partial gonadal dysgenesis, low Leydig cell number, and true hermaphroditism will usually require androgen supplement, whereas those with timing-defect do not.

Patients raised as females who have 46, XY partial gonadal dysgenesis, true hermaphroditism, or male pseudohermaphroditism will require estrogen supplementation at puberty.

Surgical Therapy

Details of the technical aspects of the reconstruction of ambiguous genitalia will be described elsewhere.

Patients Raised as Females

In these subjects, surgery to feminize the external genitalia is needed early in life (3–6 months of age). This is extremely important as it helps the family in establishing the female gender in their mind and, later, in the child. Specifically, it involves appropriate size reduction of the phallus so that it becomes inconspicuous and looks like a clitoris.

Often a second surgery will be needed to correct the shape or size of the vagina. We believe that this plastic surgery will give better results if carried out at the time the individual is ready to start her sex life.

Patients Raised as Males

The correction of ambiguous genitalia along male lines involves several steps, including release of chordee, construction of a perineal urethra, and prolongation of the urethra to the tip of the penis.

Gonads

In patients raised as males, the gonads that cannot be brought down in the scrotum must be removed because of the high risk of tumors. In patients raised as females, gonads (including streak gonads) must also be removed if the karyotype is 46,XY.

Psychological Therapy

This most important part of treatment will be discussed in another chapter. We will only mention that psychological therapy is needed not only at the time of the choice of gender, but throughout the various stages of the development of the child.

REFERENCES

1. Langman J. *Medical embryology*. 2nd ed. Baltimore: The Williams and Wilkins Company, 1969.
2. Palmer MS, Sinclair AH, Berta P, et al. Genetic evidence that ZFY is not the testis-determining factor. *Nature* 1989;342:937–9.
3. Sinclair AH, Berta P, Palmer MD, et al. A gene from the human sex determination region encodes a protein with homology to a conserved DNA-binding motif. *Nature* 1990;346:240–4.
4. Berta P, Hawkins JR, Sinclair AH, et al. Genetic evidence equating SRY and the testis-determining factor. *Nature* 1990;348:448–50.
5. Jager RJ, Anvret M, Hall K, Scherer G. A human XY female with a frame shift mutation in the candidate testis-determining gene SRY. *Nature* 1990;348:452–4.
6. Koopman P, Gubbay J, Vivian N, Goodfellow P, Lovell-Badge R. Male development of chromosomally female mice transgenic for Sry. *Nature* 1991;351:117–21.
7. Espiner EA, Veale AMO, Sands VE, Fitzgerald PH. Familial syndrome of streak gonads and normal male karyotype in five phenotypic females. *N Engl J Med* 1970;283:6–11.
8. German J, Simpson JL, Chaganti RSK, Summitt RL, Reid LB, Merkatz IR. Genetically determined sex-reversal in 46,XY humans. *Science* 1978;202:53–6.
9. Bernstein R, Koo GC, Wachtel SS. Abnormality of the X chromosome in human 46,XY female siblings with dysgenetic ovaries. *Science* 1980; 207:768–9.
10. Gessler M, Thomas GH, Couillin P, et al. A deleation map of the WAGR region on Chromosome 11. *Am J Hum Genet* 1989;44:486–95.
11. Hall BD, Spranger JW. Campomelic dysplasia: further elucidation of a distinct entity. *Am J Dis Child* 1980;134:285–9.
12. Washburn LL, Eicher EM. Sex reversal in XY mice caused by dominant mutation on chromosome 17. *Nature* 1983;303:338–40.
13. Magre S, Jost A. The initial phases of testicular organogenesis in the rat: an electron microscopy study. *Arch Anat Microsc Morphol Exp* 1980; 69:297–318.
14. Magre S, Jost A. Dissociation between testicular organogenesis and endocrine cytodifferentiation of Sertoli cells. *Proc Natl Acad Sci USA* 1984;81:7831–4.
15. Eicher EM, Washburn LL. Genetic control of primary sex determination in mice. *Ann Rev Genet* 1986;20:327–60.
16. Josso N. Physiology of sex differentiation. A guide to the understanding and management of the intersex child. In: Josso N, ed. *The intersex child*. Basel: Kager, 1981:1–13.

17. Ewing L, Brown BL. Testicular steroidogenesis. In: Johnson AD, Gomes WR, eds. *The testis, vol 4*. New York: Academic Press, 1977:239–87.
18. Josso N, Picard JY. Antimullerian hormone. *Physiol Rev* 1986;66:1038–90.
19. Siiteri PK, Wilson JD. Testosterone formation and metabolism during male sexual differentiation in the human embryo. *J Clin Endocrinol Metab* 1974;38:113–25.
20. Chan L, O'Maley BW. Mechanism of action of sex steroid hormones. *N Engl J Med* 1976; 294:1322–8.
21. O'Maley B. The steroid receptor superfamily: more excitement predicted for the future. *Mol Endocrinol* 1990;4:363–9.
22. Keenan BS, Meyer WJ III, Hadjian AJ, Migeon CJ. Androgen receptor in human skin fibroblasts; characterization of a specific 17-beta-hydroxy-5-alpha-androstan-3-one-protein complex in cell sonicates and nuclei. *Steroids* 1975; 25:535–52.
23. Migeon BR, Brown TR, Axelman J, Migeon CJ. Studies of the locus for androgen receptor: localization on the human X chromosome and evidence for homology with the Tfm locus in the mouse. *Proc Natl Acad Sci USA* 1981;78:6339–43.
24. Lubahn DB, Joseph DR, Sar M, et al. The human androgen receptor: complementary deoxyribonucleic acid cloning, sequence analysis and gene expression in prostate. *Mol Endocrinol* 1988;2:1265–75.
25. Chang C, Kohontis J, Liao S. Structural analysis of complementary DNA and amino acid sequences of human and rat androgen receptors. *Proc Natl Acad Sci USA* 1988;85:7211–5.
26. Forest MG, Sizonenko PC, Cathiard AM, Bertrand J. Hypophyso-gonadal function in humans during the first year of life. I. Evidence for testicular activity in early infancy. *J Clin Invest* 1974;53:818–28.
27. Forest MG, Ducharme JR. Hormones gonadotropes et gonadiques. In: Bertrand S, Rappaport R, Sizonenko PC, eds. *Endocrinologie pediatrique*. Paris: Payot Lausanne, 1982:91–112.
28. Migeon CJ. Diagnosis and treatment of adrenogenital disorders. In: Degroot LJ, ed. *Endocrinology, vol 2*. Philadelphia: W.B. Saunders Company, 1989:1676–704.
29. Berkovitz GB, Lee PA, Brown TR, Migeon CJ. Etiologic evaluation of male pseudohermaphroditism in infancy and childhood. *Am J Dis Child* 1984;138:755–9.
30. Pang S, Levine LS, Chow D, Sagiani F, Saenger P, New MI. Dihydrotestosterone and its relationship to testosterone in infancy and childhood. *J Clin Endocrinol Metab* 1979;48: 821–6.
31. Imperato-McGinley J, Guerrero L, Gautier T, Peterson RE. Steroid 5α-reductase deficiency in man: an inherited form of male pseudohermaphroditism. *Science* 1974;186:1213–5.
32. Walsh PC, Madden JD, Harrod MJ, Goldstein JL, MacDonald PD, Wilson JD. Familial incomplete male pseudohermaphroditism, type 2. Decreased dihydrotestosterone formation in pseudovaginal perineoscrotal hypospadias. *N Engl J Med* 1974;291:944–9.
33. Migeon CJ, Brown JT, Fichman KR. Androgen insensitivity syndrome. In: Josso N, ed. *The intersex child*. Basel: Kager, 1981:171–202.
34. Meyer WJ III, Keenan BS, De Lacerda L, Park IJ, Jones HE, Migeon CJ. Familial male pseudohermaphroditism with normal Leydig cell function at puberty. *J Clin Endocrinol Metab* 1978;46:593–603.
35. Walsh PC, Migeon CJ. The phenotypic expression of selective disorders of male sexual differentiation. *J Urol* 1978;119:627–9.
36. Brown TR, Lubahn DB, Wilson EM, Joseph DR, French FS, Migeon CJ. Deletion of the steroid-binding domain of the human androgen receptor gene in one family with complete androgen insensitivity syndrome: evidence for further genetic heterogeneity in this syndrome. *Proc Natl Acad Sci USA* 1988;85:8151–5.
37. Lubahn DB, Brown TR, Simental JA, et al. Sequence of the intron/exon junctions of the coding region of the human androgen receptor gene and identification of a point mutation in a family with complete androgen insensitivity. *Proc Natl Acad Sci USA* 1989;86:9534–8.
38. Saez JM, Peretti E de, Morera AM, David M, Bertrand J. Familial male pseudohermaphroditism with gynecomastia due to testicular 17-ketosteroid reductase defect: In vivo studies. *J Clin Endocrinol Metab* 1971;32:604–10.
39. Forest MG. Inborn errors of testosterone biosynthesis. In: Josso N, ed. *The intersex child*. Basel: Karger, 1981:133–55.
40. Bongiovanni AM. The adrenogenital syndrome with deficiency of 3β-hydroxysteroid dehydrogenase. *J Clin Invest* 1962;41:2086–92.
41. Sohval AR. The syndrome of pure gonadal dysgenesis. *Am J Med* 1965;38:615–25.
42. Federman DD. Disorders of sexual development. *N Engl J Med* 1967;277:351–60.
43. Rajfer J, Walsh PC. Mixed Gonadal Dysgenesis-dysgenetic male pseudohermaphroditism. In: Josso N, ed. *The intersex child*. Basel: Karger, 1981:105–15.
44. Scully RE. Neoplasia associated with anomalous sexual development and abnormal sex chromosomes. In: Josso N, ed. *The intersex child*. Basel: Karger, 1981:203–17.
45. Biglieri EG, Herron MA, Brust N. 17-Hydroxylation deficiency in man. *J Clin Invest* 1966; 45:1946–54.
46. New M. Male pseudohermaphroditism due to 17α-hydroxylase deficiency. *J Clin Invest* 1970; 49:1930–40.
47. Jones HW Jr. Nonadrenal female pseudohermaphroditism. In: Josso N, ed. *The intersex child*. Basel: Karger, 1981:65–79.
48. Wilkins L, Jones HW Jr, Holman GH, Stempfel RS Jr. Masculinization of the female fetus associated with administration of oral and intramuscular progestins during gestation: nonadrenal fe-

male pseudohermaphroditism. *J Clin Endocrinol Metab* 1958;18:559–85.
49. Smith DW. *Recognizable patterns of malformation.* 3rd ed. Philadelphia: WB Saunders, 1982.
50. Grumbach MM, Conte FA. Disorders of sexual differentiation. In: Wilson JD, Foster DW, ed. *Williams textbook of endocrinology.* 7th ed. Philadelphia: WB Saunders, 1985:312–401.
51. Lee PA, Mazur T, Danish R, et al. Micropenis. I. Criteria, etiologies and classification. *Johns Hopkins Med J* 1980;146:156–63.
52. Sauer MV, Lobo RA, Paulson RJ. Successful twin pregnancy after embryo donation to a patient with XY gonadal dysgenesis. *Am J Obstet Gynecol* 1989;161:380–1.
53. Amrhein JA, Klingensmith G, Walsh PC, McKusick VA, Migeon CJ. Partial androgen insensitivity: the Reifenstein syndrome revisited. *N Engl J Med* 1977;297:350–6.

Pediatric and Adolescent Gynecology,
edited by S. E. Carpenter and J. A. Rock.
Raven Press, Ltd., New York © 1992.

6

Surgical Management of Genital Ambiguity

John P. Gearhart

Department of Pediatric Urology, James Buchanan Brady Urological Institute, Department of Urology, Johns Hopkins Hospital, Baltimore, Maryland 21205

INDICATIONS

An infant with ambiguous genitalia poses a great dilemma for the parents and physician, even if the infant has a normal 46XX or 46XY karyotype. Gender assignment often is difficult and requires a full understanding of all factors involved, including chromosomal sex, hormonal sex, exogenous hormonal influence, anatomy of the internal and external genital structures, ultimate gonadal function, potential fertility, predilection of gonads for malignancy, and parental attitudes. However, in all cases, the sex of rearing should be determined as rapidly as possible after birth so that early perineal reconstruction can be performed, preferably within the first 3–6 months of life.

PREOPERATIVE MANAGEMENT

Evaluation of a newborn with ambiguous genitalia should include a careful family history, physical examination, and karyotype. Contrast studies of the urogenital system, biochemical evaluation, endoscopy, laparoscopy, and gonadal biopsy may be indicated. The history should include inquiries concerning maternal ingestion of possible androgenic substances during pregnancy. The history of an unexpected death of a sibling in the first week or two of life can pinpoint the likelihood of the adrenogenital syndrome with salt wasting. Some of these syndromes can be sex-linked recessive traits. Therefore, it may help to learn whether sterility, amenorrhea, or a hernia containing a gonad is part of the family history.

On physical examination, one should look for the following: (a) bifid scrotum, (b) labial rugae, (c) hypospadias, (d) chordee, (e) gonads above or below the inguinal ring, (f) palpation of an epididymis on the gonad, and (g) a midline uterus during the rectal examination. The presence of vaginal epithelial cells in the smear of the urethral discharge, obtained by milking the vagina during the rectal examination, is considered.

The possibility of other major associated anomalies should be considered. Karyotyping can help differentiate mixed gonadal dysgenesis (relatively common) from true hermaphroditism (rare). In addition to a karyotype, biochemical studies, including urinary ketosteroids, pregnanetriol, serum 17-hydroxyprogesterone, and electrolyte analyses, should be done to determine the presence of an enzymatic defect.

The radiologic exam at our center usually consists of a retrograde genitogram, and a pelvic ultrasound examination. There are several ways to obtain a genitogram but a surgeon should be present at the time of the study to offer technical advice and to observe the fluoroscopy personally. The main purpose of the genitogram is to confirm the presence of mullerian structures and to determine the "take off" of the vagina from the urogenital sinus. Both of these findings have significant implications in the choice of the surgical procedure for the newborn infant. Ultrasonography has been quite helpful in these infants both in identifying mullerian structures or in documenting their absence. Laparotomy and gonadal biopsy may be necessary to definitely diagnose mixed gonadal dysgenesis, male pseudohermaphroditism, or true hermaphroditism.

The choice of the sex of rearing should be based on the infant's anatomy and not on the chromosomal karyotype. Information gained with preoperative studies helps plan a surgical repair and whether it should be done from a perineal, combined perineal, or abdominal exposure, or even from a posterior sagittal approach. It is not difficult to create a vagina if one is absent, but it is difficult to create a satisfactory penis if the phallus is quite diminutive or rudimentary. Only those patients with a stretched penile length of at least 2.5 cm that will respond to testosterone should be considered for male sex of rearing. Despite major technical advances in penile reconstruction, it continues to appear that infants with a major intersex abnormality fare better psychologically and anatomically as females than as males. Thus, the general rule is that with an adequate phallus male sex assignment should be considered; otherwise, the female sex should be assigned regardless of the genetic, gonadal, or ductal sex of the individual.

SURGICAL OPTIONS

Intersex patients who require feminine reconstruction of the perineum can be divided into two groups: (a) females with extreme masculinization of the external genitalia (the adrenogenital syndrome), and (b) others with incomplete masculinization of the sexual structure (male pseudohermaphrodites, mixed gonadal dysgenesis, and some forms of true hermaphroditism) (1). Surgical repair of these infants who are to be reared as females include phallic reduction, creation of labia majora and minora, and construction of a neovagina. Originally the enlarged clitoris or diminutive phallus was managed by clitorectomy, and the entire structure was excised (2). Since that time, some conservative procedures have been implemented including excision of the corporal bodies without removal of the glans and symmetrical wedge resection of the tunica albuginea to shorten the corpora (3,4). Subsequently, methods to resect the entire corporal body while preserving innervation to the glans have been developed (5,6). A modified approach to phallic reduction has been developed by Kogan et al. (7) and has been popularized by other groups (8).

OPERATIVE TECHNIQUE

The surgical repair is similar whether the diagnosis is female pseudohermaphroditism secondary to the adrenogenital syndrome, male pseudohermaphroditism, mixed gonadal dysgenesis, or true hermaphroditism. First and most importantly, endoscopic examination of the lower genitourinary tract is performed to supplement the preoperative genital radiographs. If a vagina is present that enters the urethra or urogenital sinus distal to the external urinary sphincter, a flap vaginoplasty is performed. If construction of a neovagina is to be deferred, as in some patients whose vaginal entry is proximal to the external sphincter or those who have no vagina, phallic reduction and recession are the initial procedures of the perineal reconstruction.

Surgical repair is begun by making a circumferential incision at the phallus at the coronal level, sparing the ventral mucosal groove (Fig. 1A and B). The perineal flap is outlined and dissected carefully from the underlying tissues to insure an adequate blood supply (Fig. 2A). Any inappropriate gonads present can be removed easily through this incision at this time (Fig. 2B). Because no vagina exists in some male pseudohermaphrodites, the urethra, which may be of variable length, is opened ventrally from the meatus to the posterior bulbar area (Fig. 2C). The perineal flap is then brought into the bulbus urethra to provide a feminine appearance (Fig. 2D). Next, the dorsal skin of the prepuce is dissected from the penile shaft, starting at the glans and continuing to the base of the phallus (Fig. 3A and B). The skin is divided in the midline in preparation for construction of the labia minora (Fig. 3C). After the suspensory ligament is taken down, a 2-0 polyglycolic acid suture ligature is placed in each corporal body near the base of the penis to occlude the central corporal artery and to reduce blood flow into the erectile tissue (Fig. 3C). This maneuver minimizes the amount of bleeding during subsequent manipulation of the corporal tissues. Care is taken to avoid the neurovascular bundles.

Reduction of the phallus to a normal appearing clitoris is accomplished by making an incision into each corporal body as lateral as possible to avoid injury to the neurovascular bundles (Fig. 3C). Enough erectile tissue is removed to create a clitoris of appropriate size via these two incisions. In this manner, the phallic structure can be reduced markedly without excising the tun-

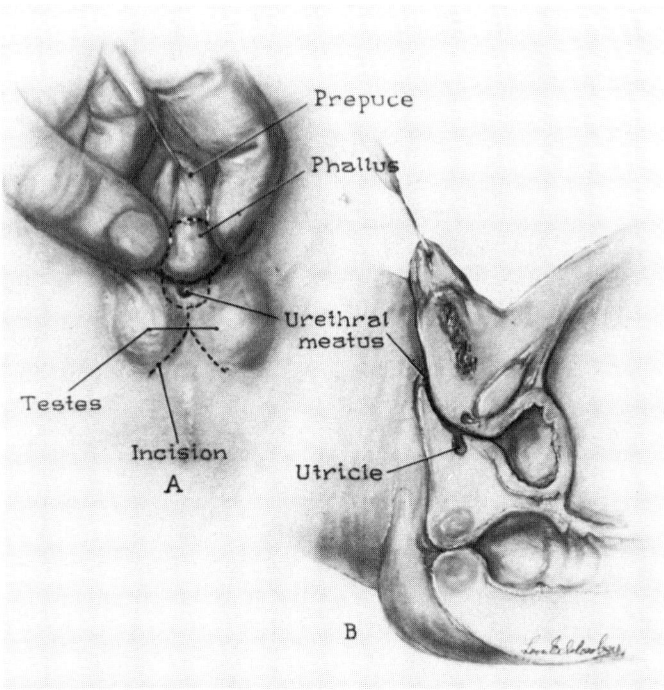

FIG. 1. A: Circumcision around the phallus and the resulting perineal flap. **B:** Lateral view.

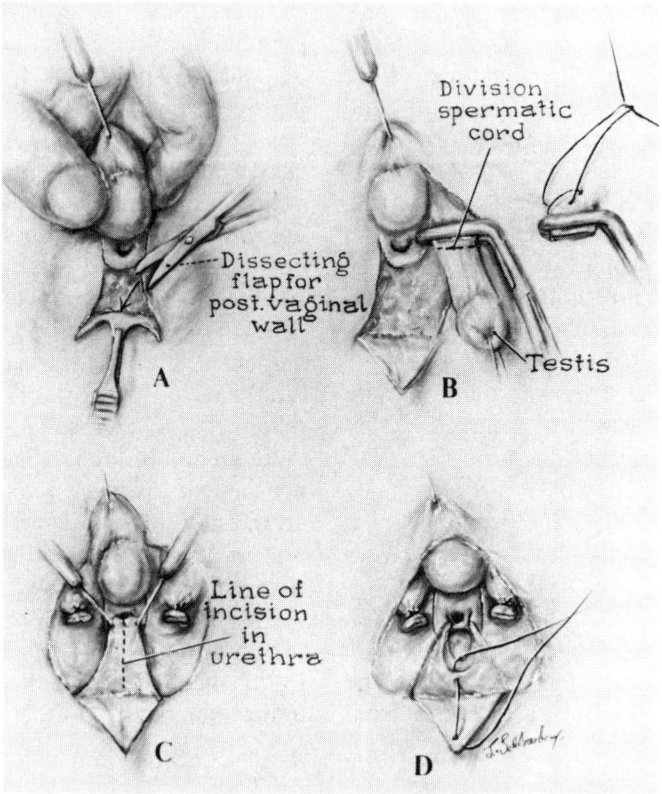

FIG. 2. A: Dissection of perineal flap. **B:** Removal of gonad via perineal flap incision. **C:** Incision into the urethral floor. **D:** Apex of perineal flap secured to floor of bulbar urethra.

ica albuginea or manipulating the neurovascular bundles supplying the glans. Sutures are placed starting at the anterior aspect of the pubic symphysis and running through the apex of the dissected dorsal skin flap to the base of the glans (Fig. 4). When they are tightened, the clitoris recesses to a concealed position near the mons pubis (Fig. 4A). In this manner, a midline scar over the mons is avoided. After excision of the erectile tissue, if the clitoris still appears to be too large it can be reduced easily before recession by excision of a dorsal wedge of tissue from the glans.

An often neglected part of the surgical reconstruction is fixation of the glans to the pubic bone. The glans must be fixed with at least two sutures to the base of the pubic bone. I usually use two sutures of 3-0 silk and sew the base of the glans to the periosteum of the pubic bone near its inferior edge, just cephalad to where the suspensory ligaments were previously cut. Care must be taken when sewing the glans to the pubis that the dorsal neurovascular bundle not be constricted in any way. Also, for cosmetic appearances, the glans should be sewn as far cephalad on the base of the pubis as possible so that the ventral mucosal strip stretches out and does not appear redundant. Also, the glans must be well fixed to the pubis so that it will remain in a normal recessed and concealed position.

The two flaps that have been created previously by dividing the phallic skin are draped around the side of the clitoris to create the labia minora (Fig. 4A and C). The

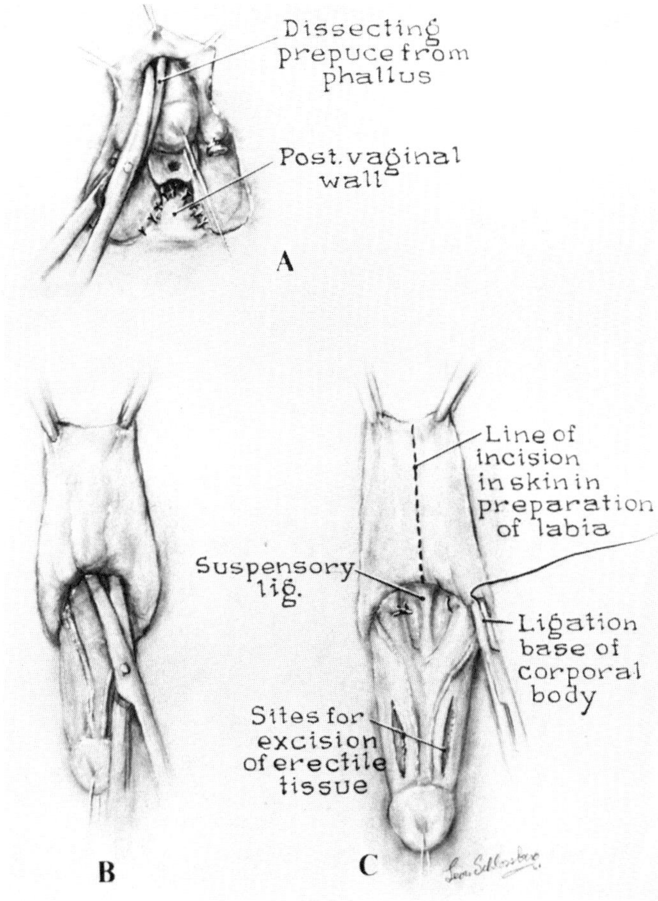

FIG. 3. A: Dorsal skin of prepuce is freed from phallic shaft. **B:** Dissection of dorsal skin is extended to base of the phallus. **C:** Ligation of each corporal body at the base of the phallus and lateral incision into the tunica albuginea.

medial edge of these flaps is sutured to the trimmed glans and to the edges of the ventral phallic urethral strip. The lateral aspect of the same dorsal skin flap is sutured to the labioscrotal folds (Fig. 4B and C). The labioscrotal flap is then extended into the angle formed by the perineal flap and the labia minora (labioscrotal Y-V plasty) to construct the labia majora (Fig. 4B and C). Some of the labioscrotal skin may have to be excised before the Y-V plasty is completed to prevent this tissue from having a rugated appearance.

The proper type of vaginoplasty performed depends on the level of the vaginal takeoff from the urogenital sinus. Although reported, the author has seen very few patients in whom a simple cut-back of the introitus would be adequate. A preoperative retrograde genitogram and cystoscopy along with vaginoscopy at that time of genital reconstructive surgery helps in proper planning of this procedure. The crucial determination that must be made at cystoscopy is whether a sufficiently large cavity lies behind the posteriorly fused labia minora. Most often in the infant coming to reconstructive surgery, a flap type vaginoplasty is carried out. The use of this perineal advancement flap along with a cli-

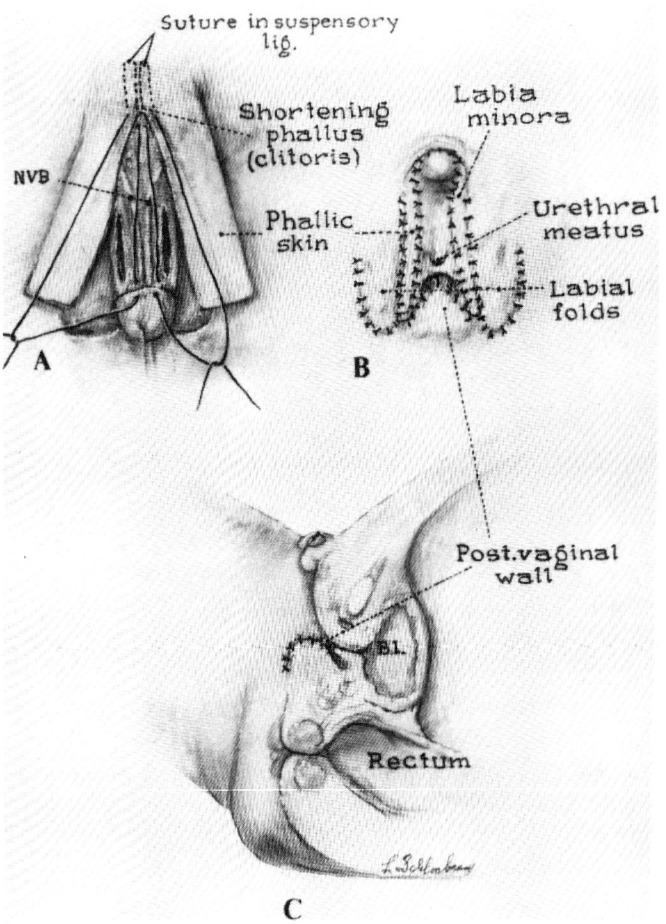

FIG. 4. A: Dissected dorsal skin and placement of phallic reduction sutures that run from the anterior pubic symphysis to the base of the glans. **B:** Completed perineal reconstruction with clitoris recessed beneath mons pubis. **C:** Lateral view of completed perineal reconstruction.

toroplasty allows most infants to have a very satisfactory cosmetic result from this unified approach. I usually place a number 12-14 sound in the urogenital sinus opening and open this structure over the sound placing marking sutures as the incision advances cephalad. The placing of these marking sutures allows the walls of the urogenital sinus to be well controlled when it is time to advance the perineal flap into the urogenital sinus and vagina. It is extremely important that the perineal flap be advanced well into the vagina so that an introitus of adequate size will be constructed so that later problems with stenosis, hematocolpos associated with the menarche or recurrent urinary tract infections be obviated. Sometimes, cystoscopy during the reconstructive procedure may be helpful to make sure that the flap is in good position and that it allows the vagina to be well drained.

A flap vaginoplasty is performed with incisions similar to those described previously (Fig. 5A and B). The urogenital sinus is opened in the midline until the posterior wall of the vagina is reached (Fig. 5A and B). Care must be taken at this juncture not to injure the rectum, which lies immediately posterior to the vagina. The posterior flap of the vagina is opened in the midline, and the perineal flap is advanced to exteriorize

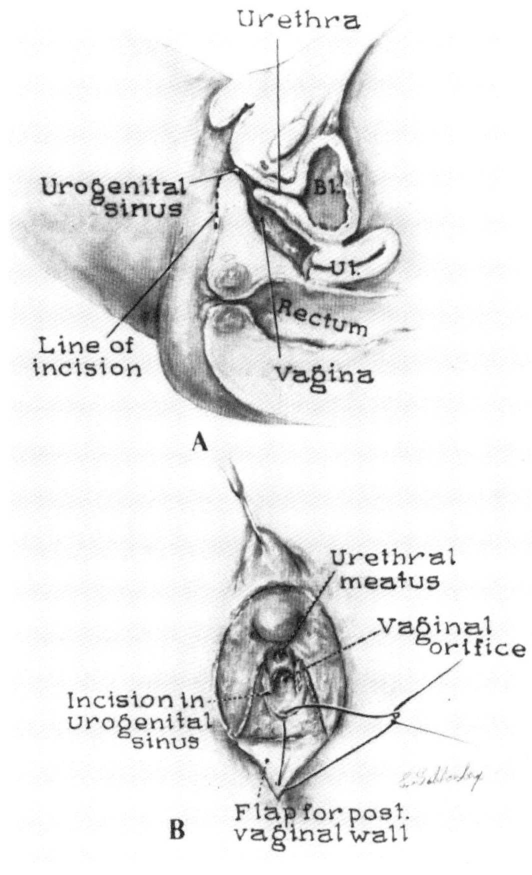

FIG. 5. **A:** Lateral view shows extent of perineal flap incision. **B:** Excision of urogenital sinus and perineal flap secured to floor of urogenital sinus to create posterior vaginal wall.

the vagina. The labioscrotal folds are sutured to the lateral borders of the urogenital sinus and vagina using the dorsal phallic skin, which has been divided previously in the midline (Fig. 4A and B). Although some recommend routine dilatation of this newly constructed vaginal orifice, in my experience this has not usually been necessary.

If the vaginal entry into the urogenital sinus is proximal to the external urinary sphincter and adequate drainage of the mullerian system is evident, the vaginoplasty is deferred to avoid injury to the sphincter and subsequent stress incontinence. In these cases, a pull-through procedure or a posterior sagittal approach is performed when the child is 18 months to 3 years of age (9–11). However, if the Müllerian tract on either side is obstructed or serves as a diverticulum for urine, a reconstructive procedure may need to be performed before 18 months. Clean intermittent vaginal catheterization may be necessary in some patients until a definitive operation can be performed. For an individual in whom the vagina is absent, creation of the neovagina is deferred until late adolescence or young adulthood. At this time, the person is mature, and regular dilatation of the vagina can be accomplished. This delay also allows time for the pelvis and perineal tissues to develop fully before reconstruction is performed.

POSTOPERATIVE MANAGEMENT AND COMPLICATIONS

The cosmetic and functional outcomes with this technique have been excellent. In all patients, the clitoris has normal sensation to pinprick. No episodes of glans sloughing, flap necrosis, urinary tract infections, or wound infections have been reported. It should also be noted that no patient has had stress incontinence as a result of this reconstruction. Of all patients in whom a flap vaginoplasty was performed at the time of the original perineal reconstruction, none has required regular dilatation to maintain an adequately sized vaginal orifice.

Most patients have had few immediate postoperative complications. A cross-shaped perineal pressure dressing is made from an adhesive elastic dressing and is left in place for 48 hr. A Foley catheter is placed at the time of surgery and left in the bladder until the dressing is removed and the wound is examined. After 5 days, the child is given sitz baths twice daily, and a blow dryer is used to dry the perineal wound after bathing. If all is well, the Foley catheter is removed and the suture lines are cleaned daily with hydrogen peroxide solution by the parent.

SUMMARY

This approach to surgical reconstruction of the perineum can be used in all patients, with ambiguous genitalia, regardless of the diagnosis, who are to be reared as females. The only aspect of the reconstruction that varies among patients is the timing of the vaginoplasty. However, in all cases, the phallic reduction, creation of the labia minora and majora, and gonadectomy (if indicated) are performed when the child is approximately 3–6 months old. Early genitoplasty insures that the appearance of the external genitalia is consistent with the female sex of rearing and relieves the parents' anxiety about the child in regard to the concerns of relatives and friends (12).

In this procedure, phallic reduction with phallic recession is described and incorporated. The erectile tissue is removed using two lateral corporal incisions without manipulation of the neurovascular bundles. The newly constructed, appropriate size clitoris is placed beneath the mons pubis without an overlying scar. In addition, the phallic foreskin is employed to create the labia minor. A labioscrotal Y-V plasty reduces the enlarged labioscrotal folds to produce normal appearing labia majora. A posterior perineal flap provides access to the vagina when present and to the urethra when absent. This unified approach is applicable to a variety of patients with different types of intersexual abnormalities.

REFERENCES

1. Donahoe PK, Hendren WH III. Perineal reconstruction in ambiguous genitalia in infants raised as females. *Ann Surg* 1984;200:363.
2. Gross RE, Randolph J, Kriggler JF Jr. Clitorectomy for sexual abnormalities: indications and technique. *Surgery* 1966;59:300.
3. Spence HM, Allen TD. Genital reconstruction in the female with adrenogenital syndrome. *Br J Urol* 1973;45:126.
4. Glassberg KI, Laungani G. Reduction clitoroplasty. *J Urol* 1981;17:604.
5. Barrett TM, Gonzalez ET Jr. Reconstruction of the female external genitalia. *Urol Clin North Am* 1980;7:455.
6. Snyder HMC III, Retik AB, et al. Feminizing genitoplasty: a synthesis. *J Urol* 1983;129:1024.
7. Kogan SJ, Smey P, Levitt SB. Subtunical total reduction clitoroplasty: a safe modification of existing techniques. *J Urol* 1983;130:746.
8. Oesterling JE, Gearhart JP, Jeffs RD. A unified approach to early reconstructive surgery of the child with ambiguous genitalia. *J Urol* 1987; 130:1079.
9. Hendren WH. Reconstructive problems of the vagina and the female urethra. *Clin Plast Surg* 1980;7:207.
10. Hendren WH, Donahoe PK. Correction of congenital anomalies of the vagina and perineum. *J Pediatr Surg* 1980;15:751.
11. Pena P, Devries P. Posterior sagittal anorectoplasty: Important technical considerations and new applications. *J Pediatr Surg* 1982;17:796.
12. Snyder HMC III. Clitoroplasty (Part II). *Dial Pediatr Urol* 1985;8:2–5.

Pediatric and Adolescent Gynecology,
edited by S. E. Carpenter and J. A. Rock.
Raven Press, Ltd., New York © 1992.

7

Psychological Aspects of Disorders of Sexual Differentiation

John Money

Johns Hopkins University and Hospital, Baltimore, Maryland 21205

SEX EDUCATION AND SEXUAL LEARNING

Most parents expect that their children, whether with or without an anatomical genital anomaly, will grow up to have normal sex lives, but all too often they leave it to chance. Even the best-intentioned parents may need assistance from a professional sexologist on how to break the taboo that forbids crossing the generation gap with explicit information on copulation and orgasm. Parental embarrassment is, to some extent, a problem of inadequate vocabulary and concepts. The story of reproduction can be simply told—in installments at the younger ages before the child can read fluently—in terms of the baby nest and baby egg; the baby tunnel or birth canal; the swimming race of the sperms, 200–300 million of them, and only one winner, with the prize of starting the baby egg to grow; the testes as sperm factories; and the fitting of the penis into the baby tunnel so that the sperms are safely delivered. Diagrams are desirable, such as can be found in *"Where Did I Come From?"* (1) or in *Sex Errors of the Body* (2). Also highly recommended are *How We Are Born* (3) and *Two Births* (4).

By the preteen years, it is the sociology of sex that becomes important in sex education. Explicitness pertains not only to "eggs, sperms, and menstrual periods," but also to erotosexual information concerning falling in love (or "limerence"), going steady, and erotic imagery in dreams and fantasies. As children become still older and move into puberty, sex education can examine being gay, straight, or in-between; erotic technique in masturbation, foreplay, and coition; contraception and abortion; protections against sexually transmitted disease (STD); and the terrible dilemma of how to begin one's sex life without running the risk of premature death from AIDS by exposing oneself to infection from a partner already carrying human immunodeficiency virus (HIV).

It is not too far-fetched to say that, in our society today, teenage sex is widely regarded not only as an evil, but also as a disease; and teenage pregnancy is overtly defined in the professional and lay literature as an epidemic. For parts of the body other than the genitalia, there are rehabilitation services and procedures, whereas even explicit audiovisual demonstrations of copulatory normality are subject to neglect, if not severe moral sanction, in most institutions. For the most part, even explicit reading or talking is avoided, particularly with teenagers. The pervasiveness of the sexual taboo affects teenagers so thoroughly that sometimes those who do have the option of explicit love and sex education are unable to accept it. Most of them become more sophisticated with age, but some remain sexologically permanently crippled.

Explicit sex education, especially during the adolescent period of growth and discovery, is needed not only to provide help in cases of sexual disorders, but to promote normal, healthy sexual development. There exists a paucity of information on love education for teenagers, but two books that make an honest and nonjudgmental approach are *Love and Sex in Plain Language* (5) and *The Facts of Love* (6).

Teenagers and adults both recognize the communicational wedge that splits them asunder. In many cases, when children have romantic and erotic questions or apprehensions that they find themselves unable to deal with through available channels (parents and/or explicit sex education classes), they may require personalized professional attention. If the case is such that the family should be involved in counseling, the child's distress will be alleviated if parents and child each have a private session first, followed by a joint interview to share information in common—though only with prior informed consent and respect for the participants' right to confidentiality.

The following Schedule of Inquiry for sexual counseling lists some of the topics with which children and their families may require help from a professional. Obviously, not all of the topics apply equally to juveniles, adolescents, and their parents: The schedules may be adapted to different age-levels and audiences as needed. Throughout the chapter, the pronoun "she" is used as the focus of inquiry here is gynecology, but most of the policies outlined in the chapter may apply to boys as well.

A SCHEDULE OF INQUIRY FOR PERSONAL SEXUAL COUNSELING

All Children

- Experience with siblings or age mates of nudity, genital inspection, genital stigmatization, childhood sexual rehearsal play, teasing, and gossip
- Social discrimination related to being too tomboyish as a girl, or not sufficiently macho as a boy
- Experience with parents or others as neglecting or providing for normal childhood sexual learning, explicitly or by diffuse assimilation, about all sexual subjects that children are likely to encounter in the media or in the experiences of their everyday lives, and the consequences of such experience relative to the child's conception of his or her genital anatomy and prognosis regarding coital adequacy
- Personal problems and/or psychopathology relative to family psychopathology, parental feuding, or parental break-up
- Concepts and fantasies regarding romantic possibilities, crushes, jealousies, love-smittenness (limerence), and love requited and unrequited

- Concepts and fantasies regarding future sex life in an adult relationship
- Concepts and uncertainties of the future status of parenthood by way of pregnancy and possible transmission of a disorder, donor insemination (sperm bank), adoption, or stepchildren
- Personal problems secondary to medication or illicit drug effects
- Knowledge and opinions regarding topics in the public domain such as STD and AIDS, gay liberation, abortion, and sexual abuse and molestation, including incest, date rape, and wife abuse

Schedule of Inquiry for Personal Sexual Counseling for Children with Genital Birth Defects

Children and adolescents with a history of a birth defect of the genitalia need, in the language of childhood, not only a cutting doctor and a needle doctor, but also a talking doctor, whose services, like those of a pediatrician or family physician, should be available on demand throughout childhood and adulthood. The talking doctor may be either a psychologist, psychiatrist, or some other specialist, provided he or she has specialty training in sexology. The frequency of demand is quite variable from one individual to another, and at different periods of the life span. The fewer the clinical and or social complications of development, the longer the interval between appointments with the talking doctor, and the greater the appropriateness of defining the visit as preventive, not therapeutic. The purpose of the visit, as defined, is to give a progress report. Progress reports are spaced preferably at intervals no longer than annually.

Items placed on the following Schedule of Inquiry are those that apply more specifically to those with birth defects of the sex organs. Expansions on some of these latter topics will be found in the sections following, in the order in which they appear in the list. With reference to these items, what applies to parents following the birth of a child with defects of the sex organs (that is, the concerns that they have, and the information that they request) will be, for the most part, what applies to patients themselves as they become adolescent and mature.

- Self-knowledge of diagnosis, prognosis, and treatment rationale
- Knowledge and explanation of the reasons for clinic visits and long-term follow-up, and clinical examinations and procedures and hospital admission experienced as nosocomial abuse
- Understanding concerning the possibilities of sterility and fertility
- Psychological adjustment to the possibility of amenorrhea
- Psychological preparation for the possibility of vaginoplasty
- Feelings about having ambiguous sexual characteristics
- The development of gender identity/role, and the unlikelihood or not of the possibility of future sex reassignment
- Overt or suspected knowledge of a history of neonatal sexual indecision and/or sex reannouncement
- Knowledge confided to or withheld from siblings, other relatives, and friends
- Academic status relative to IQ and cognitive abilities, impairment of which may be syndrome specific, as in Turner syndrome and some varieties of 46,XY hermaphroditism, whereas, by contrast, intellectual superiority may also be syndrome specific, as in 46,XX congenital virilizing adrenal hyperplasia (CVAH) hermaphroditism

KNOWLEDGE OF CONDITION

Individuals with birth defects of the sex organs are often subjected to the stigmatization and trauma of being teased as a sexual freak, or of being treated as a sexual invalid. Depriving the patient of knowledge about her condition undermines the ability to understand and defend herself against such treatment. Withholding information about the condition from the patient in order to "spare her" also creates an atmosphere of dread at the thought of the catastrophic news leaking out. This spares not the patient but rather the parents and physicians who are relieved of the need to talk about topics which are profoundly uncomfortable for them.

It is advisable to provide information progressively, in age-graded steps. In some cases however, an older patient may need to catch up on what has previously been omitted. It is important to leave ordinary channels of inquiry open and free from squeamishness and taboos. It creates unnecessary discomfort, for example, to inform a young child that her genitals are not like those of other girls, and then to evade her request to know what normal genital anatomy looks like. Rather, explicit diagrams and photographs should be used as a matter of routine.

Although openness about the diagnosis and prognosis is recommended, the information should be communicated in language designed to be therapeutic, not stigmatizing. Young people, being unsophisticated in the tradition of the doctor-patient relationship, are stigmatized by such terminology as mongolism, gargoylism, bird-headed dwarfism, and leprechaunism. Girls are stigmatized by hearing themselves referred to as male hermaphrodites, or as having testicles and male chromosomes.

EXPLAINING CLINICAL PROCEDURES

It is not uncommon for young patients to be left in the dark, or given only euphemistic or untruthful explanations regarding their frequent visits to the hospital or clinic, the procedures they undergo, and the need for medication. The taboo against the exposure of nudity in the genital examination or in medical photography may exacerbate resistance to coming into the medical environment at all. Some patients subjectively experience and misconstrue repeated genital examinations as rape, and surgical and medical procedures as nosocomial abuse. One way to alleviate this problem is to explain the procedure ahead of time. Another way is to provide terms that name the clinical procedures in such a way that a patient's various concerns can be verbalized and resolved. It is advantageous for a child to have learned and rehearsed the answers to inquiries from curious age-mates about why she is away from school, attending the clinic, or admitted for surgery. Likewise, she needs answers for the school nurse, or her future sexual partners, and so on (see below).

STERILITY AND FERTILITY

Definitive prophecies about life or death, health or sickness, and fertility or sterility are almost never warranted. Probability statements are more accurate and less stressful. For example, it is overly dramatic to tell a patient newly diagnosed as having Turner syndrome, "You won't be able to have children," when the accurate statement is about the probability of no pregnancy. There is always the possibility of misdiagnosis. Thus, there are, indeed, a few cases of Turner syndrome in which ovulation and menstruation will occur spontaneously, allowing the possibility of pregnancy. Today, there is the possibility of in vitro fertilization with a donated ovum for those who lack ovaries, but not a uterus. In the future, transplantation of a uterus may also become possible, and even an ectopic, intraabdominal pregnancy is not merely a science fiction. The very fact that such possibilities might eventuate, no matter how infinitesimal the likelihood, helps a patient to feel potentially normal or normalizable. The following case reports can be quoted in counseling.

It is normalizing for a girl with no uterus to know that there is an authentic case on record from New Zealand of a woman who delivered a normal daughter by cesarian section 9 months after she had had a total hysterectomy and oophorectomy (7). Her own fertilized egg had survived the operation and attached itself to the wall of the small intestine. In another case reported from France, a 46,XY woman with a hypoplastic uterus and streak gonads became pregnant with a donated ovum and sperm from her husband through *in vitro* fertilization (8). The cesarian birth was at 42 weeks. Most recently, in the United States, a successful twin birth at 35 weeks gestation (by cesarian section) was reported for an XY patient having a uterus but gonadal dysgenesis (9). A donated embryo was implanted in the patient, and the pregnancy was supported in the first 100 days with exogenously administered hormones.

The blow of infertility is softened if alternative forms of motherhood are mentioned, for example, adoptive motherhood, or marriage into an "instant family," of a parent with children. These alternatives provide the options of being married and being a mother, being normal, being happy, not being stigmatized, and not being discarded as a barren woman whom no man wants, so often the concerns of the patient. A girl who is told early in life of the possibility of adoption can rehearse adoptive motherhood in the "normal" fantasies and play. By the time she is ready for motherhood, no traumatic accommodation to the idea of adoption will be necessary later.

Among syndromes of birth defects of the sex organs, a few like CVAH are compatible with fertility and pregnancy. Older CVAH women may need counseling in the principles of heredity and in assessing the risk of conceiving a child with the syndrome. In counseling on the genetics of a recessive trait it may be helpful to call a heterozygous carrier a "hidden carrier," and a homozygous carrier an "open carrier." Genetic counseling may be of significance not only to the patient, but also to other members of the kinship—as in the androgen insensitivity syndrome, for example, and in other varieties of male hermaphroditism (see also below). Genetic counseling encompasses also decisions about prenatal diagnosis and abortion of an affected conceptus, and about using birth control versus having unprotected intercourse, or abstaining from sexual intercourse altogether.

AMENORRHEA

As the young, amenorrheal patient approaches the age at which she would ordinarily reach menarche, she needs to know about the monthly event she will not be experiencing, so that she will not be caught off guard in normal girlhood discussions and inadvertently reveal more than need be about her condition. Much of the common vocabulary referring to menstruation casts it in an ambivalent light. It is badge of womanhood, but also "the curse" that brings adverse physical and mood changes. This adds to the difficulty of preparing a patient for the feelings of exclusion she may encounter. Her mother commonly finds it just as disconcerting to speak with her about not having periods as about not having pregnancies.

At the younger ages, girls can be told of "the baby nest cleaning day," in accordance with the telling of the rest of the story of reproduction at their level. As they grow older, patients can learn about the physical process of the build-up of the endometrial lining and its hormonal regulation, and the shedding of the endometrium during the menses. They can be provided with a number of responses to give to inquiring agemates, such as "I've never had a problem with it," or "It never bothers me."

VAGINOPLASTY

As in the androgen-insensitivity syndrome and the Mayer-Rokitansky-Kuester syndrome, there are some patients whose vagina is a shallow dimple or blind pouch.

In some such cases, vaginal lengthening can be accomplished by self-dilation. However, overcoming childhood moral and religious rules that equate touching the genitals with masturbation may prove a major obstacle. So also may a phobia against penetration. Compliance with the regimen of self-dilation then requires supportive counseling until the obstacle is surmounted.

When surgical vaginoplasty is necessitated, the operation is usually done in midteenage, its timing decided in consultation with the patient herself. The benefits of normalizing the genitals may be under-

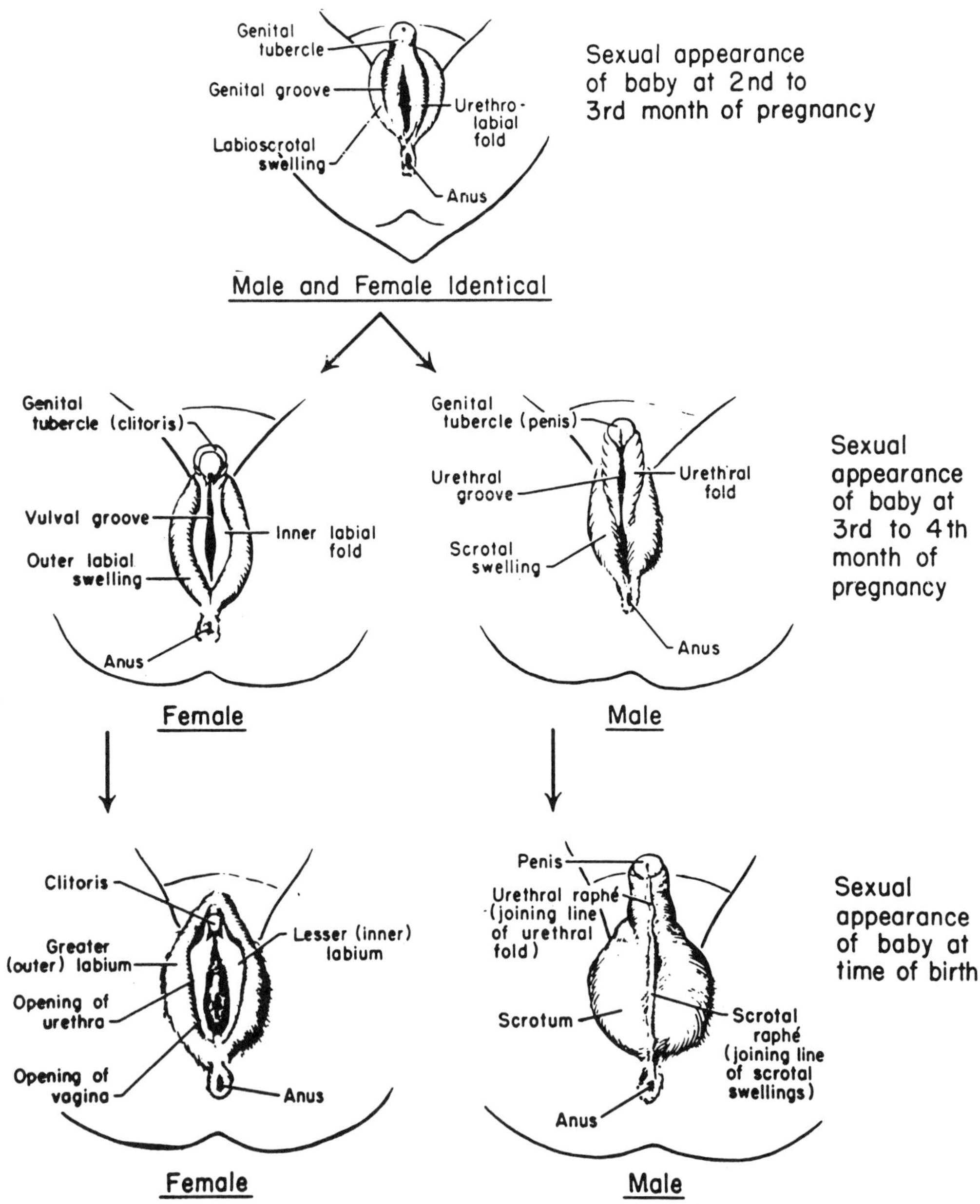

FIG. 1. Teaching diagram: differentiation of the external genitalia.

mined if the patient lacks a sense of informed consent, which may in turn lead to noncompliance with follow-up measures, and resistance to further clinical help. In discussing the operation with the patient, embryological diagrams can be used to convey how the genital apparatus of the two sexes originate in the same early structures (Figs. 1 and 2). They help a patient to understand that she is not a freak, but a girl in whom the development of the sexual organs did not proceed as expected. Explicit medical photographs of the normal vagina show what the surgical team hope to approximate.

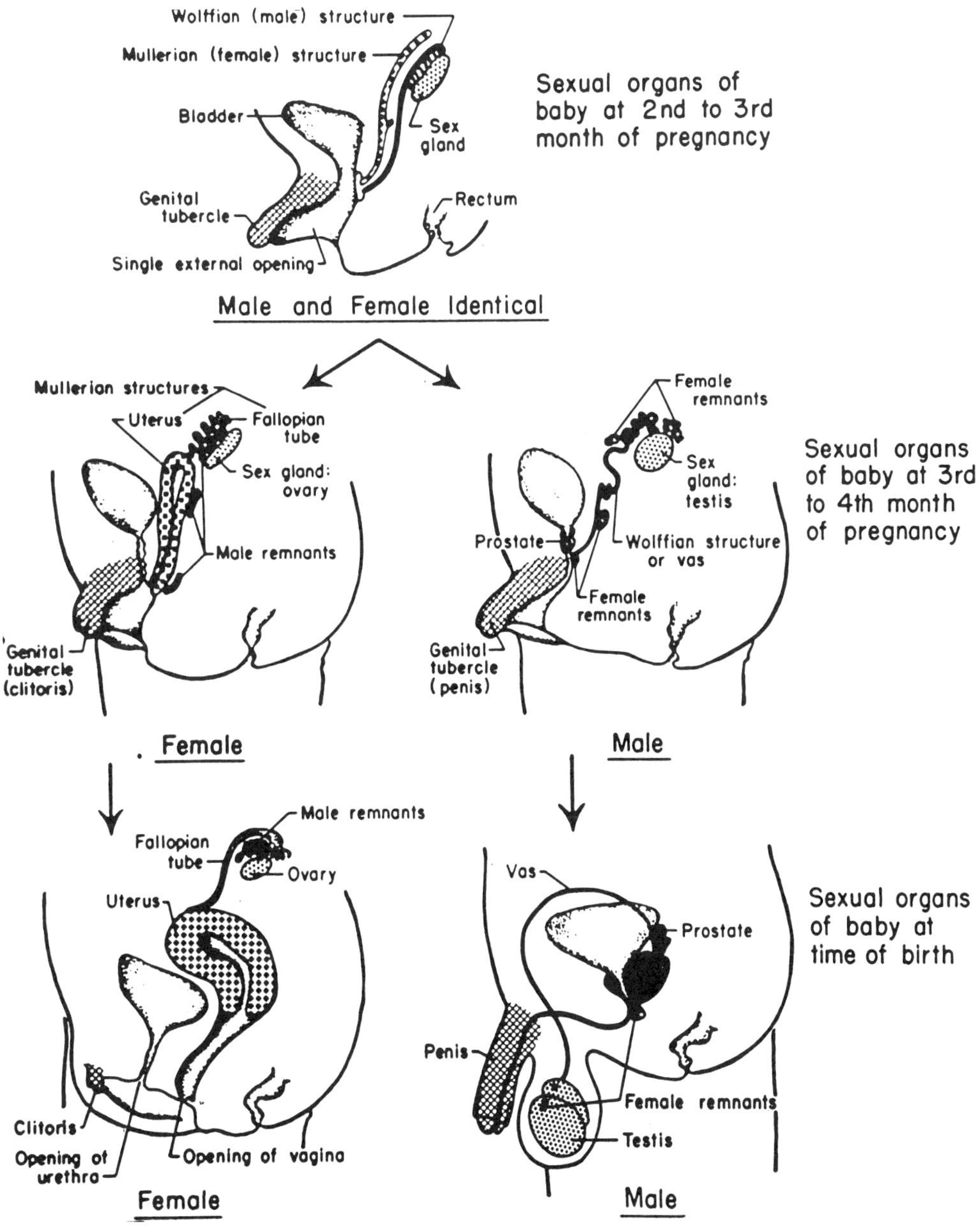

FIG. 2. Teaching diagram: differentiation of the internal genitalia.

AMBIGUOUS SEXUAL DIFFERENTIATION

There is no one single criterion of sex, but several, which can be demonstrated to both older patients and parents by opening the medical dictionary to the definition of sex. They can learn that there is the chromosomal criterion; the gonadal criterion; the external genital criterion, before and after surgery; the hormonal criterion, prenatal and postnatal; the gender identity/role (G-I/R) criterion; and the morphological, secondary sexual criterion. They learn that not even the chromosomal criterion is considered paramount: there are XY girls and women, XX boys and men, and many other chromosomal variants in both sexes, such as XXX, XXY, XYY, XO, as well as a multiplicity of mosaic combinations.

A patient with thc androgen-insensitivity (testicular-feminizing) syndrome learns that XY girls develop breasts, a female body morphology, and female romantic and erotic feelings. The cells of the body resist the influence of androgen even more than do the cells of an XX woman. In her case, the body's cells cannot be considered to be of the bona fide male type, insofar as they fail to function as authentic XY cells. One may refer to X and Y chromosomes as sometimes being sex-specific, but sometimes not, for their surface appearance under the microscope does not necessarily reveal what lies beyond. For easy understanding, one may explain that the Y is in a sense functioning as an X with two of its arms broken off. For the patient, it is very important that she not have a false concept of her cells as male, for her cells belong to her image of herself.

Rather than hearing of gonads that are named testes, XY girls may learn that there are gonads which have differentiated to appear, under the microscope, more like testicles than ovaries, but which are actually neither, as they are not able to do the complete work of one or the other. A girl can, despite the terminology of her medical record, change the word "testis" into "gonad" or "sex gland" in her own thinking and medical conversation. Similarly, the word "penis" can be changed into "genital," "sex organ," or "enlarged clitoris." The embryological diagrams of Figs. 1 and 2 are used to trace the differentiation of the sex organs from common roots. They are an invaluable aid to explanation.

HOMOSEXUALITY

For generations, folk wisdom has assumed that the morphology of the external genitalia of the neonate can be relied upon to prognosticate erotosexual development as male or female, as though male and female erotosexualism can be attributed to a preordained instinct. The term "gender role" was originally defined to designate the totalities of masculinity or femininity, which encompass not merely the copulatory roles of each but also their psychological, behavioral, social, and legal aspects: "The term 'gender role' is used to signify all those things that a person says or does to disclose himself or herself as having the status of boy or man, girl or woman, respectively. It includes but is not restricted to eroticism" (10). Later, the term "gender identity" was distinguished from gender role (11): "*Gender Identity:* the sameness, unity, and persistence of one's individuality as male or female (or ambivalent), in greater or lesser degree, especially as it is experienced in self-awareness and behavior. Gender identity is the private experience of gender role, and gender role is the public expression of gender identity."

Children with disorders of sexual differentiation typically develop the gender identity/role (G-I/R) of the sex to which they were originally assigned and in which they have been reared, and surgically and hormonally rehabilitated. Parents, however, inchoately equate homosexuality with anatomic ambiguity. They fear homosexuality as a moral disaster for which their child may be destined. Mostly their fears are unfounded. The majority of children who are born with birth defects of the sex organs, and who are brought up as girls, become romantically attracted and erotically bonded to someone not of the same sex of rearing as themselves. But there are some exceptions. In certain syndromes such as CVAH, especially in its salt-wasting (SW) form, there is an increased incidence of homosexual and bisexual orientation in adulthood (12), though not of transsexualism. It is not possible to predict ahead of time which individuals will manifest either outcome.

The issues of sexuoerotic orientation require special attention in follow-up counseling of the adolescent and young adult patient. If a homosexual or bisexual orientation does manifest itself, a patient may be relieved to learn that it is attributable to a syndrome and not to a personal moral responsibility or preference.

Mulaikal et al. (13) suggested that poorer surgical results in the salt-wasting than the simple virilizing (SV) form of CVAH lead to dissatisfaction with the vaginal introitus and avoidance of heterosexual intercourse. They mention but discount the second possibility that the higher level of androgen in SW than SV fetuses has a greater virilizing effect on the brain and hence the subsequent sexual orientation (12,14). Dittman et al. (15,24,25) hypothesize that the greater deficiency in cortisol levels in SW than in SV patients may account for a difference in fetal androgenization.

Parents assist in the development of sexological health in their daughter if they have an emancipated attitude to her sexual learning and sexual rehearsal play, as well as to her developmental need for self-knowledge concerning her clinical history and prognosis. Parents who live with the suspicion that their daughter, even though not truly a boy, is somehow a freak rather than a genuine girl may transmit their own doubt about her gender identity to their growing child.

SEX REASSIGNMENT

If a child has a well-differentiated gender identity (as is usually the case by age three), arbitrary imposition of a sex reassignment courts psychologic disaster. In some very perplexing cases, such a drastic step may be indicated, as when, for example, a child reared as a boy has a penoclitoris so small that it is functionally equivalent to a clitoris and is incapable of being surgically repaired. In most such cases, it is better to wait until the patient is older and can understand and personally endorse a program of reassignment and the surgical modification of morphological sexual characteristics.

Even at a later age, however, the pros and cons of a sex reassignment may present an extreme quandary—witness the case of two siblings concordant for 46,XY hermaphroditism. They were assigned as girls at birth, and hormonally and surgically feminized after the onset of pubertal virilization. The older of the two, after a 7-year period of sexuoerotic and vocational chaos, underwent a social self-reassignment at age 24, and lived thenceforth as a man. The younger remained satisfied with her assignment as a female and led a heterosexual love life (16).

The older sibling had been first brought to medical attention by her mother at age 5, when the mother became concerned at the appearance of the child's genitalia. The childhood diagnosis of androgen-insensitivity syndrome proved incorrect. At age 13, the girl was not feminizing, but virilizing. After a comprehensive, short-term evaluation, at age 14, she elected in favor of feminization, only to realize later the she did so under the influence of her parents' dictates, not her own. With the wisdom of hindsight, it becomes evident that the presurgical evaluation should have extended over a long-term period of the so-called Real-Life Test (17), during which the patient received both estrogen therapy and ongoing investigative psychological counseling. The insurmountable obstacle was that the patient had been referred from out-of-state with only very limited medical-assistance funding.

The difference between the two siblings in adult outcome of G-I/R may be attributable to a difference in degree of prenatal androgenization and masculinization of the bipotential fetal brain. Alternatively, differences in the postnatal social processes of gender identification and complementation may be implicated. Both siblings concurred that the older one had had a particularly close relationship with her father, which involved their sharing of "male-bonding" activities such as hunting and automobile repair. The younger sibling had been closer to her mother, and her genital anomaly remained unrecognized until age 13, so that she was not treated as sexually ambiguous while growing up.

REVEALING A HISTORY OF SEX REANNOUNCEMENT

Parents who are given nonstigmatizing and nontraumatizing explanations of the origin and nature of ambiguous genitalia are in a position to transmit the same, suitably age-graded, to their child. Beginning early in life, one mother told her daughter that she had been born with her female organs covered over with skin. Therefore, the doctors and nurses had thought at first that maybe she was a boy. Then they discovered that she was a girl. It was unnecessary for anyone in the family, or in the clinic, to be secretive with this girl about her clinical history. She was not vulnerable, for there was no secret knowledge to make her so. (For information concerning the subspecialty of counseling and neonatal sex assignment, see refs. 2, 18, and 19.)

RELEASING CONFIDENTIAL INFORMATION

In addition to having the proper vocabulary for self-knowledge of their conditions, patients (and their families) need to have counseling in the rehearsal of words and phrases that explain the condition to others without stigmatization and loss of self-respect. As already mentioned, the rehearsal may be colloquial, as in having a prepared answer for siblings or schoolmates asking about the reason for a hospital admission, or an excuse from participation in school sports. It may be medical, as in filling out a health record, or in giving a correct diagnosis to a school nurse or to a physician doing a physical examination for an employer, school, health insurer, or the military. Under some circumstances, the ability to give accurate information to a physician attending a medical or surgical emergency may be life-saving. In the case of the CVAH syndrome, for example, a patient in a salt-losing adrenocortical crisis may literally be able to save his/her own life by being able to insist on increased salt intake and increased cortisol dosage.

If the curiosity of people in the neighborhood, community, and family is satisfied at the outset, they are not only less likely to gossip, but also more likely to help in protecting the child's future integrity by not making insensitive comments about the birth history. Suitably rehearsed, and provided with diagrams of prenatal sexual differentiation (Figs. 1 and 2), some parents have found it possible to educate their friends and neighbors about the sexual anomaly of their child themselves (20). Others have enlisted the help of a community resource—a nurse, physician, teacher, or church leader.

Juvenile siblings need an explanation in terms gauged to their understanding of what is happening to their sister or brother, and why she or he is receiving so much attention. They are likely to need also to know that they too will not themselves become candidates for sexual surgery or reassignment arbitrarily. Release of information about the older patient to her relatives is subject to informed consent, not only in adulthood but also earlier, so as to prevent psychological stigmatization.

In cases where the syndrome is passed genetically, when adult siblings or other kin are preparing to have their own children, a patient may need to rehearse what information to release, especially if she was born 46,XY with testicles. Alternatively, she may bring her kinfolk to the clinic for professional counseling. The information may be of inestimable value should another baby of ambiguous sex be born within the kinship, by preventing an erroneous announcement of the new baby's sex that will later need to be changed. For the most part, the information given to her kinfolk will be the same as that given to the patient herself, including help with moral decisions surrounding birth control, prenatal testing and possible abortion of affected fetuses.

In later adolescence and early adulthood, a patient may transmit information about her condition to a lover, spouse, or intimate friend. She might well remember that information shared in confidence, especially in adolescence with even a very close friend, may backfire and become publicly disseminated. It is often wise for the patient to share information from the medical history too late rather then too soon with a lover. The stronger the pairbond between lovers, the more does love overcome obstacles. The words of one young man were, "I'm marrying you, not your uterus," when his girlfriend told him about the virtual certainty of sterility. Even if a relationship is short-lived, developmentally it is, in accordance with poetic wisdom, "better to have loved and lost, then never to have loved at all."

However, by releasing information about her condition, the patient may gain someone with whom to talk intimately about it. The benefit is personal. It is also practical in the case of a medical emergency in which the patient needs someone to speak for her. Otherwise, she may rely on registering with Medic-Alert and wearing an engraved tag that informs an examining physician where to locate the medical history.

INTERVIEWING: PARABLE AND SPORTSCASTER TECHNIQUES

In the clinic, the parable technique is a way of circumventing a communication impasse in a patient interview. The counselor narrates a story derived from the case of a person of the same age and the same diagnosis as the patient. The story may also be derived from a composite of cases. The topic of the story is presumed to be personally applicable to the listener who, even if afflicted with elective mutism, ascertains that the narrator is an informed and safe listener with whom to reopen the topic at a later date.

The great advantage of the parable technique is its nonjudgmentalism. It does not require the listener either to admit or deny the relevance of a given topic, but simply indicates that the topic is safe to talk about and be listened to, as need be. In using the parable technique, the agenda is fixed but the inquiry is open-ended and not stilted. Open-endedness allows the respondent free rein to define the topic in terms of what it means to him or her personally. An open-ended inquiry may be as straightforward as an announcement of the next topic on the standardized schedule of inquiry, for example, "Recreation: Tell me about your leisure time."

This straightforward approach is based on the premise that the topic is in the public domain and poses no threat of stigmatization, self-incrimination, or breach of confidentiality. It is when a topic is not in the public domain as far as the patient is concerned, but is taboo-ridden and potentially stigmatizing and self-incriminating, that the parable technique is especially valuable. In these instances, it may be necessary to specify, not assume, that a topic is indeed in the public domain, even though it is also partly in the private domain. For example: "The bombing of abortion clinics has been in the news recently." If the respondent indicates familiarity with this news, it is then feasible to inquire as to his or her ideas about it. Thereafter, it becomes feasible to lead into more personal references with respect to past history and future prospects regarding decisions about abortion. In this way, the inquiry becomes less and less open-ended, until eventually each particular topic may be closed with an interrogatory, employing forced-choice questions. Such questions are designed to get specific responses to specific details of chronology, prevalence, location, frequency, measurements, and so on (21).

The sportscaster technique, giving a detailed play-by-play account, is the one to use when the informant is recounting a personal experience or encounter. Otherwise, the account becomes too global and diffuse. Especially if the account involves an adversarial relationship, the raw data become lost in inferential attribution of motivation and intent, in which there is a hidden agenda, namely, to cast the interviewer in the role of juror and to win a judgment against the adversary. To establish maximum impartiality, one should interview the adversary, who also should adopt the sportscaster technique of reporting.

NONCOMPLIANCE

Two of life's great assignments come to the foreground of the agenda of teenage counseling: autonomy and sexuality. Sexuality includes falling in love, and autonomy includes preparation for economic independence. In the teenage years, responsibility for these aspects of human life is progressively transferred from the parents or guardian to the patient. Either the patient's discomfort with or her enthusiasm for this new responsibility may get in the way of clinical compliance. Thus, although problems of compliance may exist at any age, teenage noncompliance may be exceptionally trenchant.

Teenage noncompliance may also represent a so-called denial of illness—a magical sort of belief that not taking medication signifies being well. When the medication is a sex hormone, noncompliance may signify rejection of becoming sexually mature; or disavowal of genital desire and sexual sinfulness; or protest against one's hormonally induced status as male instead of female, or female instead of male.

Some adolescents have an aversion to being stigmatized as abnormal by being in the presence of a psychologist, psychiatrist, or sexologist. Some have an aversion to talking explicitly about themselves sexually. Some have an aversion to burdening their parents with a bill they know they have neither the cash nor the insurance to pay. Some, by personal decision or under the instruction of the parents, have kept their condition such a closed secret that scheduling clinic appointments becomes a major difficulty. Such patients often build a resistance to seeking help in the clinic, which stays with them in independent adult life.

If a patient fails to respond in interviews, the parable technique, which does not demand a response, provides assistance to the patient in coming to terms with her condition. Yet even this technique, except when used by phone or in writing, requires the presence of the listener in person. A teenager cannot be forced to consent to an appointment for any kind of treatment. Some do refuse, either on their own account or in complicity with one or both parents. There are many who need help but on whom compliance cannot be forced, or for whom it must be postponed until they are ready to accept the help that is available—possibly years later. The door must always be kept open.

UNIVERSAL EXIGENCIES

All teenagers can benefit from an open, sensitive exploration of what may be called the five universal exigencies of being human (22,23). These constitute a template that allows a place for all of the variables that may affect the development of an individual human life. They are as follows:

- Pairbondage, which pertains to parent-child and lover-lover bonding.
- Troopbondage, which pertains to becoming a member of a flock, herd, troop, or family.
- Abidance, which pertains to food, shelter, and clothing, and to abiding and being sustained in an ecologic niche.
- Ycleptance (a recycled Elizabethan term), which pertains to being named, nicknamed, classified, branded, labeled, or typecast.
- Foredoomance, which pertains to mortality and vulnerability to injury, defect, disease, and death, either one's own or someone else's.

These exigencies also provide a framework within which one can analyze the progress and trace the continuity of any biography in all of its components, clinical and nonclinical.

For individuals with a history of a birth defect of the sex organs, it goes without saying that, especially in adolescence and young adulthood, examining the pairbondage exigency has special clinical significance. To establish a sexual and erotic pairbond is to be confronted with questions and anxieties not only regarding one's fertility and parenthood, but also regarding the very adequacy of one's genitalia for copulation, and what to expect from sexual intercourse.

The other universal exigency that has particular significance for those counseling patients with a history of birth defect of the sex organs is ycleptance. Yclept is the past participle of the verb to clepe, meaning to name, call, or style. Human beings have named and typecast one another since recorded time. The terms range from the haphazard informality of nicknames to the systematic formality of biomedical nomenclature and diagnostic terms that prognosticate our futures and shape our lives. They affect our self-image, and all too often can be brutally stigmatizing. For example, it is brutally stigmatizing for a patient to see the diagnosis, hermaphroditism, or pseudohermaphroditism, in her medical chart, or on an insurance claim that is processed through the claims office of her place of work.

ACKNOWLEDGMENT

I thank Sara Radcliffe, M.A. for excellence in arranging, editing, and typing the manuscript.

REFERENCES

1. Mayle, P. *Where did I come from?* Secaucus, NJ: Lyle Stuart, 1973.
2. Money J. *Sex errors of the body: dilemmas, education and counseling.* Baltimore: Johns Hopkins Press, 1968.
3. Kaufman, J. *How we are born, how we grow, how our bodies work, . . . and how we learn.* New York: Golden Press, 1975.
4. Brown J, Lesser E, Mines S, Buryn E. *Two Births.* New York: Random House, 1972.
5. Johnson E. *Love and sex in plain language.* New York: Bantam Books, 1988.
6. Comfort A, Comfort J. *The facts of love.* New York: Crown Publishers, 1979.
7. Jackson P, Barrowclough IW, France JT, Phillips LI. A successful pregnancy following total hysterectomy. *Br J Obstet Gynaecol* 1980;87:353–5.
8. Frydman R, Parniex I, Fries N, Testart J, Raymond JP, Bouchard P. Pregnancy in a 46,XY patient. *Fertil Steril* 1986;50:813–4.
9. Sauer MV, Lobo RA, Paulson RJ. Successful twin pregnancy after embryo donation to a patient with XY gonadal dysgenesis. *Am J Obstet Gynecol* 1989;161:381–381.

10. Money J. Hermaphroditism, gender and precocity in hyperadrenocorticism: psychologic findings. *Bull Johns Hopkins Hosp* 1955;96:253–64.
11. Money J, Ehrhardt AA. *Man and woman, boy and girl: differentiation and dimorphism of gender identity from conception to maturity.* Baltimore: Johns Hopkins University Press, 1972.
12. Money J, Schwartz M, Lewis VG. Adult erotosexual status and fetal hormonal masculinization and demasculinization: 46,XX congenital virilizing adrenal hyperplasia and 46,XY androgen-insensitivity syndrome compared. *Psychoneuroendocrinology* 1984;9:405–14.
13. Mulaikal RM, Migeon CJ, Rock JA. Fertility rates in female patients with congenital adrenal hyperplasia due to 21-hydroxylase deficiency. *N Engl J Med* 1987;316:178–82.
14. Federman D. Psychosexual adjustment in congenital adrenal hyperplasia. *N Engl J Med* 1987;316:209–10.
15. Dittman et al. Gender-related behavior and attitudes in female salt-wasting and simple-virilizing patients. Hamburg, Germany: Psychosomatic Department, Children's Hospital, University of Hamburg (unpublished).
16. Money J, Lobato C. Matched pair of siblings concordant for 46,XY hermaphroditism with female sex assignment, and discordant for erotosexual outcome. *Psychiatry: Interpersonal and Biological Processes* 1988;51:65–79.
17. Money J, Ambinder R. Two-year, real-life diagnostic test: rehabilitation v. cure. In: Brady JP, Brodie HKH, eds. *Controversy in psychiatry.* Philadelphia: W.B. Saunders, 1978.
18. Money J. Psychologic considerations in patients with ambisexual development. *Semin Reprod Endocrinol* 1987;5:307–13.
19. Money J. Psychologic counseling: hermaphroditism. In: Gardner LI, ed., *Endocrine and genetic diseases of childhood and adolescence.* 2nd ed. Philadelphia: W.B. Saunders, 1975.
20. Money J, Potter R, Stoll CS. Sex reannouncement in hereditary sex deformity: psychology and sociology of habilitation. *Soc Sci Med* 1969;3:207–16.
21. Money J. Longitudinal studies in clinical psychoendocrinology: methodology. *J Dev Behav Pediatr* 1986;7:31–4.
22. Money J. *The psychologic study of man.* Springfield, IL: Charles C Thomas, 1957.
23. Money J. Five universal exigencies, indicatrons and sexological theory. *J Sex Marital Ther* 1984;10:229–38.
24. Dittman RW, Kappes MH, Kappes ME, Börger D, Meyer-Bahlburg HFL, Stegner H, Willig RH, Wallis H. Congenital adrenal hyperplasia II: gender-related behavior and attitudes in female salt-wasting and simple virilizing patients. *Psychoneuroendocrinology* 1991 (in press).
25. Dittmann RW, Kappes ME, Kappes MH. Sexual behavior in adolescent and adult females with congenital adrenal hyperplasia. *Psychoneuroendocrinology* 1992 (in press).

Pediatric and Adolescent Gynecology,
edited by S. E. Carpenter and J. A. Rock.
Raven Press, Ltd., New York © 1992.

8

Trauma to the Vulva and Vagina

David Dudgeon and Charles N. Paidas

Pediatric Surgery, Johns Hopkins Hospital, Baltimore, Maryland 21205

Accidental trauma to the pediatric female perineum is relatively common and occurs most often in the 4–12-year-old age group. Fortunately, most female pediatric external genitalia injuries are superficial and have a relatively low morbidity. However, because of differences in the anatomy of children and adults, relatively innocuous appearing pediatric perineal trauma can result in significant injury (1). These differences in a child's anatomy include the location of the bladder in an intraperitoneal position, the superficial location of the urogenital diaphragm, a relatively shorter distance between the perineal skin and the peritoneal cavity, and a lack of development of the perineal body with a very thin rectovaginal septum. Therefore, these differences make a penetrating wound or an otherwise insignificant laceration a potentially catastrophic injury characterized by major hemorrhage, an intraperitoneal urinary or intestinal viscus injury, or a possible rectovaginal fistula.

Vulva and vaginal trauma are the result of five mechanisms of injury. These mechanisms include "straddle," accidental penetration (including foreign bodies), sexual abuse, tearing, a tissue laceration due to sudden abduction of the lower extremities, or lacerations as a result of a pelvic fracture.

Straddle injuries account for approximately 75% of all genital injuries in young girls (1,2), however, a hymeneal injury resulting from this form of trauma is extremely rare (3). These injuries can occur as a result of straddling playground or gymnastic equipment, the center bar of a boy's bicycle, etc. The resultant trauma can appear as a small perineal ecchymotic area or a more significant hematoma with painful swelling over the labial area. The lesion is produced by the compression of the soft tissues of the vulva between the underlying bony structure and a striking object (4). The lesions may involve the mons, clitoris, urethra, and/or anterior portions of both the labia minora and labia majora. They rarely extend to the level of the vaginal opening (4). These characteristics aid in ruling out a possible intentional etiology. Hematuria, urethral trauma, and/or bloody staining of diapers or undergarments may be noted even with an apparently nonpainful periurethral lesion. Hematuria occurring as an acute symptom in the presence of a perineal lesion requires a voiding cystourethrogram to rule out bladder or urethral injury. Most blunt perineal injuries require only observation and the use of cold compresses during the acute phase (the first 6 hr) with warm sitz baths for symptomatic relief of tenderness during the recovery period. A significant urethral orifice hematoma with accompanying pain and poor urination can be treated with a urethral catheter for 2–3 days, prophylactic antibiotics, and analgesics. Subsequent strictures of the urethra or vaginal opening are rare without the presence of an associated deep laceration.

Accidental penetration is usually the result of falling on a relatively sharp object and occurs most frequently in the 2–4-year-old age group. Curiosity and self-manipulation with the use of foreign bodies such as pens and pencils are the usual culprits. These lesions can vary in appearance from a punctiform ecchymotic area to an obvious puncture wound with or without associated hemorrhage. The actual site of injury may not be obvious, and the child may present with hematuria, vaginal discharge, or bleeding. If microscopic hematuria is present, very careful urethral catheterization is indicated, since forceful insertion efforts against resistance can result in complete disruption of a partial urethral tear. Resistance to the attempted passage of a catheter is an indication for cessation of catheterization effort and a voiding cystourethrogram. Gross hematuria requires immediate cystourethrogram without a preceding catheterization effort. A perineal injury may also occur in the child who presents not with a visible puncture site or genitourinary symptoms but with rectal pain or bleeding. As previously noted, the differences in anatomy make an intraperitoneal injury in this situation much more likely in a child (1). Therefore, a thorough abdominal examination, including abdominal roentgenographs, anoscopy, and sigmoidoscopy must be performed.

An unusual form of accidental penetration is related to a high-pressure liquid injection into the vagina. A vaginal vault laceration due to this injury has been reported in a young girl held over a swimming pool fountain (5). The vaginal area most likely injured during the high pressure injection of liquids is the more distensible vault, and this injury requires a primary repair using an abdominal exposure.

Retained vaginal foreign bodies occur most frequently in the 2–4-year-old age group. Vaginal discharge, occasionally purulent but usually bloody, is the most common symptom. The patient may have genital pruritus, low grade fever, abdominal pain, or even symptoms of generalized sepsis (6). Regardless of the apparent paucity of accompanying symptoms or suggestive history, the presence of a persistent vaginal discharge in a toddler or young girl requires a vaginal examination under general anesthesia. Vaginal foreign bodies can vary from a firm wad of toilet paper to small hard objects such as buttons, coins, toys, etc. An undetected vaginal foreign body can result in peritonitis due to ascent of the purulent secretions up the fallopian tubes (6). Because of their insidious course and, thus, late diagnosis, even a spherical foreign body may be embedded in the vaginal wall and be very difficult to extirpate. Therefore, a careful examination is required after removing the foreign body to detect any residual defect in the vaginal wall. If the thin posterior rectovaginal septum has been violated, then a temporary colostomy with subsequent delayed repair of these inflamed delicate vaginal/rectal tissues is required. Antibiotic therapy should be instituted prior to removal of any suspected long standing vaginal foreign body.

The recognition of sexual abuse as the source of genital or perineal trauma, except in the case of an unstable physiologic status, demands a modified diagnostic and therapeutic approach, both to meet the emotional needs of the patient as well as the legal requirements for a successful future prosecution of the perpetrator. This difficult diagnostic and therapeutic problem is discussed in detail in the chapter by Wissow. Unfortunately, sexual abuse is common, with an incidence of approximately

90% in all pediatric female perineal injuries reported in one series (3).

Clitoral strangulation or ischemia is a rare traumatic lesion reported in infants usually as the result of a hair, from a caretaker, accidentally wrapped circumferentially about the base of the organ (1). This is a difficult diagnosis, resulting in symptoms of irritability in association with engorgement and/or cellulitis of the area. Clinical outcome, including possible auto amputation, depends on the degree of ischemia and further emphasizes the need for an early complete perineal examination in all females, regardless of age, who present with symptoms of genital irritation or trauma.

Vaginal orifice lacerations can also occur while water skiing as a result of a sudden forceful abduction of the legs. The lesion can also be produced by the same mechanism during gymnastic exercises or as a result of major motor vehicular trauma. Pain and a bloody vaginal discharge are the most prominent findings. This accidental injury, which can frequently extend posteriorly into the vaginal fornix, in a manner very similar to the lesion produced by sexual abuse, can usually be differentiated from forced penetration by the presence or absence of associated injuries and/or a suspicious patient history. The extent of these lesions should also be determined by a complete examination under general anesthesia since severe complications can result due to an undetected or underestimated injury with incomplete repair. This is a more significant lesion if involvement of the rectovaginal septum and/or extension of the laceration into the peritoneal cavity is present. Thus, appropriate therapy includes antibiotics, primary surgical repair, and a temporary colostomy if the rectum is involved.

Genitourinary injuries are common with complex pelvic fractures; however, vaginal lacerations are less common and usually only reported in adult females. Nevertheless, high-speed, high-impact vehicular injuries with massive pelvic fractures resulting in bony spicules or hip joint disruption can produce severe vaginal or combined urogenital lacerations (7,8). These lesions occur in the severely injured patient and must not be overlooked as a source of significant intraabdominal symptoms or signs, including severe hemorrhage.

MANAGEMENT PRINCIPLES

Initial resuscitation in any pediatric trauma should begin with the primary survey: stabilization of airway, breathing, circulation, neurological status, and gross bleeding. A secondary survey should complete our assessment in a head-to-toe fashion including a complete perineal examination. Performance of an initial resuscitation and assessment must be documented in writing (Fig. 1).

If the patient is neurologically and hemodynamically stable, sedation should always be used to evaluate the perineum. First, attempt to assess the origin of any bleeding site. This can be done by gently retracting the labia and looking for hematomas, gross blood, feces, etc. Next, a bimanual exam should be performed. In the prepubital female, this can be a rectal/abdominal exam. Minor nonexpanding hematomas require only supportive measures as noted. Expanding hematomas of the vulva must be opened and thus require general anesthesia for ligation of bleeding points under direct vision.

Microscopic hematuria in association with vaginal or vulva trauma should be evaluated with a computed tomography (CT) scan. Gross hematuria requires a voiding cystourethrogram and a possible CT scan as noted.

The complete perineal examination under anesthesia for a young female includes; a vaginal inspection utilizing appropriate size instruments such as a small nasal speculum for visualization in an infant or young

History and Physical
Mechanism and Time of Injury
Labs (Hematocrit, Urinalysis)
- Microscopic Hematuria - CT Scan
- Gross Hematuria - Voiding Cystourethrogram

↓

Vaginal Bleeding
Bimanual Assessment and/or Visual Assessment with Vaginal Instrumentation Under Sedation or General Anesthesia

- Vulva
  - Laceration — Repair
  - Hematoma
    - Expanding — Open, Ligate vessels
    - Nonexpanding — Observation
- Introitus
  - Laceration (Superficial) — Transvaginal Closure
  - " (Deep, perineum/rectovaginal septum) — Preoperative Antibiotics, Proximal Diverting Colostomy, Presacral Drainage, Washout of Defunctionalized Bowel, Closure Laceration
- Urethra
  - Hematoma — Urethral Catheter
  - Disruption — Suprapubic cystostomy, primary repair

FIG. 1. Approach to the patient with trauma to the vagina and/or vulva.

girl, a cystoscopic exam for suspected bladder perforation, and an anorectoscopic exam for suspected anorectal trauma. A significant penetrating wound with involvement of intraperitoneal organs requires, as noted, an exploratory laparotomy (9). Enteric injury with gross contamination and/or generalized peritonitis will require temporary intestinal bypass stomas. Repair of a bladder perforation requires either a suprapubic cystostomy or urethral catheter, depending on the location of the bladder injury. Significant urethral injuries determined by voiding cystourethrogram, should be primarily repaired and a urethral and/or suprapubic catheter placed for post operative decompression. Less severe urethral injuries, ie, no disruption, can be treated by a urethral catheter as both a stent and decompressing mechanism. Superficial vaginal lacerations may be primarily closed. Deep vaginal and/or rectal perforations due to severe trauma should be managed with preoperative antibiotics, proximal diverting colostomy, presacral drainage, washout of the defunctionalized bowel, and closure of the laceration. Postoperative complications include abscess, osteomyelitis, urethral strictures, and vaginal-rectal fistulae (10).

In summary, a high index of suspicion is necessary when evaluating trauma to the vulva and vagina in the pediatric age group. Straddle injuries, accidental penetration, sexual abuse, tearing from forced abduction, and lacerations due to pelvic fractures are the five most common mechanisms. Differences in the child's anatomy make more significant injury a distinct possibility. Management should begin with a primary and secondary survey. A decision should then be made about sedation or usually general anesthesia to evaluate the perineum. Finally, the complete evaluation should include an assessment of both the urethra and rectum, as well as the vagina.

REFERENCES

1. Sterioff S Jr, Izant RJ, Persky L. Perineal injuries in children. *J Trauma* 1969;9:56.
2. Ezell WW, Smith EI. Mechanical traumatic injury to the genitalia in children. *J Urol* 1969; 102:788.
3. Herman-Giddens ME, Frothingham TE. Prepubertal female genitalia: examination for evidence of sexual abuse. *Pediatrics* 1987;80:203.
4. West R, Davies A, Fenton T. Accidental vulval injuries in childhood. *Br Med J* 1989;298:1002.
5. Holloway GA. Vaginal vault tear following a high pressure douche. *S Afr Med J* 1987;72:886.
6. Pierce EH. Retained vaginal tampon: a unique cause of acute abdomen. *S Med J* 1973;66:640.
7. Doman AN, Hoekstra DV. Pelvic fracture associated with severe intra-abdominal gynecologic injury. *J Trauma* 1988;28:118.
8. Burrell JC, Lipinski JK. Anteromedial (perineal) dislocation of the hip: a case report. *Can J Surg* 1989;32:77.
9. Reinberg O, Uazbeck S. Major perineal trauma in children. *J Pediatr Surg* 1989;24:982.
10. Maull KI, Sachatello CR, Ernst CB. Deep perineal laceration—an injury frequently associated with open pelvic fractures: a need for aggressive surgical management. *J Trauma* 1977;17:685.

Pediatric and Adolescent Gynecology,
edited by S. E. Carpenter and J. A. Rock.
Raven Press, Ltd., New York © 1992.

9

Vulvar Disease in the Prepubertal Child

J. Donald Woodruff

Departments of Gynecologic Pathology, and Gynecology and Obstetrics, Johns Hopkins University School of Medicine, Baltimore, Maryland, 21205

The vulva in infancy and childhood is not only the area where genetic anomalies are recognized most commonly but also frequently the site of congenital and acquired diseases and tumors.

SEXUALLY TRANSMITTED DISEASES

Sexually transmitted diseases regrettably are not uncommon on the external genitalia of the child and may result from sexual molestation or maternal transmission (1).

Gonococcus

The gonococcus does not directly infect the vulva, as it does not readily affect areas of the body covered by stratified squamous epithelium. However, it does infect the thin premenarchal vaginal epithelium, and the vaginal discharge often produces a secondary irritation of the vulvar skin. Since the thin premenarchal vagina is easily infected, one of the approaches to treatment of gonococcal vaginitis in the past had been to use intravaginal estrogen suppositories. The latter produced thickening of the vaginal epithelium, and the gonococcal infection was eliminated along with the resultant dermatitis. The clinical recognition of the validity of this therapeutic maneuver is demonstrated by the spontaneous elimination of gonorrhea vaginitis at the menarche. Today, the infection is treated by antibiotics, although intravaginal estrogen was very effective and did not produce systemic reaction. The local irritation on the vulva is treated by soothing lotions or cool sitz baths with Domeboro powders. The latter not only alleviates much of the irritation but reduces any swelling that may result

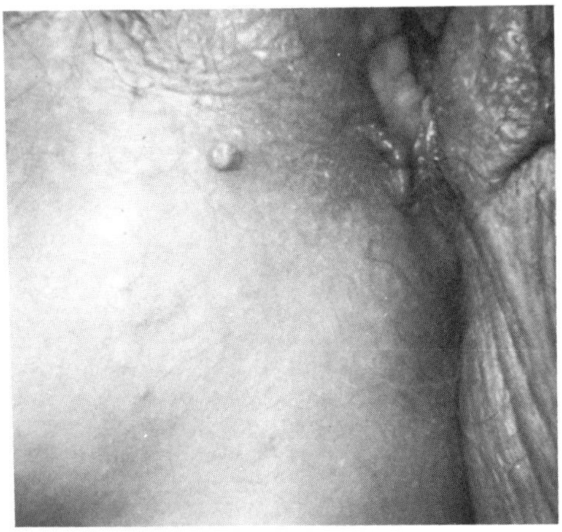

FIG. 1. Molluscum contagiosum in a 10-year-old girl—note the umbilication.

from the infection. The urethra may be irritated by such infections, and the patient may complain of discomfort on voiding. Again, local applications are usually effective. Although the gonococcus may infect the urethral meatus, it rarely produces cystitis.

Molluscum Contagiosum

Molluscum contagiosum similarly affects the vulva and produces the classic slightly elevated umbilicated nodules on the skin (Fig. 1) (2,3). These lesions are usually asymptomatic and recognized by mother or child. The diagnosis can be suspected but is only proven by biopsy. If necessary, the latter can be accomplished simply with local anesthesia and gentle pressure with the small Keys punch. Molluscum is a sexually transmitted disease, and the physician must be alert to the possible coexistence of other sexually transmitted diseases. Molluscum can be treated by curettage of the central core of each lesion under local anesthesia. However, spontaneous remission occurs within a few months. The child must be warned against scratching the lesions as this will promote their spread.

Syphilis

Syphilitic lesions on the vulva of the child are grossly confusing. Whereas the classic chancre is usually identifiable on the vulva of the adult as the asymptomatic ulcer with "rolled edges," such is not the case for the child. The lesions are frequently very superficial ulcerations, often with striking edema (Fig. 2). Again, they are classically asymptomatic, although irritative. Lymphadenitis is usually present, as in the adult, but not symptomatic. The treatment here again is local application for swelling and discomfort, and the common routine of penicillin for the treatment of the treponema infection. In the child, erythromycin may be substituted for penicillin.

The great majority of these lesions are

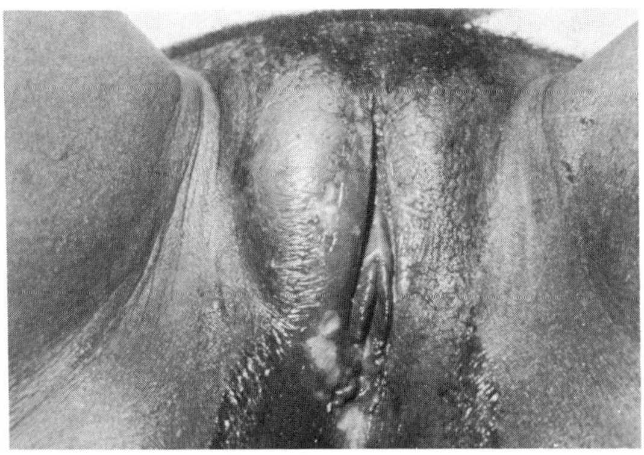

FIG. 2. Syphilis in a 14-year-old girl. Vulva and anal orifice. Multiple ulceration with marked edema.

sexually transmitted to the child by contact with the aggressive adult. Other evidence of trauma must be investigated since attempted intercourse may result in lacerations of the perineum and/or anal orifice. The psychologic impact of such sexually transmitted diseases is often of major import. Consequently, the gynecologist, the pediatrician, or the generalist should enlist the aid of the psychologist. The child's fears must be alleviated in order that in later life she will not be traumatized to any degree.

As in all sexually transmitted diseases, if one is found others must be looked for and treated.

Congenital syphilis, transmitted to the child through the infected mother, is more serious since there may not be gross demonstrable manifestations of the disease. Blood studies are necessary in order to treat the condition before it produces systemic results.

Herpes

Vulvar herpes simplex may be transmitted to the newborn through the vaginal canal, however, most adult females with herpes have been carefully followed during pregnancy because of the serious results of transmission to the fetus at the time of birth (4,5). Nevertheless, there is always this possibility that the lesions were not demonstrated during pregnancy (6). The appearance of the herpetic lesions during the first week of life suggests the possibility of maternal transmission (7–9). Conversely, herpes seen during the early years of life is a disease transmitted by sexual contact. It is of major importance to investigate the source and alleviate the child's fears. The vesicles may be small and thus may go unrecognized; nevertheless, they are usually painful. Careful inspection of the area is of major importance if the child complains of pain. The primary treatment is local applications to alleviate the discomfort. Zovirax, an antiherpetic preparation, has been used locally but does not relieve the pain. Acyclovir 200 mg four to five times a day is the program of choice for the adult; such doses have been used in the child, and reports do not relate adverse effects at the age of 3 years and older (10). In the first year of life, 30 mg of Acyclovir per kilogram of body weight every 8 hr has been proposed.

The diagnosis may be confirmed by immunofluorescence or the tzank reaction. The viral inclusions have been demonstrated on the smear; nevertheless, the gross appearance and the symptomatology are rather classic, and may provide the diagnosis relatively easily (Fig. 3). Recurrences may develop as in the adult and Acyclovir may be repeated as indicated. As a sexually transmitted disease, the origin must be identified if possible. Cultures of the mother's vagina may determine the source. Otherwise, sexual molestation must be considered and the patient studied for other sexually transmitted diseases.

As far as the author knows, herpes zoster has not been reported in the child. Whereas the herpes simplex infection is often tran-

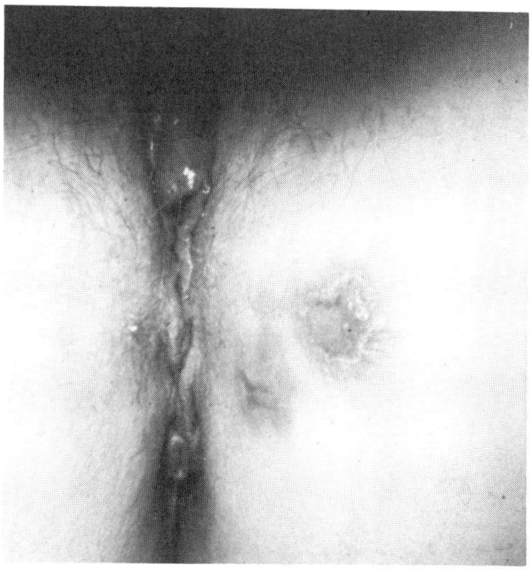

FIG. 3. Healing herpes genitalis in a prepubertal child.

sient, the zoster is painful and may last for as long as 3–4 months. Local applications are necessary, particularly in the latter situation. Classically, even in the adult, zoster is seen elsewhere on the body than the perineum, most frequently around the girdle area.

Condylomata Acuminata

Condylomata acuminata are common tumors (Figs. 4 and 5). They may be transmitted from the mother at birth or the result of molestation (11–13). Since the incubation period for condylomata is much longer than that for herpes, sometimes as long as 3–6 months, the lesions acquired during delivery may not appear until later in life. They may be present not only on the vulva but in the perianal area. It is difficult to evaluate the vagina in such situations due to the introitus, but if there is any discharge or bleeding, an evaluation should be performed. Condylomata acuminata in the child is best treated by excision (14). Specimens should be sent to the laboratory for histologic study and identification of the specific HPV if such is possible. Approximately 60 types are now identified. The common therapeutic techniques used in the adult such as the use of trichloro or bichloroacetic acid is too painful to employ in the child. The simplest treatment is to use general anesthetic and remove the lesions with a cautery tip. The fine wire is more acceptable in these situations. Laser therapy for such lesions is also useful. The entire area must be studied since "warts" may be found in the vagina, the urethra, or the perianal area. As with all such infections, the patient must be studied for other sexually transmitted diseases.

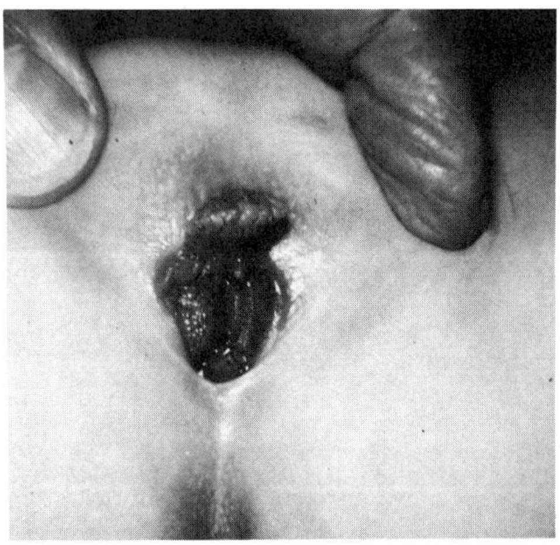

FIG. 4. Condyloma at vaginal outlet in a prepubertal child.

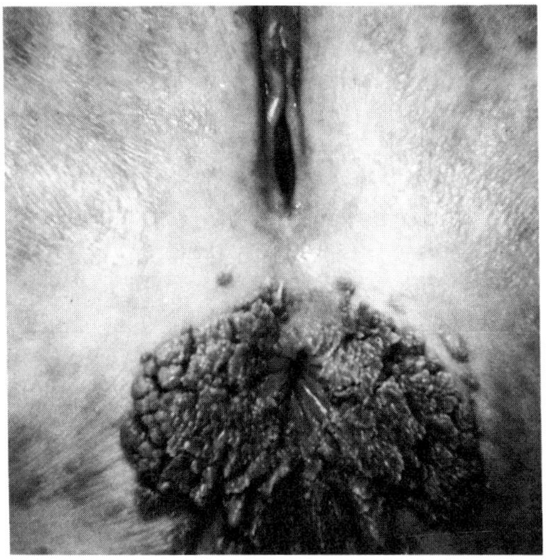

FIG. 5. Condylomata acuminata at the anal orifice in a 5-year-old girl.

Chlamydial infection in children has been reported but must be a rarity (15–17). If such truly occurs, it is a vaginal rather than a vulvar problem and is treated by estrogen suppositories or antibiotics.

BENIGN TUMORS OF THE VULVA IN CHILDHOOD

Tumors arising in the vulva during the prepubertal years are uncommon. The relatively common condylomata acuminata have been discussed under sexually transmitted diseases. Other tumors include the following.

Vascular Abnormalities

Hemangioma

Congenital hemangioma, although rare, must be recognized and treated appropriately (18). These lesions can be very extensive and cause unique concern in the family (Fig. 6). Every effort should be made to alleviate the fears of the patient and family that these lesions will distort the vulva permanently and be a deterrent to a normal adult life. The treatment for such lesions is careful neglect unless bleeding occurs. If the latter happens, local control is sufficient and accomplished by pressure, silver nitrate, or, as a last resort, cautery. In general, these lesions regress at puberty and rarely leave any distortion of the normal architecture.

Whereas the diffuse congenital hemangioma is rarely a problem unless trauma results in rupture of a vessel or vessels, the larger varices may present a major problem. These lesions vary from the large vascular dilatations (Fig. 7) that may develop in the prepuce to the small hemangioma commonly adjacent to the clitoris (Fig. 8). Again, both of these lesions should be treated expectantly unless bleeding does occur. If the lesion is extremely large and uncomfortable, cool compresses with Domeboro solution are often an adequate

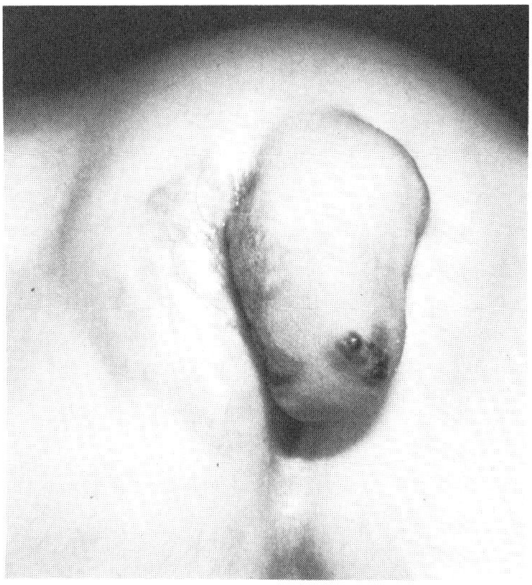

FIG. 7. Congenital hemangioma in a 3-year-old girl.

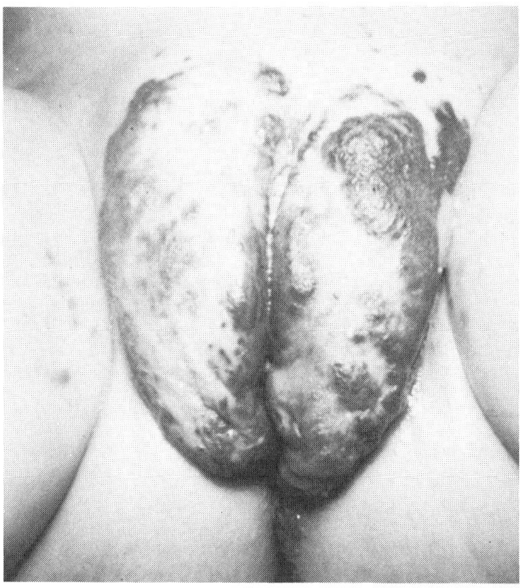

FIG. 6. Congenital hemangioma at age 3 years (resolved spontaneously at menarche).

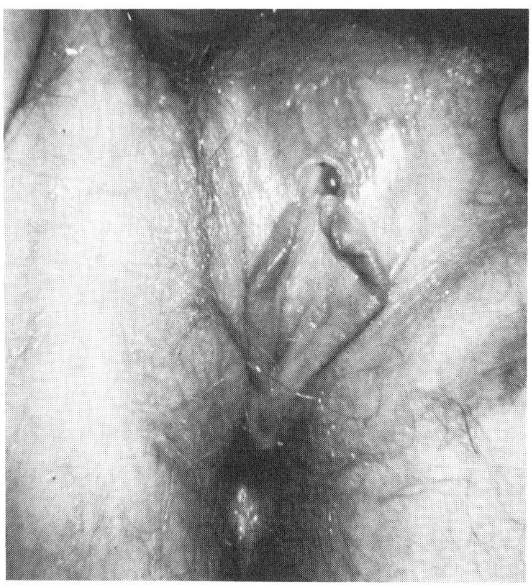

FIG. 8. Small periclitoral hemangioma in a 5-year-old girl.

answer to the associated edema. Since there is no danger of malignancy with such lesions, surgery should be avoided. If the varices occur unilaterally and bleeding becomes a problem, ligation of the vessels in the inguinal canal may be the solution to the problem. Nevertheless, it should be recognized that any vascularity below the clitoris probably involves the pudendal vessels. Most of the vascular supply to the upper external genital canal in the female comes from the pampiniform plexus in the inguinal canal, whereas that below the level of the clitoris in the female is supplied by the pudendal vessels.

On rare occasion, these major dilatations may result in discomfort to the patient. Under these circumstances, not only ligation of the vessel but plastic procedures may be considered for the prepuce. Nevertheless, great care should be taken since the clitoris may be injured and cause major problems in the future. In conclusion, all vascular dilatations in the vulva during childhood should be treated expectantly unless bleeding occurs.

Cystic Tumors

Cysts are uncommon in the prepubertal child. The common inclusion (previously sebaceous) cyst is rare since secretion of the sebaceous gland along the hair shaft is not occluded as the hair rarely appears until puberty. Similarly, the apocrine gland is inactive, as the secretion is related to cyclic ovarian hormone activity, which obviously does not occur until ovarian activity. On rare occasions, the vestibular glands secrete and a cyst may develop, as noted in Fig. 9 (19–21). Therapy is unnecessary unless discomfort or infection develops. Simple incision is sufficient if the child evidences discomfort. The insertion of a Word catheter is not appropriate at this stage of life.

Again, hydrocele is rarely recognized prepubertally since inguinal lesions are un-

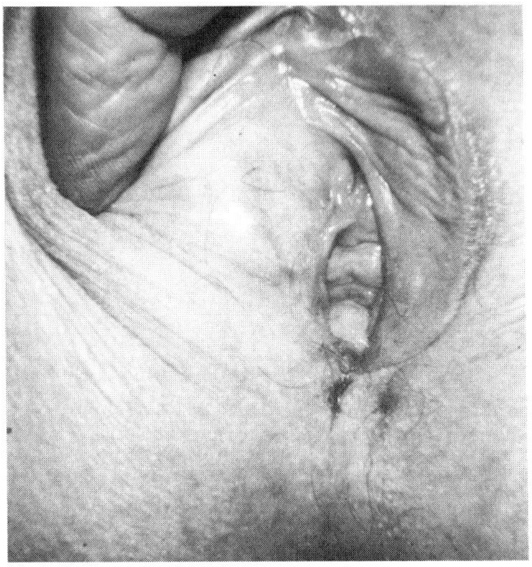

FIG. 9. Cyst of minor vestibular gland.

commonly symptomatic in the early years and fluid accumulation in the abdomen is a rarity. Nevertheless, a unilateral bulging in the vulva should make the physician aware of the possibility that such is related to a defect in the inguinal canal.

Tumors other than the hemangioma and condyloma are extremely rare in the vulva in childhood.

TRAUMATIC LESIONS

Hematomas

Hematomas develop usually in the early second decade of life and are due to injuries such as falling astride the bars of a bicycle (22,23). Such hematomas may reach magnificent proportion, and if bleeding is still active when the patient is seen in the emergency room, it may be necessary to consider ligating the offending vessel (Fig. 10). Such hematomas may extend in the fascial planes up into the lower abdomen and become large enough to occlude the urethra. If active bleeding persists, a small incision into the hematoma to evacuate most of the clot will usually identify the source of the

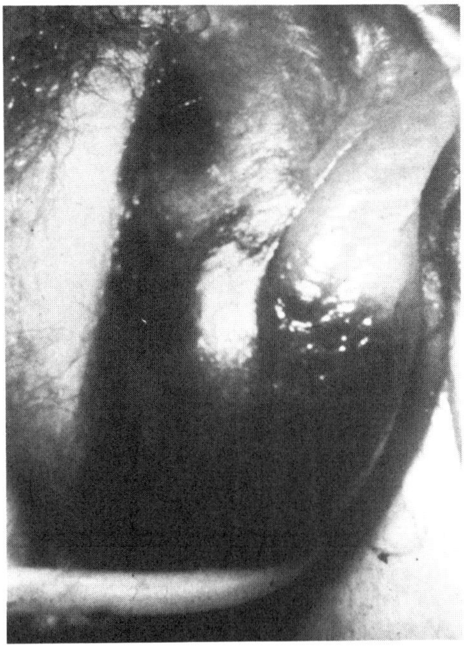

FIG. 10. Traumatic hematoma in a 12-year-old child following fall astride bicycle bar.

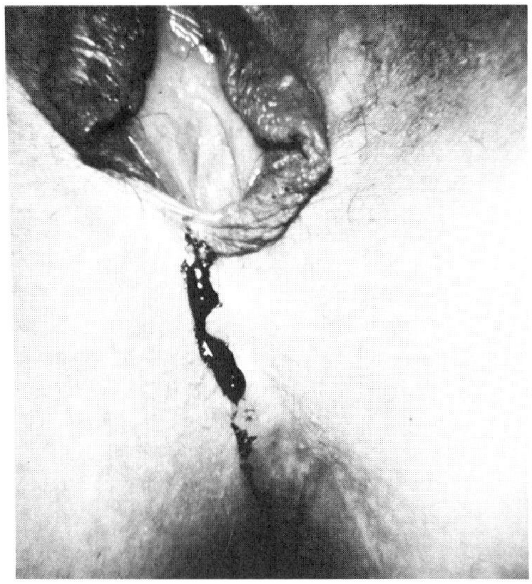

FIG. 11. Traumatic laceration at fourchette.

bleeding. Catheterization may be necessary if the hematoma continues to progress in spite of local application. Local application again is, more wisely, cool packs with Domeboro.

Posttraumatic Bleeding

Obviously, sexual molestation may produce lacerations, and these may extend very deeply into the adjacent tissue, even to the rectum (Fig. 11) (24,25). Conversely, they may be minor and necessitate only local application to control the bleeding. In the case of major lacerations, surgery should be instituted immediately to repair lacerations particularly into the rectum. Although the tissues are delicate and the area is difficult to deal with because of the smallness of the tissues, immediate repair is important.

Obviously, in these situations, the evidence of sexual molestation should be of primary concern. Attempt at coitus produces major psychologic reactions in the child. In such situations the vagina must be investigated for the presence of semen, and the psychologist should be involved in the discussion of such trauma. Although the local physical situation may be simple, the overall impact to the child may be severe.

INFLAMMATORY PROCESSES

Sexually transmitted diseases have been discussed above. Other irritations may be seen in the young child who is irritated from diapers or other close-fitting materials (26–28). The so-called diaper rash is often very irritating, producing trauma from the fingernail during scratching. Under these circumstances, a 1% hydrocortisone preparation may be applied to alleviate the itching. If the swelling is appreciable, it is wise to employ cool Domeboro compresses or have the child sit in a tub with just the buttocks and genitalia covered so that the preparation will be effective in reducing the edema. Obviously, every effort should be made to avoid the development of such irritations

(Fig. 12). Nevertheless, such do occur and appropriate local therapy is indicated, such as a cornstarch and zinc oxide mixture. Loose-fitting white cotton undergarments should be worn whenever possible. Every effort should be made to prevent the entrance of talc into the vagina as long-term irritations may result since it is a foreign body.

Dermatitis

Dermatitis may be produced by vaginal infections, and these should always be considered in the patient with persistent irritation (29). In Fig. 13, the dermatitis was related to vaginitis produced by a foreign body. Such discharge may be bloody due to the irritation of the thin vaginal epithelium. Although such problems are uncommon, it should be investigated in a persistent situation (30).

The patient with lichen sclerosus is susceptible to such irritations due to the thin parchment like skin. Under such circumstances, it has been suggested that estrogen creams be used locally. There are no estrogen receptors in the vulva, and vaginal estrogen will cause systemic effects. Thus, other agents are more appropriate. Progesterone may be used. It is preferable to use a cream base that will be absorbed rather than a greasy ointment, which often produces additional irritation. The trauma of the chronic dermatitis and local application may result in fissuring and occasional bleeding. These problems should be alleviated again by soothing lotions and cool Domeboro sitz baths.

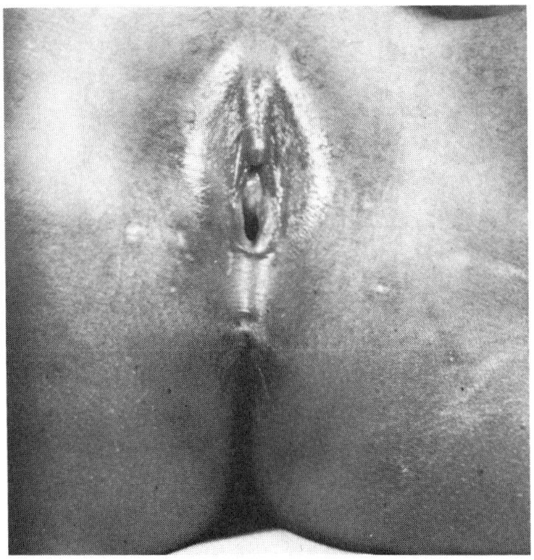

FIG. 13. Dermatitis due to a foreign body in vagina and resultant discharge.

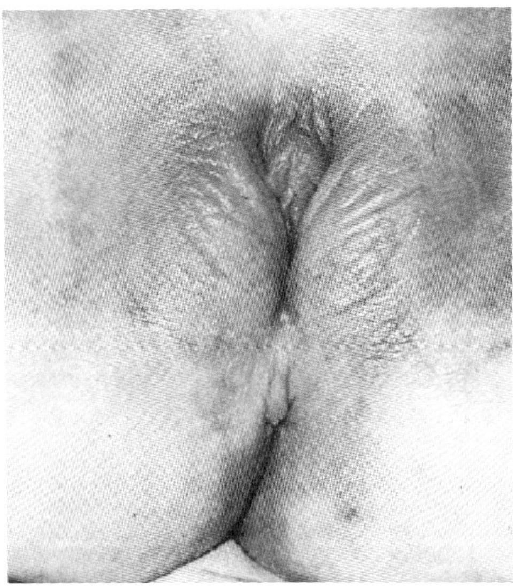

FIG. 12. Dermatitis with edema, possibly "diaper rash."

It should be appreciated that such traumas are more a problem in the prepubertal girl since she is unable to respond as well to the local irritation and thus may resort to manipulation. This only magnifies the problem since it concentrates the child on the local area. Thus, dermatitis in the child can be a major problem, and every effort should be made to identify the cause and eliminate the irritant.

Sebaceous dermatitis, common on many areas of the body, is also found on the vulva largely in the adult and relates to the greasy secretion of the sebaceous glands. Since activity of these glands is minimal in the prepubertal child, such reactions are generally uncommon, although they may be confused with the simple contact dermatitis or "diaper rash," and should be treated as such.

Other Childhood Diseases

Other childhood diseases have been reported in the literature. Chicken pox has produced rather dramatic reactions in the vagina and adjacent vulva (Fig. 14) (31). Antibiotic cream may be applied to the vulva to avoid superinfection. Generally, vulva chicken pox is associated with evidence of systemic disease. Many years ago J. Whitridge Williams reported on diphtheria of the vulva (32). In this discussion, the author noted that the "diphtheritic membrane" was not a justifiable reason to feel that the infection was true diphtheria. Specific cases of diphtheria of the vulva have not been reported in recent years to my knowledge. Nevertheless, any infectious process may affect the vulva and/or the adjacent vagina. Reaction to vaccinia has been noted and is demonstrated in Figs. 15 & 16 (33,34). This specific instance apparently was a reaction to vaccination, not an infection.

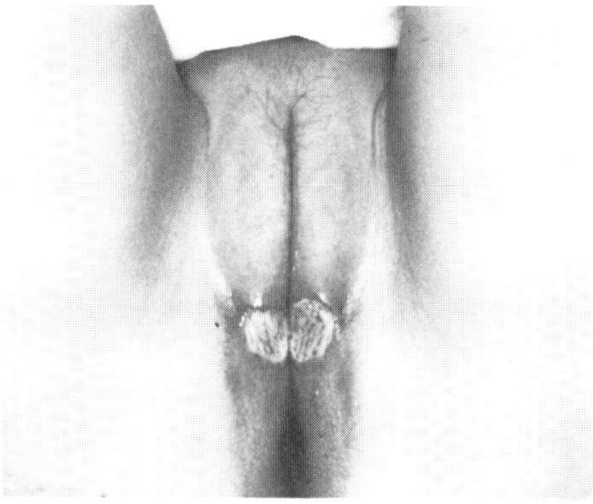

FIG. 15. Postvaccination ulcerations on vulva in an 8-year-old girl.

Candidiasis

Candidiasis is said to be a common vulvar disease in children. In the adult, it is also common but generally not a vulvar disease per se but rather a vulvovaginal problem, and treatment is directed at the vaginitis, the vulvar symptoms being secondary. Conversely, in the child, the vulva is said to be the primary site of infection. Nevertheless, whether primary or secondary, the treatment should be directed at the symptom, the pruritus, with 1–2% hydrocortisone cream as well as a topical antifun-

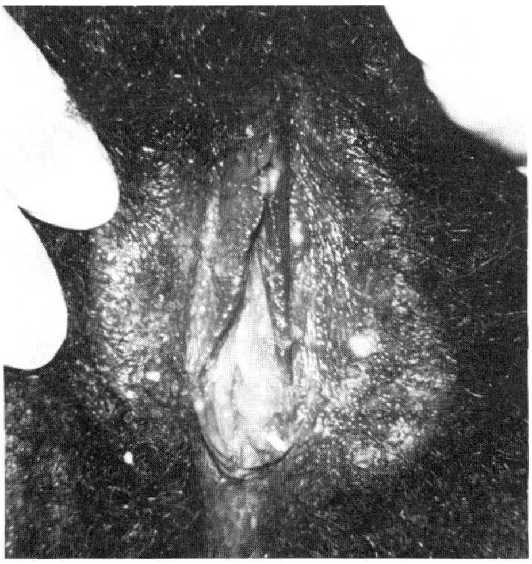

FIG. 14. Chicken pox on vulva.

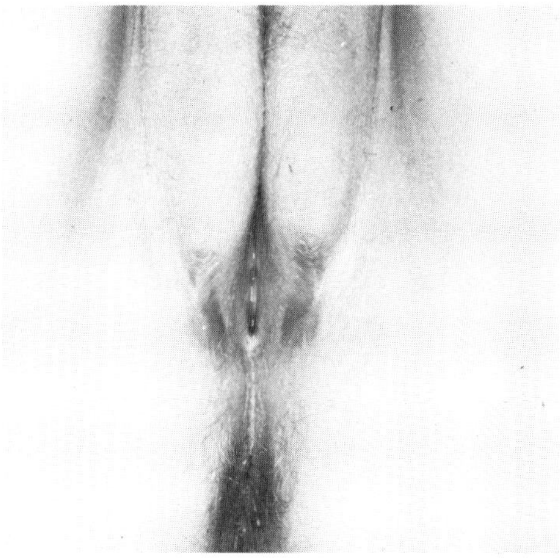

FIG. 16. Healing lesions postvaccination.

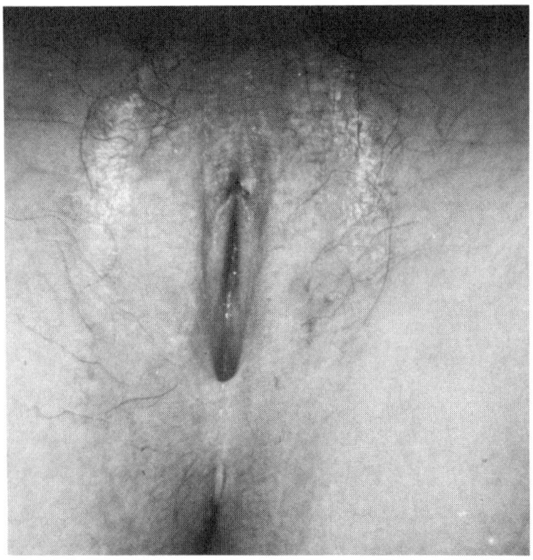

FIG. 17. Chronic eczematoid dermatitis.

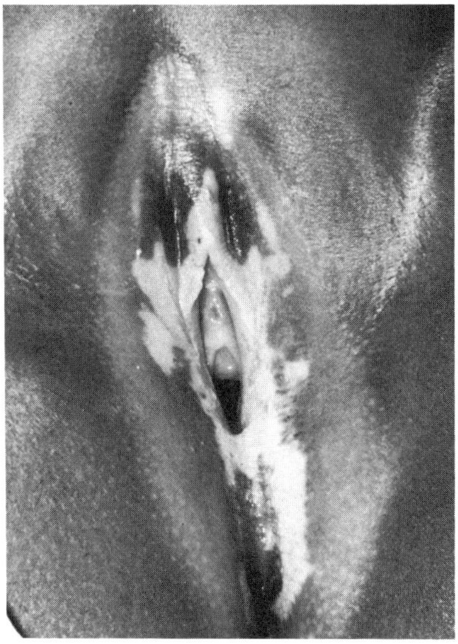

FIG. 18. Vitiligo in an 8-year-old girl.

gal agent. If there is a vaginal discharge, the cause should be identified and treated.

Nonspecific Eczema

Nonspecific eczema is usually seen in the context of local irritation (Fig. 17). As noted above, this may be related to poor hygiene commonly associated with a moist urine-soaked diaper approximating the tender skin of the perineal area. Otherwise, eczema may be a reaction to any application to the area. Various medications may produce this type of reaction. Thus, in all cases where there is an eczematoid reaction in the perineum, local irritants should be considered as the most common cause of the condition. Systemic reactions are rare.

WHITE LESIONS

White lesions may be related to congenital lack of pigment or to chronic irritative phenomenon.

Vitiligo (Fig. 18) has classically been described as a congenital lack of pigmentation. Although this is undoubtedly correct, it is interesting that classically there is no history of familial predisposition to the development of such "white patches."

Although the lesions are not uncommonly seen in any area of the body, rarely does it elicit any concern except on the vulva. Since the vulva is commonly irritated by a variety of agents, the white patches may be considered evidence of trauma or irritation. Conversely, rarely are any symptoms associated with vitiligo. The patient and mother must be made aware that this is of no clinical concern and does not relate to the development of any serious problems. Furthermore, there is no specific treatment for this problem. The use of irritants to promote the development of pigment have been totally unsuccessful and are to be condemned since they often produce additional irritation.

Microscopically there is no specific alteration except for an absence of the melanocyte, which develops from the underlying tissue, not the epithelium itself. The treatment is primarily reassurance that this condition is not related to any future problems either in the female genital canal or elsewhere.

In contrast to vitiligo is leucoderma, the acquired depigmentation of the skin. It is often related to irritative phenomenon, particularly dermatitis, which may affect the skin in any area of the body. In the adult, it must be appreciated that whitish patches may represent one of the dystrophies and under such conditions are considered to be potentially malignant but not in the child.

Neither vitiligo or leucoderma needs any specific treatment unless there is irritation associated with the phenomenon. Under such circumstances, the alleviation of the fingernail from the equation will prevent further problems. Usually, a 1% preparation of hydrocortisone will alleviate the symptom. Although malignancy is not reported on the vulva of the prepubertal child, tumors arising in the vagina may project at the outlet and cause local discharge and bleeding. Since such lesions are often malignant (i.e., sarcoma botryoides and endodermal sinus tumor), early diagnosis and treatment are of major import (Fig. 19).

Biopsy of the vulva is unnecessary unless there is a focal lesion. The latter may represent some pathologic process, for example, a wart.

Lichen Sclerosus

Lichen sclerosus, often called lichen sclerosus et atrophicus, is not uncommon in the vulva in any age (35). Although the term atrophicus has been applied to the condition because of the shrinkage that often accompanies such alterations, metabolic studies have identified the fact that this epithelium is not atrophic, but if anything is overactive.

Lichen sclerosus may be found in familial situations in which the mother or grandmother have or have had a similar condition. A specific HLA antigen has not been determined; however, the common occurrence in families suggests this possibility (36).

Lichen sclerosus is commonly asymptomatic in the child, but the parent, on discovering the pigment alteration, is often very concerned about the potentiality of more serious disease. I have seen several cases because of the parent's concern and not because of the patient's symptoms.

The condition is characterized by white alterations in the labia minora and majora. Unfortunately, many of the alterations are present in the prepuce and may result in constriction of the clitoris and paraphimosis with associated discomfort and occasionally infection (Fig. 20). Ecchymoses

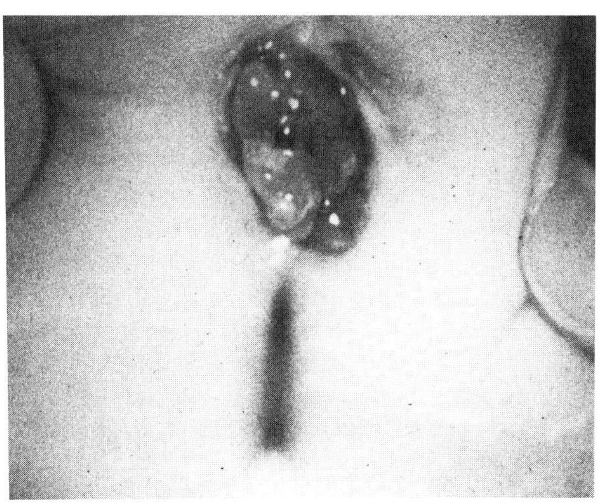

FIG. 19. Endodermal sinus tumor visible at the introitus.

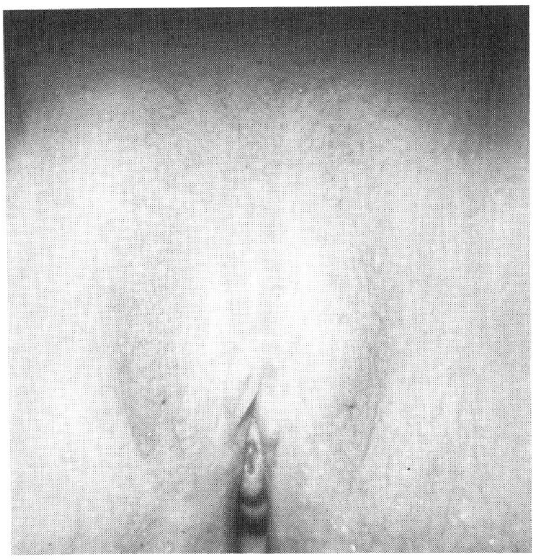

FIG. 20. Lichen sclerosis with agglutination of minor folds producing paraphimosis.

are common in lichen sclerosus and need no treatment (Fig. 21).

Every effort should be made to alleviate the parent's concern and the patient's irritation. Of major importance is the appreciation by the physician that such changes are not uncommon and that in 50% of the

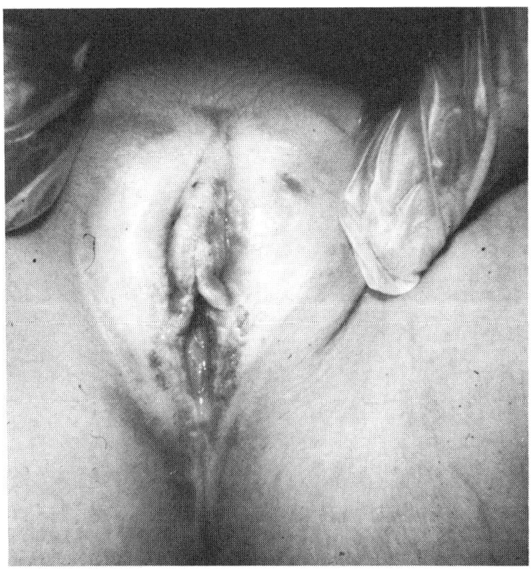

FIG. 21. Lichen sclerosis in child with ecchymoses.

cases, the condition is self-limiting or at least subsides to a major degree at the menarche.

If there is chronic irritation producing the resultant scratching, 1–2% hydrocortisone may be used. If the latter agent is prepared in a cream base there is less irritation than in the usual vaseline or petrolatum bases. Nevertheless, the preparation in cream base is commonly not available; thus, the available preparation should be used. Every effort should be made to eliminate the fingernail from the equation.

Whereas testosterone is commonly used to treat such conditions in the adult, such is not the case for the child. The use of testosterone may enlarge the clitoris and produce more irritation. Two percent preparation of progesterone in stearin lanolin may be used if the condition seems to be worsening. In contrast, if there is no evidence of distortion, it is better to allay the fears of the patient and parent, and treat the patient symptomatically.

Biopsy is unnecessary in the prepubertal child and often is traumatic. Obviously, if there are ulcerations or proliferations, these should be investigated thoroughly. Paraphimosis should be alleviated in view of the irritation and occasional infection. If circumcision becomes necessary due to infection or abscess formation, the skin removed should be minimal and the tissue at the base of the clitoris preserved to prevent discomfort.

Other Congenital Diseases

Both Hailey-Hailey's and Darier's disease have been described on the vulva but fortunately are extremely uncommon. In my experience, only one instance of the latter has been noted on the vulva in childhood (Fig. 22). Darier's disease is more commonly seen in the adult, although it is apparently an inherited disease. These conditions are extremely difficult to treat, and often biopsy is needed to establish a diag-

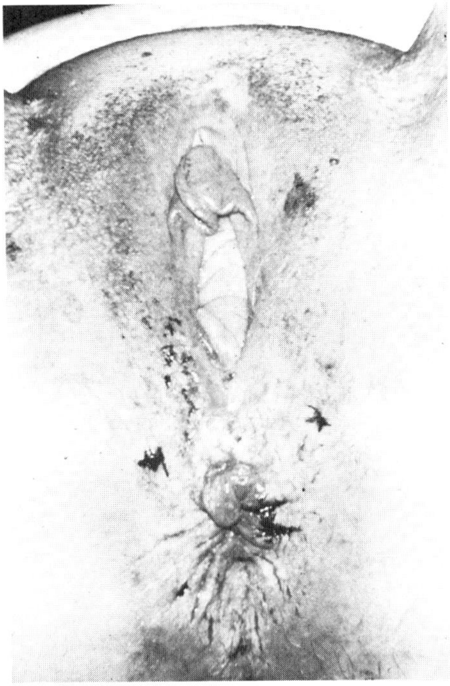

FIG. 22. Darier's disease of vulva.

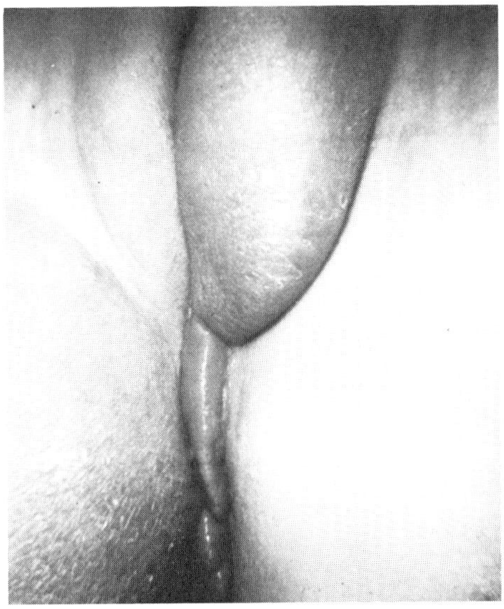

FIG. 23. Prepubertal edema.

nosis. Nevertheless, the treatment is alleviation of the symptom, which is usually pruritus. The treatment in the child, as with other pruritic diseases, should be 1–2% hydrocortisone. Again, the lesions are uncommon but should always be recognized and the familial aspect identified.

MISCELLANEOUS PROBLEMS

Edema may develop without apparent cause (Fig. 23). Obviously, any lymphatic obstruction, temporary or permanent, may produce such problems. On the other hand, the edema may be transitory and related to constriction of the prepuce, with occasionally an associated paraphimosis (Fig. 24). Thorough investigation as to any lymphatic blockage in the ileal inguinal or pelvic area should be undertaken. The treatment for such edema is local, and, again, the use of cool Domeboro soaks is recommended. Although heat has been generally used for most conditions in the perineum, it should be appreciated that cool tubs are more appropriate. Follow-up of such conditions is simply the elimination of any disease entity

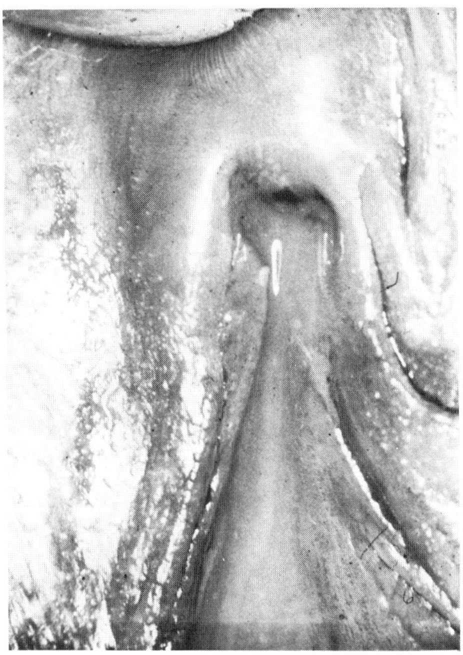

FIG. 24. Phimosis and edema of labia minora.

that may be present in the pelvis that has not been adequately identified.

Prolapse of the urethral mucosa is not uncommon in the prepubertal child and may result in bleeding due to the edematous erythematous tissue (Fig. 25) (37–39). Cool soaks, local estrogen, and systemic antibiotics may result in elimination of the everted tissue. In the case of major degrees of prolapse, ligation of the prolapsed tissue may be carried out under local anesthesia (40,41). Urination is not a problem in such cases, since the prolapse is usually focal and not circumferential. If the latter is present, cautery or laser may be used.

Tumors of the vulva in infancy and childhood are uncommon, with the exception of the inflammatory lesions, e.g., condylomata acuminata. Nevertheless, it must be appreciated that not only benign but malignant tumors have been reported. Lister (42) reported an invasive carcinoma in a 14-year-old girl, a lesion that had been present for several years. Not only carcinoma but embryonal rhabdomyosarcoma has been recorded in our laboratory in a 13-year-old girl (Fig. 26). Although rare, it is important to appreciate that abnormal swelling must be investigated if local measures fail to control the process. In the situation described above, no therapy and no investigation was carried out for 6 months although the swelling persisted and three physicians were consulted.

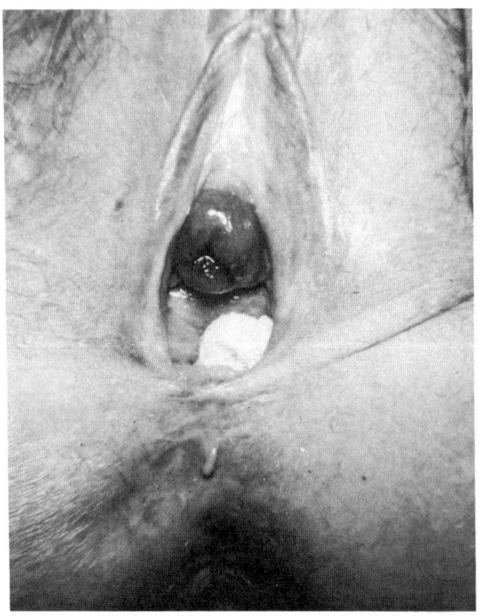

FIG. 25. Prolapsed urethral mucosa.

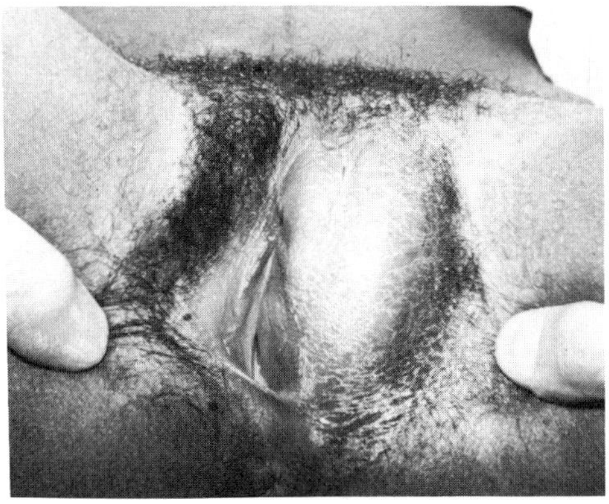

FIG. 26. Embryonal rhabdomyosarcoma of the vulva in a 13-year-old girl.

REFERENCES

1. DeJong AR. Sexually transmitted diseases in sexually abused children. *Sex Transm Dis* 1986; 13:123–6.
2. Becker TM, Blount JH, Douglas J, et al. Trends of molloscum contagiosum in the United States: 1966–1983. *Sex Transm Dis* 1986;12:88.
3. Mandel MJ, Lewis RJ. Molloscum contagiosum of the newborn. *Br J Dermatol* 1970;84:370.
4. Arvin AM, Hensleigh PA, Prober CG. Failure of antepartum maternal cultures to predict the infant's risk of exposure to herpes simplex virus at delivery. *N Engl J Med* 1986;315:796–800.
5. Prober CG, Sullender WM, Yasukawa LL. Lower risk of herpes simplex virus infections in neonates exposed to the virus at the time of vaginal delivery from mothers with recurrent genital herpes simplex virus infections. *N Engl J Med* 1987;316:240–4.
6. Nahmias AJ, Josey WE, Naib ZM. Significance of herpes simplex infection during pregnancy. *Clin Obstet Gynecol* 1972;15:929.
7. Arvin AM, Yeager AS, Bruhn FW. Neonatal herpes simplex in the absence of mucocutaneous lesions. *J Pediatr* 1982;100:715–21.
8. Mahmias AJ, Josey WE, Naib ZM. Neonatal herpes simplex infection. *JAMA* 1967;199:132.
9. Nahmias AJ, Visintine AM. Herpes simplex. In:

Remington J, ed. *Infectious diseases of the fetus and newborn infant*. Philadelphia: W.B. Saunders, 1976:156.
10. Goldberg LH, Kaufman RH, Conant MA, et al. Oral acyclovir for episodic treatment of recurrent genital herpes. *J Am Acad Dermatol* 1986;15:256–64.
11. Rock B, Zohreh N, Barnett N, et al. Genital tract papillomavirus infection in children. *Arch Dermatol* 1986;122:1129–32.
12. Stumpf PG. Increasing occurrence of condylomata acuminata in premenarchal children. *Obstet Gynecol* 1980;56:262–4.
13. Sadan O, Koller AB, Adno A, et al. Massive vulval condylomata acuminata in a 10-months-old child with suspected sexual abuse. Case report. *Br J Obstet Gynaecol* 1985;92:1201–3.
14. Stringel G, Mercer S, Corsini L. Condyloma acuminata in children. *J Pediatr Surg* 1985;20:499–501.
15. Bump RC. Chlamydia trachomatis as a cause of prepubertal vaginitis. *Obstet Gynecol* 1985; 65:384–8.
16. Rettig PJ. Pediatric genital infection with Chlamydia trachomatis: statistically nonsignificant, but clinically important. *Pediatr Infect Dis* 1984;3:95–6.
17. Schachter J, Grossman M, Holt J, et al. Infection with Chlamydia trachomatis: involvement of multiple anatomic sites in neonates. *J Infect Dis* 1979;139:232–4.
18. Knox WG, Stanley-Brown EG, Daregon HW. Surgical management of extensive hemangioma associated with severe hemorrhage in the infant. *Surgery* 1961;49:406.
19. Friedrich EG Jr. Vulvar vestibulitis syndrome. *J Reprod Med* 1987;32:110–4.
20. Marinoff SC, Turner MLC. Hypersensitivity to vaginal candidiasis or treatment vehicles in the pathogenesis of minor vestibular gland syndrome. *J Reprod Med* 1986;31:796–9.
21. Woodruff JD, Parmley TH. Infection of the minor vestibular gland. *Obstet Gynecol* 1983; 62:609–12.
22. Benrubi G, Neuman C, Nuss RC, et al. Vulvar and vagina hematomas: A retrospective study of conservative versus operative management. *South Med J* 1987;80:991–4.
23. Sheikh GN. Perineal genital hematoma. *Obstet Gynecol* 1971;38:571–2.
24. Capraro VJ. Sexual assault of female children. *Ann NY Acad Sci* 1967;142:817.
25. Woddling BA, Evans JR, Bradbury MD. Sexual assault: rape and molestation. *Clin Obstet Gynecol* 1977;20:509–30.
26. Altchek A. Pediatric vulvovaginitis. *J Reprod Med* 1984;29:359–75.
27. Paradise JE, Campos JM, Freidman HM, et al. Vulvovaginitis in premenarcheal girls: clinical feature and diagnostic evaluation. *Pediatrics* 1982;70:193–8.
28. Williams TS, Callen JP, Owen LG. Vulvar disorders in the prepubertal female. *Pediatr Ann* 1986;15:588–605.
29. Pelisse M, Hewitt J. Erythematous vulvitis en plaques. In: Friedrich EG Jr., ed. *Proceedings of the International Society for the Study of Vulvar Disease, 3rd Congress*. Milwaukee, 1976.
30. Frachtman KG. Foreign body in the vagina. *Obstet Gynecol* 1963;21:257.
31. Paryani SG, Arvin AM. Intrauterine infection with varicella-zoster virus after maternal varicella. *N Engl J Med* 1987;316:1366–70.
32. Williams JW. Diphtheria of the vulva. Paper presented at the Clinical Society of Baltimore, 1897.
33. Humphrey DC. Localized vacinia of the vulva. *Am J Obstet Gynecol* 1963;86:460.
34. Weary PE, et al. Localized accidental vaccinia. *Arch Dermatol* 1960;82:804.
35. Friedrich EG: Lichen sclerosus. In: Friedrich EG, ed. *Vulvar disease, vol. 9*. 2nd ed. Philadelphia, 1983:134–6.
36. Friedrich EG Jr, McLaren NK. Genetic aspects of vulvar lichen sclerosus. *Am J Obstet Gynecol* 1984;150:161–5.
37. Capraro VJ, Bayonit-Rivera NP, Magoss I. Vulvar tumors in children due to prolapse of the urethral mucosa. *Am J Obstet Gynecol* 1970; 108:572–5.
38. Neuwirth RS. Urethral prolapse in young girls. *Obstet Gynecol* 1963;22:290.
39. Venable DD, Markland C. Urethral prolapse in girls. *South Med J* 1981;75:951–3.
40. Friedrich EG Jr. Cryosurgery for urethral prolapse. *Obstet Gynecol* 1977;50:359–61.
41. Pearman RO. Snare for removal of urethral caruncle. *J Urol* 1960;84:779.
42. Lister WM, Akinla O. Carcinoma of the vulva in childhood. *J Obstet Gynaecol Br Comm* 1972; 79:470.

Pediatric and Adolescent Gynecology,
edited by S. E. Carpenter and J. A. Rock.
Raven Press, Ltd., New York © 1992.

10

Vaginal Discharge and Vaginal Bleeding in Childhood

Michele D. Wilson

Department of Pediatrics, Johns Hopkins Hospital, Baltimore, Maryland 21205

The genital tract of the prepubertal child is quite different from that of a woman of reproductive age. At birth, the baby's vaginal mucosa is thickened from intrauterine estrogen stimulation. After a few weeks of extrauterine life, the vaginal epithelium changes into smooth, thin, atrophic, columnar epithelium that is extremely delicate. The prepubertal vagina has a neutral pH, which provides an optimal environment for bacterial growth. Additionally, the vagina lacks antibodies that may be present later in life to help fight infection. The vagina is short, measuring 3–4 cm in length during infancy. In a child, the ratio of the size of the cervix to the size of the uterine fundus is 3:1; in an adult, the ratio is reversed to 1:3. The labia are thin, and the vaginal and vulvar tissues are sensitive. There is no visible vaginal discharge in a healthy prepubertal female.

The normal flora of the prepubertal vagina has been investigated. Hammerschlag et al. (1) obtained vaginal samples for aerobic and facultative anaerobic bacteria cultures from girls who ranged in age from 2 months to 15 years. The following bacteria were recovered in the designated percentages of individuals: diphtheroid, 78%; *Staphylococcus epidermidis*, 73%; α-hemolytic streptococci, 39%; lactobacilli, 39%; nonhemolytic streptococci, 34%; *Escherichia coli*, 34%; *Klebsiella*, 15%; *Gardnerella vaginalis*, 13.5%; group D streptococcus, 8.5%; *Staphylococcus aureus*, 7%; *Haemophilus influenzae*, 5%; *Pseudomonas aeruginosa*, 5%; and *Proteus*, 5%. Genital mycoplasma cultures showed that

6% and 27% of the girls harbored *Mycoplasma hominis* and *Ureaplasma urealyticum,* respectively. Yeast species were identified in 28% of individuals. Vaginal cultures for anaerobic bacteria were performed in a subset of the patients. *Bacteroides fragilis* and peptococci were each found in 76% of the girls; peptostreptococci and *B. melangenicus* were each recovered in 56% of the patients. Paradise et al. (2) conducted a study to examine vulvovaginitis in premenarcheal girls. As part of their study, they obtained vaginal cultures from healthy age-matched controls who had no genitourinary complaints. They found normal flora alone in 80.8% of the girls and normal flora with one or more additional isolate in 19.2% of the other girls. They considered lactobacilli, α-hemolytic streptococci and diphtheroid to be normal vaginal flora. Asymptomatic individuals also were colonized with the following organisms: bacteroides species (27.5%), β-hemolytic streptococci (not group A or B) (4%), *Escherichia coli* (8%), Group B streptococcus (2%), coagulase positive staphylococcus (2%), and yeast (4%). Both of these studies provide important information, regarding normal vaginal flora in girls.

VULVOVAGINITIS

Vulvovaginitis is the most common gynecologic problem in prepubertal girls (Table 1). Several physiologic factors contribute to the child's increased susceptibility to vulvovaginitis. A pubertal female has physical barriers that help to prevent infection. In contrast, the young girl lacks labial fat pads, she has no pubic hair, and the labia minora are relatively small. In addition, the proximity of the rectum to the vagina permits for easy fecal contamination of the vagina. All of these factors combined with suboptimal hygiene, which is frequent among young children, result in decreased protection of the vulva and vagina.

TABLE 1. *Etiologies for vaginal discharge and vaginal bleeding in childhood*

Nonspecific vaginitis
Physiologic discharge
Newborn
Physiologic leukorrhea
Sexually transmitted disease organisms
Neisseria gonorrhoea
Chlamydia trachomatis
Herpes simplex virus
Genital warts
Trichomonas vaginalis
Gardnerella vaginalis
Other infectious causes
Shigella
Yersinia enterocolitica
Staphylococcus aureus
Haemophilus influenzae
Group A β-hemolytic streptococci
Streptococcus pneumoniae
Neisseria meningitidis
Candida
Branhamella catarrhalis
Pinworms (*Enterobius vermicularis*)
Congenital anomalies
Ectopic ureter
Chemical disorders
Bubble bath, perfumes, harsh soaps, deodorants
Skin disorders
Seborrhea
Eczema
Psoriasis
Lichen sclerosus et atrophicus
Adhesive vulvitis
Systemic illness
Roseola
Varicella
Scarlet fever
Stevens-Johnson syndrome
Kawasaki syndrome
Pelvic abscess
Genital trauma
Foreign body
Urologic disorders
Urethral prolapse
Urethral polyp
Prolapsed ureterocele
Hemangioma
Physiologic vaginal bleeding in the newborn
Precocious puberty
Iatrogenic or factitious puberty
Carcinoma, sarcoma botryoides
Blood dyscrasia

Nonspecific Vulvovaginitis

Nonspecific vulvovaginitis is the single greatest cause of prepubertal vulvovaginitis, accounting for between 25% and 93% of all cases in various clinical series (2,3). When vaginal cultures are obtained in a patient with nonspecific vulvovaginitis, they will grow organisms considered to be part of normal vaginal flora, i.e., lactobacilli, diphtheroids, *Staphylococcus epidermidis*, α-hemolytic streptococci or gram negative intestinal organisms, particularly *Escherichia coli*. In spite of normal flora, vulvar irritation develops for several reasons. Frequently, poor perineal hygiene associated with wiping from the rectum anteriorly towards the vagina is the key issue. Tight fitting clothes, nylon underpants or stockings, and prolonged exposure to wet bathing suits or dancing leotards may all contribute to the problem.

Once inflammation has begun, scratching may follow, which will predispose to bacterial superinfection. Symptoms of nonspecific vulvovaginitis include vaginal discharge, genital pain, pruritus, irritation, and dysuria. The cornerstone of treatment as well as prevention of subsequent episodes of nonspecific vulvovaginitis is the institution of good perineal hygiene. Proper wiping technique, that is wiping from front to back, is essential to prevent fecal contamination of the vagina and vulva. The child should wear white cotton underwear and use white toilet paper since the dyes and perfumes used in clothing and toilet paper can act as irritants. The child should use a mild, nondeodorant, nonperfumed soap to bathe. After bathing, she or her parent should dry her vulva by patting gently with a towel, but without rubbing. Nylon stockings, ballet leotards, tight fitting clothes, and prolonged exposure to wet bathing suits or wet clothes should be avoided. The goal is to keep the genital area cool and dry. It is important to discontinue using bubble baths or harsh soaps. In the acute phase of irritation, sitz baths of warm water alone or warm water mixed with baking soda, colloidal oatmeal or cornstarch are beneficial. Wet compresses of Burow's solution may provide relief for weeping lesions. For the more persistent or severe condition, antibiotics can prove beneficial. A 10-day course of one of the following oral antibiotics is recommended: amoxicillin, amoxicillin combined with clavulanic acid (augmentin), or a cephalosporin. In persistent cases, it may be necessary to prescribe a course of low-dose antibiotics for as long as 2 months. Topical estrogen cream applied to the vulva for 2–3 weeks is efficacious when there is inadequate recovery with improved hygienic measures. Caution must be exercised in prescribing topical estrogens since prolonged use can result in iatrogenic precocious puberty.

Physiologic Discharge

A physiologic discharge frequently occurs in the newborn female due to intrauterine exposure to maternal estrogens. The discharge is characteristically white, mucoid, and without odor. It persists for approximately one week. After the first few days, the discharge may become bloody, due to withdrawal of estrogen stimulation to the endometrial lining of the uterus.

During puberty, physiologic leukorrhea begins in response to increased levels of circulating estrogens. It develops weeks to months prior to the onset of menarche and may persist for several years. It is generally described as a copious, clear-to-white colored vaginal discharge with a tenacious consistency and without odor. The discharge is composed of desquamated vaginal cells, vaginal transudate and endocervical mucus. The discharge is completely normal. Reassurance of the patient and her family is the only required treatment.

Specific Etiologies for Vulvovaginitis

In an individual with a specific etiology for vulvovaginitis, vaginal cultures will identify a pathogen. Most of these pathogens are generally categorized as respiratory, intestinal, or sexually transmitted disease organisms.

Sexually Transmitted Diseases

When a prepubertal child who is outside the newborn period is found to have a genital infection with a sexually transmitted disease agent, sexual abuse is probable. The nature of the specific organism identified and what is known about the transmission of that specific organism will determine the level of suspicion a clinician should maintain that abuse has taken place. Child sexual abuse is unfortunately a fairly frequent phenomena. It is estimated that one in four girls will be sexually molested by age 16. A study was conducted that investigated the incidence of sexually transmitted diseases in children with suspected sexual abuse. The study included 409 children under 13 years of age, of whom 360 were girls. Sexually transmitted diseases were identified in 54 (13%) children. Forty-six children had gonorrhea, six had syphilis, four had trichomonas, and three had condyloma acuminata (4).

Neisseria Gonorrhoeae

In contrast to the mature woman in whom the acidic, estrogenized vagina is inhospitable to gonorrhea and the cervix is the primary site of gonococcal infection, the vagina is the site of infection in the prepubertal child. Prior to approximately 9 or 10 years of age, the endocervix is closed, and, therefore, upper tract extension is extremely rare. Gonococcal vaginitis is usually manifested by a copious, purulent vaginal discharge. Severe vulvitis can occur secondary to irritation from the discharge. The child may complain of pruritus or dysuria. Gonorrhea is frequently asymptomatic. Microscopic examination of the urine may show polymorphonuclear leukocytes. Gram negative intracellular diplococci characteristic of *Neisseria gonorrhoeae* are sometimes detected on gram stain of vaginal secretions (5). Although the gram stain may provide support for the identification of gonorrhea, it alone is not sufficient evidence to make a definitive diagnosis in a prepubertal child. Proof of infection by a positive culture is essential. Furthermore, positive culture results for *Neisseria gonorrhoeae* in a prepubertal child must be confirmed by an appropriate laboratory. False-positive results have occurred due to misidentification of nonpathogenic *Neisseria* species and may have serious negative consequences (6). Due to the emergence of penicillinase-producing organisms, the recommended treatment for *Neisseria gonorrhoeae* is a single intramuscular injection of Ceftriaxone, 125 mg for the child weighing <45 kg, or 250 mg for those weighing 45 kg or more. The alternative regimen is a single intramuscular injection of Spectinomycin, 40 mg/kg. If the child is 8 years of age or older, she should also receive oral doxycycline, 100 mg every 12 hr for 7 days.

The American Academy of Pediatrics has stated that physicians should assume that if a child has gonorrhea, she acquired it sexually and presumably abusively (7). Gonorrhea is believed to be transmitted exclusively through sex play, sexual abuse, or sexual intercourse (8). When anogenital gonorrhea is found in a prepubertal girl, a thorough evaluation coupled with reporting to the appropriate authorities for sexual abuse must ensue. A complete search for adult contacts should be undertaken. Siblings of the index case should also be examined and cultured. It is crucial to provide for the child's safety while the investigation is proceeding.

The age-specific incidence rate for gonorrhea in 1985 for children under 9 years of age was 6.5 per 100,000 (9). Girls are overrepresented, with a female-to-male ratio of approximately 3:1 or 4:1 (10). Gonococcal infection has been diagnosed in 4–20% of sexually abused children in various series (4,11–13).

Chlamydia Trachomatis

Children acquire *Chlamydia trachomatis* genital infection either by perinatal exposure or by sexual abuse. *Chlamydia trachomatis* is increasingly recovered from sexually abused children, in whom the reported incidence rates range from 4% to 17% (12,14,15).

Although the relationship between gonococcal infection and sexual abuse is quite clear, the association between anogenital chlamydial infection in prepubertal children and sexual abuse remains controversial. Specifically, chlamydial infection acquired perinatally has been demonstrated to persist for up to 53 weeks in the vagina and perhaps longer (17). Therefore, when *Chlamydia trachomatis* is recovered from a young child, the clinician should always consider but not presume that the infection was acquired by sexual abuse. On the other hand, studies support the view that sexual abuse is more probable when *Chlamydia trachomatis* is recovered in an older child (14,18).

Because of the implications of finding a sexually transmitted disease agent in a prepubertal girl, the diagnosis of *Chlamydia trachomatis* should always be made by cell culture technique. False positive results have been reported with both enzyme immunoassay and direct fluorescent antibody tests (19). Researchers who employed direct immunofluorescent technique for detection of chlamydia found that direct immunofluorescence had a sensitivity of only 50% compared to culture technique, the gold standard (15). In summary, immunofluorescence and enzyme immunoassay techniques have not been demonstrated to be adequate for detection of *Chlamydia trachomatis* in prepubertal girls and are, therefore, not suggested for use in this population. The recommended treatment of *Chlamydia trachomatis* for a child under 8 years of age is oral erythromycin 50 mg/kg/day divided into three or four doses for 10 days. For children 8 years of age or older, the treatment is oral doxycycline 100 mg twice a day for 7 days.

Herpes Simplex Virus

Type I or II herpes simplex virus can both cause vulvovaginitis in prepubertal children. The child with an oral infection may spread it to her genital area with her hands (20). Alternatively, genital herpes simplex virus infection may be a consequence of sexual abuse. Herpes simplex virus type I has been most closely identified with oral infection and herpes simplex virus type II has been related to genital infection. Although specific serotypes of herpes simplex virus have been associated with unique sites of infection, isolation of either distinctive serotype neither proves nor excludes the possibility of sexual contact. Thus, the possibility of abuse must be explored in any child with herpes vulvovaginitis, type I or type II. Diagnosis is usually suspected by detecting the typical ulcers and should be confirmed by culture. Lesions of varicella may be mistaken for genital herpes (21). It is important to recognize that recurrences of genital herpes may occur following an episode of primary infection without repeat exposure.

Genital Warts

Genital warts are caused by the same types of human papillomaviruses that infect the anogenital area of adults. It is believed that human papillomaviruses are transmitted by perinatal exposure, by sexual abuse, or by close physical contact. The length of time after birth that perinatally acquired infection can present remains unclear. It is thought that genital warts that present within the first 1–2 years of life are likely to have been acquired perinatally. As the age at which the child is diagnosed with genital warts increases, the suspicion of sexual abuse should also rise. More than 50% of children with anal or genital warts have histories of sexual abuse (22,23).

Trichomonas Vaginalis

Trichomoniasis, an infection caused by a flagellated protozoan, rarely occurs in prepubertal girls outside the newborn period because the organism prefers an estrogenic environment (24). Diagnosis is generally made by seeing motile trichomonads on wet-mount preparation. Cultures are a more sensitive method to diagnose trichomonas and therefore may increase the yield. Wet-mount examinations are positive in only 60% of adult cases that are subsequently found to be positive by culture technique (25). In adults, wet towels have been shown to act as fomites in the spread of trichomonas. If the organism is recovered from a child, sexual abuse is extremely likely. Thus, a full evaluation and investigation for child abuse should ensue. The treatment regimen is oral metronidazole 15 mg/kg/day divided every 8 hr for a 7–10-day course.

Gardnerella Vaginalis

The association between *Gardnerella vaginalis* and sexual abuse remains uncertain. In adults, *Gardnerella vaginalis* is generally regarded as a sexually transmitted disease. In children, the role of this organism is more ambiguous since it has been recovered from girls for whom there was no suspicion of sexual abuse. *Gardnerella vaginalis* is more frequently recovered from sexually abused versus nonsexually abused girls, 14.6% vs. 4.2% in one study (26). Bacterial vaginosis, which is a mixed infection of *Gardnerella vaginalis* and anaerobes, has been diagnosed in sexually abused children. Hammerschlag et al. (27) examined 31 abused and 23 nonabused girls, aged 2½ to 13 years. The diagnosis of definite bacterial vaginosis was made if two criteria were met: (a) vaginal washings contained clue cells that are desquamated epithelial cells covered with gram-negative bacilli and (b) vaginal secretions had a fishy odor after addition of 10% solution of potassium hydroxide. A diagnosis of possible infection was made if only one of two characteristics were found. The pH was not used as a diagnostic criteria as it is for adult women because data on the normal vaginal pH for prepubertal girls does not exist. They found that four of 31 (13%) girls who were sexually abused had definite infection, and an additional four of 31 (13%) girls who were sexually abused had possible infection. In comparison, none of the 23 control subjects had definite bacterial vaginosis, and only one of 23 (4%) control subjects had possible bacterial vaginosis. These data suggest that sexual activity or abuse may have a decisive role in transmission of bacterial vaginosis. Therefore, making the diagnosis of *Gardnerella vaginalis* or bacterial vaginosis in a prepubertal girl should lead to consideration of, but not assumption of, sexual abuse.

Other Infectious Etiologies, Not Sexually Transmitted

Shigella

Shigella is an enteric pathogen that can be spread from the gastrointestinal tract to the genital region in prepubertal girls resulting in infectious vulvovaginitis. The patient typically presents with a mucopurulent and malodorous vaginal discharge. The discharge was bloody in 47% of individuals with *Shigella* vaginitis in one series (28). Concomitant vulvitis has also been described. Diarrhea is absent in the majority of patients. The recommended treatment is combination therapy with oral combined trimethoprim 8 mg/kg/day and sulfamethoxazole 40 mg/kg/day divided into two doses for 7 days.

Yersinia Enterocolitica

Rare cases of *Yersinia enterocolitica* vulvovaginitis have been reported (29).

Staphylococcus Aureus

Staphylococcus aureus may be part of the normal vaginal flora in prepubertal girls. The organism is carried by 7% of asymptomatic girls (1). In the study of Paradise et al. (2), symptomatic girls were no more likely than asymptomatic girls to be colonized with coagulase-positive *Staphylococcus*. Despite its unclear role in the etiology of vulvovaginitis, when *Staphylococcus aureus* is found in a symptomatic individual without other infectious agent, it is usually treated as a pathogen. The recommended approach is to administer oral antibiotics, specifically cephalexin 25–50 mg/kg/day for 7–10 days, oral dicloxacillin 25 mg/kg/day for 7 days, or oral augmentin 20–40 mg/kg/day for 7–10 days.

Haemophilus Influenzae

The significance of recovering *Haemophilus influenzae* type b in cultures of vaginal secretions remains unclear. *H. influenzae,* which is a respiratory organism, was found in 5% of normal girls (1). In the series of Paradise et al. (2), there were two patients with vulvovaginitis for whom *Haemophilus influenzae* was recovered from vaginal cultures. One patient improved without treatment, and the other patient did not improve despite antibiotic treatment. If *Haemophilus influenzae* is the only pathogen recovered in a symptomatic individual, a trial of oral antibiotics is indicated. The usual regimen is oral amoxicillin 20–40 mg/kg/day for 7 days.

Group A β-Hemolytic Streptococci (Streptococcus Pyogenes)

Group A β-hemolytic streptococci is an important specific cause of bacterial vulvovaginitis. Streptococcal infection may be manifested by vaginal bleeding or a blood-tinged vaginal discharge associated with distinctive fiery red vulvitis and/or with perianal involvement. Group A β-hemolytic streptococcal infection typically presents 7–10 days following a sore throat and upper respiratory tract infection. Vaginal cultures will confirm the diagnosis. The recommended treatment regimen is oral penicillin V potassium 125–250 mg four times a day for a 10 day course.

Other Respiratory Pathogens

Streptococcus pneumoniae, Pneumococcus, is a respiratory organism which is spread by the oral-digital route. It is often asymptomatic. Treatment is with oral penicillin V potassium 125–250 mg four times a day for 10 days. *Neisseria meningitidis* and *Branhamella catarrhalis* will occasionally cause vulvovaginitis.

Candida Vulvovaginitis

Candida vulvovaginitis occurs frequently in women but rarely in prepubertal girls. The child who develops *Candida* typically has one of the following risk factors: She is still in diapers, she is taking or has recently taken an antibiotic, she has diabetes mellitus, or she is immunocompromised. When *Candida* vulvovaginitis is diagnosed without a predisposing condition and particularly when an individual has recurrent bouts of infection, the clinician should consider an evaluation for diabetes mellitus or immunodeficiency. The signs and symptoms of vulvovaginal candidiasis can range from mild vulvar erythema with pruritus to severe erythema with excoriations and maceration. The discharge is white and often has the appearance of thrush. If secretions are mixed with 10% potassium hydroxide solution, hyphae and/or spores can be seen microscopically. Fungal cultures may be performed on either Sabouraud's or Nickerson's media. One should treat initially with an antifungal cream, such as mycostatin, miconazole, or clotrimazole, which is applied to the external vulva. If the initial treatment is not successful, intravaginal nystatin liquid or antifungal suppositories which have been cut to size should be gently inserted with a medicine dropper or cotton-tipped swabs.

Pinworms

Pinworm infestation, caused by *Enterobius vermicularis,* is a frequent problem in young children. Only one-fifth of girls who have pinworms develop associated vulvovaginal complaints (31). The classic symptom is perianal and vulvar itching at night when adult pinworms emerge from the rectum to lay eggs. The diagnosis is confirmed if the parents, who are asked to check with a flashlight at night, see the pinworms crawling around the rectum or if the characteristic eggs are recovered by clear cellophane tape applied to the perianal region. The treatment regimen is oral mebendazole, a single 100-mg tablet given to all members of household over 2 years of age, excluding pregnant women.

Congenital Anomalies

An ectopic ureter may open onto the perineum or into the vagina, cervix, uterus, or urethra. As a consequence, there is a discharge of clear urine or urine mixed with purulent material when the urine is infected. Urine, which appears as a chronic watery vaginal discharge, is sometimes visualized emerging from the opening. An intravenous pyelogram is often needed to make the diagnosis.

Chemical Disorders

Chemical substances including bubble baths, perfumes, or harsh soaps can act as an irritant to the exceptionally sensitive skin of the vulva and cause vulvovaginitis. Treatment involves discontinuation of use of the offending agent and institution of good perineal hygiene as described in the management of nonspecific vaginitis.

Skin Disorders

Vulvar skin may be affected by dermatologic conditions such as seborrhea, psoriasis and eczema. In contrast to vaginitis in which the primary site of skin involvement is the vagina, vestibule, and labia minora, these dermatologic conditions tend to affect the outer labia minora and labia majora. Seborrheic dermatitis may involve the vulva in addition to other areas of the body. The intertriginous regions are affected with lesions characteristic of the condition. Psoriasis is a less common condition in children that can involve the vulva. Typical lesions of eczema are dry, papular patches which cause severe pruritus. This common childhood condition can also involve the vulva. When topical steroids are used, mild, nonfluorinated types should be selected for the genital region.

Lichen sclerosus et atrophicus is a rare dermatologic disorder affecting the region surrounding the genitals, which is manifested by itching, irritation, soreness, dysuria, vaginal discharge, or bleeding. This condition has been mistaken for child sexual abuse (32). Physical examination reveals white, parchment-like skin, with vulvar atrophy. Because of vulvar and perianal involvement, the rash gives a figure-of-eight or hourglass appearance. Lichen sclerosus may be confused with vitiligo due to skin discoloration. Vesicles that bleed easily are characteristic of this disorder. It is recognized by either its distinctive appearance or, when the clinical presentation is unclear, by obtaining a skin biopsy. The best treatment for this condition is controversial. The first stage of management involves the institution of good perineal hygiene coupled with topical application of a moisturizing ointment. Antipruritic medications may be needed. If there is inadequate improvement with this regimen, topical steroids may be added. Antibiotics are indicated when superinfection ensues as a complication. Topical testosterone cream has been utilized in more recalcitrant cases of lichen sclerosus.

Adhesive Vulvitis

Adhesive vulvitis is a condition in which the labia minora fuse together, presumably secondary to chronic irritation associated with vulvitis. The peak incidence for this condition occurs between two and six years of life. The usual treatment is topical estrogen cream applied directly to the adhesion twice a day for 2–4 weeks.

Systemic Illnesses

Systemic illnesses such as roseola, varicella, scarlet fever, Stevens-Johnson syndrome, or Kawasaki syndrome may involve the vulvar skin. In addition, a draining pelvic abscess from inflammatory bowel disease may present with symptoms of vulvovaginitis.

VAGINAL BLEEDING

The prepubertal girl who presents with vaginal bleeding is a cause for concern and she requires careful evaluation (Table 1).

Genital Trauma

Genital trauma is an serious cause of vaginal bleeding. Sexual molestation, automobile and bicycle injuries, and being kicked in the pelvic area are frequent causes of injury. Straddle injuries often result from climbing over a fence or a similar structure. Blunt trauma results in a hematoma which may appear as a bluish-red mass; treatment entails the use of ice packs or ice sitz baths. If the hematoma continues to expand, evacuation and ligation of the bleeding artery may be indicated. Hymenal tears strongly suggest that the vagina has been penetrated. Lacerations may ensue and there may be internal injuries involving the bladder, intestines, and peritoneal cavity. Most extensive lacerations will necessitate sedation or general anesthesia for adequate evaluation and repair.

Foreign Body

Vaginal foreign bodies account for approximately 4% of gynecologic problems in children (33). A foreign body in the vagina may present with a foul-smelling, bloody discharge. The strong odor is often the prominent concern. Foreign bodies are discovered in a great proportion of girls with vaginal bleeding (34), and the bleeding is described as bright red in color, light in amount, and intermittent (33). In one series, girls with foreign bodies complained of vaginal bleeding more frequently than they complained of vaginal discharge (33). It is rare that the child will disclose the essential history of having inserted a foreign body in her vagina. Most foreign bodies are not radiopaque, and, consequently, x-ray studies are not beneficial. The most commonly found item is toilet paper. Large metal items are usually removed with bayonet forceps. Small items may be irrigated out using a small bladder catheter. Use of lubricant or xylocaine gel may help in the process. Sedation or general anesthesia is occasionally required.

Urologic Disorders

Urethral prolapse presents with bleeding that is generally painless. Physical exam will reveal a friable, annular, periurethral mass that is the source of the bleeding. The average age of onset for this condition is 5 years of age (35). Urethral prolapse is thought to occur after an episode of increased abdominal pressure. Treatment includes use of sitz baths. Topical estrogens may hasten the healing process. Topical antibiotics or oral antibiotics are indicated if infection occurs. Urethral prolapse generally resolves within 4 weeks. If the tissue becomes necrotic, surgery is indicated. Urethral polyps, caruncles, cysts, and prolapsed ureterocele can have similar clinical presentations.

Hemangiomas

Hemangiomas in the genital area may become irritated and bleed. At times, bleeding due to a hemangioma may be mistaken for bleeding due to sexual abuse (32).

Physiologic Vaginal Bleeding in the Newborn

In the neonate, withdrawal of maternal estrogen stimulation to the endometrial lining of the uterus may result in vaginal bleeding. This condition is self-limited and requires no treatment aside from reassurance of the parents.

Precocious Puberty

The onset of precocious puberty with menarche may first come to medical attention because of a concern about vaginal bleeding. In the individual with precocious puberty, vaginal bleeding is associated with accelerated growth and other signs of pubertal development. A rare entity known as premature menarche without other evidence of precocious puberty has also been described (36).

Iatrogenic or Factitious Precocious Puberty

Use of hormonal creams or ingestion of oral estrogens or oral contraceptives can lead to iatrogenic or factitious puberty. Treatment involves discontinuation of the offending agent.

Neoplasms

Sarcoma botryoides is the most common malignant tumor of the genital tract of young girls. The tumor can involve the vagina, uterus, bladder, or urethra. The hallmark sign of sarcoma botryoides is passage of a polypoid mass from the vagina or urethra. Other manifestations include vaginal bleeding or discharge, abdominal pain, or palpable abdominal mass on examination. The peak incidence occurs before 2 years of age; 90% of patients with sarcoma botryoides are diagnosed before age 5. The tumor is rapidly growing and very aggressive.

Blood Dyscrasia

These individuals usually present with sources of bleeding other than the vagina. Rarely, vaginal bleeding is the presenting complaint for a bleeding diathesis.

Other Disorders

Some of the entities previously described which cause vulvovaginitis may present with the chief complaint of vaginal bleeding. Vaginitis caused by group A β-hemolytic streptococci and *Shigella* often result in bleeding. Bleeding may be a predominant feature of pinworm infection if scratching and resulting excoriations are severe. Genital warts may present with bleeding. Dermatologic disorders including lichen sclerosus et atrophicus, seborrheic dermatitis, psoriasis, and atopic dermatitis, which involve the vulva, may present with vaginal bleeding.

EVALUATION OF THE PREPUBERTAL GIRL WITH SYMPTOMS OF VULVOVAGINITIS OR VAGINAL BLEEDING

History

The chief complaint may include vaginal bleeding, vaginal discharge, dysuria, itching or genital pain. The parent of a nonverbal child may state that her child scratches, rubs, or is irritable with urination and defecation. It is important to know when the problem began and if there are any associated symptoms. If a discharge is present, one should inquire about the quality, quantity, color and odor of the discharge. Has the child previously experienced a similar problem? If so, how was it treated and did the condition respond to therapy? Inquiries regarding the child's perineal hygiene are essential. Does the child use appropriate wiping technique, that is, wiping from front-to-back, and has she been exposed to any chemicals or irritants including harsh soaps, bubble baths, perfumes, or deodorants. Does the child have any underlying medical conditions such as diabetes mellitus or an immunodeficiency state that could predispose the patient to *Candida* infection? Is there a history of any skin conditions such as eczema, seborrhea, or psoriasis that is presently affecting the vulva? Has the patient had a recent upper respiratory tract infection or sore throat to suggest group A β-hemolytic streptococci or other respiratory pathogens as the etiology? It is important to inquire about recent use of medications, specifically antibiotics or hormonal preparations. The possibility of sexual abuse must be explored, and questions about who cares for the child should be posed. Family history of related medical problems such as allergic or skin disorders or diabetes mellitus may help focus the investigation.

Physical Examination

It is essential to start with a good general examination. Growth and development should be assessed and one should look for indications of puberty. The skin is inspected for any pertinent dermatologic disorder. The pharynx and cervical lymph nodes should be examined. Palpating the abdomen for masses is important. The extent of the pelvic examination should be individualized with consideration of the severity and nature of the symptoms. Inspection of the patient's underpants can provide significant information regarding any vaginal discharge or bleeding. One should inspect the perineum either in the frog-leg position, that is with the hips flexed and the soles of the feet meeting, or in the knee-chest position. Using these techniques, one can adequately visualize the lower segment, if not all of the vagina. If the discharge is purulent, persistent, recurrent, or grossly bloody, a more complete initial evaluation is indicated. In these situations, one should obtain specimens for culture and microscopy. Samples can be obtained using a moistened swab, plastic eyedropper or medicine dropper. Vaginal instrumentation in order to fully visualize the vagina is required if there is bleeding, evidence of significant trauma, suspicion of foreign body, tumor, or persistence of symptoms. Visualization may be accomplished with one of the following instruments: Cameron-Miller or Mueller vaginoscope, Huffman-Huber fibre-optic vaginoscope, or a modified Kelly air cytoscope. Depending on the child's age and level of cooperation, sedation or general anesthesia may be required to accomplish vaginal instrumentation. Rectal examination is indicated if there is persistent or purulent discharge, bleeding, or associated abdominal pain. During the rectal examination, one can milk the vagina for discharge, feel for the presence of hard foreign bodies in the vagina, palpate the cervix, and check for any adnexal masses. When pinworm infestation is being considered as a possible diagnosis, clear cellophane tape is applied to the anus. It is important to recall that a normal examination does not exclude the possibility of sexual molestation since the majority of sexually molested girls have a normal examination.

Laboratory Tests

A wet mount is prepared by mixing vaginal secretions with saline to look for trichomonads. Secretions combined with 10% potassium hydroxide solution are inspected microscopically for fungal forms. Cultures are obtained for gonorrhea, chlamydia, and aerobic organisms when indicated. The clear cellophane tape from the pinworm preparation that is applied to a glass slide is examined microscopically for the characteristic eggs.

Assessment

The qualities of the discharge help to direct the investigation. If the discharge is foul-smelling, foreign body is likely. When there is a bloody discharge, *Shigella* and group A β-hemolytic streptococci are probable causes. An odorless, bloody discharge suggests the possibility of vulvar irritation, trauma, foreign body, precocious puberty, or genital warts. A purulent discharge occurs most often with gonorrhea, chlamydia, or foreign body.

REFERENCES

1. Hammerschlag MR, Albert S, Rosner I, et al. Microbiology of the vagina in children: normal and potentially pathogenic organisms. *Pediatrics* 1978;68:57–62.
2. Paradise JE, Campos JM, Friedman HM, Frishmuth G. Vulvovaginitis in premenarcheal girls: clinical features and diagnostic evaluation. *Pediatrics* 1982;70:193–8.
3. Altchek A. Pediatric vulvovaginitis. *J Reprod Med* 1984;29:359–75.
4. White ST, Loda FA, Ingram DL, Pearson A. Sexually transmitted diseases in sexually abused children. *Pediatrics* 1983;72:16–21.
5. Wald ER. Gonorrhea: diagnosis by gram stain in the female adolescent. *Am J Dis Child* 1977;131:1094–6.
6. Whittington WL, Rice RJ, Biddle JW, Knapp JS. Incorrect identification of *Neisseria gonorrhoeae* from infants and children. *Pediatr Infect Dis J* 1988;7:3–10.
7. American Academy of Pediatrics: Committee on Early Childhood, Adoption, and Dependent Care: Gonorrhea in prepubertal children. *Pediatrics* 1983;71:553.
8. Neinstein LS, Goldenring J, Carpenter S. Nonsexual transmission of sexually transmitted diseases: an infrequent occurrence. *Pediatrics* 1984;74:67–76.
9. Gutman LT, Wilfert CM. Gonococcal diseases in infants and children. In: Holmes KK, Mardh P-A, Sparling PF, Wiesner PJ, eds. *Sexually transmitted diseases*. 2nd ed. New York: McGraw-Hill, 1990:803–10.
10. Hook EW, Holmes KK. Gonococcal infections. *Ann Intern Med* 1985;102:229–43.
11. Rimsza ME, Niggeman EH. Medical evaluation of sexually abused children: a review of 311 cases. *Pediatrics* 1982;69:8–14.
12. Ingram DS, Runyan DK, Collins AD, et al. Vaginal *Chlamydia trachomatis* infection in children with sexual contact. *Pediatr Infect Dis* 1984;3:97–104.
13. DeJong AR. Sexually transmitted diseases in sexually abused children. *Sex Transm Dis* 1986;13:123–6.
14. Ingram DL, White ST, Occhiuti AR, Lyna PR. Childhood vaginal infections: association of *Chlamydia trachomatis* with sexual contact. *Pediatr Infect Dis* 1986;5:226–9.
15. Fuster CD, Neinstein LS. Vaginal *Chlamydia trachomatis* prevalence in sexually abused prepubertal girls. *Pediatrics* 1987;79:235–8.
16. Rettig PJ, Nelson JD. Genital tract infection with *Chlamydia trachomatis* in prepubertal children. *J Pediatr* 1981;99:206–10.
17. Bell TA, Stamm WE, Kuo CC, et al. Chronic *Chlamydia trachomatis* infections in infants. In: Oriel D, Ridgeway G, Schachter J, et al., eds. *Chlamydial infections*. Cambridge: Cambridge University Press, 1986:305–8.
18. Hammerschlag MR. *Chlamydia* and suspected sexual abuse. *Pediatrics* 1988;81:600–1.
19. Hammerschlag MR, Rettig PJ, Shields ME. False positive results with the use of chlamydia antigen detection tests in the evaluation of suspected abuse of children. *Pediatr Infect Dis* 1988;7:11–4.

20. Nahmias AJ, Dowdle WR, Naib ZM, Josey WE, Luce CF. Genital infection with herpes-virus hominis types 1 and 2 in children. *Pediatrics* 1968;42:659–66.
21. Boyd M, Jordan SW. Unusual presentation of varicella suggestive of sexual abuse trauma. *Am J Dis Child* 1990;144:1319–22.
22. American Academy of Dermatology Task Force on Pediatric Dermatology. Genital warts and sexual abuse in children. *J Am Acad Dermatol* 1984;11:529–30.
23. Shelton TB, Jerkins GR, Noe HN. Condylomata acuminata in the pediatric patient. *J Urol* 1986; 135:548–9.
24. Jones JG, Yamauchi T, Lambert B. *Trichomonas vaginalis* infestation in sexually abused girls. *Am J Dis Child* 1985;139:846–7.
25. Krieger JN, Tam MR, Stevens CE, et al. Diagnosis of trichomoniasis: comparison of conventional wet-mount examination with cytological studies, culture, and monoclonal antibody staining of direct specimens. *JAMA* 1988;259:1223–7.
26. Bartley DL, Morgan L, Rimsza ME. *Gardnerella vaginalis* in prepubertal girls. *Am J Dis Child* 1987;141:1014–7.
27. Hammerschlag MR, Cummings M, Doraiswamy B, Cox P, McCormack WM. Nonspecific vaginitis following sexual abuse in children. *Pediatrics* 1985;75:1028–31.
28. Murphy TV, Nelson JD. *Shigella* vaginitis: report of 38 patients and review of the literature. *Pediatrics* 1979;63:511–6.
29. Watkins S, Quan L. Vulvovaginitis caused by *Yersinia enterocolitica*. *Pediatr Infect Dis* 1984; 3:444–5.
30. Ginsburg CM. Group A streptococcal vaginitis in children. *Pediatr Infect Dis* 1982;1:36–7.
31. Droegemueller W. Pediatric gynecology. In: Droegemueller W, Herbst AL, Mishell DR, Stenchever MA, eds. *Comprehensive gynecology*. Washington, DC: C.V. Mosby, 1987:252.
32. Bays J, Jenny C. Genital and anal conditions confused with child sexual abuse trauma. *Am J Dis Child* 1990;144:1319–22.
33. Paradise JE, Willis ED. Probability of vaginal foreign body in girls with genital complaints. *Am J Dis Child* 1985;139:472–76.
34. Droegemueller W. Pediatric gynecology. In: Droegemueller W, Herbst AL, Mishell DR, Stenchever MA, eds. *Comprehensive gynecology*. Washington, DC: C.V. Mosby, 1987:254.
35. Capraro VJ, Bayonet-Rivera NP, Magoss I. Vulvar tumors in children due to prolapse of urethral mucosa. *Am J Obstet Gynecol* 1970; 108:572–5.
36. Heller ME, Dewhurst J, Grant DB. Premature menarche without other evidence of precocious puberty. *Arch Dis Child* 1979;54:472–5.

Pediatric and Adolescent Gynecology,
edited by S. E. Carpenter and J. A. Rock.
Raven Press, Ltd., New York © 1992.

11

Precocious Puberty

Leslie Plotnick

Department of Pediatrics, Johns Hopkins University, Baltimore, Maryland 21205

Puberty involves an increase in both gonadal steroid production (gonadarche) and adrenal steroid production (adrenarche). It is initiated by changes in the sensitive negative feedback that operates between the gonad and the hypothalamus and pituitary (see the chapter by Carson).

In the majority of girls, puberty begins between the ages of 8 and 13 years. The average time from onset to completion of puberty is 4.2 years (range, 1.5–6 years). The time from breast buds to menarche is 2.3 ± 1.0 years. If a girl shows signs of pubertal development before age 8 years, this is considered precocious and an evaluation is warranted. The timing of progression is also important. Pubertal changes that progress too rapidly require evaluation as do heterosexual changes (i.e., virilization).

Puberty is initiated as the gonadostat begins to lose its sensitivity to negative feedback by sex hormones. This change allows increasing pulsatile gonadotropin releasing hormone (GnRH) secretion from the hypothalamus. There is increased sensitivity of the pituitary to GnRH leading to increased LH and FSH secretion, detectable first during sleep. The gonads also develop increased sensitivity to LH and FSH secretion, grow in size and produce increases in levels of sex steroids. These events are synergistic leading to accelerated change. With further maturation, a positive feedback system develops which enables the LH surge necessary for ovulation (see the chapter by Carson) (1).

PRECOCIOUS SEXUAL MATURATION

Table 1 lists the causes of precocious or inappropriate sexual maturation (2,3).

Puberty is generally considered precocious when it begins before the age of 8 years in girls.

It is important initially to distinguish between true or central precocious puberty which is central gonadotropin mediated, and puberty that is independent of pituitary gonadotropins.

TRUE (OR CENTRAL) PRECOCIOUS PUBERTY

In girls, the vast majority of cases of precocious puberty are central in origin, due to

TABLE 1. *Precocious or inappropriate sexual development in girls*

True (or central) precocious puberty (central gonadotropin mediated)
Idiopathic
CNS tumor
Hamartomas
Other
Other CNS disorders
Trauma
Hydrocephalus
Postinfectious
Cranial irradiation
Independent of pituitary gonadotropins
Exposure to exogenous estrogens
Estrogen-secreting tumors (adrenals or ovaries)
Ovarian cysts
McCune-Albright syndrome
Primary hypothyroidism
Heterosexual development
Congenital adrenal hyperplasia
Androgen-secreting tumors (adrenals or ovaries)
Exposure to exogenous androgens
Variations of normal puberty
Premature thelarche
Premature adrenarche

early maturation of hypothalamic GnRH secretion. In many cases, this is idiopathic; i.e., no organic lesion can be found. With idiopathic central precocious puberty, the pattern of development and timing of progression is normal although the onset is at an early age.

CNS tumors, particularly hypothalamic hamartomas, are known causes of central precocious puberty. Gliomas, neurofibromas and others are also seen. Central precocious puberty may also occur with hydrocephalus (with or without associated meningomyelocele), after head trauma (4), or after CNS infections (encephalitis, meningitis) or CNS irradiation.

Girls with central precocious puberty have an acceleration in their linear growth velocity, advancement in skeletal age, pubertal levels of gonadotropins (LH and FSH) and sex steroids. Since LH and FSH levels fluctuate, single samples may not be helpful in making this diagnosis. Multiple samples, for example at 20-min intervals for several hours, particularly at night, and/or an infusion of GnRH with LH and FSH levels measured at regular intervals may, therefore, be important in making this diagnosis.

Once the diagnosis of central precocious puberty is made, CNS imaging [with CT (5) or MRI] is indicated to look for an underlying CNS abnormality.

Knowledge of the importance of the frequency of GnRH pulses for pituitary LH and FSH secretion has led to development of long-acting GnRH agonists. These agonists produce down-regulation of pituitary GnRH receptors, desensitize pituitary gonadotrophs and inhibit LH and FSH release. This treatment stops progression of puberty, and secondary sex characteristics often regress. Specifically, there is reduction in breast size, and, on ultrasound examination, decrease in ovarian and uterine size may be seen.

Thus, treatment with GnRH analogs produces a prepubertal hormonal state which causes cessation of growth acceleration, bone age advancement and pubertal progression. Although use of a GnRH agonist is the treatment of choice in central precocious puberty, none are currently FDA-approved for this purpose. Subcutaneous, intranasal and depot IM preparations are available (6–12).

The decision to treat central precocious puberty rests on several factors. The girl's age and her psychosocial adjustment to her degree of pubertal maturation must be considered. A 2-year-old girl, for example, clearly needs treatment, whereas a $7\frac{1}{2}$-year-old girl may be well able to psychologically handle the changes. Rapidity of progression also must be considered. In older girls with precocious puberty, a major issue in decisions about treatment is the degree of bone age advancement and its speed of progression, the degree of compromise of adult stature and calculated decreases in predicted adult height.

In order to assess adequate suppression in a girl on treatment with a GnRH agonist, it may be useful to do a GnRH infusion test to be sure LH and FSH levels remain suppressed after this stimulus.

PRECOCIOUS PUBERTY INDEPENDENT OF PITUITARY GONADOTROPINS

Girls with precocious puberty independent of pituitary gonadotropins have an independent source of estrogen as the cause of their sexual maturation. A search must be made for an exogenous estrogen source, for example, in medications (e.g., oral contraceptives) or in certain skin creams. There have been some cases where ingestion of meat of an estrogen-treated animal, especially with poultry, has been implicated in producing estrogenization in a child.

Ovarian (13) or adrenal estrogen-producing tumors must also be considered. These tumors are likely to present with rapid onset and progression of pubertal changes as well as have high levels of estradiol. Ovarian estrogen-producing tumors are uncommon. They may be palpable with careful bimanual examination. Ultrasound (14,15) will usually demonstrate the ovarian mass. Adrenal estrogen-producing tumors are rare and may be associated with increased levels of adrenal androgens in addition to high estrogen levels. MRI or CT should visualize the adrenal mass. Treatment involves surgical removal of the tumor, and if malignant, appropriate additional treatment. Tumor excision will produce regression of sexual precocity.

Ovarian cysts associated with increased estradiol levels are another cause of gonadotropin-independent precocious puberty (16). These may be recurrent. Ultrasound imaging will identify these cysts and their regression, progression or recurrence. Because of the incidence of recurrence, surgical excision may not affect the child's long-term clinical course. These cysts may produce recurrent episodes of breast development, and vaginal bleeding may also occur. Estradiol levels may be high. Treatment with medroxyprogesterone acetate may be considered. This medication inhibits ovarian steroidogenesis and FSH release and therefore, cyst regression may occur. Testolactone, which blocks estrogen synthesis by inhibiting aromatase may also be considered.

McCune-Albright syndrome is a syndrome of irregular café-au-lait spots, polyostotic fibrous dysplasia and GnRH independent precocious puberty. In girls, breast development and vaginal bleeding, which may be periodic, are associated with intermittent increases in estradiol levels in association with one or more ovarian cysts. LH and FSH levels are prepubertal. Excessive hormone production by other endocrine glands (e.g., thyroid, adrenal, parathyroid) may occur. The etiology of this syndrome may be a basic defect of cellular regulation (17). Treatment of the sexual precocity in McCune-Albright syndrome involves use of medroxyprogesterone acetate and testolactone (18).

With the above causes of gonadotropin independent precocious puberty, prolonged or repeated estrogen exposure of the CNS may lead to central precocious puberty. In this situation, after the specific estrogen source is removed or treated, central puberty will progress. Treatment with GnRH analogs is useful in this situation.

Severe and prolonged primary hypothyroidism has also been associated with sexual precocity probably through formation of multicystic ovaries. Also, the clinical coinciding of primary hypothyroidism and precocious puberty has been associated with pituitary enlargement and galactorrhea. In this clinical situation, bone age and growth velocity are typically subnormal. Treatment with thyroxine reverses the precocious puberty.

HETEROSEXUAL DEVELOPMENT

In girls, heterosexual development, or virilization, is caused by excess androgen production from the adrenal in congenital adrenal hyperplasia, or by androgen production from adrenal or ovarian tumors.

Adrenal enzyme deficiencies (21-hydroxylase, 11-hydroxylase, and 3β-hydrosteroid dehydrogenase) may produce genital ambiguity in a female neonate but may also present in later childhood. Plasma levels of sex steroids including androgen precursors must be measured in girls with virilization and diagnostic imaging (ultrasound, CT, or MRI) done to identify tumors. As with other forms of gonadotropin-independent precocious puberty, treatment or removal of the excess androgen may, if the bone age is accelerated enough, be associated with progression of central (gonadotropin-dependent) precocious puberty. If this occurs, treatment with GnRH analogs is effective.

Exposure to exogenous androgens must also be considered, especially with the current abuse of anabolic steroids in the athletic community.

VARIATIONS OF NORMAL PUBERTY

Premature thelarche occurs commonly in girls, most frequently between the ages of 1 and 4. Breast enlargement is seen, often without development of the nipple or areolae. There is no sexual hair development and no acceleration of linear growth nor of bone age. No progression occurs on follow-up. Laboratory evaluation shows prepubertal gonadotropin dynamics, prepubertal or mildly increased estradiol levels and incomplete estrogenization of the vaginal mucosa.

Possible causes include ovarian cysts and transient, nonprogressive secretion of pituitary gonadotropins. No treatment is necessary. However, since the early stages of precocious puberty may be clinically identical to premature thelarche, close follow-up is important (19).

Premature adrenarche is defined as the appearance of sexual hair (pubic and/or axillary) before the age of 8 years in girls. The pubic hair often begins on the labia. Premature adrenarche is due to early activation of adrenal androgen secretion. Height and bone age are often slightly greater than the mean but are usually within 2 SD. Adrenal androgen levels are in the early pubertal range, as are urinary 17-ketosteroids (androgen metabolites). It is not uncommon for children with neurologic problems to have premature adrenarche.

Late onset adrenal hyperplasia may have a similar presentation and measurement of 17-hydroxyprogesterone (and 17-hydroxypregnenolone) is indicated, especially in those girls with bone age advancement. Dynamic testing with ACTH is helpful to evaluate for these adrenal enzyme deficiencies.

REFERENCES

1. Rosenfield RL. The ovary and female sexual maturation. In: Kaplan SA, ed. *Clinical pediatric endocrinology.* Philadelphia: WB Saunders, 1990;259–323.
2. Plotnick LP. Puberty and gonadal disorders. In: Oski FA, ed. *Principles and practice of pediatrics,* Philadelphia: Lippincott, 1990:1799–803.
3. Kaplan SA, Grumbach MM. Clinical review 14. Pathophysiology and treatment of sexual precocity. *J Clin Endocrinol Metab* 1990;71:785–9.
4. Sockalosky JJ, Kriel RL, Krach LE, Sheehan M. Precocious puberty after traumatic brain injury. *J Pediatr* 1987;110:373–7.
5. Rieth KG, Comite F, Dwyer AJ, Nelson MJ, Pescovitz O, Shawker TH, Cutler GB, Loriaux DL. CT of cerebral abnormalities in precocious puberty. *Am J Roentgenol* 1987;148:1231–8.
6. Boepple PA, Mansfield MJ, Wierman MF, et al. Use of a potent long acting agonist of gonadotropin-releasing hormone in the treatment of precocious puberty. *Endocrinol Rev* 1986;7:24–33.
7. Lin TH, LePage ME, Henzl M, Kirkland JL. Intranasal nafarelin: an LH-RH analogue treatment of gonadotropin-dependent precocious puberty. *J Pediatr* 1986;109:954–8.
8. Manasco PK, Pescovitz OH, Feuillan PP, et al. Resumption of puberty after long term luteinizing hormone-releasing hormone agonist treat-

ment of central precocious puberty. *J Clin Endocrinol Metab* 1988;67:368–72.
9. Kappy M, Stuart T, Perelman A, Clemons R. Suppression of gonadotropin secretion by a long-acting gonadotropin-releasing hormone analog (leuprolide acetate, Lupron Depot) in children with precocious puberty. *J Clin Endocrinol Metab* 1988;69:1087–9.
10. Lee PA, Page JG. Effects of leuprolide in the treatment of central precocious puberty. *J Pediatr* 1989;114:321–4.
11. Manasco PK, Pescovitz OH, Hill SC, et al. Six-year results of luteinizing hormone releasing hormone (LHRH) agonist treatment in children with LHRH-dependent precocious puberty. *J Pediatr* 1989;115:105–8.
12. Parker KL, Lee PA. Depot leuprolide acetate for treatment of precocious puberty. *J Clin Endocrinol Metab* 1989;69:689–91.
13. Biscotti CV, Hart WR. Juvenile granulosa cell tumors of the ovary. *Arch Pathol Lab Med* 1989;113:40–6.
14. Fleischer AC, Shawker TH. The role of sonography in pediatric gynecology. *Clin Obstet Gynecol* 1987;30:735–46.
15. Salardi S, Orsini LF, Cacciari E, et al. Pelvic ultrasonography in girls with precocious puberty, congenital adrenal hyperplasia, obesity, or hirsutism. *J Pediatr* 1988;112:680–7.
16. Case records of the Massachusetts General Hospital. Weekly clinicopathological exercises. Case 47-1989. A six-year-old girl with sexual precocity. *N Engl J Med* 1989;321:1463–71.
17. Lee PA, Van Dop C, Migeon CJ. McCune-Albright syndrome. Long-term follow-up. *JAMA* 1986;256:2980–4.
18. Feuillan PP, Foster CM, Pescovitz OH, et al. Treatment of precocious puberty in the McCune-Albright syndrome with the aromatase inhibitor testolactone. *N Engl J Med* 1986;315:1115–9.
19. Pescovitz OH, Hence KD, Barnes KM, Loriaux DL, Cutler GB Jr. Premature thelarche and central precocious puberty: the relationship between clinical presentation and the gonadotropin response to luteinizing hormone-releasing hormone. *J Clin Endocrinol Metab* 1988;67:474–9.

Pediatric and Adolescent Gynecology,
edited by S. E. Carpenter and J. A. Rock.
Raven Press, Ltd., New York © 1992.

12

Menstrual Cycle

Eugene Katz

Department of Obstetrics and Gynecology, Division of Reproductive Endocrinology, University of Maryland, Baltimore, Maryland 21201

The menstrual cycle with its periodic desquamation of the endometrium is unique to the primate. Its occurrence is a result of a delicate interaction between the hypothalamus, the pituitary gland, and the ovaries. This dynamic relationship is manifested in the cyclic stimulation of the ovaries to develop and extrude an oocyte (gametogenesis) and to release into the general circulation among other hormones, estrogen throughout the cycle and progesterone after ovulation (steroidogenesis). The close proximity between the gametes and the steroidogenic apparatus suggests that the two elements communicate with each other, resulting in a perfect coordination between them. In addition to modulating the hypothalamic pituitary function, estrogens promote the growth of the endometrium, whereas progesterone prepares the tissue for the eventual implantation of a zygote (Fig. 1).

The completion of a normal ovulatory menstrual cycle is the culmination of a maturational process which begins prior to the appearance of the first external signs of puberty. This process is first evident by the appearance of nocturnal pulsatile secretion of the gonadotropins, a reflection of pulsatile secretion of hypothalamic gonadotropic releasing hormone (GnRH). The gonadotropins promote estrogen biosynthesis which in turn promote the development of secondary sexual characteristics (i.e., thelarche) and endometrial proliferation. The latter explains the fact that irregular menses, product of anovulatory cycles, occur during the first year of puberty. Maturation is completed when the hypothalamus displays continuous pulsatile secretion of GnRH and all the feed-back mechanisms within the hypothalamic-pituitary-ovarian axis are operational. This will result in the cyclic activity of the system made evident externally by the appearance of regular ovulatory menstrual cycles. This chapter describes how, given a mature hypothalamus and an intact pituitary, the ovary modulates the hypothalamic-pituitary-ovarian axis to maintain normal ovulatory cycles.

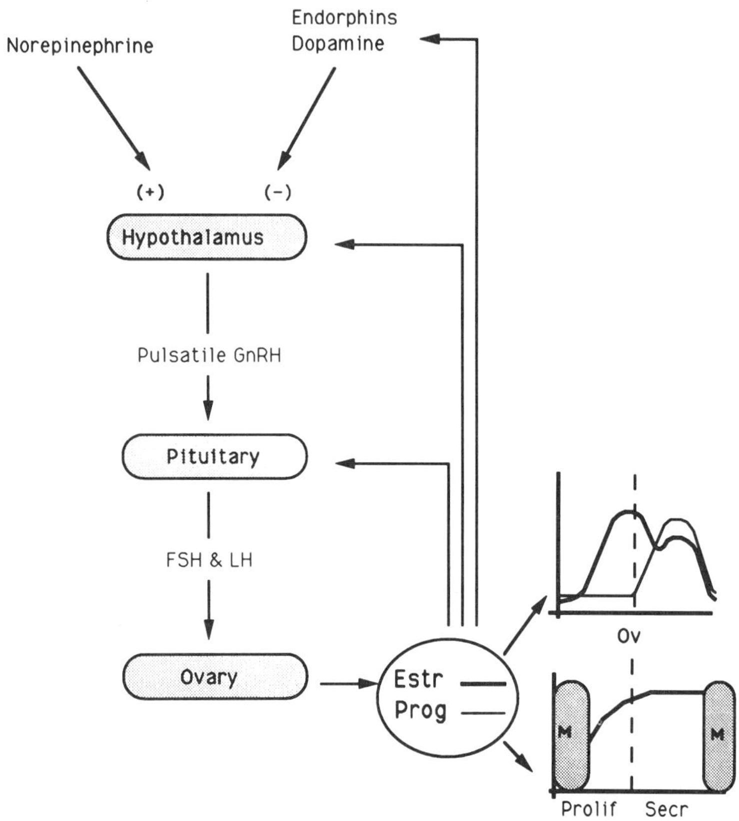

FIG. 1. The hypothalamic-pituitary-ovarian axis. Its final products, estrogen and progesterone, promote endometrial proliferation and secretion respectively. GnRH, gonadotropin releasing hormone; FSH, follicle stimulating hormone; LH, luteinizing hormone; Estr, estrogen; Prog, progesterone; Ov, ovulation; M, menses; Prolif, proliferative phase; Secr, secretory phase.

Ovulation divides the menstrual cycle in two phases: follicular and luteal. The follicular or proliferative phase is characterized by follicular development, increasing estrogen secretion, and oocyte maturation. Proliferative refers to the estrogen effect on the endometrium. During ovulation, the follicle undergoes rupture while the oocyte resumes meiosis and is extruded. The luteal or secretory phase is characterized by the production of progesterone by the newly formed corpus luteum. Progesterone promotes endometrial glandular secretion (secretory phase) and stromal changes (decidualization) that will allow the implantation of the embryo.

FOLLICULAR PHASE

The follicular phase lasts 10–14 days. During this phase, a dominant follicle selected from a cohort of primordial follicles reaches final maturity (Fig. 2). The follicle, the functional unit of the ovary, contains a germinal cell surrounded by granulosa cells. The origin of this structure can be traced to the identification of germ cells as early as the third week of gestation. The primordial germ cells migrate from the yolk sac toward the genital ridge to induce and sustain gonadal development. The number of germ cells reaches a maximum of 20 million at 20 weeks of gestation. The prolifer-

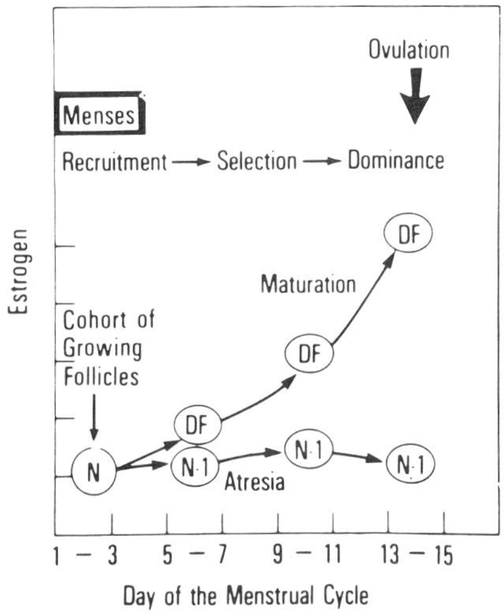

FIG. 2. Representation of the fate of a cohort of follicles (N) initiating growth during the follicular phase of the cycle. With the exception of the dominant follicle destined to rupture (ovulation), the remaining follicles (N – 1) suffer atresia. (From ref. 33, with permission.)

ation of the local coelomic germinal epithelium provides cells that surround the germ cells giving birth to a "primordial follicle." The oocyte, arrested in the diplotene stage of prophase of the first meiotic division, is surrounded by a single layer of flattened pregranulosa cells. From that stage, the tendency of primordial follicles is toward involution or atresia. This process appears to be gonadotropin-independent and occurs throughout life. Thus, 1–2 million germ cells are present at birth, and merely 300,000 remain at puberty; although only one follicle reaches maturity during each menstrual cycle, few germ cells remain in the ovary at menopause.

Escape from this fate is gonadotropin-dependent. Thus, follicle stimulating hormone (FSH) promotes the maturation of a cohort of follicles, a process that has been termed "recruitment." It takes place not later than the first day of the cycle, and it extends to the fourth day of the cycle. The continuous stimulation by FSH transforms the primordial follicle into a primary follicle. It is characterized by a primary oocyte surrounded by a single layer of now cuboidal granulosa cells. The latter are surrounded in turn by a basement membrane that separates the granulosa cells from the theca cells of stromal origin. In addition, FSH increases the number of granulosa cells (mitogenic effect) and therefore the overall number of FSH receptors. The follicle surrounded by several layers of granulosa cells is now called "secondary or preantral follicle" (Fig. 3). Meanwhile, the oocyte is surrounded by a translucent mucopolysaccharide material called the zona pellucida.

In addition to its mitogenic action, FSH stimulates aromatase activity which catalyzes the conversion of androgens, mainly (androstenedione) provided by the theca cells into estrogens (Fig. 4). Functionally and anatomically, the follicle contains two compartments: the theca cell compartment, which produces androgens, mainly androstenedione, and the granulosa cell compartment, which produces estrogens by aromatizing the theca cell androgen precursors. This model is known as a two-cell theory. Early in the cycle, the capacity of the preantral follicles to aromatize androgens is limited. Because an environment dominated by androgens promotes atresia, further maturation depends on the capacity to acquire aromatization capabilities. Estrogens, the product of androgen aromatization, promote further increase in follicular FSH and estrogen receptors, an important paracrine effect. In addition, estrogens, the most important marker of follicular maturation, further promote mitosis of granulosa cells and amplify FSH-dependent aromatase induction. Estrogens also stimulate the formation of "gap junctions" between granulosa cells. The relevance of the action of estradiol is exemplified in women unable to synthesize sex steroids due to a 17-hydroxylase deficiency in whom despite high circulating levels of gonadotropins there is no follicular development.

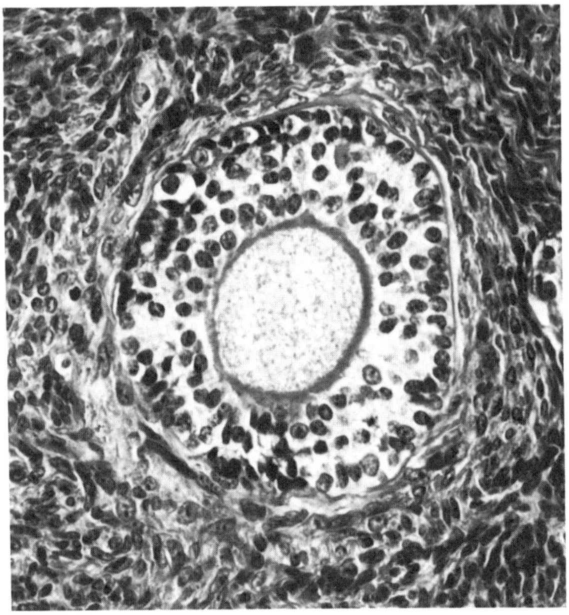

FIG. 3. Secondary or preantral follicle. The oocyte is surrounded by several layers of granulosa cells separated from the stroma by a basement membrane. (From ref. 34, with permission.)

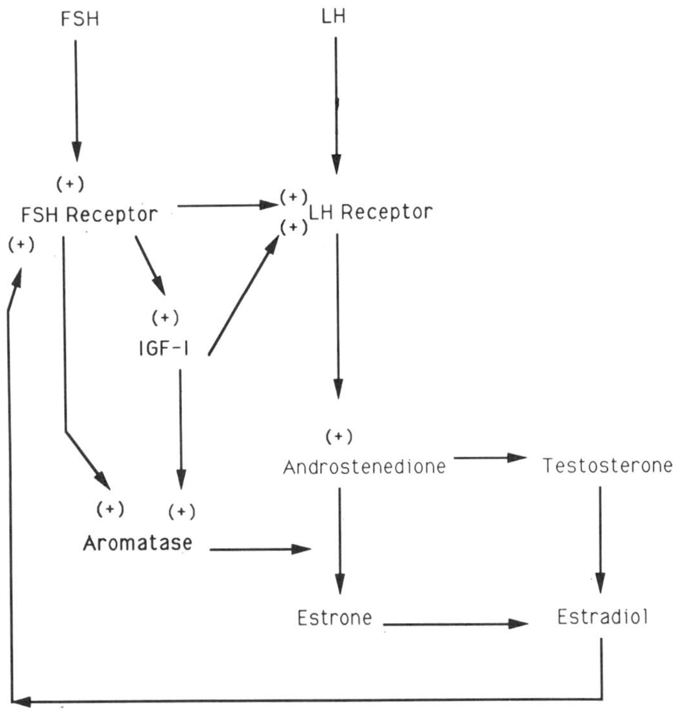

FIG. 4. Schematic events occuring as a result of the stimulation of the ovaries by gonadotropins (see text).

During its development, the follicle secretes follicular fluid which accumulates in a cavity or "antrum." The resultant structure becomes a "tertiary or antral follicle" (Fig. 5). The oocyte within the follicle remains in an eccentric position surrounded by granulosa cells in what is called the cumulus oophorus.

Recruitment is followed by "selection" (Fig. 2). From the initial cohort of follicles recruited, a dominant follicle is chosen, a process that takes place on day 5–7 of the menstrual cycle. The selection of a particular follicle depends on its intrinsic capacity to synthesize estrogen. Indeed, by day 5–7, the ovary containing the dominant follicle can be shown to secrete more estradiol than the contralateral ovary (1). Furthermore, its follicular fluid milieu is characterized by a high estrogen/androgen ratio.

Estrogens in conjunction with FSH induce LH receptors. The two-cell theory assigns specific roles to the two compartments of the follicular apparatus. Thus, LH stimulates theca cells to take up cholesterol carried in the circulation in low-density lipoproteins (LDL) and to convert the precursors into androstenedione and testosterone. Meanwhile, FSH stimulates the aromatization of these androgens into estrone and estradiol respectively. The final product, estradiol, in turn increases FSH receptors, amplifies FSH action and assists FSH in inducing more LH receptors not only in the theca cells but also in the granulosa cell compartment (Fig. 4). The lack of adequate LH receptors induced prior to ovulation will result in impaired steroidogenic function of the corpus luteum.

Other substances may play a role in folliculogenesis. Much attention has been given to insulin-like growth factors (IGF), specifically to IGF-I formerly called somatomedin-C. Although traditionally associated with the growth promoting effect of growth hormone, this 70-amino-acid-long peptide whose most abundant source is the liver has been found in many other tissues including the ovary. Both the granulosa and theca cells possess receptors for IGF-I, but the IGF-I gene is expressed only in the former. Thus, intrafollicular concentrations

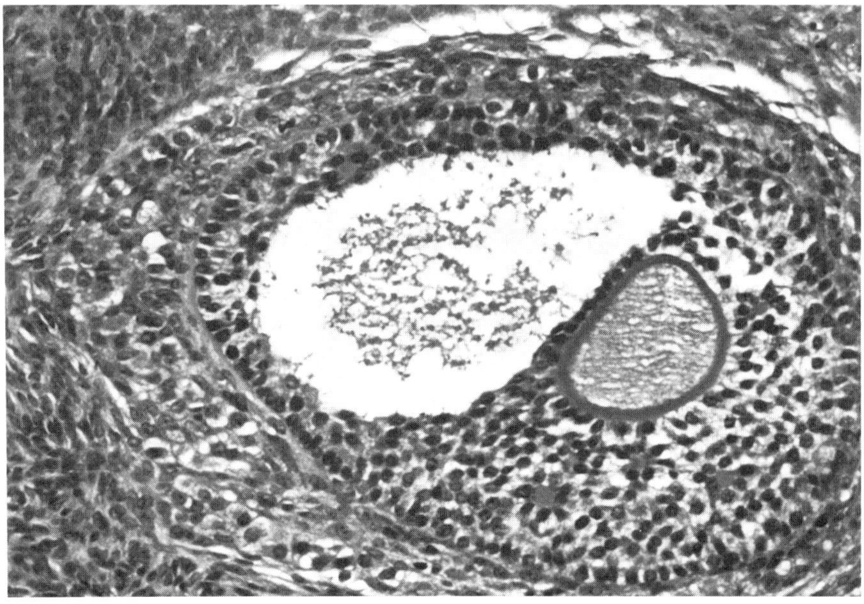

FIG. 5. Antral follicle. (From ref. 34, with permission.)

of immunoreactive IGF-I are substantially higher in dominant follicles (2). Granulosa cell derived IGF-I may be FSH- and estrogen-dependent, but the role of growth hormone in its stimulation is not entirely clear. For instance, FSH and LH upregulate granulosa cell IGF-I binding, an effect augmented by growth hormone (3). IGF-I increases FSH-induced estrogen and progesterone synthesis as well as FSH-mediated steroid biosynthesis and acquisition of LH receptors (4) (Fig. 4). In addition to this autocrine effect, IGF-I may exert a paracrine effect on the theca-intersticial cell compartment by increasing ovarian androgen which is subsequently aromatized into estrogens (5).

Several growth factors other than IGF-I may have a role in folliculogenesis. For instance, granulosa cell of larger follicles appear to secrete endotheliotropic factors that may explain the richer vascular network surrounding the dominant follicle (6,7). Such network may further facilitate growth by increasing access to gonadotropins.

It appears that the preovulatory follicle secretes proteins that inhibit the response of the follicle to gonadotropin stimulation (8). Furthermore, as follicles mature, they secrete increasing amounts of estradiol which inhibit gonadotropin secretion via a negative feed-back mechanism. Moreover, maturation of the follicles is accompanied by increasing granulosa cell production of inhibin (9). This peptide is composed of two subunits, "α" and "β." The β subunit determines the type of inhibin. Thus, bound to the α-subunit, Inhibin A includes a β_A-subunit (α-β_A) and Inhibin B a β_B-subnit (α-β_B). In addition to the negative feedback of estradiol on the pituitary secretion of FSH, circulating inhibin further inhibits FSH secretion at the pituitary level. However, at the local level, inhibin enhances LH-stimulated androstenedione production which serves as a substrate for aromatase (10). Interestingly, follicular fluid also contains "activin" a dimmer of the β-subunit, either a homodimmer $\beta_A\beta_A$ or a heterodimmer $\beta_A\beta_B$. Although there is no evidence that this peptide enters the circulation, activin displays a stimulatory action on FSH-induced estrogen production by rat granulosa cells (11). In an environment in which circulating estradiol and inhibin decrease circulating FSH, the follicle with the highest number of gonadotropin receptors continues to thrive, whereas the remaining follicles in the cohort initially recruited, unable to maintain and estrogenic microenvironment, become atretic.

In general, the process of selection represents a victory of a follicle over the natural tendency to become atretic. Once selection is completed on day 7–8 of the cycle the dominant follicle continues to mature until ovulation. Meanwhile, lesser follicles are unable to aromatize and therefore accumulate androgens. Androgens reduce estrogen receptors, inhibit cell mitosis, and aromatase activity arresting development of the follicle and leading it to atresia. This last phenomenon culminates with the replacement of the follicles by fibroblasts and scarring. Theca cells, however, become part of the ovarian stroma, thus retaining potential function.

PREOVULATORY PERIOD

Increasing circulating estradiol levels and inhibin reduce pituitary FSH secretion. This negative feedback mechanism is operational since childhood. At puberty, a positive feedback phenomenon between estradiol and gonadotropins becomes functional. Indeed, increasing estradiol levels elicit a positive LH response from the pituitary. With the surge of LH, the follicle having acquired LH receptors induced by estradiol and FSH, display secretion of 17-hydroxyprogesterone and progesterone (12,13). Progesterone appears to assist in the gonadotropin response, particularly in the midcycle FSH rise (14).

The mature follicle measuring 18–20 mm in diameter by producing high persistent circulating estradiol levels, triggers the acute pituitary release of LH and FSH, thereby controlling its own fate (15). The LH surge precedes follicular rupture by 32–26 hr (Fig. 6). Circulating LH peaks in 14 hr and lasts 48 hr. It is accompanied by a rapid fall in estradiol levels (13,16). This surge affects the oocyte, the follicular wall and the granulosa cells by triggering resumption of meiosis and formation of the first polar body, and by inducing rupture (ovulation) and luteinization respectively.

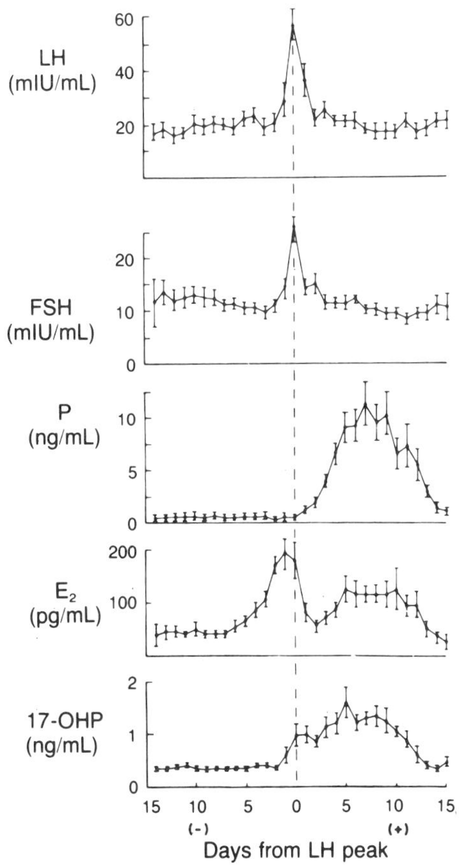

FIG. 6. Levels of circulating LH, FSH, progesterone (P), estradiol (E_2), and 17-hydroxyprogesterone (17-OHP) during the menstrual cycle. (From ref. 12, with permission.)

OVULATION

During ovulation, the dominant follicle protrudes from the ovarian cortex. This is followed by a gentle release of the oocyte surrounded by the cumulus granulosa cells. Several hypotheses have been formulated to explain follicular rupture.

Increased Follicular Pressure

Changes in the composition of the antral fluid namely proteoglycans may result in increases in the colloid-osmotic pressure and further growth of the antral cavity. Although an increase in intrafollicular pressure has not been detected in the primate, drugs known to inhibit smooth muscle contraction (calcium antagonists, prostaglandin synthetase inhibitors) inhibit follicular rupture and extrusion of the oocyte (17).

Enzymatic Rupture of the Follicular Wall

Both LH and FSH stimulate the production of plasminogen activator by granulosa cells (18). This results in the conversion of plasminogen activator into plasmin which increases fibrinolytic activity thereby producing a breakdown of the follicular wall. LH may play an additional role by increasing prostaglandin E which also increases plasminogen activator. Moreover, prostaglandin $F_{2\alpha}$ induces the appearance of lysosomes under the follicular wall, which may further enhance proteolytic activity.

LUTEAL PHASE

Luteinization refers to a morphologic and metabolic shift of the theca and granulosa cells induced by luteinizing hormone (LH). Although endogenously synthesized cholesterol may be employed in steroid hormone synthesis, circulating LDL constitute the most abundant source of this precursor.

Following ovulation, vascular capillaries cross the basement membrane invading the granulosa cell compartment greatly increasing the availability of LDL-bound cholesterol. At the same time LH stimulates the binding of LDL to its ovarian receptors (19). Moreover, LH increases 3-β-hydroxysteroid dehydrogenase activity thus directing the cholesterol-derived pregnenolone towards the production of progesterone.

Although estrogens continue to be produced, the luteal phase is characterized by the marked secretion of progesterone. Progesterone induces endometrial maturation and suppresses follicle maturation in the ipsilateral ovary (20). Clinically, the hormone displays a thermogenic activity evident by increased basal body temperatures an effect of the steroid on the hypothalamic thermoregulatory center. In the laboratory, luteinization is assumed to have occurred when circulating progesterone levels exceed 3 ng/dl (21). Peak progesterone levels occur 7–8 days into the luteal phase (Fig. 6). The luteal phase lasts 14 days, although some variation (±2 days) may occur.

The corpus luteum is sustained by LH secretion; however, it soon loses sensitivity to gonadotropins, and luteolysis ensues. The resultant decline in circulating hormones brings about the desquamation of the endometrium (menses). In the late luteal phase, the reduction of estrogen and progesterone allows gonadotropin to rise, the first stimulus for a new recruitment cycle (22).

Luteolysis is inevitable unless pregnancy occurs and the trophoblast rescues the corpus luteum by secreting high amounts of human chorionic gonadotropin (hCG). The regressed corpus luteum becomes the "corpus albicans," an avascular scar.

HYPOTHALAMIC ROLE IN THE MENSTRUAL CYCLE

So far, the cycle has been described in terms of the interplay between the ovary, its compartments with each other, and the pituitary. However, the pituitary function is GnRH dependent.

GnRH activity is first evident at puberty. Nocturnal pulsatile activity induces a similar release of gonadotropins which in turn initiate and maintain the secretion of estradiol. The continuous pulsatile release of GnRH induces the appearance of increased GnRH receptors in the gonadotroph (self-priming effect). Whereas small pulses display a priming effect, longer ones result in release of gonadotropins.

The pulsatile secretion of GnRH depends on the activity of a pulse generator with intrinsic rhythmicity located in the arcuate nucleus of the mediobasal hypothalamus (23). Each pulsatile episode of LH results from a corresponding hypothalamic discharge of GnRH (24). Experimentally, the loss of GnRH pulsatility (i.e., continuous administration of GnRH) results in down-regulation of pituitary GnRH receptors and inhibition of pituitary secretion of gonadotropins (25).

The release of GnRH is modulated by external neural signals as well as by steroid hormones directly and indirectly via neurotransmitters. For instance, dopamine and β-endorphins decrease GnRH activity while norepinephrine stimulates GnRH release (Fig. 1). Progesterone and testosterone each reduce GnRH pulse frequency a phenomenon mediated in part by the opioidergic system (26). On the other hand, estradiol increases pulse frequency and amplitude in normal preovulatory primates, but it exerts the opposite effect in castrated ones (27). During the follicular phase, GnRH pulses occur hourly. During the luteal phase while estrogen and progesterone reduce the pulse frequency to one pulse every 90 min, amplitude is increased (28). Although GnRH, gonadotropins and circulating steroids modulate GnRH release, the importance of the modulation of the "pulse generator" by these hormones has not been clearly defined. In fact, ovulation can be induced in women with hypothalamic failure

by administering GnRH in a fixed pulsatile fashion. In this respect, more important is the regulation of pituitary function by ovarian steroids.

Estrogens exert both a negative and a positive feedback action at the level of the pituitary gland. To explain this apparent paradox, the existence of two pools of gonadotropins in the pituitary gland has been postulated, namely a "releasable gonadotropin pool" reflecting "sensitivity" to a discrete GnRH stimulus and a "reserve" pool which becomes apparent when the pituitary is exposed to large and more prolonged GnRH stimulation. In this scenario, the two pools are stimulated the resulting secretion reflecting both pools or the total "capacity" of the gonadotrophs (29,30).

Estrogen appears to stimulate both but preferentially the reserve pool. Therefore, during the follicular phase the negative feedback action of estrogen on the pituitary is exerted on release rather than synthesis or reserve pool. Late in the follicular phase, higher and sustained estradiol levels promote the transfer of LH from the reserve into the acute release pool resulting in the acute discharge of LH (positive feedback). The small preovulatory increase in circulating progesterone increases the LH response. In the clinical settings, some patients undergoing ovulation induction with gonadotropins display a premature LH surge induced by the high estradiol levels. Such surges can be avoided by downregulating pituitary GnRH receptors with long-acting GnRH agonists. The above not withstanding a steroid induced pre-ovulatory GnRH surge may play a role in the generation of the LH surge (31).

It is evident from the description of the events that the follicle controls the cycle by modulating the pituitary response directly and indirectly through the hypothalamus. The intraovarian regulation is complex and may include roles for vasopressin, oxytocin, relaxin, aromatase inhibitors, and other substances for which the physiologic role has not been clearly delineated. This regulatory mechanism governing the ovarian and higher centers appears optimum because it makes use of both intraovarian signals to coordinate steroidogenesis and oogenesis locally and of extraovarian messengers to modulate gonadotropin secretion distally.

REFERENCES

1. DiZerega GS, Hodgen GD. Folliculogenesis in the primate ovarian cycle. *Endocrinol Rev* 1981;2:27–49.
2. Eden JA, Jones J, Carter GD, Alaghband-Zadeh J. A comparison of follicular fluid levels of insulin-like growth factor-I in normal dominant and cohort follicles, polycystic and multicystic ovaries. *Clin Endocrinol* 1988;29:327–36.
3. Adashi EY, Resnick CE, Svoboda ME, Van Wyck JJ. Follicle-stimulating hormone enhances somatomedin-C binding to cultured rat granulosa cells: Evidence for cAMP-dependence. *J Biol Chem* 1986;261:3923–6.
4. Adashi EY, Resnick CE, D'Ercole AJ, et al. Insulin-like growth factors as intraovarian regulators of granulosa cell growth and function. *Endocrinol Rev* 1985;6:400–20.
5. Hernandez ER, Resnick CE, Svoboda ME, et al. Somatomedin-C/insulin-like growth factor I (Sm-C/IGF-I) as an enhancer of androgen biosynthesis by cultured rat ovarian cells. *Endocrinology* 1987;122:1583–92.
6. Zeleznik AJ, Schuler HM, Reichert LE. Gonadotropin-binding sites in the rhesus monkey ovary: role of the vasculature in the selective distribution of human chorionic gonadotropin to the preovulatory follicle. *Endocrinology* 1981; 109:356–62.
7. Katz E, Rone JD, Garcia J, Goodman AL. Evidence for the production of a non-steroidal endotheliotropic factor by human granulosa cells in culture. *Fertil Steril* (in press).
8. DiZerega GS, Goebelsman V, Nakamura RM. Identification of a protein(s) secreted by the preovulatory ovary which suppresses the follicle response to gonadotropins. *J Clin Endocrinol Metab* 1982;54:1091–6.
9. Chaning CP, Anderson LD, Hoover DG, et al. The role of nonsteroidal regulators in control of oocyte and follicular maturation. *Recent Prog Horm Res* 1982;38:331–40.
10. Hsue AJW, Dahl KD, Vaughan J, et al. Heterodimmers and homodimmers of inhibin subunits have different paracrine action in the modulation of luteinizing hormone-stimulated androgen biosynthesis. *Proc Natl Acad Sci USA* 1987;84: 5082–6.
11. Burger HG, Findlay JK. Potential relevance on inhibin to ovarian physiology. *Semin Reprod Endocrinol* 1989;7:69–78.

12. Thorneycroft IH, Mishell DR Jr, Stone SC, Kharma KM, Nakamura RM. The relation of serum 17-hydroxyprogesterone and estradiol-17 β levels during the human menstrual cycle. *Am J Obstet Gynecol* 1971;111:947–51.
13. Thorneycroft IH, Sribyatta B, Tom WK, Nakamura RM, Mishell DR Jr. Measurement of serum LH, FSH, Progesterone, 17-hydroxy-progesterone and Estradiol-17 β levels at 4-hour intervals during the periovulatory phase of the menstrual cycle. *J Clin Endocrinol Metab* 1974;39:754–8.
14. March CM, Goebelsmann U, Nakamura RM, et al. Role of estradiol and progesterone in eliciting the midcycle luteinizing hormone and follicle stimulating hormone surges. *J Clin Endocrinol Metab* 1979;49:507–13.
15. Hackeloer J, Fleming R, Robinson HP et al. Correlation of ultrasonic and endocrinologic assessment of human follicular development. *Am J Obstet Gynecol* 1979;135:122–8.
16. World Health Organization Task Force Investigators. Temporal relationships between ovulation and defined changes in the concentration of plasma estradiol 17-β, luteinizing hormone, follicle-stimulating hormone, and progesterone. *Am J Obstet Gynecol* 1980;138:383–90.
17. Katz E, Dharmarajan AM, Suoka K, Ghodgaonkar RB, Dubin NH, Wallach EE. Effects of systemic administration of indomethacin on ovulation, luteinization, and steroidogenesis in the rabbit ovary. *Am J Obstet Gynecol* 1989;161: 1361–6.
18. Strickland S, Beers WH. Studies on the role of plasminogen activator in ovulation. *J Biol Chem* 1976;251:5694–702.
19. Golos TG, Soto EA, Tureck RW, Strauss JF III. Human chorionic gonadotropin and 8-bromo adenosine 3′-5′ monophosphate stimulate [^{125}I] low density lipoprotein uptake and metabolism by luteinized human granulosa cells in culture. *J Clin Endocrinol Metab* 1985;61:633–8.
20. DiZerega GS, Hodgen GD. The interovarian progesterone gradient: a spatial and temporal regulator of folliculogenesis in the primate ovarian cycle. *J Clin Endocrinol Metab* 1982;54:495–9.
21. Israel R, Mishell DR Jr, Stone SC, et al. Single luteal phase serum progesterone assay as an indicator of ovulation. *Am J Obstet Gynecol* 1972;112:1043–6.
22. Ross GT, Cagrille CM, Lipsett MB, et al. Pituitary and gonadal hormones in women during spontaneous and induced gonadal cycles. *Recent Prog Horm Res* 1970;26:1–62.
23. Kessner JS, Kaufmann JM, Wilson RC, Knobil E. On the short-loop feedback regulation of the hypothalamic luteinizing hormone releasing hormone "pulse generator" in the rhesus monkey. *Neuroendocrinology* 1986;42:109–11.
24. Neill JD, Patton JM, Dailey RA, et al. Luteinizing hormone releasing hormone (LHRH) in pituitary stalk blood of rhesus monkeys: relationship to level of LH release. *Endocrinology* 1977;101:430–4.
25. Belchetz PE, Plant TM, Nakai Y, et al. Hypophyseal responses to continuous and intermittent delivery of hypothalamic gonadotropin-releasing hormone. *Science* 1978;202:631–2.
26. Plan TM. Gonadal regulation of hypothalamic gonadotropin-releasing hormone release in primates. *Endocrinol Rev* 1986;7:75–88.
27. Djahanhakhch O, Warner P, McNeilly AS, Baird DT. Pulsatile release of LH and estradiol during the pre-ovulatory period in women. *Clin Endocrinol* 1984;20:579–89.
28. Reame N, Sauder SE, Kelch RP, et al. Pulsatile gonadotropin secretion during the human menstrual cycle: evidence for altered frequency of gonadotropin-releasing hormone secretion. *J Clin Endocrinol Metab* 1984;59:328–37.
29. Yen SSC, Lein A. The apparent paradox of the negative and positive feedback control system on gonadotropin secretion. *Am J Obstet Gynecol* 1976;126:942–54.
30. Hoff JD, Lasley BL, Wang CF, Yen SSC. The two pools of pituitary gonadotropins: regulation during the menstrual cycle. *J Clin Endocrinol Metab* 1977;44:302–12.
31. Levine JE, Normal RI, Gliessmann FR, et al. In vivo gonadotropin-releasing hormone release and serum luteinizing hormone measurements in ovariectomized estrogen-treated rhesus monkeys. *Endocrinology* 1985;117:711–21.
32. Filicori M, Flamigni C, Campaniello E, et al. Evidence for a specific role of GnRH pulse frequency in the control of the human menstrual cycle. *Am J Physiol* 1989;257:E930–6.
33. Hodgen GD. Physiology of follicular maturation. In: In-vitro fertilization. Edited by HW James Jr., GS Jones, GD Hodgen, Z Rosenwaks. Williams Co., Baltimore, 1986. p. 11.
34. Clement PB. Anatomy and hystology of the ovary. In Balustein's pathology of the female genital tract. Edited by R.J. Kurman. Springer-Verlag, New York, 1987. p. 446.

Pediatric and Adolescent Gynecology,
edited by S. E. Carpenter and J. A. Rock.
Raven Press, Ltd., New York © 1992.

13
Adolescent Amenorrhea

G. William Bates

Department of Obstetrics and Gynecology, Greenville Hospital System, Greenville, South Carolina 29605

Amenorrhea is absence or cessation of menses. If menstruation does not begin by age of 16 years in the presence of female secondary sexual maturation or does not begin by 14 in the absence of secondary sexual maturation, the condition is classified as primary amenorrhea. If menstruation occurs, then ceases, and does not resume within 6 months, the condition is classified as secondary amenorrhea. This classification, however, gives no insight into the etiology of the amenorrhea or the prognosis for future ovulation and menstruation. In this chapter, the classification of primary and secondary amenorrhea is not absolute but is referred to as a marker for timing the onset of amenorrhea. An understanding of amenorrhea is developed that is based on the physiology of puberty and the physiology of ovulation.

PHYSIOLOGY OF PUBERTY

Puberty is held in abeyance until about age 10 in girls. The hypothalamic-pituitary axis does not secrete the pituitary gonadotropin, follicle-stimulating hormone (FSH), and luteinizing hormone (LH) in pulsatile bursts that will stimulate the ovarian follicles until about age 10. The mechanism(s) for restraining puberty and the endocrine events that initiate the onset of secondary sexual maturation are unknown. The hypothalamic-pituitary-gonadal axis functions during fetal life and during the first few weeks following birth. Then, the hypothalamic-pituitary-gonadal axis becomes quiescent.

Around age 8 in girls and boys, the adrenal glands begin to secrete increasing quantities of dehydroepiandrosterone; approxi-

mately 2 years later, the gonads begin secreting sex-steroid hormones. Sex-steroid hormones stimulate growth and development of the breasts, the genital tract, sexual hair, and the adult body habitus. After the secondary sexual characteristics are developed, menstruation and the process of ovulation is initiated. The process of secondary sexual maturation occurs in an orderly, predictable sequence. The sequence of secondary sexual maturation in girls was described by Marshall and Tanner (1) and is presented in Table 1.

These events are predictable and reflect the secretion and action of the hypothalamic peptide hormones (gonadotropin-releasing hormone and corticotropin releasing hormone), anterior pituitary protein hormones (FSH, LH, adrenocorticotropic hormone), adrenal steroid hormones (dehydroepiandrosterone, androstenedione, and cortisol) and ovarian sex-steroid hormones (progesterone, androstenedione, testosterone, and estradiol). An alteration in the hormonal events that lead to secondary sexual maturation results in an alteration in secondary sexual maturation including amenorrhea. In their description of the sequence of secondary sexual maturation, Marshall and Tanner (1) reported that approximately 10% of girls will have sexual hair growth as the first sign of puberty. However, if sexual hair growth occurs prematurely or leads other developmental events by more than a few months, this should not be considered normal and provides clues to the cause of abnormal puberty and amenorrhea.

In response to the increasing secretion of gonadotropin releasing hormone (GnRH) that occurs with the initiation of puberty, there is progressive rise in the secretion of FSH and LH several months or years before the physical manifestations of secondary sexual maturation. Boyar et al. (2) and Katz et al. (3) described the changing pattern of gonadotropin secretion during the pubertal years that leads to sexual maturation. These data are presented in Fig. 1. Gonadotropin secretion stimulates the ovarian follicles to secrete estradiol thus giving hormonal stimulation to the estrogen-dependent cells in the breasts and genital tract that allows for their development. The endometrium is stimulated by estradiol to the point that any estrogen withdrawal will cause endometrial sloughing. The first menstrual period is usually the result of estrogen withdrawal, not the result of ovulation. Ovulation is established within a few months of the first menstrual period in most girls.

As soon as the menstrual cycle is established, it remains constant in most women for the remainder of their prime reproductive years. The menstrual cycle begins to change as a women approaches menopause. Subtle changes in the cycle begin some 5–7 years prior to menopause.

Frisch and Revelle (4) proposed a theory that girls must attain a critical body weight before puberty begins. According to this theory, breast budding, growth spurt, and menarche occur as there is a change in the lean-to-fat ratio. In prepubertal girls, the lean-to-fat ratio is 5:1. With the onset of

TABLE 1. *Sequence of sexual maturation in girls*

Event	Age (years)	Hormone(s)
Breast budding	10–11	Estradiol
Sexual hair growth	10.5–11.5	Androgens
Growth spurt	11–12	Growth hormone
Menarche	11.5–13	Estradiol
Adult breast development	12.5–15	Progesterone
Adult sexual hair pattern	13.5–16	Androgens

From ref. 1.

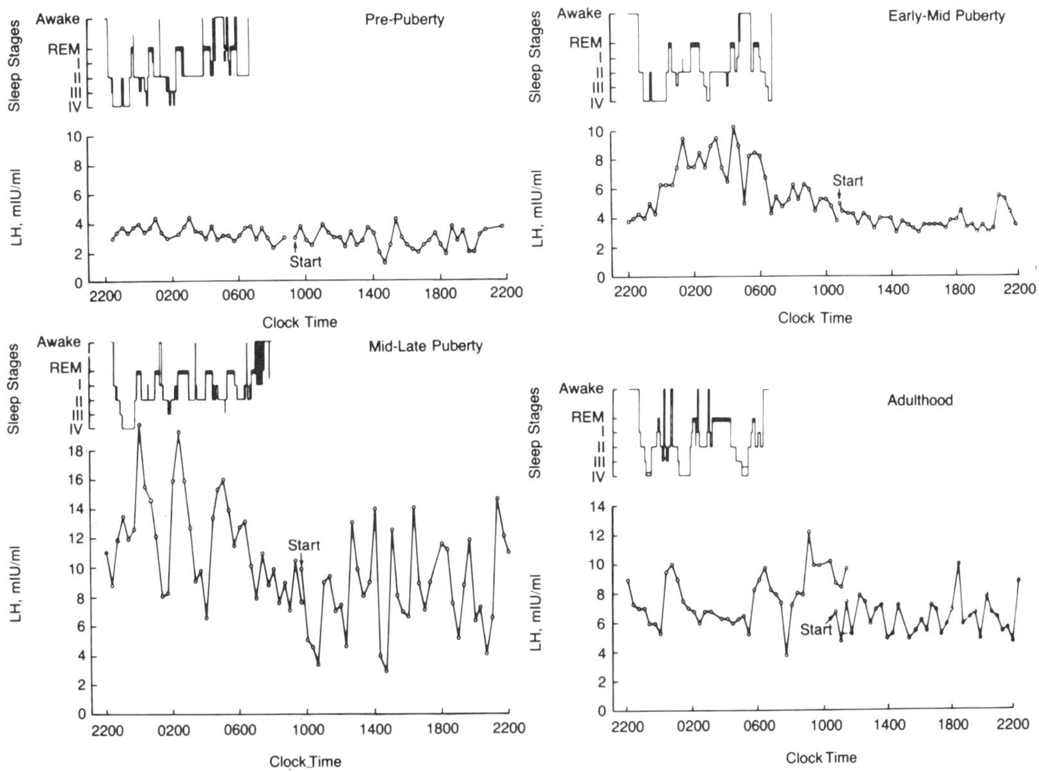

FIG. 1. Changes in LH secretion during various stages of puberty and in adulthood (3).

puberty, the lean-to-fat ratio decreases to 3:1 and is maintained at that level as ovulatory cycles are established. Menarche occurs when the percentage of body mass as body fat reaches 21%; ovulatory cycles are established and maintained when body mass is 24% body fat.

In clinical practice, the observation is made frequently that plump girls begin breast development early and that slender girls have delayed breast development. Moreover, plump—but not morbidly obese girls—may have early menarche; slender girls may have delayed menarche.

Several clinical conditions seen in adolescent girls who present with amenorrhea can be related to alterations in body weight that interfere with the physiologic secretion of GnRH by the hypothalamus and gonadotropin by the anterior pituitary gland.

How does body fat alter the neuroendocrine mechanism(s) that triggers hypothalamic-pituitary function? There is accumulating evidence that body fat plays a direct and indirect role in sex-steroid hormone metabolism. When Fishman et al. (5) infused radiolabeled estradiol into three groups of women (obese women, women of normal body weight, and women with anorexia nervosa), they found differences in the metabolism of estradiol among the three groups. Obese women excreted estriol as the major metabolite of estradiol, whereas women with anorexia nervosa excreted 2-hydroxyestradiol (a catechol estrogen) as the major metabolite of estradiol. Thus, in women with a low percentage of body fat, the pathway for estradiol metabolism is directed toward the production of catechol estrogens. Adashi et al. (6) found that the administration of catechol estrogens to hypogonadal women results in a decrease in the amplitude and pulse frequency of pituitary gonadotropin secretion.

Systematic evaluation of an adolescent woman with amenorrhea must include a history of the occurrence and sequence of the developmental events of secondary sexual maturation, and a history of the accumulation of body fat during childhood and adolescence.

PHYSIOLOGY OF OVULATION

Ovulation is the final event in the process of secondary sexual maturation. Usually, menarche—the first menstrual period—will occur several months before ovulation is initiated and established as a periodic event.

Ovulation depends upon the cyclic interaction of hypothalamic GnRH, pituitary FSH and LH, and ovarian estradiol and progesterone (7,8). These hormones have positive and negative regulating effects on one another. These regulating effects are presented in Table 2.

The secretion of FSH and LH is dependent upon the pulsatile release of GnRH from the hypothalamus. Under physiologic conditions, the hypothalamus secretes GnRH at intervals of approximately 90 min (9). If this pulse frequency is altered, the secretion of FSH and LH is altered, and the signal to stimulate ovarian follicular maturation is altered as well. Anovulation and amenorrhea result. The pulse frequency of GnRH secretion can be altered by low body weight, stress, excessive physical exercise, and marijuana use.

Pituitary gonadotropin secretion also depends upon ovarian estradiol and progesterone. If the ovaries fail to secrete these sex-steroid hormones in a cyclic manner, anovulation and amenorrhea result. Moreover, the pituitary secretion of gonadotropin can be altered by other hypothalamic, pituitary, and sex-steroid hormones such as thyrotropin-releasing hormone, prolactin, androstenedione, testosterone, and dehydroepiandrosterone. When these hormones are secreted in abnormal ways, pituitary gonadotropin secretion is altered. Anovulation and amenorrhea result.

The evaluation of amenorrhea must include an evaluation of the cyclic interactions between the hypothalamus, anterior pituitary gland, and the ovaries. To establish a specific diagnosis of the etiology of amenorrhea, the physiology of ovulation must be clearly understood.

The menstrual cycle is divided into three phases: the follicular phase, the phase of the LH peak (ovulation), and the luteal phase. A composite of these events and their effects on the ovarian follicles, endometrium, vaginal epithelium, and cervical mucous is presented in Fig. 2.

The follicular phase usually lasts 14 days but may be as short as 7 days or as long as 21 days. At the beginning of the follicular phase, the plasma concentrations of estradiol and progesterone are low. This causes increased release of FSH to stimulate a new cohort of follicles in order that one follicle will be ovulated. With follicular stimulation by FSH, one follicle becomes dominant and secretes maximal estradiol. Estradiol has positive feedback on the pituitary secretion of LH, which triggers the LH surge. Once the LH surge is triggered, the follicular phase ends and ovulation occurs. The primary physical manifestation of the follicular phase of the menstrual cycle is the change that occurs in the secretion of endocervical mucous. The mucous in the late follicular phase of the cycle becomes abun-

TABLE 2. *Hormonal interrelationships*

Hormone	Effects on other reproductive hormones
FSH	Stimulates follicular maturation (estradiol production)
LH	Triggers ovulation (stimulates androgen production)
Estradiol	Stimulates LH; downregulates FSH
Progesterone	Downregulates LH and FSH

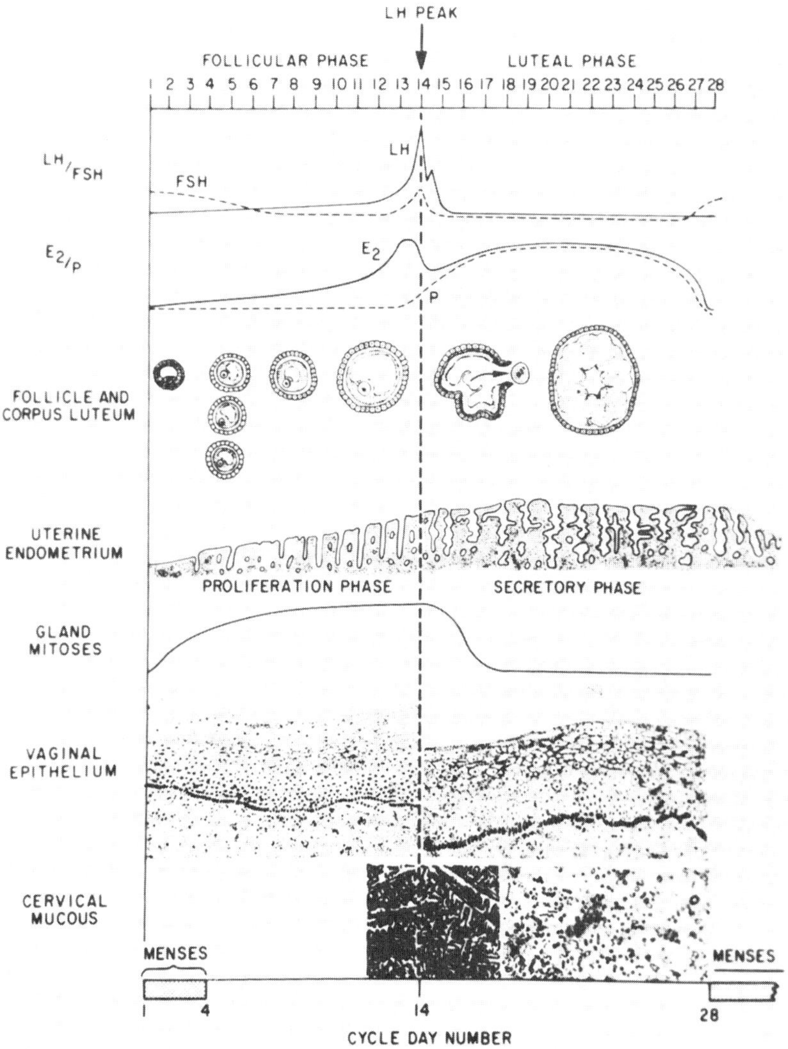

FIG. 2. Pictorial presentation of some of the events during a menstrual cycle (7).

dant in amount, thin in viscosity, clear in color, and watery in consistency.

The mechanism for ovulation is unknown and the mechanism for ovum pickup by the fallopian tube is unknown. The LH peak and time of ovulation is short. The transition from the follicular phase of the cycle to the luteal phase of the cycle consists of 36–48 hr. There is no good physical manifestation of ovulation. Many women, however, will report a sensation of unilateral lower abdominal pain in the ovarian area at the time of ovulation.

The luteal phase is the time of the cycle between ovulation and the onset of menstruation. The luteal phase, unlike the follicular phase, tends to be fixed at 14 days. Progesterone is the dominant hormone of the luteal phase. It has its obvious physical effects on the breasts, the endocervix, and the endometrium. The breasts become rounded in the lateral quadrants during the late luteal phase of the cycle, the endocervical mucous becomes opaque, thick, and inelastic, and the endometrium is converted into a secretory endometrium that has specific histologic characteristics depending on the day of the luteal phase.

These changes that occur in hormone secretion and physical manifestations are useful in evaluating women with amenorrhea (10). The application of these changes will be discussed subsequently in the diagnosis of amenorrhea and specific causes of amenorrhea.

EVALUATION OF THE ADOLESCENT WITH AMENORRHEA

The adolescent young woman with menstrual abnormalities is usually brought to the physician by her mother (11). By the time a menstrual abnormality is recognized by the young woman and her parents, the adolescent has a concept of secondary sexual development, menstruation, and reproductive function. These concepts are well-established, even if the adolescent presenting with menstrual failure has not initiated puberty. It is important that the physician communicate with the adolescent young woman! Too often, the parent(s) becomes the focus of the discussion and the adolescent simply becomes the subject of the discussion.

History of Secondary Sexual Development

The young woman should provide as much of the history as possible. If communication is conducted through the parent(s), the patient becomes a third party to the conversation, who can provide yes and no answers with interspersed grunts. This can be avoided by allowing the patient to provide the history.

The physician obtaining the history should be comfortable inquiring about breast development, sexual hair growth, development of libidinal desire, and menstruation. If the physician is uncomfortable asking these questions of adolescents (in private with the adolescent or in the presence of the adolescent and her parents), the adolescent will feel ill at ease as well. Open communication at the time of the initial visit will allow for further open communication later with the adolescent girl, the physician, and the parents.

The physician begins obtaining the history by inquiring about the stages of secondary sexual development (12). By following the expected stages of secondary sexual development, the history is logical for the physician to formulate a cause for the amenorrhea, and makes the line of reasoning logical for the patient as she knows what is happening to her peers and the sequence of those happenings. Inquire about breast development first, followed by the onset of sexual hair growth, the growth spurt, menstruation, established cycles and the effects of cycles on breasts, skin, mood, and affect.

If no secondary sexual development has occurred by age 13–14 years, this fact suggests that the hypothalamic-pituitary axis has failed to secrete GnRH and/or gonadotropins, or that the ovaries have failed to respond to the hypothalamic-pituitary signal.

If secondary sexual development has occurred partially—i.e., breast development has begun but not completed, and sexual hair growth has begun but not completed—this suggests that the pubertal process was initiated but interrupted prior to completion of sexual maturation.

If menstruation has occurred but cyclic menses have not developed, this suggests that hypothalamic-pituitary-ovarian function was interrupted before ovulation was fully established.

If fully sexual maturation has occurred—i.e., there is full breast development with full sexual hair growth—and if there is history of menstrual molimina (cyclic breast fullness, cyclic mood changes, cyclic acne, cyclic bloating), it is likely that the young woman has adult sexual maturation with an obstruction of the genital outflow tract or absence of the uterus.

Libidinal desire stems from cyclic sex-steroid hormone secretion and is usually established with ovulation. The presence or absence of libidinal desire is helpful in developing a differential diagnosis of the etiology of amenorrhea.

Since many adolescents are sexually active, it is important to obtain a sexual history as pregnancy is the most common cause of amenorrhea. Moreover, adolescent girls may be utilizing oral contraceptives which can produce alterations in the menstrual cycle as oligomenorrhea or amenorrhea.

Illicit drug use—especially the use of marijuana—can alter hypothalamic-pituitary function to produce cessation of ovarian function (13). Other illicit drugs have less effect on the menstrual cycle.

Alterations in body weight, both rapid weight gain and rapid weight loss interfere with estrogen metabolism to produce amenorrhea. Body weight alterations can result from both caloric intake and exercise. These issues must be covered when the history is obtained.

Physical Examination

A thorough physical examination should be performed with special reference to the development of secondary sexual characteristics, the integument, the senses, and vital signs. No effort should be made to avoid performing a pelvic examination; if this is the first pelvic examination for a young woman, it must be performed with reassurance and sensitivity.

The general body habitus should be evaluated first. Obesity and slimness are associated with amenorrhea. Excessively tall adolescent women may have a 46,XY karyotype; excessively short women may have a 45,X karyotype (Turner syndrome) or a 46,XX/45,X mosaic karyotype. Abnormalities in the shape of the skull, scoliosis, limb defects, and spacing of the nipples can be found in association with amenorrhea.

When the vital signs are obtained, be aware that hypertension in an adolescent with delayed sexual maturation is associated with the enzyme defect, 17α-hydroxylase deficiency. Hormonal studies are required to establish this diagnosis, but the finding of hypertension makes this a likely cause of sexual infantilism and amenorrhea.

Abnormalities of specific cranial nerves are associated with conditions of amenorrhea. The history of poorly developed senses of taste and smell, and the physical finding of anosmia or hyposmia is a clue to the condition of Kallman syndrome (DeMosier syndrome in women). This will be described in more detail. A history of high frequency hearing loss or dysfunction is associated with partial deletion of the long-arm (q) of one X-chromosome. In this condition, there is premature ovarian failure which may present as complete lack of secondary sexual characteristics with amenorrhea, partial secondary sexual development with amenorrhea, or the establishment of complete secondary sexual maturation with ovulation and secondary amenorrhea due to premature ovarian failure. A history of visual field disturbances can be associated with pituitary adenomas or other benign tumors which impinge on the optic chiasma. In patients with prolactin secreting pituitary adenomas, amenorrhea may be secondary; in patients with hamartomas or craniopharyngiomas, amenorrhea may be primary. In patients with visual field disturbances, the presenting symptom may be difficulty driving an automobile. Severe visual field defects may be detected by gross evaluation of visual fields; subtle visual field defects must be elicited by special visual field testing.

Changes in the integument may give clues to the etiology of amenorrhea. Young women with acne and hirsutism likely have an underlying androgen excess disorder.

Women with absence of sexual hair or sparse sexual hair and presence of breast development may have a 46,XY chromosomal karyotype with a deficiency of androgen receptors. Hypopigmented skin can be associated with pituitary failure or adrenal gland failure; vitiligo (patchy areas of depigmented skin) may be associated with immunologic ovarian failure. Hyperpigmented skin can be associated with cortisol excess when the adrenal glands are hyperstimulated by excess adrenocorticotrophic hormone. Sallow skin color can be found in young women with chronic diseases while skin with a yellow cast may be associated with anorexia nervosa. Acanthosis nigricans is found in areas of skin folds (on the posterior neck, between the breasts, in the intertriginous areas of the thighs, and on the elbows and knees). The finding of acanthosis nigricans is associated with androgen excess and insulin-resistant diabetes mellitus.

The thyroid gland must be palpated as a routine in evaluation of young women with amenorrhea. Both hypothyroidism and hyperthyroidism can present with amenorrhea as a feature. It is difficult to differentiate these two conditions on the basis of the consistency of the thyroid gland alone. However, in hyperthyroidism, the gland may be pulsatile and elicit bruits to auscultation. In thyroiditis, the thyroid gland may be tender to palpation. Thyroiditis can be associated with immunologic premature ovarian failure.

Breast examination is essential to understanding the causes of amenorrhea. Breast development is dependent upon estrogen production and progesterone production. Estrogens stimulate the ductal elements of breasts, whereas progesterone stimulates the acinar elements of the breasts. Estrogens alone produce tubular appearing breasts; progesterone produces rounding of the breasts. A deficiency in estrogen exposure causes breast underdevelopment. Truncated or delayed breast development is often found in adolescent women with premature ovarian failure, failure of breast development is often found in women with hypothalamic-pituitary dysfunction. The physical characteristics of the nipples and areola provide clues to the hormonal environment to which they have been exposed. The nipples and areola are rich in estrogen receptors; conditions of estrogen excess lead to protuberance of the nipples and areola while conditions of estrogen deficiency lead to small, pale nipples and areola. This is especially seen in anorexia nervosa.

Few abnormalities of the heart and lungs coexist with conditions of amenorrhea. Adolescent women with Turner syndrome may have coarctation of the aorta with its characteristic auscultatory changes. However, this diagnosis is obvious from other physical findings.

On abdominal examination, pay particular attention to the inguinal canals. Inguinal hernia in an adolescent female may be a clue to the diagnosis of androgen insensitivity syndrome.

Examination of the external and internal genitalia is essential to evaluate amenorrhea. Is pubic hair present? Absence of pubic hair with breast development is found in androgen insensitivity syndrome. If pubic hair is excessive and the clitoris is enlarged, then there is usually an androgen excess condition. In the androgen insensitivity syndrome, the external genitalia appear female. Yet, on careful inspection, the labia majora and labia minora are hypoplastic. In conditions of estrogen deficiency, the vaginal mucosa is pale, thin, dry, and lacks rugation. In conditions of estrogen excess, the vaginal mucosa is pink, thick, moist, and has full rugation. The cervical mucous is absent in conditions of estrogen deficiency; the cervical mucous is abundant in conditions of estrogen excess.

In genital tract anomalies, the hymen may appear imperforate. When imperforate hymen is the cause of amenorrhea, the hymen will be bulging. When the vagina (and usually the uterus) is absent, the hymen will be flat. This is an important point for clinical differentiation.

The remainder of the physical examination has few correlative findings.

Laboratory Evaluation of Amenorrhea

The physician should quickly establish the role of the hypothalamus, pituitary gland, and the ovaries in conditions of amenorrhea. The best method to isolate the roles of these glands is to measure FSH and LH. If the problem is hypothalamic-pituitary dysfunction, FSH and LH will be in the low range; if the problem is ovarian failure, FSH and LH will be in the menopausal range. Adolescent women with ovarian failure who have never been exposed to estrogens will not have hot flushes, and adolescent women with hypothalamic-pituitary dysfunction will not have hot flushes. Therefore, this is not necessarily a useful clinical clue in differentiating between these causes of amenorrhea.

Some authors (14) recommend a progestin challenge test as the first step in the diagnostic evaluation of amenorrhea. The response to the progestin challenge test is dependent on previous estrogen exposure by the endometrium. If the endometrium has been stimulated previously by estrogen, the administration of progestins will produce a withdrawal bleed by the endometrium. However, if the endometrium has not been previously exposed to estrogen prior to progestin administration, there will be no withdrawal bleed. The progestin challenge test provides information only about previous endometrial estrogen exposure. The knowledgeable clinician can predict the response to the progestin challenge test by evaluating the cervical mucous. If the mucous is abundant, thin, clear, and watery, there will be a positive response to progestin withdrawal. On the other hand, if the cervical mucus is scant, the progestin challenge test will be negative.

Prolactin measurement should be a routine part of the laboratory evaluation of amenorrhea. Hyperprolactinemia, in the absence of galactorrhea, can exist as the cause of amenorrhea. In conditions of hyperprolactinemia, FSH and LH are suppressed from providing an adequate signal to stimulate ovarian function.

Primary hypothyroidism is a rare cause of adolescent amenorrhea. In this condition, there may be hyperprolactinemia. I do not obtain thyroid function studies (TSH, T3, T4) as a routine part of the evaluation of amenorrhea.

If there is clinical evidence of androgen excess (hirsutism, excessive acne, anatomical alterations of the genitalia), then androstenedione, testosterone, and dehydroepiandrosterone sulfate should be obtained as a part of the initial laboratory evaluation.

Imaging studies, chromosomal studies, and stimulation studies should be reserved until the initial studies have been obtained and interpreted. The rush to be complete at time of initial evaluation may cause the physician to order expensive, irrelevant tests.

If the adolescent woman with amenorrhea has hypogonadotropic hypogonadism (low FSH and LH) or hyperprolactinemia, it is appropriate to follow up with a lateral skull film to evaluate the sella turcica and suprasellar area of the skull. Lesions such as craniopharyngioma, hamartoma, and prolactin-secreting pituitary adenomas may produce abnormal calcification of the suprasellar region or erosion of the sella turcica on lateral skull film. If these lesions are still suspected despite a normal lateral skull film, the next study obtained should be a magnetic resonance image of the hypothalamic-pituitary area of the brain.

Chromosomal studies should be obtained in adolescent women with premature ovarian failure and in adolescent women who are suspected of having an intersex problem. Particular attention should be paid to the X chromosomes. Deletion of a fragment of the long arm of one X chromosome can result in premature ovarian failure with resultant amenorrhea. The presence of a Y chromosome in a person raised as a female denotes an intersex problem.

It is difficult for the clinician to distinguish hypothalamic dysfunction from pituitary dysfunction when the differential diagnosis has placed the cause of amenorrhea in this area. The differential diagnosis can be further elucidated by the intravenous injection of a bolus of GnRH (100 μg) and measuring FSH and LH at 10-min intervals for 60 min. In conditions of hypothalamic dysfunction, there will be a rise in FSH and LH; in conditions of pituitary dysfunction, FSH and LH will remain at the basal level. This test is rarely indicated in the evaluation of amenorrhea.

CAUSES OF AMENORRHEA

Hypothalamic-Pituitary Dysfunction

Hypothalamic-pituitary dysfunction occurs with increasing frequency as a cause of primary and secondary amenorrhea (15). The gonadotropin signals from the pituitary gland are inadequate to produce follicular maturation with subsequent sex-steroid hormone secretion. The causes of hypothalamic-pituitary dysfunction are presented in Table 3.

TABLE 3. *Hypothalamic-pituitary dysfunction*

Functional causes
Low body weight
Exercise-induced amenorrhea
Marijuana-induced amenorrhea
Stress
Pituitary failure (primary and secondary)
Isolated GnRH deficiency
Sheehan syndrome
Kallman syndrome
Neoplastic disorders
Craniopharyngioma
Pituitary prolactinoma

Kallman syndrome is a condition of hypoplasia of the olfactory tracts with coexisting dysfunction of the arcuate nucleus of the hypothalamus (16). The hypothalamus cannot secrete GnRH. Because of the olfactory tract hypoplasia, the patient cannot smell and has an absent or poorly developed sense of taste. In this condition, there is little or no secondary sexual development. The diagnosis can be made in the ambulatory setting by challenging the patient to recognize common odors such as coffee, rubbing alcohol, or ether. A young woman with Kallman syndrome is presented in Fig. 3A-B.

Sheehan syndrome is rare in adolescent women. This condition occurs when the pituitary gland sustains infarction and loses the ability to secrete pituitary tropic hormones (17). In addition to ovarian dysfunction, thyroid and adrenal dysfunction usually exist as well. Pituitary infarction is most likely to occur in association with obstetrical hemorrhage leading to shock.

Craniopharyngioma is a benign neoplasm located between the hypothalamus and pituitary gland that interferes with portal blood flow between the hypothalamus and pituitary gland (18). This diagnosis is suspected by the finding of calcification in the area described on lateral skull film (Fig. 4). Follow-up evaluation is made by magnetic resonance imaging. Secondary sexual development can be initiated and completed by the administration of exogenous sex-steroid hormones and ovulation can be induced by the administration of human menopausal gonadotropin (hMG) when pregnancy is desired. Since the tumor must be removed surgically, the physician must proceed with caution in advising surgery. Unless the patient is suffering from chronic, debilitating headache, surgical removal may not be necessary.

Isolated gonadotropin deficiency is a rare condition, similar to Kallman syndrome, in which the hypothalamus does not secrete GnRH. It may be a variant of Kallman syn-

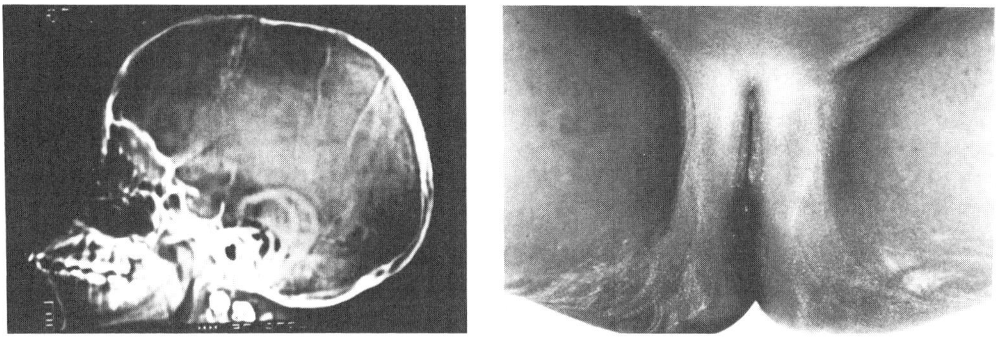
A B

FIG. 3. An example of craniopharyngioma in a 17-year-old adolescent girl with sexual infantilism. **A:** The lateral skull film demonstrates a suprasellar calcification with enlargement of the sella turcica. **B:** The perineum shows lack of secondary sexual development.

drome. The diagnosis is made by priming the pituitary gland with exogenous estrogens, and injecting later a bolus of GnRH. A person with this disorder will respond by secreting FSH and LH from the pituitary gland. Isolated gonadotropin deficiency presents as sexual infantilism. There is usually no breast development and only sparse pubic hair.

Low body weight, exercise-induced amenorrhea, and stress-induced amenorrhea can be grouped together because the pathophysiology is similar (19–21). In each of these conditions there is interference with the pulsatile release of GnRH—both amplitude and pulse frequency are altered—such that gonadotropin release from the pituitary gland does not adequately stimulate follicular development. There are varying degrees of ovarian dysfunction in these dis-

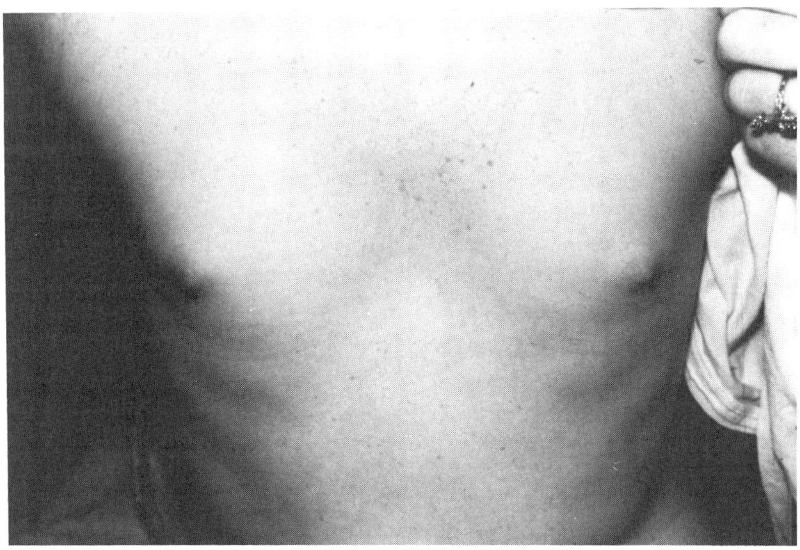

FIG. 4. A 19-year-old woman with Kallmann syndrome. Note the lack of breast development due to no ovarian secretion of estradiol.

orders ranging from a short luteal phase of an ovulatory reproductive cycle to amenorrhea. The mechanism(s) for these alterations are poorly understood. When low body weight, exercise induced amenorrhea, or stress-induced amenorrhea is suspected, the adolescent woman should be counseled to change behavior or alter coping skills in order to restore cyclic reproductive function.

Problems with low body weight are seen with increasing frequency in clinical practice. Young women should be encouraged to attain and maintain their ideal body weight.

Marijuana use is widespread in modern society. Marijuana finds its way into high schools and junior high schools, so it cannot be assumed that adolescent women with amenorrhea, delayed sexual development, or incomplete sexual development do not use the drug. Marijuana blocks release of GnRH. Thus, gonadotropin stimulation of the ovaries (and testicles in adolescent men) is truncated or absent. The effects of marijuana on reproductive function are self-limiting. When drug use is discontinued, cyclic reproductive function is restored (13).

Hyperprolactinemia rarely is associated with delayed sexual maturation and primary amenorrhea, but must be considered in the adolescent with secondary amenorrhea (22). Galactorrhea may or may not be a clinical finding. The diagnosis is established by the finding of prolactin excess in plasma. If the plasma prolactin exceeds 100 ng/ml, imaging studies of the sella turcica are warranted. An example of a pituitary microadenoma demonstrated by magnetic resonance imaging is presented in Fig. 5.

Treatment of hypothalamic-pituitary dysfunction must be directed to the underlying cause. Women with Kallman syndrome, craniopharyngioma, Sheehan syndrome, and isolated gonadotropin deficiency, require exogenous hormone replacement to establish secondary sexual development (if it has failed to occur) and will require replacement with pulsatile GnRH or ovarian stimulation with hMG to induce ovulation for the purpose becoming pregnant.

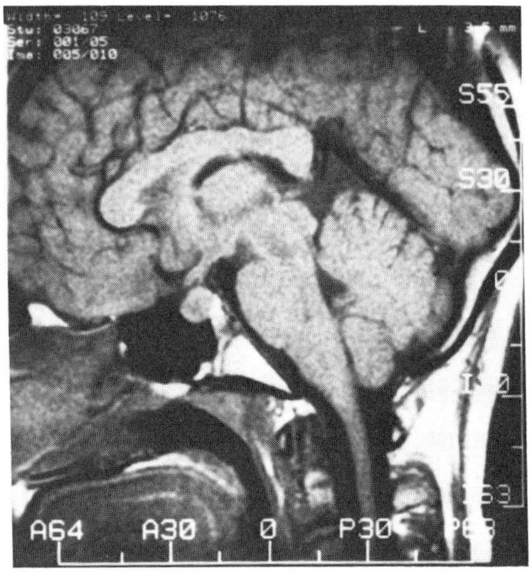

FIG. 5. A weighted MRI scan of the sella turcica reveals a 1-cm lesion in the mid-pituitary gland that is consistent with a prolactin secreting pituitary adenoma. This study was performed on a 17-year-old girl with secondary amenorrhea.

Women with low body weight, exercise-induced amenorrhea, and stress-induced amenorrhea will have spontaneous resumption of hypothalamic-pituitary function when they change behavior and lifestyle. The problem is self-limiting. However, it is often difficult to convince adolescent women and their parents that lifestyle and behavior can produce hypothalamic-pituitary dysfunction and be the cause of amenorrhea. Women with these conditions are at risk for the development of osteoporosis. Women with excercise-induced amenorrhea—especially ballerinas, competitive runners, and gymnasts—are at increased risk for fractures of the vertebral column and calcaneus (23,24). Consideration must be given to exogenous estrogen replacement for protection from osteoporosis. Yet, the underlying causes cannot be allowed to go ignored.

Marijuana-induced amenorrhea is self limiting and is reversed promptly after drug use is discontinued. It is the skillful physician who can elicit the history of marijuana use and counsel the adolescent to stop the practice of drug use.

Ovarian Failure

Ovarian failure in adolescents is most commonly the result of chromosomal deletions, especially deletions of the X-chromosome or fragments of the long-arm of the X-chromosome. Less common causes of ovarian failure in adolescents result from the toxic effects of alkylating chemotherapy on the ovarian follicular membranes when administered for the treatment of childhood and adolescent neoplasms, and the rare gonadotropin-resistant ovary syndrome (Savage syndrome). These conditions will be discussed in this section.

Turner's syndrome (45X gonadal dysgenesis) is the most frequent cause of premature ovarian failure (25). The defect results from the absence of one of the two X-chromosomes. The short arm of the X-chromosome (designated p) carries somatic information necessary for full adult height, development of the skeletal system, and cardiovascular system. The long-arm of the X-chromosome (designated q) carries information necessary for maintenance of the ovarian follicles in an arrested state for future for subsequent maturation and ovulation. In Turner's syndrome the absence of an X-chromosome causes both skeletal abnormalities and premature atresia of ovarian follicles. At birth, girls with Turner syndrome have characteristic physical findings of lymphedema, shield chest, and cubitus valgus (increased carrying angle of the arms). Most have ovarian failure at birth. The oocytes which normally migrate to the ovarian stroma by midgestation do migrate in girls with Turner's syndrome. However, these oocyte—due to lack of the long-arm of the X-chromosome—undergo atresia prior to birth. Gonadotropin are in the menopausal range at birth. The physical characteristics that distinguish Turner's syndrome are recognized prior to puberty. Therefore, the failure to undergo secondary sexual maturation can be anticipated, and exogenous hormone administration initiated at the appropriate time to prevent embarrassing delay in breast development and sexual hair growth. Since short stature is a feature of Turner's syndrome, estrogen administration must be initiated at a low dosage level of avoid premature epiphyseal closure. By giving estradiol-17 at a rate of 0.5 mg/day for 6–9 months before increasing the dosage to one larger to stimulate breast development, maximal height can be attained.

Other X-chromosomal disorders include the mosaic Turner's syndrome (45,X/46,XX karyotype) where some of the cell lines have a normal chromosomal complement. In the mosaic Turner's syndrome, there may be partial or even full secondary sexual maturation before ovarian failure occurs. There are some case reports of pregnancy in women with mosaic Turner's syndrome. In the mosaic Turner's syndrome, women are usually short of stature but not as short as Turner's syndrome.

A variant of the Turner's syndrome is Sweyer's syndrome (46,XY karyotype). These individuals have female external and internal genitalia. The testicles are dysgenetic during embryogenesis resulting in failure to secrete Müllerian duct inhibiting factor and testosterone. At birth, the sexual assignment is female. At the expected time of puberty, there is no secondary sexual development which leads to the diagnosis. When the diagnosis is established, the dysgenetic testicles should be removed because of the high incidence (>25%) of developing gonadoblastoma. Management is otherwise the same as in other adolescent women with ovarian failure.

Long-arm deletion of the X-chromosome (46,XXq−) is a variant of gonadal failure where the extent of deletion of the long-arm of the X-chromosome determines the extent of the ovarian failure (26). If all of the long-arm is deleted, there will be ovarian failure at birth as in Turner's syndrome. On the other hand, if there is fragmentary deletion of the long-arm, then secondary sexual maturation may be complete. Pregnancies occur commonly in women with small fragmentary deletions.

Alkylating chemotherapy administered for childhood leukemia, lymphoma, and other childhood and adolescent neoplasms has a toxic effect on the follicular membrane of the ovarian follicles (27). Many young women and men have gonadal failure following several courses of alkylating chemotherapy.

Gonadotropin-resistant ovary syndrome is rare in adolescent women but is seen with increasing frequency in adult women (28). In this poorly understood disorder, the ovarian follicles are present within the ovarian stroma but do not bind FSH. Thus, FSH and LH are elevated in the menopausal range despite the presence of ovarian follicles. There is no known associated chromosomal abnormality with the gonadotropin-resistant ovary syndrome. The diagnosis is made by histologic confirmation of ovarian follicles within ovarian stroma. However, ovarian biopsy is not recommended as it can produce periovarian adhesion formation and compromise later reproduction. In the gonadotropin-resistant ovary syndrome, a number of case reports of pregnancy have appeared to women receiving exogenous estrogen replacement treatment.

The diagnosis of ovarian failure can be suspected when an adolescent woman complains of hot flushes. However, many do not have this complaint until they have first received exogenous estrogen replacement and had estrogen withdrawn. A combination of hypergonadotropic hypogonadism with estrogen exposure seems to be prerequisite for hot flushes.

Ovarian failure is treated by estrogen and progestin replacement. If left untreated, adolescent women with ovarian failure will develop early, profound osteoporosis. This can be prevented by timely administration of estrogen. Moreover, estrogen is necessary to stimulate breast development, facilitate sexual hair growth, stimulate uterine and endometrial growth, and initiate menses. After secondary sexual maturation has reached that compatible with an adolescent woman ready to establish cyclic ovulatory cycles, progesterone should be added to the hormone replacement regimen.

Ovarian failure formally carried a hopeless prognosis for pregnancy. With the advances in assisted reproductive technology, oocyte donation and embryo transfer open new vistas for adolescent women with ovarian failure and adult women with premature ovarian failure. This technology can be applied even in women with Sweyer's syndrome.

Anatomical Causes of Amenorrhea

The internal genital tract forms from the fusion and canalization of the Mullerian ducts during the first 8–12 weeks of fetal life. Failure of formation, fusion, and/or canalization of the Müllerian ducts, failure of canalization of the urogenital sinus will result in primary amenorrhea. Anatomical defects of the genital tract have no effect on ovarian function. Thus, in adolescent women with genital tract abnormalities, there will be no interference with secondary sexual maturation. In some adolescent women, ovulatory cycles may be established before the diagnosis of genital tract atresia or obstruction is made.

The most common anatomical defects of the genital tract are imperforate hymen and Müllerian agenesis (Rokitansky-Küster-Hauser syndrome) (29). The imperforate hymen presents with a history of cyclic pelvic pain and a bluish bulge at the perineum. These symptoms begin once cyclic menses are established. The diagnosis is simple to make.

Müllerian agenesis is most often painless

since the uterus and vagina are congenitally absent (Fig. 6). On rare occasion (10% of cases), the uterus will be present and the vagina absent. In this situation, the adolescent woman presents with cyclic abdominal pain and an abdominal mass. In total Müllerian agenesis, there is full secondary sexual maturation with cyclic ovulation (Fig. 7). Because menstruation has not occurred, the adolescent woman and her parents present for evaluation.

Treatment of the imperforate hymen requires only a simple hymenotomy. Treatment of vaginal agenesis is controversial. Some advocate pressure dilatation of the genital tract to create a vagina (Frank procedure and Ingram procedure), whereas others advocate the creation of a neovagina by transplanting a split-thickness skin graft from the hip to the vaginal space. The vaginal space is opened at the time the skin graft is taken, and the graft is placed around a vaginal prosthesis. After several months, the neovagina takes on the secretory characteristics of natural vaginal epithelium (30).

In the rare situation where the uterus is present, if the cervix is present, a neovagina can be surgically created and connected to the uterus. A recent report by Hampton et al. (31) describes such a case that resulted in a term birth of a healthy child.

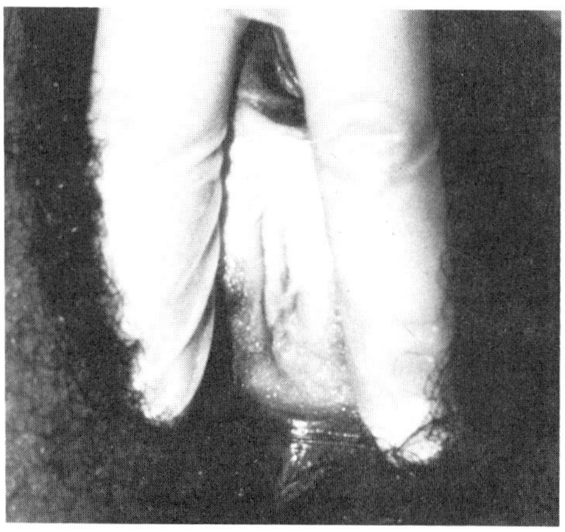

FIG. 6. Perineum in the patient in Fig. 7 with Mullerian agenesis.

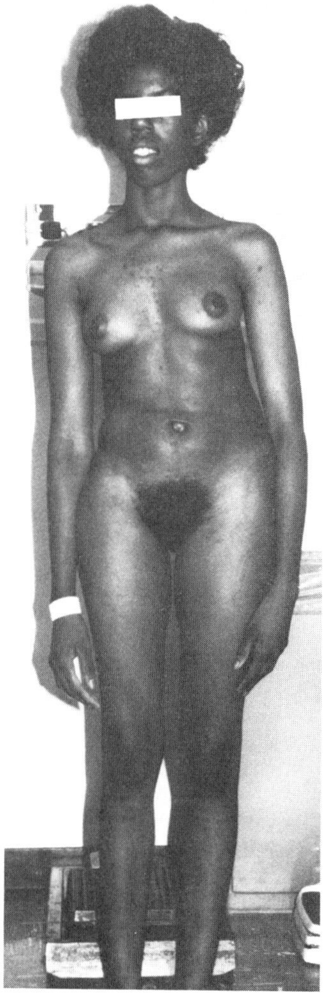

FIG. 7. A 16-year-old girl with primary amenorrhea due to Mullerian agenesis. Note the full secondary sexual maturation. Scoliosis occurs in about 25% of women with this disorder.

Intrauterine adhesions (Asherman syndrome) is usually an acquired condition which results following curettage of the endometrial cavity (32). Intrauterine adhesions have been reported in association with tuberculous endometritis. These are very rare occurrences in adolescent women.

Pregnancy

Pregnancy should always be considered in adolescent women with secondary amenorrhea. Pregnancy can occur prior to menarche but this is extremely rare. Early symptoms of pregnancy include breast fullness, morning sickness, chloasma, and a change in body habitus. Pregnancy is confirmed by positive hCG pregnancy test.

Intersex Problems

Male pseudohermaphrodites present with primary amenorrhea. There are other clues to the diagnosis of male pseudohermaphroditism in addition to amenorrhea.

Male pseudohermaphroditism results either from inadequate testosterone synthesis or inadequate testosterone action (33). If testosterone synthesis is absent (e.g., 17-αhydroxylase deficiency, 20,22-desmolase deficiency), there will be no secondary sexual development at the expected time. Physical examination will reveal absence of the uterus and vagina since the fetal testis secreted Mullerian duct inhibiting factor. If testosterone receptors are absent, there will be breast development but no sexual hair growth. Moreover, the uterus and usually the vagina will be absent. The absence of pubic hair and a vagina and uterus with the presence of breasts distinguishes Müllerian agenesis from androgen insensitivity syndrome (complete testicular feminization).

Incomplete male pseudohermaphroditism is likely to be suspected at birth because of genital ambiguity. In this condition there is either partial secretion of testosterone by the testicles during fetal life and at the time of puberty, or partial androgen receptor activity resulting in partial masculinization.

Male pseudohermaphrodites raised as females will require removal of the testicles due to the high risk of development of gonadoblastoma and will require exogenous estrogen replacement along with surgical reconstruction of the perineum and vagina.

Other Conditions

Polycystic ovarian disease and late-onset adrenal hyperplasia do not conveniently fit into the other classifications. These disorders do not often present as primary amenorrhea but may present to the physician as secondary amenorrhea (34).

Polycystic ovarian disease is characterized by a chronic state of estrus and a chronic state of androgen excess (35). The adolescent woman with polycystic ovarian disease will complain of irregular menses or amenorrhea associated with hirsutism and acne (Fig. 8). Obesity is a common feature. Hormonal evaluation reveals an increased LH:FSH ratio, elevated androstenedione, and testosterone at the upper limits of normal or slightly elevated.

The treatment of choice is to administer a combined estrogen-progestin oral contraceptive for indefinite duration to suppress the excess androgens being secreted by the ovaries. When pregnancy is desired, ovulation induction is usually required.

Late-onset adrenal hyperplasia (36) is another condition not uncommon to adolescence women that presents with irregular cycles or secondary amenorrhea. In the common form of this disorder, there is deficiency of the enzyme, 21-hydroxylase that catalyzes the conversion of progesterone to deoxycorticosterone. Due to this enzyme deficiency, there is an accumulation of adrenal androgens that produces acne, mild hirsutism, and menstrual irregularities (Fig. 9). In women who express this deficiency prior to the onset of puberty, sexual hair growth may precede breast development. This fact may be an important clue to the diagnosis.

Late-onset adrenal hyperplasia can be difficult to distinguish from polycystic ovarian disease. The clinical manifestations are

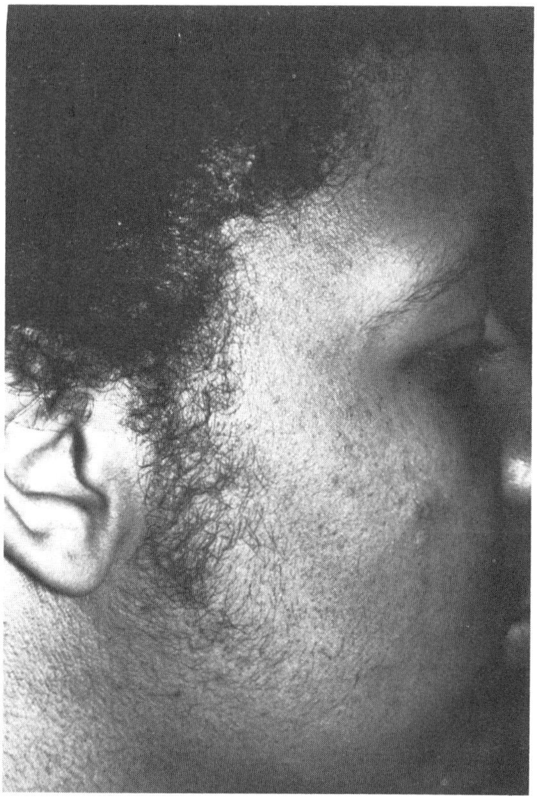

FIG. 8. A 17-year-old girl with polycystic ovarian disease. Note facial hair and acne due to excess androgens.

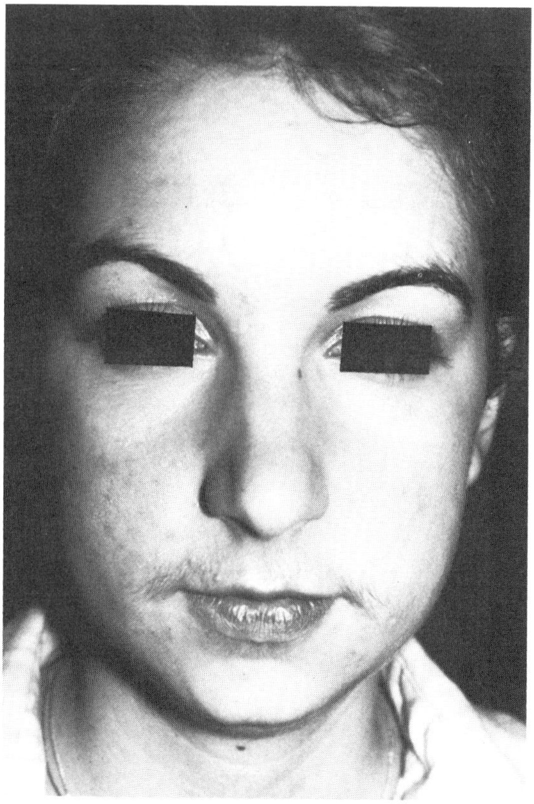

FIG. 9. Acne and hirsutism in an 18-year-old woman with late-onset adrenal hyperplasia. Her problem was resolved when she was placed on glucocorticoid replacement therapy.

similar. The differential diagnosis is established by the finding of an elevated dehydroepiandrosterone sulfate and an exaggerated response to the injection of a known amount of ACTH. Treatment for late-onset adrenal hyperplasia is the administration of small amounts of glucocorticoid (prednisone, 2.5 mg/day).

SUMMARY

Amenorrhea is a symptom of altered function of the hypothalamic-pituitary axis, the ovarian response to gonadotropins, the integrity of the genital outflow tract, or the mechanisms of sexual differentiation. The diagnosis of the etiology of amenorrhea should be based on an understanding on the physiology of puberty, the physiology of the female reproductive cycle, and the hormonal interactions between the hypothalamus, pituitary gland, and the ovaries. Physical examination should provide clues to the etiology. Laboratory studies should be held to a minimum to establish the etiology. A comprehensive laboratory evaluation should not be undertaken as a routine part of the evaluation. Rather, complex laboratory studies should be carefully selected based on initial history, physical findings, and initial laboratory studies. Treatment of amenorrhea should be directed to correct the underlying pathophysiology. Estrogen replacement is essential for adolescent women with ovarian failure, and may be warranted for those with hypothalamic-pituitary dysfunction.

REFERENCES

1. Marshall WA, Tanner JM. Variations in the pattern of pubertal changes in girls. *Arch Dis Child* 44;1969:291.
2. Boyar RM, Finkelstein JW, David R, et al. Twenty-four hour patterns of plasma lutinizing hormone and follicle stimulating hormone in sexual precocity. *N Engl J Med* 1973;289:282.
3. Katz J, Boyar RM, Finkelstein JW, et al. Weight and circadian luteinizing hormone secretory pattern in anorexia nervosa. *Psychosom Med* 1978;40:549.
4. Frisch RE, Revelle R. Height and weight at menarche and a hypothesis of critical weights and adolescent events. *Science* 1970;169:397.
5. Fishman J, Boyar RM, Hellman L. Influence of body weight gain on estradiol metabolism in young women. *J Clin Endocrinol Metab* 1975; 41:988.
6. Adashi EY, Rakoff J, Divers W, et al. The effect of acutely administered 2-hydroxyestrone on the release of gonadotropins and prolactin before and after estrogen priming in hypogonadal women. *Life Sci* 1979;25:2051.
7. Marshall JC, Odell WD. The menstrual cycle—Hormonal regulation, mechanisms of anovulation, and responses of the reproductive tract to steroid hormones. In: DeGroot LJ, ed. *Endocrinology*. Philadelphia: W.B. Saunders, 1989:1940.
8. Abraham GE, Odell WD, Swerdloff RS, et al. Simultaneous radioimmunoassay of plasma FSH, LH, progesterone, 17-hydroxyprogesterone and estradiol-17 during the menstrual cycle. *J Clin Endocrinol Metab* 1972;34:312.
9. Knobil E, Plant TM, Wildt L, Belchetz PE, Marshall G. Control of the rhesus monkey menstrual cycle: permissive role of the hypothalamic gonadotropin-releasing hormone. *Science* 1980; 207:1371.
10. Bates GW, Garza DE, Garza MM. Clinical manifestations of hormonal changes in the menstrual cycle. *Obstet Gynecol Clin North Am* 1990; 17:289.
11. Neinstein LS. Menstrual problems in adolescents. *Med Clin North Am* 1990;74:1181.
12. Bates GW. Disorders of puberty. *Contemporary Ob/Gyn* 1982;19:165.
13. Asch RH, Smith GC, Siler-Khodr TM, Pauerstein CJ. Effects of δ^9-tetrahydrocannabinol during the follicular phase of the Rhesus monkey (*Macaca mulatta*). *J Clin Endocrinol Metab* 1981;52:50.
14. Speroff L, Glass RH, Kase NG. *Clinical gynecologic endocrinology and infertility*. 4th ed. Baltimore: Williams & Wilkins, 1989:171.
15. Vigersky JRA, Anderson AE, Thompson RH et al. Hypothalamic dysfunction in secondary amenorrhea associated with simple weight loss. *N Engl J Med* 1977;297:1141.
16. Kallmann FJ, Schoenfeld WA, Barrera SE. The genetic aspects of primary eunuchoidism. *Am J Ment Defic* 1944;48:203.
17. Sheehan HL. Simmonds's disease due to postpartum necrosis of the anterior pituitary. *Q J Med* 1940;32:277.
18. Banna M, Hoare RD, Stanley P, Till K. Craniopharyngioma in children. *J Pediatr* 1980;83:781.
19. Bates GW. The hypothalamus. In: Aiman EJ, ed. *Infertility: diagnosis and management*. New York: Springer-Verlag, 1984:31.
20. Warren MP. The effect of exercise on pubertal progression and reproductive function in girls. *J Clin Endocrinol Metab* 1980;51:1150.
21. Axelrod J, Reisine TD. Stress hormones: their

interaction and regulation. *Science* 1984; 224: 452.
22. Quigley ME, Judd SJ, Gilliland GB, Yen SSC. Functional studies of dopamine control of prolactin secretion in normal women and women with hyperprolactinemic pituitary microadenoma. *J Clin Endocrinol Metab* 1980;50:994.
23. Warren MP, Brooks-Gunn J, Hamilton LH, Warren LF, Hamilton WG. Scoliosis and fractures in young ballet dancers. Relation to delayed menarche and secondary amenorrhea. *N Engl J Med* 1986;314:1348.
24. Drinkwater BL, Nilson K, Ott S, Chesnutt CH. Bone mineral density after resumption of menses in amenorrheic athletes. *JAMA* 1986;256: 380.
25. Turner HH. A syndrome of infantilism, congenital webbed neck, and cubitus valgus. *Endocrinology* 1938;23:566.
26. Krauss CM, Turksoy RN, Atkins L, McLaughlin C, Brown LG, Page DC. Familial premature ovarian failure due to an interstitial deletion of the long arm of the X chromosome. *N Engl J Med* 1987;317:125.
27. Siris ES, Leventhal BG, Vaitukiatis JL. Effects of childhood leukemia and chemotherapy on puberty and reproductive function in girls. *N Engl J Med* 1976;294:1143.
28. Aiman J, Smentek C. Premature ovarian failure. *Obstet Gynecol* 1985;66:9.
29. Griffin JE, Edwards C, Madden JD, Harrod MJ Wilson JD. Congenital absence of the vagina. The Mayer-Rokitansky-Kuster-Hauser syndrome. *Ann Intern Med* 1976;85:224.
30. Wiser WL, Bates GW. Surgical management of vaginal agenesis. A review of 92 cases. *Surg Gynecol Obstet* 1984;159:108.
31. Hampton HL, Meeks GR, Bates GW, Wiser WL. Pregnancy after successful vaginoplasty and cervical stenting for partial atresia of the cervix. *Obstet Gynecol* 1990;76(S):900.
32. Asherman JG. Amenorrhoea traumatica (Atretica). *J Obstet Gynecol Br Emp* 1948;55:23.
33. Bates GW, Wiser WL. Problems of sexual differentiation: Diagnosis and management. *Urol Ann* 1988;2:21.
34. Bates GW. Hirsutism and androgen excess in childhood and adolescence. *Pediatr Clin North Am* 1983;28:513.
35. Rebar RW. Hirsutism, hyperandrogenism, and polycystic ovarian syndrome. In: DeGroot LJ, ed. *Endocrinology*. Philadelphia: W.B. Saunders, 1989:1982.
36. White PC, New MI, Dupont B. Congenital adrenal hyperplasia. *N Engl J Med* 1987;316:1519.

Pediatric and Adolescent Gynecology,
edited by S. E. Carpenter and J. A. Rock.
Raven Press, Ltd., New York © 1992.

14

Abnormal Uterine Bleeding

Donald E. Pittaway and Jeffrey L. Deaton

Department of Obstetrics and Gynecology, Section on Reproductive Endocrinology, Bowman Gray School of Medicine, Winston-Salem, North Carolina 27157

Abnormal vaginal bleeding is a presenting complaint for many gynecologic and nongynecologic conditions, and is a common problem encountered by physicians providing health care for adolescents. Possible etiologies include (a) organic causes such as pregnancy complications, infections, trauma, cancer lesions and tumors of the genital tract, blood dyscrasias, and endocrine and systemic disorders; (b) abnormal consequences of contraceptive methods such as oral contraceptives and intrauterine devices; and (c) dysfunctional uterine bleeding (DUB), which refers to abnormal uterine bleeding for which no demonstrable organic cause can be found.

In the adolescent, DUB is the most common cause of abnormal bleeding, comprising about 48–97% of the causes (1–4). The underlying problem is anovulation or oligoovulation with the maturational process of the hypothalamic-pituitary-ovarian (H-P-O) axis often taking 2–5 years to complete (5–7). Menarche, which occurs at an average age of 12.8 years in the United States, is an anovulatory bleeding episode, and as many as 82% of the cycles in the first postmenarcheal year (5,6) and up to 28% of the cycles in the fifth postmenarcheal year are anovulatory (6). However, most adolescents having irregular bleeding in the first and second postmenarcheal year do not require long-term management (2,8). Yet, when irregular bleeding persists after 4 years from the onset of bleeding, serious gynecologic sequelae such as problematic uterine bleeding, reduced fertility potential, and a high rate (1.3%) of endometrial cancer in women under 40 years of age were observed (8).

Normal variations in bleeding patterns are important to understand in order to establish when to consider the bleeding as abnormal. The mean amount of blood loss in a normal cycle is about 35 ml (range, 20–60 ml). Chronic blood loss of >80 ml/cycle results in a high frequency of iron deficiency anemia (9). Outside of research protocols, estimating the amount of blood loss is difficult at best, and frequently the perception of how much blood has been lost is not reliable (10). Even using estimates based on

TABLE 1. *Classification of abnormal uterine bleeding in the adolescent*

Menorrhagia (Hypermenorrhea): Excessive uterine bleeding in either the amount or the duration of flow, which occurs at the normal intervals of regular menses. Etiologies may include blood dyscrasias, endometrial polyps, hypothyroidism, chronic endometritis, or submucus myoma.

Polymenorrhea: Regular episodes of uterine bleeding occurring at intervals of <24 days due to either a proliferative phase of <10 days or a secretory phase of <12 days. Endocrine, systemic or metabolic disorders, or psychogenic causes may be found.

Metrorrhagia: Uterine bleeding occurring at irregular intervals, which may range from spotting to a normal menstrual-like flow. Some causes include anovulation, oligoovulation, blood dyscrasias, complications of pregnancy, breakthrough bleeding with oral contraceptives, benign or malignant pelvic conditions, and thyroid disorders.

Menometrorrhagia: Irregular and frequent bleeding, which may be excessive in amount and/or prolonged induration. Causes are similar to metrorrhagia.

Oligomenorrhea: Irregular bleeding episodes occurring at intervals of >42 days. The most frequent causes are anovulation, recurrent functional ovarian cysts, and pregnancy.

Intermenstrual Bleeding: Episodes of uterine bleeding occurring between regular menstrual periods. Ovulatory dysfunctional uterine bleeding, and benign or malignant pelvic conditions are frequent causes.

Postcoital Bleeding: Bleeding occurring after sexual intercourse, which frequently indicates a cervical problem such as cervicitis, eversion, erosion, polyp, or cancer.

Hypomenorrhea: Decreased amount of uterine bleeding occurring at regular intervals. Causes include premature ovarian failure, cervical stenosis, intrauterine adhesions (Asherman's syndrome), and endocrine and oral contraceptive effects.

the number of well-soaked regular perineal pads such as eight or the number of tampons such as 12 as upper limits of normal may not correlate with actual blood loss when pads and tampons are frequently changed or blood clots are present (10). The duration of flow averages 3–7 days with >7 days considered prolonged. The frequency of bleeding occurs between 24 and 36 days in normal cycles. However, cycle lengths as short as 21 days and as long as 40 days may be normal. In general, an adolescent's established menstrual pattern can serve as a reference to determine how the problematic bleeding differs from her "normal" menstrual flow, but in the absence of previously regular menstrual bleeding, these values may be used as guidelines.

Bleeding abnormalities may be classified according to the amount of flow, the duration of flow, and the regularity or interval between bleeding episodes. Certain descriptive terms such as "menorrhagia" (hypermenorrhea), "metrorrhagia," and "menometrorrhagia" may be used to classify the types of bleeding and assist in establishing a differential diagnosis. These terms and others are defined in Table 1, and some of the possible etiologic conditions are included. With the inherent difficulties in assessing irregular bleeding in the adolescent, and the numerous organic causes that must be excluded before DUB can be designated as the etiology, the health care provider is faced with a significant diagnostic challenge. In addition, the physician must be aware of both the treatment options in order to individualize the management as well as the potential psychoemotional impact of the problem on the adolescent and her parents.

MENSTRUAL CYCLE

Before one can understand the abnormalities of the adolescent cycle, a thorough understanding of the normal cycle is needed. Except for the extremes of reproductive life, the menstrual cycle has a median duration of 28 days due to a 14-day follicular phase and a 14-day luteal phase (11). The cyclic expression of the H-P-O axis leads to functional and structural changes in several target tissues, particularly the endometrium. In the absence of a conception, the demise of the corpus luteum leads to the withdrawal of ovarian steroids from the endometrium, which in turn leads to an orderly withdrawal menses. Any aberration in this orderly sequence of events can lead to asychronous development and shedding of the endometrium with subsequent abnormal uterine bleeding.

The actual event that is responsible for the initiation of puberty and subsequent maturation of the hypothalamus is unknown. Prior to the onset of puberty, insufficient hypothalamic gonadotropin-releasing hormone (GnRH) stimulation to the pituitary causes low gonadotropin levels and subsequent absent follicular development (7). As the hypothalamus begins to mature, sleep-induced LH pulses are seen which disappear after puberty (12,13). In early adolescence, follicular recruitment and episodic estrogen secretion leads to development of the endometrium, but this is often followed by an inability of the immature hypothalamus to respond with an LH surge (14). This leads to the frequent occurrence of anovulation and dysfunctional uterine bleeding, as described below.

The human menstrual cycle can be divided into three distinct phases. The follicular phase, which probably begins in the preceding luteal phase, is characterized by the selection of a dominant follicle and growth of the endometrium under the influence of estrogen. The ovulatory phase, which begins with the onset of the luteinizing surge, is characterized by a dramatic switch from estrogen to progesterone production and final release of the oocyte. The luteal phase, which lasts 13–14 days after ovulation, is characterized by preparation of the endometrium for implantation under the influence of the corpus luteum. The H-P-O axis and the endometrial changes for each phase will be described in the following section. The hormone pattern of the adult human menstrual cycle is shown in Figs. 1 and 2.

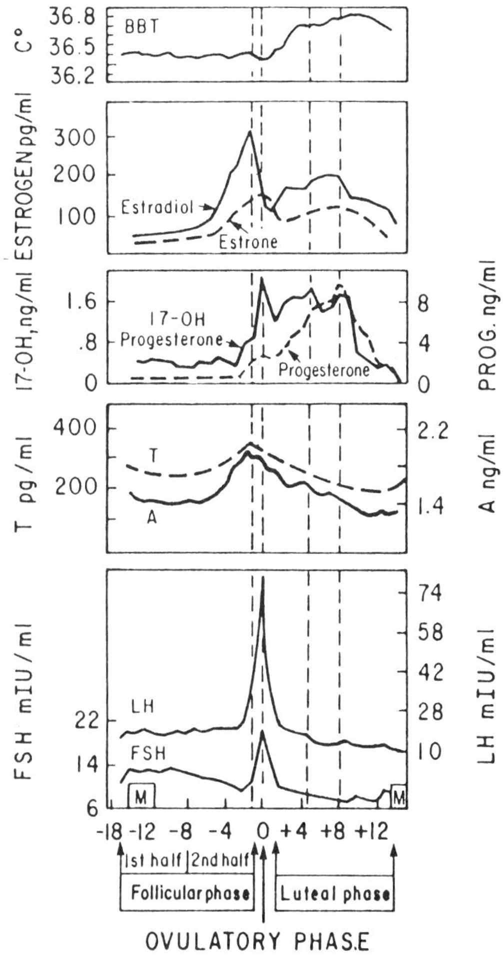

FIG. 1. The cyclic hormone pattern of the adult human menstrual cycle centered on the day of the LH peak (day 0). Basal body temperatures (BBT) are shown on the top, ovarian steroids are shown in the center, and gonadotropin levels are shown on the bottom. (From ref. 32, with permission.)

Follicular Phase

Hypothalamic-Pituitary-Ovarian Axis

Knobil has shown that gonadotropin output by the pituitary is directly controlled by the GnRH pulse generator located in the arcuate nucleus of the hypothalamus (15). Administration of a GnRH agonist leads to rapid pituitary gonadotropin suppression which is quickly reversed upon discontinuation of the drug (16). In the absence of either implantation or exogenous hCG, there is demise of the corpus luteum followed by a fall in serum progesterone. This declining steroid output by the ovary causes an alteration in the GnRH pulse generator, leading to more frequent pulses of

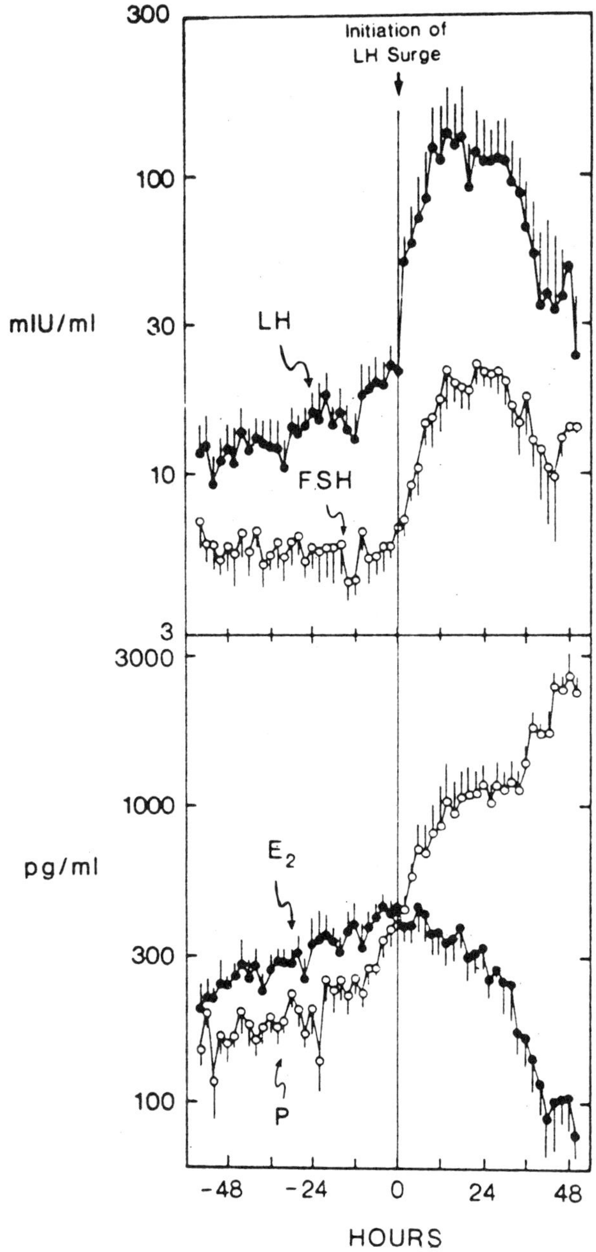

FIG. 2. Mean (±) luteinizing hormone, follicle stimulating hormone, estradiol, and progesterone levels measured every 2 hr for 5 days at midcycle in seven studies. Data are centered around the initiation of the gonadotropin surge. Note that the hormone concentrations are plotted on a logarithmic scale. (From ref. 29, with permission.)

GnRH. Falling serum steroid levels combined with a change in the pulse generator causes a rise in pituitary FSH output, which can be detected 1–2 days before menses (17). It is this rise in serum FSH that is believed to initiate the subsequent follicular phase.

The first half of the follicular phase is marked by selection of the dominant follicle. At the start of each cycle, there exists a cohort of follicles destined for either atresia or ovulation (18). During the early follicular phase, all follicles show growth up to 10 mm; however, after selection of the dominant follicle, the remaining follicles show a decrease in size (19). The selection of the dominant follicle is dependent on both its microenvironment and its capacity for estrogen synthesis (20).

Although LH has multiple target sites, FSH appears to act only on the granulosa cells. Prior to selection of the dominant follicle, increasing levels of FSH causes an increase in the number of FSH receptors and induces granulosa cells to convert androgens to estrogens via an aromatizing enzyme (21). These two actions lead to an increase in estrogen within the follicle. Estrogen is then able to increase the number of its own receptors. The follicle that is best able to utilize this synergistic relationship between FSH and estrogen is destined to change from an androgenic microenvironment to an estrogenic microenvironment and thus selection as the dominant follicle.

Once the dominant follicle has been selected (day 7), the next half of the follicular phase is marked by growth of the dominant follicle and preparation for ovulation. Declining serum levels of FSH, probably secondary to inhibin production from the dominant follicle (22,23), leads to a withdrawal of support from the secondary follicles. This ensures that only one oocyte will be ovulated each cycle. During the early part of the cycle, FSH has no effect on LH receptors. However, after exposure to increasing levels of estrogen, there is induction of LH receptors in the granulosa cells of the dominant follicle. Although LH stimulation of the theca interna is responsible for androgen production (which is subsequently aromatized to estrogen in the dominant follicle), it is the appearance of LH receptors in the granulosa cells that is responsible for subsequent progesterone production (24,25).

Endometrium

The anatomic changes that occur in the endometrium in response to ovarian steroids has been extensively studied in the human (26). The early follicular phase endometrium (i.e., menstrual endometrium) is marked by tissue breakdown in the form of necrosis, white cell infiltration, and glandular disruption. It is composed primarily of a nonfunctioning basalis component, which is left after the majority of the endometrium has sloughed. If the breakdown is secondary to a programmed withdrawal of progesterone, then the loss is orderly and complete and occurs in all segments of the endometrium.

Once estrogen levels start to rise in response to follicular recruitment, the process of growth and healing begins in the endometrium. The two structures that respond dramatically to the estrogen are the glands and spiral arterioles. During the next several days, the endometrium will grow from 0.5 up to 5 mm due to an increase in the number and size of the glands. In stimulated cycles, the number of glands is positively correlated to the serum estrogen level (27). The glandular epithelium, marked by mitosis and pseudostratification, extends to form an epithelial lining facing the endometrial cavity. The spiral vessels also extend through the stroma.

Estrogen has been shown to have a significant effect on endometrial blood vessels (28). When estrogen levels fluctuate, changes can be seen in vessel permeability and fragility. Therefore, in an estrogen-primed endometrium, fluctuations in estrogen levels that are seen in the typical anovulatory cycles during adolescence lead to vessel fragility and incomplete and disorderly endometrial breakdown. This disorderly endometrial breakdown leads to the classic anovulatory uterine bleeding seen in early adolescence.

Ovulatory Phase

Hypothalamic-Pituitary-Ovarian Axis

The increasing amounts of estrogen produced by the dominant follicle exert a positive feedback on the hypothalamic-pituitary axis (29). The onset of the mid-cycle gonadotropin surge (LH and FSH) is related to the peak estradiol level and lasts roughly 48 hr as shown in Fig. 2. The LH surge is characterized by a rapid ascending limb (accompanied by a rapid decline of serum estradiol) followed by a longer descending limb. The shift in steroidogenesis begins roughly 12 hr before the onset of the LH surge, when progesterone levels start to rise and estradiol levels begin to plateau. During the 48 hr of the LH surge, progesterone abruptly rises as estradiol continues to decline. An abnormal LH surge is often seen in adolescence where the hypothalamic-pituitary axis is unable to respond to the rising estradiol levels (14).

In addition to a shifting of steroidogenesis from estrogen to progesterone in the granulosa cells, the LH surge serves two other important functions. First, it causes resumption of meiosis, and, second, it causes an alteration in the follicular environment, which leads to the physical process of ovulation (29). Tissue levels of cAMP rise in the preovulatory follicle and are followed by digestion of the follicular wall (30). Follicular fluid levels of prostaglandins are highest at ovulation (31) and appear to be involved in the actual process of ovulation, although the precise mechanism is unclear. The role of follicular fluid oxytocin and FSH are also unknown at this time.

Endometrium

During the 48 hr of the LH surge, the switch to progesterone fixes the height of the endometrium and begins the process of moving glandular secretions to the lumen of the glands. The early secretory endometrium is remarkable for movement of the intracellular vacuoles from the sub-nuclear region into the lumen. This is most prominent from days 16–19. Due to continued growth in a fixed structure, the glands and spiral vessels begin to coil, and as long as steroid output by the corpus luteum is adequate then the vessels will maintain their structure.

Once follicular recruitment begins and estrogen levels start to rise in early adolescence, the endometrium responds by growth and development of the glands and arterioles. In the absence of an LH surge and subsequent progesterone production, estrogen levels begin to fluctuate which leads to vessel fragility in the endometrium. This causes incomplete breakdown of the endometrium and prolonged dysfunctional uterine bleeding.

Luteal Phase

Hypothalamic-Pituitary-Ovarian Axis

As the most steroidogenically active tissue in the body, the corpus luteum produces about 25 mg of progesterone per day as shown in Table 2 (32). This progestogenic dominance serves to slow the GnRH pulse generator, thereby preventing further recruitment of follicles. The corpus luteum progesterone also serves to prepare the endometrium for implantation. Serum progesterone levels reach a peak roughly 8 days after the LH peak, and there is a parallel

TABLE 2. *Production rate of sex steroids in women during the early follicular and midluteal phase*

Sex steroids	Daily production rate[a]	
	Early follicular	Midluteal
Progesterone	1.000	25.000
17-Hydroxyprogesterone	0.500	4.000
Androstenedione	2.600	3.400
Testosterone	0.200	0.170
Estrone	0.050	0.250
Estradiol	0.036	0.250

[a]Expressed as mg/24 h.
From ref. 32.

increase seen with 17-hydroxyprogesterone, estradiol, and estrone levels.

The health of the corpus luteum appears to be dependant on the preceding follicular phase (i.e., the development of LH receptors on the granulosa cells) (33,34). Selective suppression of FSH during the follicular phase results in a decreased luteal cell mass and a decreased progesterone production by the corpus luteum (35). The health of the corpus luteum also appears to be dependant on proper vascularization and the delivery of cholesterol for progesterone synthesis (36).

Pituitary LH is vital for the survival of the corpus luteum. This has been demonstrated by several studies. First, in hypophysectomized women, ovulation induction with gonadotropins is followed by low progesterone levels and a short luteal phase (37). Second, administration of a potent GnRH agonist or antagonist in the luteal phase results in a dramatic decline of progesterone (38). Cell culture experiments have shown that luteinized granulosa cells produce large amounts of progesterone which peaks on day 3 of culture and is greatly increased in the presence of hCG (39). Thus, even though the GnRH pulse generator is slowed, pituitary LH is the vital luteotropic hormone in adult women.

Without hCG or LH stimulation, the lifespan of the human corpus luteum is generally 13–14 days. Although the precise mechanism of luteolysis has yet to be determined in humans, prostaglandins are thought to play a major role (40). With the demise of the corpus luteum, there is a dramatic fall in serum progesterone and estradiol with a resultant increase in pulses from the GnRH pulse generator. This increase in GnRH pulse frequency leads to a rise in serum FSH levels and initiation of the next follicular phase.

Endometrium

During the luteal phase the endometrium continues to prepare for implantation. The vacuoles have moved into the lumen of the glands, the glands have become exhausted, and the stroma has become edematous. Although the precise role of the glandular secretions is unknown, a teleologic view would hold that they provide nourishment for the embryo. The glandular secretions are prominent at a time when the embryo is in the endometrial cavity and preparing for implantation, between 4 and 7 days postovulation.

Progesterone also has an effect on endometrial stroma cells, leading to edema, decidualization, and prolactin production (41). Around day 22–23, the spiral arterioles acquire a cuff of pseudodecidualized stromal cells. This is the earliest predecidual change. Pseudo-decidualized stromal cells extend to beneath the epithelium by day 25 and by day 27 the endometrium appears as solid sheets of pseudodecidualized cells (26). Prostaglandin $F_{2\alpha}$ ($PGF_{2\alpha}$), which is felt to be important in the process of both implantation and menstruation, rises in late luteal endometrium (42) and appears to be decreased by the addition of progesterone (43).

Inadequate progesterone production following estrogen priming of the endometrium leads to a thin endometrium without stromal edema or decidualization (44). Treatment during the follicular phase with an antiestrogen leads to lower levels of cytoplasmic progesterone receptors in the luteal endometrium (45). This could be a factor leading to lower conception rates in these cycles. Progesterone also has an effect on endometrial vessels and probably acts synergistically with estrogen to maintain an intact endometrium (46). Administration of an antiprogesterone during the early luteal phase results in decreased glandular secretory activity, vascular changes, and accelerated degenerative changes (47). Furthermore, administration of an antiprogesterone during the late luteal phase leads to a prompt withdrawal menses and shortening of the luteal phase (48). Although the precise role of decidualization and endometrial prolactin production is unclear, they may serve a role in the initial establishment of an intact feto-maternal unit. Women who have delayed or abnormal decidualization show an increased incidence of both infertility and recurrent pregnancy loss (49,50). Furthermore, embryos implanted in tissue other than the endometrium show both an abnormal amount of trophoblastic invasion (51) and abnormal development (51,52).

In the absence of implantation and subsequent hCG, there is demise of the corpus luteum and waning estrogen and progesterone levels. The withdrawal of steroids from the endometrium leads to vessel fragility and spiral arteriole constriction. Tissue necrosis, white cell migration, and menstruation follows. The edematous stoma of the spongiosum is sloughed, leaving behind the basalis and a residual spongiosum. The progesterone withdrawal also leads to an alteration in the GnRH pulse generator and a subsequent rise in FSH levels. This serves to initiate the next follicular phase and aid in the healing process of the endometrium. Menstrual flow stops due to prolonged vasoconstriction, platelet aggregation, and estrogen induced vessel stability and healing.

CAUSES OF ABNORMAL UTERINE BLEEDING

Anovulatory dysfunctional uterine bleeding is the most frequent cause of abnormal bleeding in the adolescent, but requires the exclusion of many disorders (Table 3) before arriving at this diagnosis. Less commonly observed is ovulatory DUB, which may present as polymenorrhea, periovulatory (mid-cycle) bleeding, or premenstrual spotting. Mid-cycle bleeding may be attributed to the decrease in estrogen prior to ovulation and occasionally may be due to uterine polyps or fibroids. Premenstrual spotting may be seen with luteal phase inadequacy and decreased progesterone effect on the endometrium, although a fairly high association with endometriosis has been observed (53).

The frequency of the other causes of abnormal bleeding is different depending on the presentation. Extremely heavy menses requiring transfusions and beginning with or shortly after menarche is likely to be due to a coagulation disorder. One review of acute adolescent menorrhagia found 19% of the patients with a coagulation abnormality (1). Primary and secondary thrombocytopenia were the most common blood dyscrasias observed. Many of the coagulation disorders are familial and a positive family history of bleeding problems may be frequently elicited. Leukemia may present

TABLE 3. *Causes of abnormal uterine bleeding*

- Dysfunctional uterine bleeding
  - Anovulatory
  - Ovulatory
- Blood dyscrasia
  - Idiopathic thrombocytopenia
  - Von Willebrand's disease
  - Leukemia
  - Thrombocytopenia
  - Drug-induced
  - Thalassemia major
  - Fanconi's anemia
  - Glanzmann's disease
  - Hemophilia
  - Anticoagulants
- Complications of pregnancy
  - Spontaneous or induced abortion
  - Ectopic pregnancy
  - Hydatidiform mole
- Disorders of the cervix
  - Cervicitis
  - Polyps
  - Condylomata
  - Erosion
  - Sarcoma botyroides
  - Mixed mesodermal sarcoma
- Disorders of the vagina
  - Vaginitis
  - Foreign body
  - Coital trauma
  - Sexual abuse
  - Septum
  - Adenosis
  - Clear cell carcinoma
- Disorders of the uterus
  - Congenital anomalies
  - Endometritis
  - Neoplasia
  - Polyps
  - Fibroids
  - Cancer
- Disorder of the ovary
  - Polycystic ovarian disease
  - Neoplasia (benign or malignant)
  - Premature ovarian failure
- Disorders of the Adrenal Gland
  - Congenital adrenal hyperplasia
  - Cushings disease
  - Addison's disease
  - Neoplasia (benign or malignant)
- Neoplasia of the central nervous system
  - Prolactinoma
  - Nonsecreting pituitary tumor
  - Craniopharyngioma
- Pelvic inflammatory disease
- Weight disorder
  - Malnutrition
  - Excessive exercise
  - Anorexia nervosa
  - Bulimia
  - Obesity
- Thyroid disease
  - Hyperthyroidism
  - Hypothyroidism
- Chronic illness
  - Cancer
  - Organ failure (heart, lung, liver, kidney)
- Psychogenic factors

with either menorrhagia or menometrorrhagia usually as a result of decreased plasma fibrinogen.

Adolescent pregnancy is an all too common occurrence in the United States. As many as 70% of women have sexual intercourse by age 19, and only half used contraception during their first intercourse (54). Consequently, a high index of suspicion of a possible pregnancy complication such as a threatened or spontaneous abortion is required when evaluating abnormal bleeding.

Infections as a cause of abnormal bleeding are more likely in acute episodes although chronic endometritis may present with menorrhagia. Cervicovaginitis, including trichomoniasis, gonorrhea, herpes, condylomata, and chlamydia, may cause vaginal bleeding, and when painful bleeding is observed, pelvic inflammatory disease must be considered as a possible cause. Local irritation and trauma from a foreign body left in the vagina may present with a bloody, malodorous discharge and requires differentiation from an infection. Atrophic vaginitis from premature ovarian failure may be seen rarely in the adolescent presenting with spotting and vaginal discharge.

Sexual intercourse and/or abuse may present with vaginal trauma and bleeding, and requires a thorough history and examination for legal documentation when identified or suspected. We have seen one adolescent presenting with an acute, heavy vaginal bleeding after insertion of a tampon which partially avulsed a vaginal septum.

Neoplasms of the cervix, vagina, uterus and ovaries are fortunately rare causes of bleeding in the adolescent, but because of the often more serious nature of both benign and malignant tumors, a physician should always be concerned about these etiologies when performing an examination.

Endocrine causes most often present with recurrent abnormal bleeding with thyroid disorders most commonly found. Hypothyroidism often is associated with hypermenorrhea, whereas hyperthyroidism usually results in hypomenorrhea. Signs of hyperandrogenism in the adolescent with abnormal bleeding may occur with polycystic ovarian disease, congenital adrenal hyperplasia, androgen secreting neoplasms of the ovary or adrenal glands and Cushing's disease, and anovulatory uterine bleeding frequently results from these endocrinopathies as is also the case with weight disorders, chronic illnesses and psychogenic causes.

TABLE 4. *Evaluation of abnormal bleeding in the adolescent*

- I. Essential evaluation
  - A. Careful history
    1. Pubertal events/menstrual history
    2. Sexual history
    3. Coagulation disorders
    4. Extremes of weight/exercise
    5. Sexually transmitted diseases
    6. Contraceptive use
    7. Sexual abuse/trauma
    8. CNS tumors (headache, visual changes, weight loss)
    9. Medications
  - B. Physical examination
    1. Systemic signs of chronic illness
    2. Systemic signs of a coagulopathy
    3. Systemic signs of an endocrinopathy
    4. Exact source of bleeding
    5. Vaginal, cervical, or pelvic abnormalities
  - C. Laboratory testing
    1. Complete blood count
    2. Coagulation screen—platelet count, PT, PTT, bleeding time
    3. Pregnancy test
    4. PAP smear
    5. Endometrial biopsy in selected cases
- II. Additional laboratory studies if clinically indicated
  - A. Further endocrine work-up if anovulatory bleeding persists or clinically indicated
    1. Thyroid studies
    2. Prolactin level
  - B. Blood glucose
  - C. Screen for sexually transmitted disease
    1. Cervical cultures
    2. Erythrocyte sedimentation rate
  - D. Evaluation of hirsutism
    1. DHEA-S
    2. Testosterone
    3. 17-OH progesterone
- III. Additional evaluation if clinically indicated
  - A. Pelvic ultrasound
  - B. CT scan of the pituitary
  - C. Hysteroscopy/dilatation and curettage (last resort)
  - D. Consultation
    1. Hematologist
    2. Endocrinologist
    3. Psychiatrist
    4. Oncologist

DIAGNOSIS AND EVALUATION

As noted in Table 3, the causes of abnormal bleeding in adolescence are numerous. Even though the majority of cases represent anovulatory uterine bleeding, the more serious causes need to be excluded. The investigation of the adolescent with abnormal bleeding consists of three initial phases—history, physical examination, and laboratory tests. Table 4 outlines the essential evaluation and additional tests in the evaluation of adolescent bleeding.

As with most presenting complaints, a careful history will enable the clinician to make the diagnosis in the majority of cases. The history should be obtained with and without the patient's parent in the room. Reviewing the sequence of pubertal events and a detailed menstrual history are important. The absence of secondary sexual characteristics along with uterine bleeding should alert the physician to some of the more unusual and rare causes of abnormal bleeding since menarche is the final event in puberty and therefore DUB should occur only after the development of secondary sexual characteristics. Symptoms of systemic progesterone (breast tenderness, mood swings, bloating) should alert the physician to ovulatory cycles and the probable diagnosis of dysfunctional uterine bleeding. Even though teenagers are poor at estimating the amount of blood loss, an attempt should be made to determine if the blood loss is excessive.

The remainder of the history should be directed toward the possibility of pregnancy and its complications, coagulation defects, sexually transmitted disease, sexual abuse or trauma, diet and/or exercise extremes, drug and/or medication use, and central nervous system tumors. After a thorough history, the physical exam is performed with the above disorders in mind. An initial height and weight will help determine pubertal events, diet abnormalities, and overall health. The general physical exam may reveal systemic signs of a coagulation defect (petechiae or ecchymoses), an endocrinopathy (hirsutism, hair changes, galactorrhea, virilization, striae), a CNS tumor (visual changes), or chronic illness. The pelvic exam, which may need to be performed under anesthesia in the very young patient, may reveal the exact site of bleeding and help rule out infection, cervicitis, sexually transmitted diseases, sexual abuse, trauma, and a foreign body. A PAP smear should be performed at this time.

Following a careful history and physical exam, laboratory tests should be ordered. The essential laboratory evaluation of acute adolescent bleeding should include a complete blood count which provides an indication of the severity of the bleeding in both acute and chronic losses, and screens for an infectious etiology. Due to the importance of pregnancy complications, a pregnancy test should always be performed. Since many adolescents will have an underlying coagulation defect, blood should be sent for a platelet count, prothrombin time, partial thromboplastin time, and bleeding time especially in cases of either acute hemorrhage or where the hemoglobin is less than 10 g/dl. This coagulation screen, if normal, will rule out all but the most unusual forms of coagulation defects, and, if abnormal, indicate additional studies and consultation with a hematologist.

In addition to the essential workup as outlined above, other laboratory studies such as endocrine testing may be obtained if clinically indicated. Since the majority of anovulatory uterine bleeding in early adolescence will resolve with maturation of the H-P-O axis, these further tests are also indicated in non-acute cases where the anovulatory uterine bleeding persists long after menarche. Additional testing to evaluate anovulatory uterine bleeding may include thyroid studies, prolactin level, evaluation of hirsutism, and radiologic evaluation of the pituitary. A blood glucose, pelvic ultrasound, or screen for sexually transmitted disease should be obtained when clinically indicated.

Due to the low yield and potential harm, surgical evaluation in the form of hysteroscopy, and dilatation and curettage is seldom necessary in the evaluation of an adolescent and should be used as a last resort when medical treatment fails. This is especially true when anovulatory uterine bleeding is the working diagnosis. Surgical evaluation may be useful in cases where a neoplasm or trauma is suspected. It may also be useful in certain pregnancy complications.

In the cases where anovulatory uterine bleeding does not appear to be the diagnosis, a consultation with a specialist may be appropriate. The expertise of a hematologist, a reproductive endocrinologist, or a psychiatrist may be useful in the evaluation of the adolescent with abnormal bleeding refractory to treatment.

TREATMENT

Frequently the evaluation and the treatment of uterine bleeding are being performed concurrently and do overlap signif-

TABLE 5. *Management of abnormal uterine bleeding*

- I. Chronic/recurrent episodes of mild to moderate bleeding
    - Rule out pregnancy
    - Examination
    - Endometrial sampling, selected cases
    - Observation
    - Iron replacement
    - Prostaglandin synthetase inhibitors
- II. Chronic/recurrent episodes of heavy bleeding
    - Rule out pregnancy
    - Examination
    - Endometrial sampling (if not on hormonal medication)
    - Hormonal
        - Oral estrogen/progestin
        - Oral progestin
            - Periodic
            - Continuous
        - Danazol
        - GNRH agonists
        - Depo-Progestin
    - Prostaglandin synthetase inhibitors
    - Antibiotics
    - Iron replacement
    - Dilatation and curettage (if significant bleeding persists on medical therapy)
    - Hysteroscopy
- III. Acute heavy bleeding
    - Rule out pregnancy
    - Examination
    - Endometrial sampling
    - Hormonal
        - Progesterone in oil, intramuscular
        - Oral progestin
        - Oral estrogen/progestin
        - Oral estrogen
    - Correction of coagulation abnormalities
    - Antinauseants
    - Antibiotics
    - Dilatation and curettage (if significant bleeding persists after 24–48 hr)
- IV. Acute hemorrhage
    - Rule out pregnancy
    - Hospitalization
    - Intravenous fluid
    - Blood replacement
    - Correction of coagulation abnormalities
    - Hormonal
        - Oral estrogen
        - Oral estrogen/progestin
        - Intravenous estrogen
    - Antibiotics
    - Antinauseants
    - Observation
    - Dilatation and curettage (if significant bleeding persists after 24 hr)

icantly. Once specific organic causes and blood dyscrasias have been excluded, a designation of DUB may be made. Since the underlying problem is hormonal in DUB, the bleeding can be managed primarily with hormonal preparations and secondarily with adjunctive measures.

With organic causes, endocrine causes such as hypothyroidism or congenital adrenal hyperplasia, and blood dyscrasias, correcting or treating the disorder is foremost whenever possible, with hormonal treatments reserved for control of heavy, refractory uterine bleeding in appropriate cases.

The most common clinical situation which will be seen in adolescents by health care providers is an irregular interval of bleeding which is neither heavier nor longer than a normal menstrual flow. Reassurance, observation, and recording the days and amount of bleeding (menstrual calendar) are sufficient in these individuals unless a progression to problematic bleeding is observed. Chronic or recurrent episodes of mild to moderate bleeding (Table 5) are the next most common presentation followed, in decreasing frequency, by chronic or recurrent episodes of heavy bleeding, acute heavy bleeding, and acute hemorrhage.

In each presentation of abnormal bleeding, excluding pregnancy is a necessary prerequisite to initiating therapy. In addition, an endometrial sampling should be performed with heavy bleeding whether acute or chronic once a pregnancy has been ruled out. Frequently, a physician may decide to forego endometrial sampling when the history strongly suggests DUB or the adolescent cannot be examined adequately. However, use of intravenous sedation may sufficiently reduce apprehension to allow performance of both the examination as well as endometrial sampling in an office setting. In rare instances, examination under general anesthesia may be required when organic causes are strongly suspected. The value of endometrial sampling lies in both assisting in the immediate management by assessing the quantity of tissue obtained and evaluating pathologic changes causing the bleeding. Very little tissue suggests a relatively atrophic endometrium or chronic bleeding with only basal endometrium remaining which would best respond to estrogen initially. A large amount of tissue is consistent with an unopposed estrogenic milieu and anovulation which generally responds well to progestin therapy.

Long-term management of bleeding may require iron supplementation to prevent iron deficiency anemia, and may include a prostaglandin synthetase inhibitor to reduce blood loss with each episode (55–57). When the amount of bleeding is heavy initially or after a period of observation, then hormonal treatment may also be prescribed.

ACUTE BLEEDING

There are several regimens of hormonal therapy that have been used in acute episodes of heavy bleeding, but data comparing the various approaches are lacking. Consequently, the following discussions on hormonal therapy should be viewed as guidelines to be individualized by the health care provider, not necessarily exclusive of alternative regimens. In adolescents with suspected anovulatory type bleeding from their menstrual histories, with more than usual amounts of endometrial tissue when sampled, or who have been receiving estrogenic preparations, progestin therapy to produce a secretory change of the endometrium and ultimately a progestin withdrawal bleed should be the initial hormonal intervention.

Progestin therapy may be accomplished using (a) progesterone in oil, 100–200 mg, intramuscular injection followed by 10–14 days of oral progestin; (b) medroxyprogesterone acetate (MPA) 10–20 mg orally per day for 10–14 days; or (c) norethindrone acetate 5–10 mg orally per day for 10–14 days.

Progesterone in oil offers an immediate progestational effect on a bleeding endometrium with a decrease in bleeding usually occurring within 12–24 hr, but must be followed by 10–14 days of an oral progestin. Common errors of progestin therapy are inadequate duration of treatment which should be a minimum of 10 days, and failure to counsel patients to anticipate bleeding after completing the prescribed course of the progestational agent. Following control of the acute bleeding, periodic progestin therapy for 10–14 days each month should be given for up to 6 months before observing the bleeding pattern without medication, and is also the treatment of choice for chronic or recurrent bleeding due to anovulation in an adolescent who has withdrawal bleeding when progestins are administered. The periodic administration of progestational agents has less suppressive effects on the H-P-O axis, and does not impede the maturational process which is frequently incomplete.

In adolescents with prolonged bleeding, decreased amount of tissue on endometrial sampling or suspected hypoestrogenism, estrogen therapy to cause proliferation of an otherwise atrophic or "thinned out" endometrium should be used. Initial regimens of estrogen therapy include (a) conjugated estrogens 0.625–1.25 mg every 4–6 hr orally, (b) conjugated estrone 0.625–1.25 mg every 4–6 hr orally, and (c) estradiol 1–2 mg every 4–6 hr orally.

Once significant bleeding has been stopped, reduction of the dose to a daily or b.i.d. schedule may be tried. Because of the greater potential for thromboembolic sequelae with high dose synthetic estrogens such as ethinyl estradiol, the above regimens are preferable. Also, intravenous use (58) of conjugated estrogens (25 mg) should be reserved for acute hemorrhage and attempts to control such serious bleeding in a rapid manner, or in those individuals unable to tolerate oral preparations. Although very rare, deaths have occurred with high dose intravenous estrogen preparations due to thromboembolic complications.

Once the acute episode of bleeding has been controlled, periodic withdrawal bleeding can be achieved with the progestin regimens previously described while continuing a maintenance dose of the estrogen preparation. Although oral contraceptives containing 30–50 μg of a synthetic estrogen can be administered orally every 4–6 hr and do successfully control bleeding in most cases, three potential problems raise concerns with this approach more so than with estrogen and/or progestin regimens. These include the risk of thromboembolic complications both with acute and long term therapy with high dosages; the potential suppression of the H-P-O axis and risk of recurrent anovulatory bleeding after the discontinuation of the oral contraceptives; and the difficulty ascertaining the reason for treatment failures, i.e., insufficient estrogenic effect versus insufficient progestin effect. Nevertheless, in the sexually active adolescent, oral contraceptives may address both the bleeding and the contraceptive needs.

Other important measures in the management of uterine bleeding may be beneficial such as: the correction of significant abnormalities in coagulation factors when feasible; the use of antinauseants to improve toleration of high-dose hormonal therapies; and the use of antibiotics when prolonged bleeding, moderate to severe dysmenorrhea, or a tender uterus are noted. Chronic endometritis may present with menorrhagia (59) and an ascending secondary infection may occur in heavy prolonged bleeding, resulting in the loss of local hemostatic mechanisms in an inflamed or infected endometrium.

Dilatation and curettage are rarely required in the adolescent and should be performed only after failure of hormonal therapies either acutely or after longer term treatments, or when a high index of suspicion for an organic cause exists. When curettage is to be performed to identify or exclude a suspected intrauterine lesion, hysteroscopy may offer a higher sensitivity than curettage for the identification of intrauterine pathology, but the overall efficacy in this age group has not been reported.

Long-term suppression of menses may be advantageous in the adolescent who has moderate to severe anemia because of heavy bleeding due to a blood dyscrasia, chronic illness, or DUB. Danazol, 200–800 mg daily, has been effective in producing an atrophic endometrium and an amenorrheic state (59). However, the cost and the androgenic side effects frequently limits its use. Recently, GnRH agonists have become available to the clinician and produce a reversible hypoestrogenic state, and amenorrhea in most individuals. Hot flushes occur in most individuals but can be alleviated with norethindrone acetate 2.5 mg (half of 5 mg tablet) daily. Because of loss of calcium from bone, GnRH agonists have been limited to 6 months of use at present. Norethindrone acetate 5 mg daily (half tablet, b.i.d.) may also be used to achieve long-term suppression of uterine bleeding.

The intramuscular depot form of MPA may produce prolonged suppression of the H-P-O axis and, therefore, should only be used in limited situations in the adolescent, such as mentally retarded or chronically ill individuals with problematic bleeding. This approach generally produces amenorrhea, overcomes any compliance or absorption problems of oral preparations, and does provide contraception. Initially, 100–150 mg of depo-MPA is given intramuscularly on a weekly basis for a month; then, monthly for 3–4 months; and, then every 2–4 months as required to suppress uterine bleeding completely.

There is no single method or approach which will control problematic bleeding in every adolescent. Consequently, in order to achieve optimal results, thoroughness in evaluating the numerous causes, development of a comprehensive, individualized therapeutic plan, and close surveillance of the responses to treatment are required. Nevertheless, the health care provider should also remember the importance of being informative, caring, and supportive to the adolescent and her parents during this often frightening and frustrating process.

REFERENCES

1. Claessens EA, Cowell CA. Acute adolescent menorrhagia. *Am J Obstet Gynecol* 1981;139: 277–80.
2. Demanest CB. When the teen has irregular periods. *Patient Care* 1984;18:151–63.
3. Pepe F, Iachello PM, Panella M. Dysfunctional uterine bleeding in adolescents. *Clin Exp Obst Gyn* 1987;14:182–4.
4. Giowani GP. Vaginal bleeding in adolescents. *J Reprod Med* 1984;29:417–20.
5. Apter D, Viinkka L, Vihko R. Hormonal pattern of adolescent cycles. *J Clin Endocrinol Metab* 1978;47:944–54.
6. McDonough PG, Gantt P. Dysfunctional bleeding in the adolescent. In: Barwin BN, Belisle S, eds. *Adolescent gynecology and sexuality*. New York: Masson Publishing, 1982.
7. LeMarchand-Beraud T, Zufferey M, Reymond M, et al. Maturation of the hypothalalamo-pituitary-ovarian axis in adolescent girls. *J Clin Endocrinol Metab* 1982;54:241–6.
8. Southam AL, Richart RM. The prognosis for adolescents with menstrual abnormalities. *Am J Obstet Gynecol* 1966;94:637–45.
9. Hallberg L, Hogdahl AM, Nelsson L, et al. Menstrual blood loss—a population study. *Acta Obstet Gynecol Scand* 1966;45:320–51.
10. Fraser IS, McCannon G, Markham R. A preliminary study of factors influencing perceptum of menstrual blood loss volume. *Am J Obstet Gynecol* 1984;149:788–93.
11. Treloar AE, Boynton RE, Benn BG, et al. Variation of human menstrual cycle through reproductive life. *Int J Fertil* 1967;12:77–126.
12. Boyar R, Finkelstein JW, David R, et al. Twenty-four hour patterns of plasma luteinizing hormone and follicle-stimulating hormone in sexual precocity. *N Engl J Med* 1973;289:282–6.
13. Boyar RM, Finkelstein J, Roffward H, et al. Twenty-four-hour luteinizing hormone and follicle-stimulating hormone secretory patterns in gonadal dysgenesis. *J Clin Endocrinol Metab* 1973;37:521–5.
14. Fraser IS, Michie EA, Wide L, et al. Pituitary gonadotropins and ovarian function in adolescent dysfunctional uterine bleeding. *J Clin Endocrinol Metab* 1973;37:407–14.
15. Knobil E. The neuroendocrine control of the menstrual cycle. *Recent Prog Horm Res* 1980; 36:53–88.
16. Bider D, Ben-Rafeal Z, Shalev J, et al. Pituitary and ovarian suppression rate after high dosage of gonadotropin-releasing hormone agonist. *Fertil Steril* 1989;51:578–81.
17. Midgley AR Jr, Jaffe RB. Regulation of human gonadotropins: IV. Correlation of serum concentrations of follicle-stimulating and luteinizing hormones during the menstrual cycle. *J Clin Endocrinol Metab* 1968;28:1699–703.
18. diZerega GS, Hodgen GD. Folliculogenesis in the primate ovarian cycle. *Endocr Rev* 1981;2: 27–49.
19. Pache TD, Wladimiroff JW, De Jong FH, et al. Growth patterns of nondominant ovarian follicles during the normal menstrual cycle. *Fertil Steril* 1990;54:638–42.
20. Hillier SG, Reichert LE Jr, Van Hall EV. Control of preovulatory follicular estrogen biosynthesis in the human ovary. *J Clin Endocrinol Metab* 1981;52:847–56.
21. Dorrington JH, Armstrong DT. Effects of FSH on gonadal functions. *Recent Prog Horm Res* 1979;35:301–42.
22. Marrs RP, Lobo R, Campeau JD, et al. Correlation of human follicular fluid inhibin activity with spontaneous and induced follicle maturation. *J Clin Endocrinol Metab* 1984;58:704–9.
23. McLachlan RL, Robertson DM, Healy DL, et al. Circulating immunoreactive inhibin levels during the normal human menstrual cycle. *J Clin Endocrinol Metab* 1987;65:954–61.
24. Welsh TH Jr, Zhuang L-Z, Hsueh AJW. Estrogen augmentation of gonadotropin-stimulated progestin biosynthesis in cultured rat granulosa cells. *Endocrinology* 1983;112:1916–24.
25. McNatty KP, Makris A, DeGrazia D, et al. The production of progesterone, androgens and estrogens by human granulosa cells, thecal tissue and stromal tissue from human ovaries in vitro. *J Clin Endocrinol Metab* 1979;49:687–99.
26. Noyes RW, Hertig AW, Rock J. Dating the endometrial biopsy. *Fertil Steril* 1950;1:3–25.
27. Bonhoff A, Johannisson E, Bohnet HG. Morphometric analysis of the endometrium of infertile patients in relation to peripheral hormone levels. *Fertil Steril* 1990;54:84–9.
28. Schmidt-Matthiesen H. Die vaskularisierung des menschlichen endometriums. *Arch Gynaek* 1962;196:575–84.
29. Hoff JD, Quigley ME, Yen SSC. Hormonal dynamics at midcycle: a reevaluation. *J Clin Endocrinol Metab* 1983;57:792–6.
30. Nilsson L, Hillensjo T, Ekholm C. Preovulatory changes in rat follicular cyclic AMP and sensitivity to gonadotropins. *Acta Endocrinol (Copenh)* 1977;86:384–93.
31. LeMaire WJ, Leidner R, March JM. Pre- and post-ovulatory changes in the concentration of prostaglandins in rat Graffian follicles. *Prostaglandins* 1975;9:221–9.
32. Yen SCC. The menstrual cycle. In: Yen SCC, Jaffe RB, eds. *Reproductive endocrinology*. 2nd ed. Philadelphia: W. B. Saunders, 1986:200–36.

33. Goodman AL, Hodgen GD. The ovarian triad of the primate menstrual cycle. *Recent Prog Horm Res* 1983;39:1–73.
34. DiZerega GS, Hodgen GD. Luteal phase dysfunction infertility: a sequel to aberrant folliculogenesis. *Fertil Steril* 1981;35:489–99.
35. Stouffer RL, Hodgen GD. Induction of luteal phase defect in rhesus monkeys by follicular fluid administration at the onset of the menstrual cycle. *J Clin Endocrinol Metab* 1980;51:669–71.
36. Carr BR, Sadler RK, Rochell DB, et al. Plasma lipoprotein regulation of progesterone biosynthesis by human corpus luteum tissue in organ culture. *J Clin Endocrinol Metab* 1981;52:875–81.
37. VandeWiele R, Bogumil J, Dyrenfurth I, et al. Mechanisms regulating the menstrual cycle in women. *Recent Prog Horm Res* 1970;26:63–103.
38. Yen SSC. Clinical applications of gonadotropins-releasing hormone and gonadotropin-releasing hormone analogs. *Fertil Steril* 1983;39: 257–66.
39. Greenberg LH, Stouffer RL, Brenner RM, et al. Are human luteinizing granulosa cells a site of action for progesterone and relaxin? *Fertil Steril* 1990;53:446–53.
40. Korda AR, Shutt DA, Smith ID, et al. Assessment of possible luteolytic effect of intraovarian injection of prostaglandin F in the human. *Prostaglandins* 1975;9:443–9.
41. Maslar IA, Riddick DH. Prolactin production by human endometrium during the normal menstrual cycle. *Am J Obstet Gynecol* 1979;135: 751–4.
42. Brumsted JR, Chapitis J, Deaton JL, et al. Prostaglandin $F_{2\alpha}$ synthesis and metabolism by luteal phase endometrium in vitro. *Fertil Steril* 1989;52: 769–73.
43. Abel MH, Baird DT. The effect of 17β-estradiol and progesterone on prostaglandin production by human endometrium maintained in organ culture. *Endocrinology* 1980;106:1599–606.
44. Good RG, Moyer DL. Estrogen-progesterone relationships in the development of secretory endometrium. *Fertil Steril* 1969;19:37–49.
45. Molina R, Castilla JA, Vergara F, et al. Luteal cytoplasmic estradiol and progesterone receptors in human endometrium: in vitro fertilization and normal cycles. *Fertil Steril* 1989;51:976–9.
46. Kaiser IH. Newer concepts of menstruation. *Am J Obstet Gynecol* 1948;56:1037–47.
47. Li T-C, Dockery P, Thomas P, et al. The effects of progesterone receptor blockade in the luteal phase of normal fertile women. *Fertil Steril* 1988;50:732–42.
48. Roseff SJ, Kettel LM, Rivier J, et al. Accelerated dissolution of luteal-endometrial integrity by the administration of antagonists of gonadotropin-releasing hormone and progesterone to late-luteal phase women. *Fertil Steril* 1990;54: 805–10.
49. Wentz AC. Endometrial biopsy in the evaluation of infertility. *Fertil Steril* 1980;33:121–4.
50. Jones GS. The luteal phase defect. *Fertil Steril* 1976;27:351–6.
51. Kirby DRS. The influence of the uterine environment on the development of mouse eggs. *J Embryol Exp Morph* 1962;10:496–506.
52. Kirby DRS. The development of mouse blastocysts transplanted to the scrotal and cryptorchid testis. *J Anat* 1963;97:119–30.
53. Wentz AC. Premenstrual spotting: its association with endometriosis but not luteal phase inadequacy. *Fertil Steril* 1980;33:605–7.
54. Alan Guttmacher Institute. *Teenage pregnancy: the problem that hasn't gone away.* New York: AGI, 1981.
55. Fraser IS, Sherman RP, McIlveen J. Efficacy of mefenamic acid in patients with a complaint of menorrhagia. *Obstet Gynecol* 1981;58:543–51.
56. Hall P, MacLachlan W, Thom W, et al. Control of menorrhagia by the cyclo-oxygenase inhibitors naproxen sodium and mefenamic acid. *Br J Obstet Gynecol* 1987;94:554–8.
57. Vargyar JM, Campeau JD, Mishell DR. Treatment of menorrhagia with meclofenamate sodium. *Am J Obstet Gynecol* 1987;157:944–50.
58. DeVore GR, Owens O, Kase W. Use of intravenous Premarin® in the treatment of dysfunctional uterine bleeding—a double-blind randomized study. *Obstet Gynecol* 1982;59:285–91.
59. Fraser IS. Treatment of dysfunctional uterine bleeding with danazol. *Aust NZ J Obstet Gynecol* 1985;25:224–6.

Pediatric and Adolescent Gynecology,
edited by S. E. Carpenter and J. A. Rock.
Raven Press, Ltd., New York © 1992.

15
Dysmenorrhea

John S. Hesla

Department of Gynecology and Obstetrics, Division of Reproductive Endocrinology, The Johns Hopkins University School of Medicine, Baltimore, Maryland 21205

Dysmenorrhea, or painful menstruation, is the most common gynecologic complaint of young women (1). This disorder has been traditionally divided into two basic types. Primary dysmenorrhea is defined as pelvic pain that is experienced during menstruation in the absence of gross underlying pelvic pathology. In contrast, the discomfort of secondary dysmenorrhea can be ascribed to the presence of physical alterations in normal pelvic anatomy (Table 1). Hence, direct visualization of the peritoneal structures may be necessary for establishment of the etiology of the pain and appropriate categorization of the disorder.

The first dysmenorrheic symptoms typically develop 1–3 years following menarche in those girls who have established ovulatory menstrual cycles (Fig. 1). Spasmodic suprapubic pain usually begins within 1–4 hr after the onset of menstrual flow and lasts for 24–48 hr. Less commonly, the pain may be present 1–2 days prior to menstruation and continue to 2–4 days following the onset of flow. The pelvic cramping may radiate to the back and along the inner aspects of the thighs and is accompanied by one or more systemic symptoms in greater than 50% of patients, including nausea and vomiting (89%), fatigue (85%), lower backache (60%), diarrhea (60%), and headache (45%) (2). Rarely, the severity of pain may cause syncope and collapse. Menstrual pain that arises more than 3 years after menarche is more likely to be caused by an associated pathologic condition such as infection or endometriosis rather than the biochemical alteration present in primary dysmenorrhea.

Classification systems that label the de-

TABLE 1. *Causes of secondary dysmenorrhea*

Endometriosis
Pelvic inflammatory disease
Ovarian cysts
Intrauterine device
Congenital malformations of the müllerian system
Cervical strictures
Uterine myomas, uterine polyps[a]
Adenomyosis[a]
Complications of early pregnancy[b]

[a]Rare in adolescents.
[b]Associated with irregular bleeding and pain.

gree of disability associated with primary dysmenorrhea vary somewhat among published studies. Nevertheless, the definition of general terms facilitates discussion of the disorder. Dysmenorrhea may be considered mild if pain occurs only on the first day of menstruation, has little or no associated systemic symptoms, and does not inhibit the daily activities of the adolescent (3,4). Moderate dysmenorrhea is typically experienced during the first 2–3 days of menses and is frequently accompanied by diarrhea, headache, and fatigue. Some restriction in the daily routine may be necessary during the time period of peak discomfort, although absenteeism from school is infrequent. Intense, spasmodic pain may develop prior to the onset of flow and last 2–7 days in patients with severe dysmenorrhea. This pain and associated gastrointestinal symptoms may significantly impinge upon the adolescent's ability to carry out her normal activities.

PREVALENCE

Although there is some variation in the definition and analysis of subjective pain symptoms among epidemiologic studies, a consistently high prevalence of dysmenorrhea has been found to exist irrespective of socioeconomic status and cultural and geographic background. Of 2,699 menarcheal adolescents questioned in The National Health Examination Survey, 59.7% reported some degree of menstrual pain (5). The pain was described as mild by 49%, moderate by 37%, and severe by the remaining 14%. Fourteen percent of the girls reported frequent school absenteeism during the time of menstruation, whereas data extracted from teachers' reports suggested that 25% of all excessive school absences among female pupils were due to dysmen-

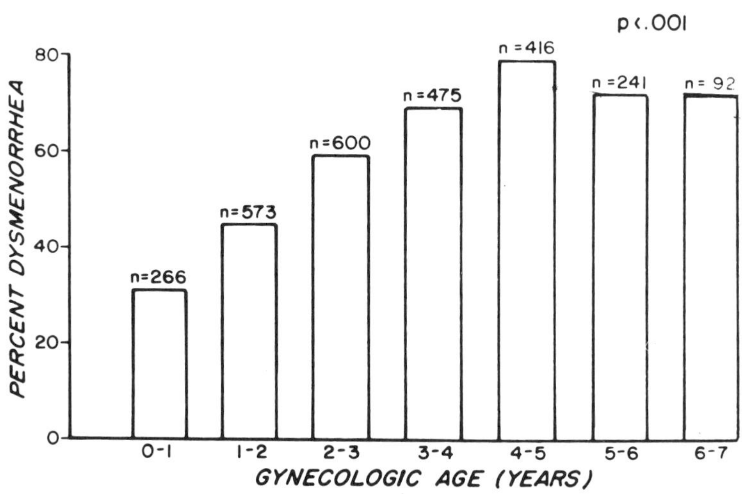

FIG. 1. Prevalence of dysmenorrhea in adolescents by gynecologic age. (From ref. 5, with permission.)

orrhea. These statistics are confirmed by several other studies, where the prevalence of dysmenorrhea among females aged 10–20 years ranged from 43–72.7% (3,6,7,8,9).

The prevalence of dysmenorrhea increases with age and reaches its peak during early adulthood. Widholm (7), in a 1979 study of Finnish adolescents aged 13–20 years, reported a 36.2% incidence of occasional or recurring dysmenorrhea during the first gynecologic year as compared to a 64.7% incidence during the fifth gynecologic year. The lower incidence in the younger age group has been attributed to an increased proportion of anovulatory cycles during the first years after menarche. Menstrual pain is most commonly experienced between the ages of 20 and 24 years but then declines after age 25 as well as after the birth of a child (10).

As one of the leading if not the greatest single cause of lost working hours and school days among young women, dysmenorrhea presents a significant problem from an individual and public health perspective (11). It has been estimated that 140 million hours are lost annually because of the abdominal pain, vomiting, nausea, headache, and other discomfort associated with primary dysmenorrhea (5). In addition, dysmenorrheic women receive lower grades and have more school adjustment problems than do nondysmenorrheic women (12).

ETIOLOGY OF PRIMARY DYSMENORRHEA

The etiology of severe incapacitating pain in the absence of obvious pathology was a matter of great debate until the latter part of this century. Hippocrates believed that cervical obstruction and stagnation of menstrual blood were responsible for dysmenorrhea. This theory persisted for centuries; it was recognized only recently that dilatation and curettage for presumed cervical stenosis is an ineffective and inappropriate treatment for primary dysmenorrhea (13). Prior to the discovery of prostaglandins, painful menstruation was frequently thought to be due to a psychosomatic derangement in which the woman was rejecting her femininity. Nonanalytical psychologic factors that were proposed to explain this complaint include patient suggestibility, a self-fulfilling prophecy, imitation of the mother, and the benefits of secondary gain. In addition, primitive taboos and lack of education were felt to contribute to an overly negative attitude toward menstruation on the part of the patient and society (14). Dysmenorrhea has been historically associated with severe depression, increased suicide rates, neuroticism, and general maladjustment (15). In accordance with these theories, past treatment regimens included psychotherapy, narcotics, exercise, vitamins, and surgery, including hysterectomy.

Evidence has existed since the 1950s to support the concept that dysmenorrhea arises through the active expulsion of degenerating endometrium during menstruation and that this activity is related to a substance released by the menstrual endometrium into the circulating blood. Pickles was the first investigator to extract a lipid-like smooth muscle stimulant from menstrual fluid in 1957 (16); this substance was later identified as the 20-carbon-chain prostaglandins E and F (17). Elevated levels of prostaglandin $F_{2\alpha}$ and its metabolites have been found in the menstrual fluid of dysmenorrheic women; the concentration of these substances in the menstrual effluvium and plasma correlate well with the presence of pain (18,19). Direct measurement of prostaglandins in the endometrium and jet-washings of the uterus have also shown increased concentrations in dysmenorrheic women as compared to those who do not experience painful menses (20,21). In addition, there is a striking similarity between the symptoms of primary dysmenorrhea and the clinical effects created by the administration of exogenous prostaglandin via differing routes for the induction of labor or abortion (11).

The mechanisms by which menstruation, prostaglandin production, and pelvic pain are associated are still being clarified. It appears that a decline in progesterone secretion by the corpus luteum during the perimenstrual time period leads to breakdown of endometrial cell lysosomes and release of phospholipase A_2. This enzyme converts fatty acids into arachidonic acid, a precursor of prostaglandins via the cyclooxygenase enzyme pathway. Arachidonic acid is also a precursor of leukotrienes by the 5-lipoxygenase pathway. Increased production of prostaglandins and leukotrienes results in a rise in resting tone of the uterus and a greater frequency and dysrhythmia of uterine contractions. The intensity of these contractions may be 1.5–3 times greater than the peak pressures experienced during labor. The resultant uterine ischemia promotes a heightened sensitivity of pain fibers to the action of bradykinin and other physical stimuli (22,23). Hence, arachidonic acid metabolites modulate blood flow, smooth muscle tone, contractile responses of the uterus, and pain receptor sensitivity.

The posterior pituitary hormone vasopressin has been ascribed an important etiological role in the myometrial hyperactivity, reduced uterine blood flow, and pain of primary dysmenorrhea. Some preliminary data suggest that there may be an increase in circulating vasopressin levels in this group of women at the time of menstruation (24). If this rise is not accompanied by a proportional increase in oxytocin concentration, dysrhythmic uterine contractions may ensue (25). Nevertheless, serial changes in vasopressin concentrations for an individual patient have not been analyzed over the course of the perimenstrual period. One pilot study did reveal that parenteral administration of a short-acting vasopressin antagonist was significantly more effective in relieving moderate to severe dysmenorrheic symptoms than placebo (24).

Epidemiologic Associations

The severity of dysmenorrhea that is experienced by the patient is significantly correlated with the duration and amount of menstrual flow (3). The physiological basis for this association may be explained by recognizing the action of prostaglandins in both the regulation of menstruation and the rise in pain (2). Epidemiologic studies have also revealed that indicators of unhealthy behavior and poor self-rated health status are almost as strongly associated with a high prevalence of pain as the duration of menstrual flow and gynecologic age of the patient (26). Girls who smoked daily, consumed alcohol occasionally or frequently, and engaged in little physical activity were found to be at increased risk of severe dysmenorrhea. Nevertheless, a dose-response relationship between smoking and dysmenorrhea could not be demonstrated, and the association between the two became statistically insignificant when alcohol consumption was controlled. Furthermore, in one Swedish survey nineteen year old smokers had significantly less menstrual pain than nonsmokers (3).

Wood and colleagues attempted to clarify the association between alcohol intake and pelvic pain symptomatology by proposing that alcohol may be used to dull menstrual pain or, alternatively, alcohol may worsen the pain by interfering with the breakdown of prostaglandins (27). Teperi and Rimpelä (26) did find increased alcohol consumption in patients who described severe dysmenorrhea; nevertheless, the perception of pain by this subgroup of teenagers did not vary as their consumption of alcohol increased. Moreover, the frequency of alcohol use is low in adolescent girls, minimizing the importance of this relationship. Although caffeine intake has also been linked with premenstrual symptomatology, the consumption of beverages containing caffeine has not been demonstrated to heighten dysmenorrhea (30).

Studies linking psychological attributes to perimenstrual distress have shown that patients with more pain complaints also score higher on measures of depression and anxiety. Metheny and Smith (28), in a multivariate analysis, reported that women experiencing higher levels of stress also described more severe menstrual discomfort. The effect of stress on symptom severity overshadowed the influences of optimism and mood. Women who expressed more severe dysmenorrhea generally felt more overwhelmed by life experiences. In addition, subjects with negative expectations about menstruation and a traditional view of the female role report higher perimenstrual distress than those with opposing views (29). A history of maternal or sibling dysmenorrhea does appear to be an important characteristic of adolescents with dysmenorrhea, perhaps due to an inherited increased production of prostaglandins by the menstrual endometrium along with psychological conditioning by the family unit (3,14).

SECONDARY DYSMENORRHEA

Endometriosis and pelvic inflammatory disease are the most frequent causes of secondary dysmenorrhea and chronic pelvic pain in adolescence. Goldstein et al. (31) diagnosed endometriosis in 47 of 140 (47%) of postpubertal girls with chronic pelvic pain who underwent diagnostic laparoscopy. Postoperative adhesions and pelvic inflammatory disease were discovered in 18 (13%) and 10 (7%), respectively. Of 47 adolescent females aged 11 to 19 years undergoing laparoscopy for chronic pelvic pain in Milan, 19 (40.4%) had no detectable pelvic abnormalities and 18 patients (38.3%) were found to have endometriosis (32). The majority of these patients had minimal disease, and many of the lesions were nonpigmented or nonclassic in appearance.

Acquired dysmenorrhea is the most prominent symptom of adolescent patients with laparoscopically confirmed endometriosis. Twenty-two of 28 girls in one surgical series noted such discomfort; even mild and moderate stages of disease may be associated with severe, disabling pelvic pain (33). Whether these cramps are secondary to the early development of endometriosis or whether the greater uterine contractility associated with menstrual pain predisposes these patients to endometriosis is not known. Genetic factors have been established in its development, as Simpson et al. (34) reported a 6.9% rate of endometriosis in first-degree relatives of women with the disease as compared to only 1% of control relatives.

The pain symptoms of endometriosis may be cyclic or acyclic in nature, with the most severe symptoms occurring just prior to and during the menses. In one study, 64% of girls with endometriosis had cyclic pain and 36% had acyclic pain that initially developed at an average of 2.9 years following menarche (35). The pain tends to increase in severity over time and may begin to occur throughout the month. Rectal pressure and dyspareunia are occasionally reported. Although oral contraceptives and antiprostaglandin agents may ameliorate the discomfort, the pain is usually not totally relieved by these medications and will begin to increase in intensity over subsequent cycles.

Mild to moderate tenderness may be the only positive finding on physical examination in the adolescent with endometriosis; this sign is most frequently elicited in the late luteal phase of the menstrual cycle. Uterosacral nodularity and pelvic masses are rare in this age group; in fact, 20–30% of patients in Goldstein's series who were diagnosed with endometriosis had a completely normal pelvic examination at initial assessment (35).

Most adolescents with endometriosis have minimal or mild stages of disease; however, girls with obstructing genital tract malformations have a high rate of severe endometriosis, even in the immediate postmenarcheal years (36). The patient with complete obstruction of the lower genital tract presents with primary amenorrhea and cyclic pelvic pain caused by reflux menstruation that begins two to three years after the onset of breast development. Presumably, endometriotic foci form through peritoneal implantation of the large volumes of refluxed menstrual tissue, as initially hypothesized by Sampson in the 1920s.

Imperforate hymen and complete transverse vaginal septum, two müllerian fusion defects associated this disorder, are readily diagnosed on pelvic examination. Hematocolpos formation may cause severe pain and a bulging of the introitus. Cervical atresia in conjunction with a functioning endometrium results in hematometra development.

Vertical fusion defects that yield unilateral müllerian obstruction with patency of the contralateral outflow tract are more difficult to detect by physical examination and are typically associated with cyclic menses and increasing dysmenorrhea. The blockage may occur in the lower genital region, such as unilateral vaginal atresia associated with uterus didelphys, or higher as with a noncommunicating rudimentary uterine horn. Palpation of a vaginal or adnexal mass in the patient with a suggestive history is virtually diagnostic of this category of anatomic abnormality.

Other Causes of Secondary Dysmenorrhea

Pelvic adhesions may develop due to previous surgery or an inflammatory process such as salpingitis. Cyclic discomfort at the time of menstruation is unlikely to be caused by mere adhesive disease. Ascending pelvic infections most commonly originate during or shortly after menstruation and may be characterized by increasing pelvic pain despite the resolution of menstrual flow, irregular bleeding, and the development of fever.

The occasional young woman with an intrauterine device may note increased dysmenorrhea after placement, particularly if it is not a progesterone-containing system. An inflammatory-like response and a heightened production of $PGF_{2\alpha}$ develop in the endometrium immediately adjacent to the device within 1 to 5 months after its insertion (2).

Adenomyosis, endometrial polyps, and uterine leiomyomas are rare in adolescents. Onset of pain with these conditions usually begins after the age of 20 and has been associated with increased levels of endometrial prostaglandins.

EVALUATION OF THE DYSMENORRHEIC PATIENT

The adolescent patient may spontaneously raise the issue of dysmenorrhea during a routine office visit. Its detection may also be the result of a systematic inquiry that should be a part of the medical history of any postmenarcheal patient.

A complete menstrual history includes the age of menarche, approximate date of the first day of the last menstrual period, regularity of menses, duration and amount of flow, and presence or absence of cramps or other associated symptoms. If dysmenorrhea is present, the patient should be questioned as to when the painful periods began, whether the pain develops before, coincident with, or after the onset of flow, the location and quality of the pain, and whether or not it is associated with other symptoms such as those involving the gastrointestinal, musculoskeletal, and urinary systems. The degree of disruption of daily routine, including school and social activities, should be elicited. The names, dosages, and treatment schedules of medications used in the past must be obtained; in addition, the adolescent should be asked of any behavior that ameliorates or exacerbates the symptoms. The family and social history, as well as the association of the pain episodes with stressful events, should be detailed. A history of maternal or sibling dysmenorrhea or endometriosis should be noted. An accurate sexual history is essential, including contraceptive method employed, if applicable.

Some adolescent girls will be found to have disability related to menstrual cramps that seems out of proportion to the severity of the pain. Occasionally, an underlying psychosocial problem, such as school phobia, sexual abuse, or other serious personal or family problem may be identified as contributing to the decreased pain tolerance and heightened anxiety centered around the menses.

The diagnosis of dysmenorrhea secondary to pelvic disease depends on recognition of an atypical history or abnormal pelvic examination, such as lateralization of symptoms or signs. Pain onset more than 3 years after menarche, dysfunctional uterine bleeding or change in menstrual pattern, and history of pelvic surgery may suggest secondary etiologies. Pelvic inflammatory disease should be suspected in dysmenorrheic adolescents with a fever as well as those patients whose pelvic pain increases as the menses end. Pelvic infection and abnormal pregnancy are possible causes of acute pain associated with vaginal bleeding in the sexually active young woman.

Examination

The physical examination of the patient with cyclic pain is helpful in excluding causes of secondary dysmenorrhea and will allow the physician to reassure the adolescent of the normality of her genital organs. The abdomen is carefully palpated in search of tenderness, masses, or organomegaly. It is often helpful to ask the patient to point with one finger to the location of the pain. The physician can then attempt to reproduce the pain by gentle palpation.

The approach for the evaluation of the pelvic organs may vary depending upon the patient's symptoms and history of sexual activity. If the patient is virginal and her pain is mild and typical of primary dysmenorrhea, a trial of nonsteroidal antiinflammatory drugs (NSAID) therapy may be prescribed without examination of the genital tract. Virginal adolescents who have moderate or severe pain that is otherwise characteristic of primary dysmenorrhea should be more thoroughly evaluated. After inspection of the vulva and vaginal introitus, bimanual rectoabdominal examination is performed in the lithotomy position to assess for abnormal pelvic masses or tenderness. If the hymen is not intact, the patient may tolerate a vaginal speculum examination and vaginoabdominal bimanual palpation. This will allow a greater appreciation of the uterine size and shape, the presence of cervical or adnexal tenderness, and the identification of adnexal masses or thickening. All adolescents with atypical symptomatology suggestive of secondary dysmenorrhea should have a complete examination, including evaluation of the internal genital tract. Administration of anesthesia may be necessary in some circumstances to ensure patient comfort. Pelvic sonography is helpful to confirm the presence of a mass when the pelvic examination is not completely satisfactory, to identify the presence of free fluid in the cul de sac, and to localize a suspected pregnancy; magnetic resonance imaging can be used to better characterize a mass or suspected müllerian anomaly.

All dysmenorrheic adolescent women with a history of sexual activity should undergo speculum examination to exclude the presence of congenital abnormalities and to take cervical cultures for *C. trachomatis* and *N. gonorrhoea*. A Pap smear is also recommended. Bimanual palpation may reveal abnormalities suggestive of associated disease states. Cervical motion tenderness is typical of pelvic inflammatory disease. Adnexal masses, decreased mobility of pelvic structures, and cul de sac nodularity may be detected in cases of tubo-ovarian abscess, hydrosalpinx, ovarian cyst, or endometriosis.

The basic laboratory evaluation of the patient with dysmenorrhea of moderate or severe intensity should include a complete blood count with differential, erythrocyte sedimentation rate, urinalysis, urine culture, pregnancy test, and cervical cultures for gonorrhea and chlamydia.

The finding of leukocytosis or an elevated sedimentation rate suggests the presence of either an infectious or inflammatory process. Less frequently, tissue ischemia that occurs with adnexal torsion or bowel obstruction may cause these hematologic abnormalities. An ectopic pregnancy or abnormal intrauterine pregnancy may present with pain and irregular bleeding.

Diagnostic Laparoscopy

The timely use of laparoscopy for the evaluation of undiagnosed pelvic complaints in young women provides a convenient, minimally traumatic and often definitive method of establishing a diagnosis and at times permits correction of various abnormalities without recourse to major abdominal surgery. Laparoscopy should be considered in the patient with dysmenorrhea unresponsive to the usual therapy with antiprostaglandin agents or ovulation suppression as well as for the confirmation or exclusion of clinically suspected endometriosis, chronic pelvic inflammatory disease, pelvic adhesions, ovarian cysts, and appendiceal disease. Any areas suspicious for endometriosis should be biopsied during laparoscopy. Endometriosis implants may be clear red, black, grey, blue, yellow, and white in color and may range in appearance from macular to papular to nodular with subperitoneal penetration (33,37). Many of the early lesions are small and atypical in appearance; lack of tissue biopsy results in a failure to diagnose the disease in a significant proportion of cases (35).

THERAPY FOR PRIMARY DYSMENORRHEA

Nonsteroidal antiinflammatory drugs (NSAIDs) have effectively alleviated symptoms of primary dysmenorrhea in 64% to more than 95% of patients studied, although these response rates may be influenced by large variations in methodology and the relatively high placebo response noted in pain therapy (38). These drugs act at 2 different sites in the arachidonic acid cascade to inhibit prostaglandin synthetase. Type I inhibitors suppress the action of cyclic endoperoxide synthetase at the cyclooxygenase enzyme level, whereas Type 2 inhibitors affect the cyclic endoperoxide cleavage enzymes after the formation of cyclic endoperoxides. Most of the marketed prostaglandin synthetase inhibitors act on cyclooxygenase; Type II inhibitors are less efficacious because they do not significantly suppress the production of cyclic endoperoxides which are potent uterotonic substances.

Smith and Powell studied one such NSAID, meclofenamate, by correlating uterine activity assessed by intrauterine pressure measurements, plasma drug levels, and subjective scoring of pain intensity (38). They demonstrated that a reduction in intrauterine pressure and uterine activity during drug treatment results in a reduction in pain associated with primary dysmenorrhea. All parameters which reflected uterine work showed statistical greater effect of NSAID over placebo. Sixty-three percent of the patients receiving this antiprostaglandin agent experienced a reduction in the number of uterine contraction waves to below 20% of their pretreatment levels. In addition, the intensity of the contractions was diminished and the uterine tonus remained at the basal level for a greater proportion of time as compared to nontreated patients. Other studies that examined the effect of flurbiprofen and naproxen sodium described a similar reduction in active pressure, frequency of the pressure cycles and the area under the curve after the oral administration of these NSAIDs (39). Hence, drug therapy acts to prevent pain rather than merely to ameliorate pain.

NSAID Classifications

The nonsteroidal antiinflammatory agents may be broadly grouped into several categories according to their chemical structures. These include benzoic acid derivatives (aspirin), butyrophenones (phenylbutazone), indoleacetic acid derivatives (indomethacin), fenamates (mefenamic acid, meclofenamate), oxicams (piroxicam), and arylpropionic acid derivatives (ibuprofen, ketoprofen, naproxen) (Table 2).

Aspirin and acetaminophen-containing analgesics, while only marginally effective, constitute very common therapy for the adolescent patient population, primarily because of their ready availability. A double-blind crossover study of 32 dysmenorrheic women comparing the analgesic benefit of aspirin, naproxen sodium, and placebo showed no superiority of aspirin to placebo in reducing dysmenorrhea (40). Other published data support these findings, although one study which used a menstrual distress questionnaire noted that pain scores and school absenteeism were significantly lower in patients who took aspirin 600 mg four times a day as compared to placebo (41).

Enolic acid derivatives include phenylbutazone and piroxicam and act by inhibition of the isomerase/reductase step in the production of PGE_2 and $PGF_{2\alpha}$. Due to the high incidence of adverse effects, phenylbutazone is not prescribed for the treatment of dysmenorrhea. Piroxicam, however, has been shown to be efficacious in alleviating symptoms. Single daily doses of piroxicam 20 mg and 40 mg are as effective as ibuprofen 400 mg four times daily for the relief of primary dysmenorrhea (32). In addition, the incidence of side effects for patients treated with piroxicam 40 mg for two days has not been found to be greater than that experienced with ibuprofen.

Indomethacin and other indoles cause gastrointestinal distress in a significant proportion of patients and therefore are not usually prescribed for the treatment of dysmenorrhea.

The most obvious advantage of ibuprofen is that it is available in the United States without a prescription. The dose must be repeated every 6 hr to maintain effective in-

TABLE 2. *Pharmokinetic parameters/dosage recommendations of NSAIDS*

	Time to peak levels (hr)[a]	Half-life (hr)	Usual starting dose	Maximum recommended daily dose (mg)	Frequency
Flurbiprofen	1.5	5.7	50 mg qid	300	bid–qid
Ibuprofen	1–2	1.8–2.5	400 mg q 4–6 h	3,200	q 4–6 h
Ketoprofen	0.5–2	2–4	25–50 mg q 6–8 h	300	tid–qid
Naproxen	2–4	12–15	250 mg q 6–8 h[c]	1,500	q 6–8 h
Naproxen sodium	1–2	12–13	275 mg q 6–8 h[c]	1,375	q 6–8 h
Meclofenamate	0.5–1	2(3.3)[b]	100 mg tid	400	tid–qid
Mefenamic acid	2–4	2–4	250 mg q 6 h[c]	1,000	q 6 h
Piroxicam	3–5	30–86	20 mg qd	40	qd

[a]Food decreases the rate of absorption and may delay the time to peak levels.
[b]Half-life with multiple doses.
[c]Recommended initial loading dose is two times the maintenance dose.

hibition of prostaglandin synthetase activity. Ketoprofen and ibuprofen have equivalent duration of action and time to onset of analgesia (43). Ketoprofen exhibits inhibitory effects on both prostaglandin and leukotriene synthesis, antibradykinin activity, and lysosomal membrane-stabilizing action.

Naproxen sodium has the dual advantages of being very rapidly absorbed and having a relatively long half-life. This allows a twice per day dosage schedule which is often easier for adolescents to follow than a briefer interval between dosing. Naproxen sodium, the sodium salt, is more rapidly absorbed and reaches peak plasma levels sooner than naproxen.

Mefenamic acid and related drugs have the theoretical advantage in pharmacologic action of both inhibiting prostaglandin synthetase and blocking myometrial receptor sites for already formed prostaglandins (44). The rapid onset of action for these drugs may be useful in patients who experience acute onset of severe discomfort, although mefenamic acid and meclofenamate are not recommended in children less than 14 years of age.

Medication selection should be based on clinical experience, patient convenience, side effects, and cost. If the therapeutic response with one medication is not satisfactory, substitution of a different drug is reasonable option. Nevertheless, the psychological impact of frequent alterations of therapy must be considered. Hulka et al. (45) reported that the greater the number of drugs prescribed by a physician, the greater the number of drugs discarded by patients and the greater the number of nonprescription drugs taken by patients.

When to Begin NSAID

Since prostaglandin synthesis by the endometrium may occur *de novo,* effective suppression of menstrual prostaglandins can be achieved with rapidly absorbed NSAIDs even when therapy is initiated at the onset of flow. Chan et al. (46) demonstrated that introduction of therapy on Cycle Day 1 was as effective in relieving pain as beginning the drug three days prior to the expected onset of the menses. If, during the first cycle of use, some degree of uterine cramping persists following the initial ingestion of drug, the starting dose should be increased by 50–100% with the next cycle. Alternatively, a nonsexually active patient with severe cramps accompanied by early vomiting may often benefit from starting the drug 1 or 2 days before the onset of her menses. Nevertheless, a careful medication history must be elicited since the patient may have taken inadequate doses of the drug previously, particularly if it was a nonprescription item.

The NSAID selected for administration should be taken continuously throughout the first 48 hr of menstrual flow in order to correct the biochemical derangement in excessive production and release of menstrual fluid prostaglandins. A higher failure rate is more likely to be observed if medication is ingested on an as-needed basis rather than regularly during this time period.

Due to the potential placebo effect of any medical regimen introduced for the alleviation of pain, the response of the patient must be followed over the initial cycles of therapy in order to fully appreciate its efficacy. Fedele et al. (47) reported that 84% of dysmenorrheic patients noted a favorable response to placebo during the first menstrual cycle of therapy; this was not statistically significant from patients receiving nonsteroidal antiinflammatory agents. Nevertheless, the response rate fell to 29% in the second, 16% in the third, and 10% in the fourth placebo treatment cycle. Conversely, the efficacy of antiprostaglandin agents was maintained throughout the course of study. Psychological theories suggest that deterioration of the placebo response may be attributed to deconditioning of the patient. Hence, a single preliminary cycle of NSAID may not distinguish responders from nonresponders. An adjustment of the type and/or dosage of drug over a three to six month period is reasonable prior to consideration of ovulatory suppression with oral contraceptives or diagnostic laparoscopy to exclude secondary causes of dysmenorrhea.

Side Effects of NSAIDs

Epigastric distress, nausea, vomiting, and diarrhea are occasional side effects of NSAID therapy and are probably caused by suppression of the protective effect of prostaglandins on the gastric mucosa (48). The incidence of such toxicity is highest with aspirin, indomethacin, and phenylbutazone, although these reactions may exist with fenamates and arylpropionic acid derivatives. Other side effects include constipation, anorexia, headache, dizziness, vertigo, and, less commonly, visual disturbances, melena, hearing disturbances, irritability, depression, drowsiness, skin rash, edema, bronchospasm, hepatotoxicity, and nephrotoxicity (49). All NSAIDs can interfere with platelet function and prolong bleeding time and therefore should be avoided in patients with hematologic disorders or in those who are scheduled for surgery. In addition, NSAIDs are contraindicated in patients with a history of aspirin allergy or aspirin-induced bronchospasm.

Acetaminophen in combination with small doses of codeine may be prescribed for girls who cannot take NSAIDs. Dizziness and nausea are frequently experienced by adolescents who take codeine-containing medications.

Leukotrienes and NSAID Nonresponders

Preliminary results from ongoing research indicate that the activity of the 5-lipoxygenase pathway is increased in a subgroup of women with primary dysmenorrhea who do not have increased production and release of uterine prostaglandins. In vitro culture of endometrial tissues obtained from these patients have demonstrated an increased biosynthesis of leukotrienes (50). These potent hydrocarbons cause vasoconstriction and induce uterine muscle contractions. Since NSAIDs are essentially cyclooxygenase blockers, they may be unable to completely relieve dysmenorrhea in patients with an increased activity of the 5-lipoxygenase pathway. Meclofenamate and the other fenamates do inhibit the activity of 5-lipoxygenase, but the clinical importance of the inhibition of leukotrienes has not been clearly established.

Oral Contraceptives

Prostaglandin synthetase inhibitors have certain distinct advantages over the alternative option of hormonal manipulation of the dysmenorrheic patient with oral contraceptives, since the former are taken only during 2–3 days of the menstrual cycle, lack significant suppression of the pituitary-gonadal axis, and do not carry the metabolic effects of the birth control pill, which has to be taken for at least 21 of every 28 days. Nevertheless, NSAIDs are not universally effective, and oral contraceptives offer dual benefits in the sexually active, dysmenorrheic adolescent who wishes to prevent conception.

Menstrual fluid prostaglandin levels are reduced to below normal during oral contraceptive therapy. This may occur via two mechanisms. Combination steroid contraceptives suppress endometrial growth and therefore reduce menstrual fluid volume. In addition, the anovulation induced by oral contraceptive therapy creates an endocrine milieu that is not favorable for the production of prostaglandins. The endometrium must be exposed to luteal phase levels of progesterone after it has been adequately estrogenized in order to produce and release $PGF_{2\alpha}$ and PGE_2 in amounts that result in the development of primary dysmenorrhea (11).

Initiation of oral contraceptive therapy in patients with a history of primary dysmenorrhea has been shown to suppress spontaneous uterine activity as reflected by the frequency and amplitude of contractions. In addition, intravenous injections of vasopressin or prostaglandin $F_{2\alpha}$ were found to induce less pain after study subjects began taking oral contraceptives, presumably by lessening the uterine sensitivity to these agents which promote tissue ischemia (51). Ninety percent or more of women with primary dysmenorrhea experience symptom relief following initiation of combination oral contraceptive therapy. Maximal benefit is noted after 2–3 months of use. If the patient has not experienced relief after 3–4 months of pill therapy, a NSAID may be added.

The sexually active adolescent with severe dysmenorrhea usually prefers to continue on oral contraceptives for a long-term period. However, if contraception is unnecessary, the medication may be discontinued after 3–6 months of use. The patient may continue to have relief from cramps for several additional, possibly anovulatory cycles before the baseline menstrual discomfort recurs.

Other Medical Therapies

Calcium antagonists such as nifedipine and verapamil have been shown to reduce prostaglandin-induced uterine hypercontractility and by doing so relieve menstrual pain (52). Oral intake of a sigle dose of 30–40 mg nifedipine markedly reduced or abolished uterine contractions in the majority of healthy and dysmenorrheic patients as objectively verified by intrauterine pressure recordings. An improvement in pain symptoms occurred simultaneous with a decrease in uterine activity, typically within 15–20 min of drug intake. Nevertheless, headaches are a troublesome side effect of these preparations; in addition, a slight fall in blood pressure may be measured. Dawood (2) has noted that, in his experience, nifedipine has been efficacious when utilized in a limited number of intractable cases of dysmenorrhea without pelvic pathology. However, the prescription of this class of drug is not recommended on a routine basis because of a lack of sufficient clinical trials documenting efficacy and adverse effects.

Ulmsten administered 30 mg of oral nifedipine to 12 patients ranging in age from 14–22 years and noted an alleviation of pain in nine subjects (53). Two of the remaining three were found to have a secondary cause for dysmenorrhea on subsequent laparoscopy and the third patient failed to experience any of the usual peripheral vasodilatory side effects of the medication, perhaps due to incomplete gastrointestinal absorption of the drug. These findings suggest that short term administration of nifedipine may be a tool to delineate disorders of primary versus secondary dysmenorrhea (53).

The therapeutic benefits of β-adrenergic receptor agonists in alleviating primary dysmenorrhea have also been investigated. Terbutaline and related drugs are only partially effective (54), and the results of double-blind studies suggest that they are not significantly better than placebo and carry considerable side effects (11). Their use in dysmenorrhea, therefore, is currently limited and perhaps reserved for only those women in whom more proven methods of therapy have failed or are contraindicated.

Behavioral Therapy

Relaxation training is a common component of all behavioral treatments and has been used successfully in the management of spasmodic pain associated with menstruation (55). In addition, activity scheduling has been shown to reduce symptom severity (56). This operant approach to pain management consists of increasing activity levels through reinforcement principles, reducing pain medications, and increasing social reinforcement for well behavior by family members. Although emotional distress seems to exacerbate perimenstrual symptoms (57), alternative behavioral treatments such as biofeedback have demonstrated limited utility (55).

Regular exercise decreases stress, improves mood, and even lifts depression; nevertheless, the direct effect of exercise on dysmenorrheic symptoms is controversial (26). Although Prior et al. (58) reported that habitual physical exercise decreased the severity of some premenstrual symptoms presumably by altering hormonal physiology, Metheny and Smith (28) found that complaints of menstrual discomfort were generally increased in those subjects who exercised regularly. Undoubtedly, the impact of physical activity on the symptoms associated with dysmenorrhea is complex and individualized.

Alternative Treatments

In traditional Chinese medicine, acupuncture has long been utilized during labor and at delivery as well as in the treatment of various gynecologic disorders, including amenorrhea, menorrhagia, dysmenorrhea, and infertility. The peripheral sensory, central, and autonomic nervous systems mediate the activity of acupuncture inputs through dermatomal nerve radiation influences and a complex combination of cutaneovisceral, visceromotor, and viscerocutaneal reflexes, perhaps by activating the endogenous opioid system. Helms (59) recently reported that 10 of 11 subjects treated with acupuncture for relief of dysmenorrhea showed an improvement in symptoms, compared with four of 11 of women treated with placebo acupuncture. In addition to decreasing cramping pain, acupuncture resulted in an amelioration in the extragenital symptoms of nausea, headache, and backache, and in premenstrual symptoms of fluid retention and breast tenderness. The physiologic mechanisms involved in this pain relief are unknown.

Transcutaneous electrical nerve stimulation (TENS) has also been found to be an effective and safe method for relieving the pain of primary dysmenorrhea. In a randomized, four-cycle crossover study comparing TENS treatment with sham TENS (placebo) or ibuprofen, Dawood and Ramos found that one-third of patients treated with TENS did not require any sort of supplemental pain medication (60). Among those who required backup ibuprofen, the doses needed were significantly lower than those in placebo TENS cycles or cycles treated with ibuprofen alone. Furthermore, the use of TENS temporally delayed the need for rescue medications. TENS significantly reduced the occurrence of diarrhea, fatigue, menstrual flow, and clot formation as compared with placebo TENS. Only a small fraction of patients noticed side effects of muscle vibrations, change in stimulation with movement, tightness, headaches after use, or a slight redness or a burning sensation with TENS treatment (60). Although TENS alone was effective, TENS plus ibuprofen provided the best overall pain relief.

Most patients treated with TENS in a study by Lundeberg et al. (61) reported that the best site for stimulation was the painful area on the back (T10–L1). A smaller proportion of patients preferred an abdominal location. About 70% of subjects in this investigation experienced pain reduction when treated with high frequency (100 Hz) TENS. Low-frequency (2 Hz) TENS was clearly less effective, relieving only about 45%.

Smith and Hentzel recently reported that high frequency TENS therapy in 3 patients led to a successful subjective improvement in symptoms at the same time that intrauterine pressure parameters remained steady or showed signs of worsening (62). These results suggest that there is a fundamental difference in the mechanism of action between TENS and drug therapy, for with NSAIDs the perception of pain is inextricably linked to the process that causes the pain.

TENS relieves primary dysmenorrhea through two likely mechanisms. With continuous TENS, the preganglionic fibers are bombarded with impulses that saturate the nerve cells of the dorsal horn and therefore block propagation of pain impulses along these fibers. The nerve stimulation may also stimulate endorphin release from these nerve cells which may additionally contributes to the relief of pain. None of the patients in the series by Lundeberg consistently experienced any inhibition of pain reduction with the administration of naloxone, suggesting that the mode of action was not through the release of endogenous opioids (61).

TREATMENT OF SECONDARY DYSMENORRHEA

Endometriosis

Treatment of the less advanced stages of endometriosis, that which is usually encountered in the adolescent patient, includes laparoscopic ablation of lesions with laser, electrocautery, or thermocoagulation, and/or hormonal suppression with oral contraceptives, progestational agents, gonadotropin releasing hormone analogs, or danazol. A NSAID should not be the agent of first choice for managing dysmenorrhea and pelvic pain in the patient with endometriosis. Laparotomy with resection of endometriosis and possible presacral neurectomy are recommended for most cases of severe disease. Goldstein et al. (31) treated adolescent endometriosis patients with surgery alone or surgery with or without subsequent ovulation suppression and followed them postlaparoscopy from 1 to 58 months. Of those with endometriosis as the sole pathologic finding at surgery, 71% experienced pain relief with their initial treatment, while the remaining 29% reported pain persistence or recurrence.

Ultrasonography, magnetic resonance imaging, examination under anesthesia, laparoscopy, and hysterosalpingography are useful in defining the anatomy of the young woman with a suspected müllerian anomaly so that appropriate reconstruction can be carried out. Excision of the rudimentary blind horn or creation of a permanent outflow tract in the case of a lower genital obstruction may prevent the development of endometriosis by eliminating menstrual reflux. Complete and spontaneous regression of endometriosis has been documented following the creation of an outlet for the menstrual effluvium away from the peritoneal cavity.

Other Categories of Secondary Infertility

In patients experiencing dysmenorrhea in association with IUD usage, NSAIDs can effectively suppress the induced prostaglandin production to normal or below-normal levels and thereby minimize the discomfort.

Patients who are diagnosed with pelvic inflammatory disease should have cervical cultures taken for potential pathogens followed by introduction of broad spectrum antibiotic therapy. Hospitalization is frequently necessary in order to administer parenteral antibiotics. Therapy for other causes of secondary dysmenorrhea is oriented toward correction of the underlying disease state.

CONCLUSION

Despite the high frequency of occurrence of dysmenorrhea in adolescent females of all backgrounds, only a fraction have an appropriate understanding of the pathophysiology of their condition and the medications available to relieve their symptoms. Over the counter aspirin and acetaminophen preparations are the most commonly used medications, even though the antiprostaglandin action of these drugs is minimal. Only 14.7% of girls in one American survey could name a nonsteroidal antiinflammatory agent besides aspirin as potentially effective for dysmenorrhea; 46% of these students were unaware that certain medications existed that could relieve cramps (8). In another study completed prior to the availability of nonprescription ibuprofen, 49% of dysmenorrheic subjects took medication to relieve symptoms, but only 10% of these used a prescription drug (9).

A mere 15% or so of dysmenorrheic girls in the United States seek consultation with a physician or nurse for their symptoms. This percentage increases to approximately 26–29% for young women with more severe conditions resulting in a greater absenteeism from school or work (5,8). When dysmenorrhea is ignored, underlying medical problems and gynecologic diseases such as pelvic infection and endometriosis may be left untreated, leading to potential long term disability. Hence, this subject should be raised during each health care visit of the adolescent girl.

Education concerning the pathophysiology of primary dysmenorrhea and the availability of antiprostaglandin medications may dispel any misperceptions and lessen the possibility that the patient will fear menstruation or begin to view herself as ill or handicapped. NSAIDs interfere with the pathogenic process, may be limited in administration to the time when an individual suffers the pain, are highly effective and without undue side effects, and have a prompt onset of analgesic action.

The adolescent with primary dysmenorrhea should be seen initially every 3 or 4 months to evaluate the effectiveness of the medication. Such visits also facilitate the doctor-patient rapport that is essential in the treatment of this problem. Those patients with persistent symptoms after this time period despite the introduction of antiprostaglandin agents and/or oral contraceptives should be considered for diagnostic laparoscopy.

REFERENCES

1. Alvin PE, Litt IF. Current status of the etiology and management of dysmenorrhea in adolescence. *Pediatrics* 1982;70:516–25.
2. Dawood MY. Etiology and treatment of dysmenorrhea. *Semin Reprod Endocrinol* 1985;3:283–94.
3. Andersch B, Milsom I. An epidemiologic study of young women with dysmenorrhea. *Am J Obstet Gynecol* 1982;144:655–60.
4. Coupey SM, Ahlstrom P. Common menstrual disorders. *Pediatr Clin North Am* 1989;36:551–71.
5. Klein JR, Litt IF. Epidemiology of adolescent dysmenorrhea. *Pediatrics* 1981;68:661–4.
6. Svanberg L, Ulmsten U. The incidence of primary dysmenorrhea in teenagers. *Arch Gynecol* 1981;230:173–7.
7. Widholm O. Dysmenorrhea during adolescence. *Acta Obstet Gynecol Scand* 1979;87(suppl):61–6.
8. Johnson J. Level of knowledge among adolescent girls regarding effective treatment for dysmenorrhea. *J Adolesc Health Care* 1988;9:398–402.
9. Wilson C, Emans SJ, Mansfield J, Podolsky C, Grace E. The relationships of calculated percent body fat, sports participation, age and place of residence on menstrual patterns in healthy adolescent girls at an independent New England high school. *J Adolesc Health Care* 1984;5:248–53.
10. Svennurud S. Dysmenorrhea and absenteeism. *Acta Obstet Gynecol Scand* 1959;38(suppl 2):1–88.
11. Ylikorkala O, Dawood MY. New concepts in dysmenorrhea. *Am J Obstet Gynecol* 1978;130:833–47.
12. Frisk M, Widholm O, Hortling H. Dysmenorrhea: psyche and soma in teenagers. *Acta Obstet Gynecol Scand* 1965;44:339–47.
13. Cholst IN, Carlon AT. Oral contraceptives and dysmenorrhea. *J Adolesc Health Care* 1987;8:121–8.
14. Widholm O, Kantero R-L. Correlations of menstrual traits between adolescent girls and their mothers. *Acta Obstet Gynecol Scand* 1971;50(suppl 14):30–6.
15. Dawood MY. Nonsteroidal anti-inflammatory drugs and changing attitudes toward dysmenorrhea. *Am J Med* 1988;84:23–9.
16. Pickles VR. A plain-muscle stimulant in the menstruum. *Nature* 1957;180:1198–9.
17. Pickles VR, Hall WJ, Best FA, Smith GN. Prostaglandins in endometrium and menstrual fluid from normal and dysmenorrhoeic subjects. *J Obstet Gynecol Br Commonwealth* 1965;72:185–92.

18. Lundström V, Green K. Endogenous levels of prostaglandin F_2 and its main metabolites in plasma and endometrium of normal and dysmenorrheic women. *Am J Obstet Gynecol* 1978; 130:640–6.
19. Chan WY, Dawood MY. Prostaglandin levels in menstrual fluid of nondysmenorrheic and of dysmenorrheic subjects with and without oral contraceptive or ibuprofen therapy. *Adv Prostaglandin Thromboxane Leukotriene Res* 1980; 8:1443–7.
20. Willman EA, Collins WP, Clayton SG. Studies in the involvement of prostaglandins in uterine symptomatology and pathology. *Br J Obstet Gynaecol* 1976;83:337–41.
21. Halbert DR, Demers LM, Fontana J, Jones DED. Prostaglandin levels in endometrial jet wash specimens in patients with dysmenorrhea before and after indomethacin therapy. *Prostaglandins* 1975;10:1047–56.
22. Csapo AI, Pulkkinen MO, Henzl MR. The effect of naproxen sodium on the intrauterine pressure and menstrual pain of dysmenorrheic subjects. *Prostaglandins* 1977;13:193–9.
23. Åkerlund M. Pathophysiology of dysmenorrhea. *Acta Obstet Gynecol Scand* 1979;(suppl)87: 27–32.
24. Haukttsson A, Åkerlund M, Forsling ML, Kindahl H. Plasma concentrations of vasopressin and a prostaglandin $F_{2\alpha}$ metabolite in women with primary dysmenorrhoea before and during treatment with a combined oral contraceptive. *J Endocrinol* 1987;115:355–61.
25. Åkerlund M. Can primary dysmenorrhea be alleviated by a vasopressin antagonist? Results of a pilot study. *Acta Obstet Gynecol Scand* 1987; 66:459–61.
26. Teperi J, Rimpelä M. Menstrual pain, health and behaviour in girls. *Soc Sci Med* 1989;29:163–9.
27. Wood C, Larsen L, Williams R. Social and psychological factors in relation to premenstrual tension and menstrual pain. *Aust NZ J Obstet Gynecol* 1979;19:111–5.
28. Metheny WP, Smith RP. The relationship among exercise, stress, and primary dysmenorrhea. *J Behav Med* 1989;12:569–86.
29. Aubuchon PG, Calhoun KS. Menstrual cycle symptomatology: the role of social expectancy and experimental demand characteristics. *Psychosom Med* 1985;47:35–45.
30. MacKay Rossingnol A. Caffeine-containing beverages and premenstrual syndrome in young women. *Am J Publ Health* 1985;75:1335–7.
31. Goldstein DP, deCholnoky C, Emans SJ, Leventhal JM. Laparoscopy in the diagnosis and management of pelvic pain in adolescents. *J Reprod Med* 1980;24:251–6.
32. Vercellini P, Fedele L, Arcaini L, Bianchi S, Rognoni MT, Candiani GB. Laparoscopy in the diagnosis of chronic pelvic pain in adolescent women. *J Reprod Med* 1989;34:827–30.
33. Chatman DL, Ward AB. Endometriosis in adolescents. *J Reprod Med* 1982;27:156–60.
34. Simpson JL, Elias S, Malinak LR, Buttram VC Jr. Heritable aspects of endometriosis: I. Genetic studies. *Am J Obstet Gynecol* 1980; 137:327–31.
35. Goldstein DP, DeCholnoky C, Emans SJ. Adolescent endometriosis. *J Adolesc Health Care* 1980;1:37–41.
36. Olive DL, Henderson DY. Endometriosis and mullerian anomalies. *Obstet Gynecol* 1987;69: 412–5.
37. Jansen RPS, Russell P. Nonpigmented endometriosis: clinical, laparoscopic, and pathologic definition. *Am J Obstet Gynecol* 1986;155: 1154.
38. Smith RP, Powell JR. Simultaneous objective and subjective evaluation of meclofenamate sodium in the treatment of primary dysmenorrhea. *Am J Obstet Gynecol* 1987;157:611–8.
39. Milson I, Andersch B, Sundell G. The effect of flurbiprofen and naproxen sodium on intra-uterine pressure and menstrual pain in patients with primary dysmenorrhea. *Acta Obstet Gynecol Scand* 1988;67:711–6.
40. Rosenwaks Z, Jones GS, Henzl MR, Dubin NH, Ghodgaonkar R, Hoffman S. Naproxen sodium, aspirin, and placebo in primary dysmenorrhea. Reduction of pain and blood levels of Prostaglandin $F_{2\alpha}$ metabolite. *Am J Obstet Gynecol* 1981;140:592–8.
41. Klein JR, Litt IF, Rosenberg A, Udall L. Effect of aspirin on dysmenorrhea in adolescents. *J Pediatr* 1981;98:987–90.
42. Pasquale SA, Rathauser R, Dolese HM. A double-blind, placebo-controlled study comparing three single-dose regimens of piroxicam with ibuprofen in patients with primary dysmenorrhea. *Am J Med* 1988;84(suppl 5A):30–4.
43. Mehlisch DR. Ketoprofen, ibuprofen, and placebo in the treatment of primary dysmenorrhea: a double-blind crossover comparison. *J Clin Pharmacol* 1988;28:529–33.
44. Budoff PW. Use of mefenamic acid in the treatment of primary dysmenorrhea. *JAMA* 1979; 241:2713–6.
45. Hulka BS, Cassel JC, Kupper LC, Burdette JA. Communication, compliance, and concordance between physicians and patients with prescribed medications. *Am J Public Health* 1976;66:847–53.
46. Chan WY, Dawood MY, Fuchs F. Prostaglandins in primary dysmenorrhea. *Am J Med* 1981;70:535–41.
47. Fedele L, Marchini M, Acaia B, Gargiola U, Tiengo M. Dynamics and significance of placebo response in primary dysmenorrhea. *Pain* 1989; 36:43–7.
48. Henzl MR, Massey S, Hanson FW, Buttram VC Jr, Rosenwaks Z, Pauls FD. Primary dysmenorrhea, the therapeutic challenge. *J Reprod Med* 1980;25:226–35.
49. Dawood MY. Dysmenorrhea. *Clin Obstet Gynecol* 1990;33:168–78.
50. Demers LM, Hahn DW, McGuire JL. Newer concepts in dysmenorrhea research: leukotrienes and calcium channel blockers. In: Dawood MY,

McGuire JL, Demers LM, eds. *Premenstrual syndrome and dysmenorrhea*. Baltimore: Urban and Schwarzenberg, 1985:205–20.
51. Hauksson A, Ekstrom P, Juchnicka E, Laudanski T, Åkerlund M. The influence of a combined oral contraceptive on uterine activity and reactivity to agonists in primary dysmenorrhea. *Acta Obstet Gynecol Scand* 1989;68:31–4.
52. Andersson D-E, Ulmsten U. Effects of nifedipine on myometrial activity and lower abdominal pain in women with primary dysmenorrhea. *Br J Obstet Gynaecol* 1978;85:142–8.
53. Ulmsten U. Calcium blockade as a rapid pharmacological test to evaluate primary dysmenorrhea. *Gynecol Obstet Invest* 1985;20:78–83.
54. Åkerlund M, Andersson KE, Ingemarsson J. Effects of terbutaline on myometrial activity, uterine blood flow and lower abdominal pain in women with primary dysmenorrhea. *Br J Obstet Gynaecol* 1976;83:673–8.
55. Denny Dr, Gerrard M. Behavioral treatments of primary dysmenorrhea: a review. *Behav Res Ther* 1981;19:303–12.
56. Sigmon ST, Nelson RO. The effectiveness of activity scheduling and relaxation training in the treatment of spasmodic dysmenorrhea. *J Behav Med* 1988;11:483–95.
57. Logue CM, Moos RH. Perimenstrual symptoms: prevalence and risk factors. *Psychosom Med* 1986;48:388–414.
58. Prior JC, Vigna Y. Conditioning exercise and premenstrual syndrome. *J Reprod Med* 1987; 32:423–8.
59. Helms JM. Acupuncture for the management of primary dysmenorrhea. *Obstet Gynecol* 1987; 69:51–6.
60. Dawood MY, Ramos J. Transcutaneous electrical nerve stimulation (TENS) for the treatment of primary dysmenorrhea: a randomized crossover comparison with placebo TENS and ibuprofen. *Obstet Gynecol* 1990;75:656–60.
61. Lundeberg T, Bondesson L, Lundström V. Relief of primary dysmenorrhea by transcutaneous electrical nerve stimulation. *Acta Obstet Gynecol Scand* 1985;64:491–7.
62. Smith RP, Heltzel JA. Interrelations of analgesia and uterine activity in women with primary dymenorrhea. A preliminary report. *J Reprod Med* 1991;36:260–4.

Pediatric and Adolescent Gynecology,
edited by S. E. Carpenter and J. A. Rock.
Raven Press, Ltd., New York © 1992.

16

Premenstrual Syndrome

*Carol A. Wilson and †William R. Keye, Jr.

**School of Health, Physical Education, and Recreation, University of Nevada, Las Vegas, Nevada 89154-3007; †The Beaumont Hospital Fertility Center, Royal Oak, Michigan, 48072*

Adolescent health advocates have asked, "Who speaks for the female adolescent?" (1). Henceforth, we ask, "Who speaks for the female adolescent who suffers with premenstrual syndrome (PMS)?" Although recognized in adult women and often referred to as "the mid-thirties syndrome" (2), PMS has been largely unrecognized in adolescents. Adolescent premenstrual symptomatology and rebellious or rapidly changing behavior has often been labeled "just adolescence," or "changing hormones," a trivialization or denial of PMS. On the other hand, severe premenstrual symptomatology has often been referred to as "periodic psychosis of puberty." Because of this, many adolescents with premenstrual symptoms have been ignored or misdiagnosed and thus, inappropriately evaluated and treated. Unfortunately, years of untreated premenstrual symptoms often results in unnecessary suffering and psychosocial complications such as decreased self-esteem and assertiveness, loss of self-confidence, disturbed relationships, unfinished education, and loss of employment (3). Thus, it is imperative that PMS in the female adolescent be recognized and treated.

Ironically, there has been controversy over whether or not PMS is experienced by adolescents. A common assumption has been that adolescents suffer only with dysmenorrhea and older, premenopausal women suffer with PMS (4–9). Many health care providers believe this is true for several reasons. First, researchers such as Golub et al. found and reported that normal adolescents did not experience increased anxiety or depression during the premenstrual phase of the menstrual cycle. Second, early assays on PMS by such pioneers in reproductive medicine as Israel (10) claimed that premenstrual tension occurs in women between the ages of 20 and 40. Finally, few adolescents complain to their pediatrician, family doctor or gynecologist about premenstrual symptoms.

However, there is abundant evidence that PMS exists in the female adolescent.

Researchers have reported that many women with PMS retrospectively trace the genesis of their symptoms to adolescence (11–13; Deneris, 1987, unpublished observations). In addition, other researchers have reported, from retrospective assessments, that PMS is a disorder of adolescence (14–17). Furthermore, Wilson et al. reported that 44% of a group of adolescent girls (n = 88) perceived that premenstrual symptoms affected academic performance, 17% reported class absenteeism as a result of those symptoms, and depression was reported by 42% of the adolescent women. In addition, there was no significant difference between the prevalence of premenstrual symptoms and the prevalence of dysmenorrhea.

Recently, Wilson et al. (18,19) found PMS in the adolescent daughters of adult women with PMS. In this prospective study, they found that adolescents whose mothers experienced premenstrual syndrome were more likely to experience premenstrual symptoms than daughters of mothers without premenstrual syndrome. Thus, doubt as to the existence of premenstrual syndrome in adolescents continues to exist only in the minds of the uninformed or inexperienced clinicians and researchers.

DEFINITION AND DIAGNOSTIC CRITERIA

Premenstrual syndrome is diagnosed as a combination of time-delineated physical, emotional, and behavioral symptoms that occur before menstruation but after ovulation (luteal phase) and regress or disappear during menstruation; not solely the result of environmental stress, the occurrence of which interferes with the quality of life. A multiplicity of more than 150 symptoms representing every organ system have been reported as part of the syndrome of PMS (20,21)—symptoms that are overwhelmingly numerous, diverse, complex and diagnostically nonspecific (22). Unfortunately, this conceptual definition is of little help to the health care provider in the usual clinical setting.

Fortunately, there are several sets of specific diagnostic criteria available to aid the clinician. For example, diagnostic criteria for PMS are now listed in the revised version of the Diagnostic Statistical Manual for Mental Disorders (DSM-IIIR). The criteria included in this manual include the requirement that specified symptoms, some of which are listed on the Utah PMS Calendar II (Appendix), are present and occur in the week prior to menses. In addition, these symptoms disappear within a few days of the onset of menses. Furthermore, the criteria state that these symptoms cause "marked distress or marked impairment in social or occupational function." PMS is present when there is evidence of symptoms during the premenstrual (luteal) phase of the menstrual cycle with significantly fewer or no symptoms during the postmenstrual (follicular) phase. Criteria also require that these symptoms are confirmed by daily prospective self-ratings in at least two symptomatic cycles (23). Although the National Institute of Mental Health (24) has suggested that there should be at least a 30% increase in symptom severity in the five days prior to menses compared with the 5 days following menses, adolescents and women with severe premenstrual syndrome frequently will note at least a doubling of the severity of their symptoms during the premenstrual (luteal) phase of the menstrual cycle.

However, we have used the following diagnostic criteria in our clinical work:

1. Patients between the ages of menarche and menopause.
2. Evidence of ovulatory menstrual cycles.
3. A history of premenstrual (luteal) but not follicular (postmenstrual) symptoms.
4. A premenstrual (luteal) pattern of symptoms obtained prospectively on the Utah PMS Calendar II with an increase of at least 100% from the follicular (post-

menstrual) to the premenstrual (luteal) phase.
5. The absence of chronic physical or psychiatric disease.
6. The absence of environmental stresses that occur periodically and coincide with the premenstrual (luteal) phase of the menstrual cycle.

The utility of these diagnostic criteria will be illustrated in this chapter in our discussion regarding the evaluation of possible causes of premenstrual syndrome.

Premenstrual syndrome in the adolescent is characterized by recurring physical, emotional and behavioral symptoms or changes during the premenstrual (luteal) part of the menstrual cycle. Common premenstrual physical symptoms include: bloating, breast tenderness, headache, weight gain, joint pain, palpitations and fatigue. Common emotional symptoms among adolescents include anxiety, irritability, depression, paranoia, increased sensitivity, decreased self-confidence, altered and negative body image, and loneliness. Finally, the behavioral changes that are common in adolescents with premenstrual syndrome include: social withdrawal, emotional or physical abuse, binge eating or consumption of alcoholic beverages, increased sexual activity, and suicidal gestures.

Adolescent premenstrual symptoms are essentially no difficult than those that occur in adult women, but when superimposed upon the stresses of adolescence, they often cause interpersonal and social crises. In addition, because menstrual periods in adolescents are commonly irregular, the association between these symptoms and behavior changes and the premenstrual (luteal) part of the menstrual cycle may not be obvious. As a result, parents and other persons in authority positions, unaware of the underlying cause of the behavior, may either ignore the behavior or react negatively. This can lead to obvious personal and social complications that may in and of themselves become problematic. Not frequently, the adolescent with severe behavioral changes will have faced severe criticism from parents, teachers or law enforcement officers.

ETIOLOGY OF PMS

Beginning with Frank's (25) description of premenstrual syndrome in 1931, there has been a succession of authors and researchers who have proposed various etiologies for premenstrual syndrome. The etiologies tend to fall into three groups: medical, psychological or social.

Common medical theories regarding the etiology of premenstrual syndrome include deficiencies or excesses of estrogen and progesterone, imbalances in the ratio of estrogen and progesterone, excess in the production of various other hormones including prolactin or prostagladins, and deficiencies in such hormones as beta-endorphin or thyroxin. Nonhormonal medical theories include infection with various bacteria or yeast, vitamin deficiencies, alteration in the metabolism of essential fatty acids, or abnormalities in neurotransmitter metabolism (26).

Psychological explanations for premenstrual syndrome in adolescents include a rejection of the female role or a variation of common affective disorders. Social explanations for the existence of premenstrual syndrome include the mimicking of the behavior of other significant females in the life of the adolescent, social expectations, or pressure from others in the social environment of the adolescent (27).

Unfortunately, none of these theories have proven to explain premenstrual syndrome in all situations and none of them have withstood close and careful scientific scrutiny. Recent research findings suggest that the hormones of the premenstrual (luteal) phase of the menstrual cycle, while normal in their nature and amounts, act as triggers to stimulate the development of premenstrual symptoms in women who are predisposed to develop PMS. However, this biological stimulus appears not to be sufficient for the development of premenstrual syndrome.

Therefore, we have constructed a biopsychosocial model of premenstrual syndrome. This biopsychosocial model is a methodologic tool, germane to all illnesses, all disciplines, and all types of health care professionals. It has been utilized to recognize and investigate PMS because the syndrome involves the convergence of endocrinology, chronobiology, behavioral phenomenology, social psychology, neurobiology and their interactions (28). This model assumes that premenstrual syndrome is a result of reciprocal ongoing interactions of the following factors: biological (atoms, molecules, organelles, cells, tissues, organs, organ systems), psychological (personal), and social (family, community, culture, and society). In addition, it recognizes that psychosocial factors are equally—if not more important—than biomedical factors in determining the nature and severity of premenstrual syndrome (29).

The biopsychosocial model as seen in Fig. 1 states that the hormone changes of the premenstrual (luteal) phase of the menstrual cycle—that is the increase in estradiol and/or progesterone that occur in the premenstrual (luteal) phase, trigger premenstrual symptoms in women who are biologically or psychologically predisposed to develop PMS (30). Although these hormonal changes appear to be necessary for the development of premenstrual syndrome, they may not be sufficient. It appears that whether or not an individual develops premenstrual symptoms in response to the hormonal change of the menstrual cycle depends upon past and present biological, psychological or social conditions that may have predisposed the individual to develop premenstrual syndrome. Therefore, one may have a biological predisposition but experience no premenstrual symptoms because the psychological and social conditions that are necessary for the development of premenstrual symptoms have not been present. The benefit of the biopsychosocial model is that it encourages clinicians and health care providers to recognize the contribution to PMS by biological, psychological and social factors and provides a logical approach to therapy, including medical, psychological and social therapy and support (12,31).

The biopsychosocial model, as used in the evaluation and treatment of premenstrual syndrome, is consistent with the recommendation that an adolescent should be viewed within the parameters of a biopsychosocial framework. Coupey (32) claimed that adolescent health care is unique in that it demands of its practitioners the integration of the biology, psychology and sociology of each individual as a "whole" person every time there is a health problem to be solved. Katchadourian (33) claimed, "Ultimately, understanding the developmental events after the second decade, or for that matter any other decade of life, depends on our comprehension of the interactional patterns between biological and psychosocial variables." These variables are recogniz-

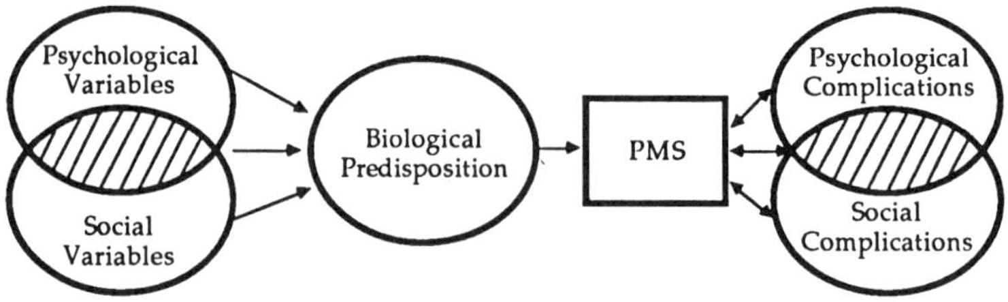

FIG. 1. Biopsychosocial model.

able in theories that are specific to adolescence. Hill's (34) framework identified the following changes: biological: puberty; psychological: changes in reasoning and cognition; social: societal norms for behavior. The psychosocial issues of adolescent development, identity, achievement, sexuality, intimacy, autonomy, and attachment are labeled secondary changes (35).

EVALUATION OF THE FEMALE ADOLESCENT FOR PMS

Many professionals find that providing health care to adolescents—although rewarding—is frustrating, difficult, challenging, and time consuming. The adolescent is in transition between childhood and adulthood, between dependence and independence—never static in her physical, cognitive and social growth. Thus, the diagnostic evaluation of the adolescent and treatment of PMS poses a dual challenge: the enigmatic complexity of PMS combined with the equally complex nature of adolescent development.

As a preface, it is helpful to realize that adolescent development precipitates a normative crisis in family-life development (36,37). For example, the onset of menses is a significant biological event for the female adolescent (38,39). In addition, marked changes occur in cognition (38,40) and thought organization (38,40,41); maturity in interests and attitudes (42,43); and acceptance of female role and sexuality (38,44). However, research by Peterson (45) has indicated that although the biological events of puberty are unavoidable, not all adolescents experience the "storm." Rather, social and environmental factors play a significant role. These factors include the death of a parent or divorce of parents; a change in schools that may have other ramifications: disruption of peer-group structure and different achievement expectations. It is again in consideration of these factors that health care providers are forced to evaluate adolescents with premenstrual symptoms.

In the assessment of adolescent PMS, the practitioner should realize that the most important need of the adolescent is private and confidential care. At least part of the interview and physical examination should be private. Findings should be discussed with both the adolescent and parents, if possible. However, if the adolescent requests confidentiality, it is important that the health care provider or practitioner respect this confidence in order to maintain trust and communication. At times, it may be necessary that the practitioner insure that the parents are aware of a problem if it involves a serious health risk. This is best done with the adolescent's permission, told to the parents with the adolescent present, or more ideally, by the adolescent herself (46). In addition, the initial evaluation is performed most effectively at the time when the adolescent is not suffering from premenstrual symptoms.

The practitioner should be flexible and understanding of adolescent life experience that differs from the adult. For example, whereas the adult woman may be angry that her mother-in-law is visiting her or devastated over a recent divorce, the adolescent may be angry that her brother ate her cereal for breakfast or devastated that she didn't win a position on the cheerleading squad.

In order to assess and diagnose PMS, the following four-step procedure is recommended:

Initial Assessment and Interview

The patient is asked at the time of the initial interview to describe her physical, emotional and behavioral symptoms and changes. She is also asked to describe her menstrual period, including the age at which she first menstruated, the interval between her menstrual periods, the duration of her periods, the regularity, and the presence or absence of pelvic pain during her menstrual periods. She is asked to relate the timing of her symptoms to the onset of her menstrual periods to determine if she perceives a premenstrual occurrence of her symptoms. In addition, her general medical, family and social history should be obtained. Finally, any previous therapies and their outcomes should be discussed with the patient.

In addition to evaluating the specific symptoms, it is also important to determine the impact of behavioral changes and symptoms on the patient's self-esteem, self-image, assertiveness, and relationships with family, friends, co-workers, and fellow students. Adolescence that is complicated by premenstrual syndrome is often a perplexing issue and may lead to a variety of social problems that need to be considered.

After the physical symptoms have been described by the patient, it is important to perform a physical examination to rule out underlying diseases. Pelvic examination for the adolescent is indicated under the following circumstances: (a) menstrual abnormalities, (b) abdominal pain, (c) sexual activity, (d) vaginal discharge, (e) maternal history of DES exposure during pregnancy, (f) teenagers desire to know that she is "normal," and (g) rape (47).

Utah PMS Calendar II

A premenstrual history of symptoms needs to be confirmed by a prospective gathering of data (23,24). We have found the Utah Calendar II (Fig. 2) to be an extremely useful and easy tool for obtaining prospective data. This calendar (appendix) is a grid that makes it possible for the adolescent or adult woman suffering from premenstrual symptoms to record each day, on a single sheet of paper, the presence and severity of symptoms that she may experience. To facilitate statistical research analysis, we have asked our patients to rate the severity of the symptoms on a Likert scale of 1–7, with 1 representing mild symptoms and 7 representing severe symptoms. However, for simplicity, a 3 point rating scale of symptoms may be more practical for patients who are not research subjects: 1 = mild, 2 = moderate, and 3 = severe.

The adolescent should record her daily weight. If there is a question of whether or not she is ovulating, her basal body temperature should be taken upon awakening in the morning and recorded on the calendar. In addition, she can record on the calendar the use of medication and the presence of other significant events in her life that may influence the presence of symptoms. After 2 months of charting information on the calendar, the patient is interviewed again. The calendar is then evaluated to determine if there is a premenstrual pattern to her symptoms.

It is important to realize that not all of the symptoms that the adolescent reports are necessarily related to premenstrual syndrome. It is not uncommon for an adolescent or an adult woman to experience some symptoms premenstrually and some symptoms throughout the menstrual cycle that may be exacerbated premenstrually. A premenstrual pattern of symptoms is displayed in the sample calendar in this chapter.

Psychosocial Evaluation

It is essential that a psychosocial evaluation be performed in the adolescent who displays or complains of marked behavioral changes or emotional symptoms in the premenstrual (luteal) phase of the menstrual cycle. Although we have used the Minnesota Multiphasic Personality Inventory (MMPI) (18,19,48–51), scoring its 566 items is often laborious for the adolescent. Therefore, simpler psychometric tests that are designed to evaluate the presence or absence of depression or anxiety, such as the Spielberg State Trait Anxiety Scale or the Beck Depression Inventory, may be more practical. Alternatively, an interview by a trained social worker or psychologist may be very useful.

It is necessary to note, however, that psychometric or psychosocial evaluations need to be performed at each of the phases of the menstrual cycle. That is, the psychometric tests or interviews should be performed once during the follicular (postmenstrual) phase of the menstrual cycle and once during the premenstrual (luteal) phase of the menstrual cycle. If one interviews or evaluates a woman or adolescent with premenstrual syndrome during only one of these phases, one will be left with the impression that either the individual is completely free of any emotional distresses or that she indeed suffers from a chronic affective disorder or other significant psychiatric illness. In addition to determining that there is a significant change in the psychological status from the follicular (postmenstrual) or premenstrual (luteal) phase, the psychometric tests and/or interview should be designed to determine the severity of any psychosocial complications that may have occured as a result of recurring premenstrual symptoms.

Review and Diagnostic Session

At the conclusion of the evaluation, it is useful to sit down with the adolescent and her parents (if appropriate), to review the results of the findings from previous visits and evaluations. It is also important that this diagnostic session be held during the follicular (postmenstrual) phase of the menstrual cycle because the patient may be angry, depressed, or confused during the premenstrual (luteal) phase of the menstrual cycle and unable to cooperate or concentrate during the session. It is during this time that the findings are reviewed, the diagnosis is discussed, and a practical approach to the management of PMS is established.

Therapy of Premenstrual Syndrome in the Adolescent

Validation

The therapy of premenstrual syndrome in the adolescent begins with the process of evaluation. Often the adolescent is unable to understand why she engages in socially unacceptable behavior such as rapidly-changing, destructive mood swings. As a result, she may begin to feel inadequate and have self-doubts, feelings that are reinforced by authority figures within her life. By evaluating her behavior and her feelings in medical terms, the burden of guilt is often removed from the shoulders of the adolescent. Ultimately, if premenstrual syndrome is diagnosed, the self-worth and emotional strength of the adolescent female is validated. Therefore, her improved self-image may singularly decrease the severity of her premenstrual symptoms.

Reassuring the adolescent that her experiences are real and that she is not "going crazy" can have a powerful therapeutic effect. In addition, if a psychometrist, social worker, or psychologist demonstrate through standardized psychometric tests that the adolescent is suffering from premenstrual syndrome but is emotionally stable and healthy during most of the days of the month, the adolescent with PMS will begin the long process of healing and recovery.

Education

It is important that the female adolescent with PMS—and her family—be educated that certain behaviors and feelings are due to premenstrual syndrome. However, there are other times when negative or unpleasant emotional feelings are appropriate and represent the healthy, normal range of human feelings. Thus, the adolescent should be educated as to the importance of appropriately expressing her feelings under certain circumstances, rather than suppressing them. In addition, neither the adolescent nor family and friends should use premenstrual syndrome as a scapegoat for unacceptable feelings and behavior.

Preventive Care

Premenstrual syndrome is often amenable to a number of self-help measures that require adequate rest and sleep, stress management, aerobic exercise and good nutrition (3). Many of the daily activities of the adolescent tend to aggravate the severity of her premenstrual symptoms. For example, long periods of fasting in an attempt to maintain or lose body weight, may aggravate the symptoms of PMS. Although there is little scientific evidence to document the value of adequate nutrition in the treatment of premenstrual syndrome, many adolescent and adult women relate that they experience fewer and less severe premenstrual symptoms if they follow a modified hypoglycemic diet that includes frequent, small meals to avoid fasting; the incorporation of complex carbohydrates; a decrease in the amount of simple sugars, salt, caffeine and alcohol; and the avoidance of fat diets which can create metabolic abnormalities that may aggravate the symptoms of premenstrual syndrome. There is clinical evidence that anorexia and bulimia are increasing among female adolescents (52) and recent clinical observations suggest that the amenorrhea that follows anorexia may act as a precipitating event for PMS (13).

Aerobic exercise has been shown to reduce the severity of premenstrual symptoms (53). Whether this is due to the fact that the woman is distracted from her emotional feelings or because the exercise increases the beta-endorphins is uncertain. However, again, many women report anecdotally that 20–30 minutes of aerobic exercise 3–7 days a week during the premenstrual (luteal) phase of the menstrual cycle is beneficial. By teaching the adolescent female how to manage her symptoms through diet and exercise, she is learning how to manage her life instead of being victimized by her health. This principle is one that the adolescent female may find helpful in other areas of her daily life.

Achieving Cooperation

The adolescent who is diagnosed with premenstrual syndrome and is given medication or a variety of self-help measures to decrease the severity and frequency of her symptoms may find it difficult to be compliant if she does not have the support and acceptance of her family, friends and school authority figures. There are many instances in which family members or friends have undermined or sabotaged the success of the patient's therapy and have discouraged her from complying with the recommendations of the health care professional. It is important to educate those in the immediate family so that they can be supportive of the adolescent and make it easier for her to comply with medical recommendations.

Eliminating Contributing Factors

Often the severity of premenstrual syndrome is influenced by the psychosocial milieu such as the psychological and social dysfunction within the family unit. An adolescent who experiences premenstrual symptoms but has to live in a household dominated by an alcoholic or abusive father will probably continue to have significant premenstrual symptoms in addition to other psychophysiologic reactions. Therefore, it is important to identify and attempt to help the adolescent control those negative social and psychological forces in her life. It may be necessary to recommend that the family seek counseling or therapy for issues unrelated to premenstrual syndrome so that the adolescent can recover in a relatively stress-free environment.

Medical Therapy

The therapies available to the adolescent with PMS can be divided into three categories: (a) symptomatic therapies (b) therapies of yet unproven value, and (c) therapies that cause anovulation and amenorrhea.

Symptomatic Therapies

Among the symptomatic therapies, there are a number of over-the-counter medications that are available and promoted for the reduction of symptoms of premenstrual syndrome. Commonly, they contain a diuretic, analgesic and antihistamine. Women and adolescents with mild premenstrual symptoms and premenstrual molimina may experience relief of their premenstrual symptoms when using these symptomatic medications. For the adolescent who has a single specific premenstrual symptom, symptomatic therapy may also be beneficial. For example, if premenstrual headaches are experienced, the use of appropriate analgesics or antiprostagladins is recommended after a thorough neurological evaluation has ruled out underlying disease. However, we attempt to avoid the use of antidepressants and anzeolitic medications when these symptoms are present only for a few days of each month. If severe mastalgia (breast tenderness) is experienced, bromocryptine 2.5 mg at bedtime once a day during the premenstrual (luteal) phase of the menstrual cycle is suggested. Those who experience the sensation of bloating may benefit from periodic premenstrual (luteal) phase administration of Spirolactone in doses of 50–100 mg a day. However, the long-term use of diuretics in the adolescent or adult woman should be discouraged.

Therapies of Yet Unproven Value

The second category of medical therapies include those unproven therapies that are documented in the literature and are usually based on the clinical observations of physicians. While they may be unproven in scientific studies, they nonetheless may help reduce the frequency and severity of symptoms in many adolescents.

Among these approaches to therapy are combination multiple vitamins that are rich in Vitamin B_6 and magnesium. However, the use of megadoses of vitamins should be discouraged because significant side effects have been found to occur. A common example of this is the neurologic symptoms that have occurred in women using doses of 200 mg or more of Vitamin B_6 for premenstrual symptoms. Nutritional supplementation of Oil with Evening Primrose, which is rich in gamma linolenic acid, may also be helpful, although controlled scientific studies have been contradictory. Finally, progesterone has been endorsed for the treatment of adolescent premenstrual symptoms by Dr. Katharina Dalton in England. In her vast experience, she has noted and reported significant reduction of premenstrual symptoms in the adolescent following the administration of progesterone. There have been a number of double-blind placebo-controlled crossover studies that have been inconsistent. The vast majority of studies using vaginal suppositories have failed to demonstrate a benefit of progesterone over placebo. However, a single study using oral micronized progesterone by Dr. Dennerstein has demonstrated an effect of the progesterone that cannot be accounted for by the placebo. One hundred milligram capsules of micronized progesterone can be prepared by a local pharmacy upon request by a physician and administered in doses of 1–300 mg a day. The dose that has been demonstrated to be effective in the literature is 100 mg in the morning followed by 200 mg in the evening in the adult woman.

Smaller doses may be beneficial for the adolescent.

Anovulatory Therapy

The third approach to therapy creates anovulation. The most common medication used to create anovulation in the adolescent are birth control pills. While approximately two-thirds of adult women are intolerant of birth control pills, adolescents with premenstrual symptoms tend to have a positive response. Therefore, the administration of any combination of oral contraceptive for 21 days of each month will not only regulate the sometimes irregular menstrual periods of the adolescent but may also reduce the severity of her symptoms. Alternatively, medroxyprogesterone acetate 10 mg three times a day continuously will cause anovulation and amenorrhea and the reduction of premenstrual symptoms. Unfortunately, some women have significant fluid retention and may experience mild headache or depression while on medroxyprogesterone acetate and therefore, discontinue its use. The use of large doses of Danazol or of GnRH agonists is useful only for a brief duration of time and are not useful for long-term therapy.

In addition to these therapies, there are a number of alternative medical therapies based on alternative theories of premenstrual syndrome. These include the use of antibiotics, antifungal agents, immunotherapy, nutritional therapies, or muscle and joint manipulations. The value of these alternative therapies is yet unproven.

Dealing with the Impact of PMS

The patient, family and friends should realize that ignoring PMS can cause a series of spiraling multi-dimensional programs that may impact health and quality of life. The patient may lose self-confidence and experience a decrease in her self-esteem. She may develop an altered body image while feelings of inadequacy amplify, and she may lose assertiveness, a characteristic much needed to resist peer pressure. Second, relationships with significant others may deteriorate, and additional close relationships may become strained or non-existent. Third, the PMS sufferer's functional level can retrogress and deteriorate if she is unable to cope emotionally, maintain a job, or pursue educational goals, particularly if she becomes withdrawn or socially isolated (3).

CONCLUSION

The biopsychosocial model, as a methodological tool for the evaluation of PMS in adolescents, demonstrates the dynamic complexity of the etiology and pathophysiology of premenstrual syndrome. However, this complexity will be minimized when validated standardized tools are used to assess PMS. In addition, diagnostic criterion should be standardized based on the recommendations and guidelines of the Diagnostic and Statistical Manual for Mental Disorders (DSM-III). Controversy may exist over these criterion and assessment tools but acceptance is necessary in order to create uniformity in diagnostic and therapeutic methodology. Furthermore, research demands controlled, well-designed studies, free of flawed methodology (28,30, 54–56).

Practitioners and health care providers need to be understanding and sensitive to the physical, psychological and social dynamics of the adolescent. As medicine becomes more specialized, the practitioner often loses sight of the "whole" person. Thus, it is often necessary for the practitioner to network with professionals who are trained in different disciplines in order to provide needed multidisciplinary care. The appropriate support team may consist of physician assistants, health educators, nurses, social workers, gynecologists, psychiatrists and psychologists.

Confidential, empathetic, entrusted care for the adolescent is essential. Health education is critical. The female adolescent with PMS has an opportunity to learn healthy lifestyle habits that may control her PMS or prevent it from worsening. The woman in her mid-thirties who has not exercised or applied preventive care to her lifestyle has an extremely difficult time changing her behavior. However, the adolescent is flexible and teachable and adverse habits are usually not well established.

Adolescent female health care providers face the challenge of understanding, preventing, detecting, and treating premenstrual syndrome. Hopefully, the enigmatic controversies surrounding the etiology and pathophysiology of premenstrual syndrome will be unraveled as we focus on the female adolescent. The reward will be manifested in the women of the future—women who will suffer less—women who will live happier, healthier, more productive lives.

APPENDIX

INSTRUCTIONS

The PMS Calendar II is essential for the diagnosis of PMS (Fig. 2A,B). In addition, it is the only way to monitor your response to treatment. The PMS Calendar II should be completed according to the following instructions.

1. Mark the date of the first day of your menstrual period that corresponds to the first day of your cycle (the first day of bleeding). If you do not have periods simply begin with the first day of each month.
2. Each morning before arising, take your temperature orally with an oral thermometer. With a red pencil put a dot below the appropriate date and opposite the temperature.
3. Weigh yourself unclothed each morning before you eat or drink and after you empty your bladder and, if possible, your bowels. Record the results.
4. Note any medications taken or dietary changes made under the heading, "Treatment." Write the name and dose of medication (e.g., progesterone suppositories, 200 mg). Note the number of times that medication was taken on a given day by writing the appropriate number in the box opposite the medication and below the date.
5. Choose the most common physical, emotional; and/or social symptoms that you experience with PMS from the symptom lists below and write them in the blanks on the PMS Calendar II. (Remember, the list below is not complete. Add to your calendar any other recurring symptoms you can identify.)
6. Note at the end of each day if you have experienced any of the physical, emotional or social symptoms during that day. If you have experienced a symptom, estimate the severity of that symptom from 1 (mild) to 7 (severe) and write the number in the box opposite the symptom and below the appropriate date.
7. Bring this calendar with you to each appointment.
8. Also, bring or send a written description of how severe your PMS was during the month, how effective the treatment was and suggestions or any questions you wish to have answered.

Physical Symptoms

- Abdominal bloating
- Acne
- Accidents
- Backache
- Breast swelling
- Breast tenderness
- Chest pain
- Constipation
- Craving for sweets or salty foods
- Decreased alcohol tolerance
- Dizziness
- Fainting spells
- Headache
- Heart palpitations
- Herpes "cold sores"
- Hives or rash
- Incoordination "clumsiness"
- Increased appetite
- Increased alcohol consumption
- Increased thirst
- Irritated eyes
- Itching
- Joint pain
- Leg cramps
- Leg heaviness or swelling
- Nasal congestion
- Seizures
- Sensitivity to light
- Sensitivity to noise
- Sharp one-sided ovarian pain
- Sinusitis

Mental Symptoms

- Anger
- Anxiety
- Apathy
- Decreased self-esteem
- Depression
- Fatigue
- Fear
- Forgetfulness
- Guilt feelings
- Hostility
- Inability to cope
- Change in sex drive
- Indecision
- Inefficiency
- Insecurity
- Insomnia
- Intolerance
- Loneliness
- Mania
- Mental aggression
- Panic
- Paranoia
- Physical aggression
- Physical violence
- Poor concentration or distractability
- Poor Judgement
- Sense of being out of control
- Suicidal thoughts
- Tearfulness
- Tension
- Weakness

Social Symptoms

- Absence from work
- Abuse alcohol
- Abuse drugs
- Allow friends to make decisions
- Argue with significant other
- Argue with family or friends
- Cannot discuss sex
- Desire to leave home
- Desire to stay home
- Dislike being a girl
- Family cares about me when I'm sick or don't feel well
- Family listens to me when I'm sick or don't feel well
- Feeling that no one understands or supports me
- Few close friends
- Few or no recreational or athletic habits
- Inability to say "no"
- Inability to form close relationships
- Inability to verbally express feelings
- Need to be alone
- Negative feelings about menstruation
- Poor personal hygiene
- Poor relationship with significant other
- Poor relationship with family or friends
- Special attention when sick or don't feel well
- Strained family relations
- Verbally abuse family or friends
- Verbally abuse significant other
- Withdrawal from people

UTAH PMS CALENDAR II

Name ______________________ Month ______________

Date																															
Day of Menstrual Cycle	1	2	3	4	5	6	7	8	9	10	11	12	13	14	15	16	17	18	19	20	21	22	23	24	25	26	27	28	29	30	31
Weight																															
Treatment																															
1. ______																															
2. ______																															
Physical Symptoms																															
1. ______																															
2. ______																															
3. ______																															
4. ______																															
5. ______																															
6. ______																															
7. ______																															
Emotional Symptoms																															
1. ______ 98.8																															
2. ______ 98.6																															
3. ______ 98.4																															
4. ______ 98.2																															
5. ______ 98.0																															
6. ______ 97.8																															
7. ______ 97.6																															
Social Symptoms																															
1. ______																															
2. ______																															
3. ______																															
4. ______																															
5. ______																															
6. ______																															
7. ______																															

A

FIG. 2. Utah PMS Calendar II. **A:** Blank form. **B:** Sample form.

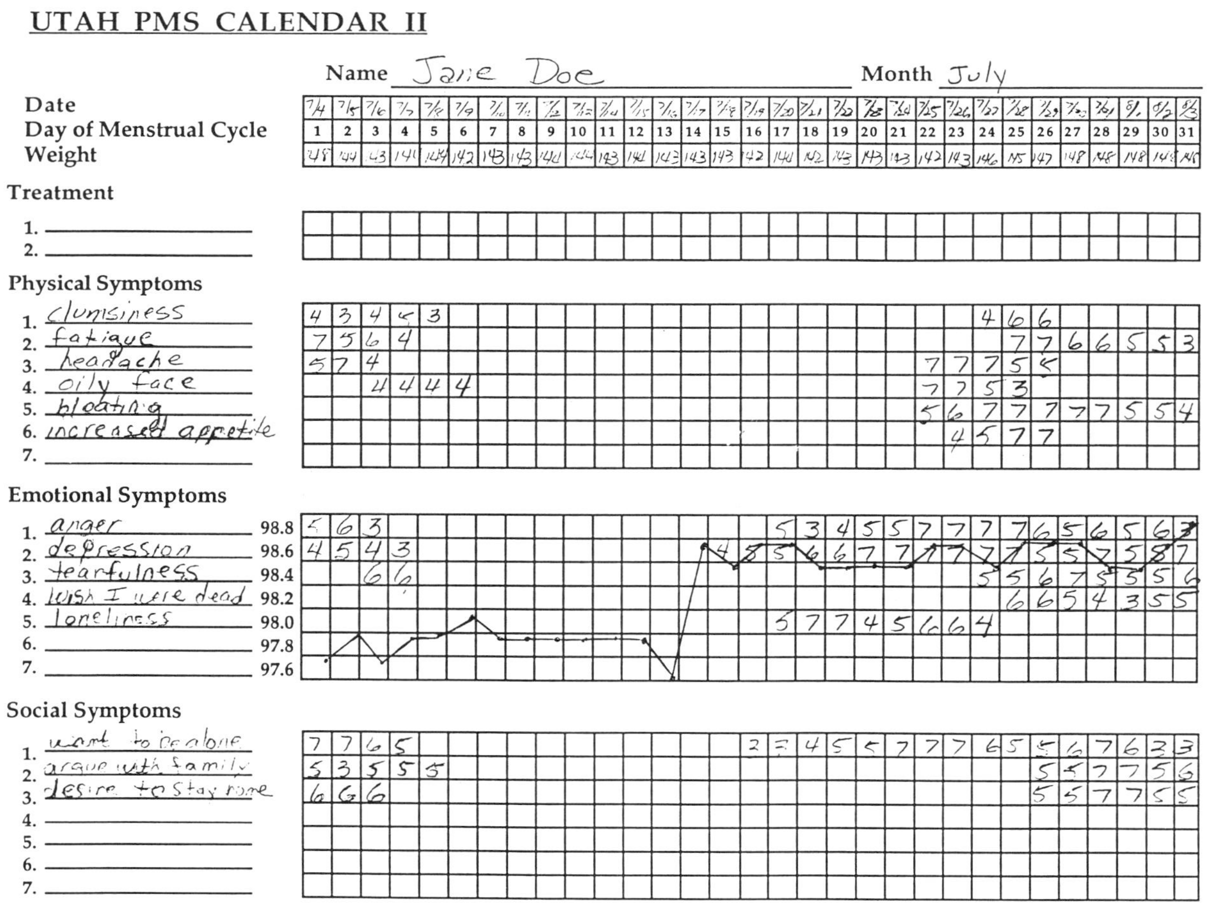

B

FIG. 2. *Continued.*

REFERENCES

1. Golub S. Who speaks for the female adolescent? *Women Health* 1984;9:xiii–xvi.
2. Lloyd TS. The mid-thirties syndrome. *Va Med* 1963;90:51.
3. Wilson CA, Keye WR Jr. A survey of adolescent dysmenorrhea and premenstrual symptom frequency: A model program for prevention, detection and treatment. *J Adolesc Health Care* 1989;10:317–22.
4. Golub S, Harrington D. Premenstrual and menstrual mood changes in adolescent women. *J Pers Soc Psychol* 1981;41:961–5.
5. Logue C, Moos R. Premenstrual symptoms: prevalence and risk factors. *Psychosom Med* 1986;48:388–414.
6. Moos RH. Typology of menstrual cycle symptoms. *Gynecology* 1969;103:390–402.
7. Rosenwaks Z, Seegar-Jones G. Menstrual pain: its origin and pathogenesis. *J Reprod Med* 1980;25:207–12.
8. Rubinow D, Roy-Byrne P. Premenstrual syndrome: overview from a methodologic perspective. *Am J Psychol* 1984;141:29–38.
9. World Health Organization. A cross-cultural study of menstruation: Implications for contraceptive development and use. *Stud Fam Plann* 1981;12:3–16.
10. Israel SL. Premenstrual tension. *JAMA* 1938; 110:1721–1723.
11. Dalton K. *Once a month*. New York: Hunter House, 1983.
12. Keye WR Jr. Premenstrual symptoms: Evaluation and treatment. *Compr Ther* 1988;14:19–26.
13. Norris SV, Sullivan C. *PMS*. New York: Rawson Associates, 1983.
14. Fisher M, Trieller RN, Napolitano B. Premenstrual symptoms in adolescents. *J Adolesc Health Care* 1989;10:369–75.
15. Widholm O. Dysmenorrhea during adolescence. *Acta Obstetr Gynecol Scand* [*Suppl*] 1979;87:61.
16. Widholm O, Kantero RL. Menstrual patterns in adolescent girls according to the chronological gynecological ages. *Acta Obstetr Gynecol Society* [*Suppl*] 1971;14:19–29.
17. Wilson C, Emans S, Mansfield J. The relationship of calculated percent body fat, sports participation, age, and place of residence on menstrual patterns in healthy adolescent girls at an independent New England high school. *J Adoles Health Care* 1988;5:248–53.
18. Wilson CA, Turner C, Keye WR Jr. Firstborn adolescent daughters and mothers with and without premenstrual syndrome: a comparison. *J Adolesc Health Care* 1990 (in press.)
19. Wilson CA, Turner C, Reagan P, Keye WR Jr. Premenstrual symptoms in mother-daughter dyads: mothers diagnosed with and without premenstrual syndrome. 1990 (submitted).
20. Dalton K. *The premenstrual syndrome*. Springfield: Charles C. Thomas, 1964.
21. Moos RH. The development of a menstrual distress questionnaire. *Psychosom Med* 1968;30: 853–67.
22. Rubinow D, Hoban C, Grover G. Medical and psychiatric perspectives. In: Keye WR Jr, ed. *The premenstrual syndrome*. Philadelphia: W. B. Saunders, 1988:27–43.
23. American Psychiatric Association. *Diagnostic and statistical manual of mental disorders*. 3rd ed. Washington DC: APA, 1987.
24. National Institute of Mental Health. *Workshop on premenstrual syndrome*. Rockville MD: NIMH, 1983.
25. Frank, RT. The hormonal causes of premenstrual tension. *Arch Neur Psych* 1937;26: 1053–7.
26. Reid, R. Etiology: medical theories. In Keye, WR Jr ed. *The premenstrual syndrome*. Philadelphia: WB Saunders, 1988;66–93.
27. Abplanalp J. Psychosocial theories. In: Keye WR Jr, ed. *The premenstrual syndrome*. Philadelphia: WB Saunders, 1988:94–112.
28. Rubinow D, Hoban C, Roy-Bryne P, Grover G, Post R. Premenstrual syndrome: past and future research strategies. *Can J Psychiatry* 1985;30: 469–73.
29. Keye WR Jr, Trunnell E. A biopsychosocial model of premenstrual syndrome. *Int J Infertil* 1986;31:259–62.
30. Trunnell E, Turner C, Keye WR Jr. A comparison of the psychological and hormonal factors in women with and without premenstrual syndrome. *J Abnorm Psychol* 1988;97:1.
31. Trunnell EP, White GL. Pedersen DM, Keye WR Jr. Biopsychosocial model for premenstrual syndrome *Physician Assist* 1989;13:45–52.
32. Abplanalp J, Haskett R, Rose R. The premenstrual syndrome. *Psychiatr Clin North Am* 1980;3:327–47.
33. Katchadourian H. *The biology of adolescence*. San Francisco: W. H. Freeman, 1977.
34. Hill JP. *Understanding early adolescence: a framework*. Carrboro, NC: Center for Early Adolescence, 1980.
35. Jenkins R. Future directions in research. In: Brooks-Gunn J, Peterson A, eds. *Girls at puberty: biological and psychological perspectives*. New York: Plenum Press, 1983:325–38.
36. Blos P. *On adolescence: a psychoanalytic interpretation*. New York: Free Press, 1971.
37. Erikson EH. *Identity and the life cycle*. New York: International Universities Press, 1959.
38. Koff E, Rierdan H, Silverstone E. Changes in representation of body image as a function of menarcheal status. *Dev Psychol* 1978;14:635–42.
39. Danza R. Menarche: Its effects on mother-daughter and father-daughter interactions. In: Golub S, ed. *Menarche*. Lexington: Lexington Books, 1983.
40. Kestenberg J. *Menarche in adolescents—psychoanalytic approach to problems and therapy*. New York: Harper and Brothers, 1961.
41. Whisant L, Zegans L. A study of attitudes toward menarche in white middle-class American adolescent girls. *Am J Psych* 1975;132:809–14.

42. Davis BL. Attitudes toward school among early and late maturing adolescent girls. *J Genet Psychol* 1977;131:261–6.
43. Stone CP, Barker RG. The attitudes and interests of premenarcheal and postmenarcheal girls. *J Genet Psychol* 1939;54:27–71.
44. Lambert G, Rothchild B, Altand R, Greer L. *Adolescence*. Monterey: Brooks/Cole, 1972.
45. Peterson AC. Those gangly years. *Psychol Today* Sept. 1981:28–34.
46. Coupey SM. The challenge of providing health care to adolescents. *Women Health* 1984;9:1–14.
47. Hein K. The first gynecologic examination. *Diagnosis* 1981;3:32–52.
48. Hathaway Sr, McKinley JC. *Manual for administration and scoring MMPI*. Minneapolis: University of Minnesota Press, 1983.
49. Keye Wr Jr, Hammond C, Strong T. Medical and psychologic characteristics of women presenting with premenstrual symptoms. *Obstet Gynecol* 1986;68:634–7.
50. Hammond DC, Keye WR Jr. Premenstrual syndrome. *N Engl J Med* 1985;312:920.
51. Hammond CD. The psychosocial consequences. In Keye WR Jr, ed. *The premenstrual syndrome*. Pennsylvania: WB Saunders, 1988:128–41.
52. Morgan BLG. Nutritional needs of the female adolescent. *Women Health* 1984;9:15–28.
53. Prior JC, Vigna Y, Sciarreta D. *Conditioning exercise decreases premenstrual symptoms: a prospective, controlled 6-month trial. Fertil Steril* 1987;47:402–8.
54. Abplanalp J, Haskett R, Rose R. The premenstrual syndrome. *Psychiatr Clin North Am* 1980;3:327–47.
55. Dennerstein L, Abraham SF. Affective changes and the menstrual cycle. In: Beaumont PJV, Burrows GD, eds. *Handbook of psychiatry and endocrinology*. New York: Elsevier Biomedial, 1982:367–400.
56. Dennerstein L, Spencer-Gardner C, Burrows GD. Mood and the menstrual cycle. *J Psychiatr Res* 1984;18:1–12.

Pediatric and Adolescent Gynecology,
edited by S. E. Carpenter and J. A. Rock.
Raven Press, Ltd., New York © 1992.

17

Hirsutism in the Pediatric or Adolescent Patient

Ricardo Azziz

Department of Obstetrics and Gynecology, University of Alabama, Birmingham, Alabama 35294

Following we will outline the normal pubertal development and metabolism of androgens; the normal physiology and pathophysiology of hair growth; and the differential diagnosis, work-up, and treatment of hirsutism in the pediatric and adolescent patient.

NORMAL ANDROGEN METABOLISM

Androgens are C-19 steroids (containing 19 carbons) derived from cholesterol, and secreted by the adrenal cortex and ovaries. Androgens may also be derived (not secreted) from the conversion of other steroids by the liver and some peripheral tissues (e.g. adipose tissue, muscle, skin, etc.). Principle circulating androgens include testosterone (T) and its metabolite dihydrotestosterone (DHT), androstenedione (A), and dehydroepiandrosterone (DHA) and its metabolite dehydroepiandrosterone sulfate (DHEAS) (Fig. 1). Androgens act through a specific cytoplasmic/nuclear intracellular receptor.

Following puberty, T originates approximately 25% from the ovary, 25% from the adrenal, and 50% from the peripheral conversion of A (1). T and A are metabolized to DHT, the most potent of androgens, through the action of the enzyme 5-α reductase in the liver and skin. Androstenedione is produced equally from the ovary and the adrenal cortex. Approximately 90% of DHA and 99% of DHEAS are produced by the adrenal cortex. DHA, DHEAS and A exhibit a circadian rhythm similar to that of cortisol, with peak serum concentrations in early morning and the nadir in late evening

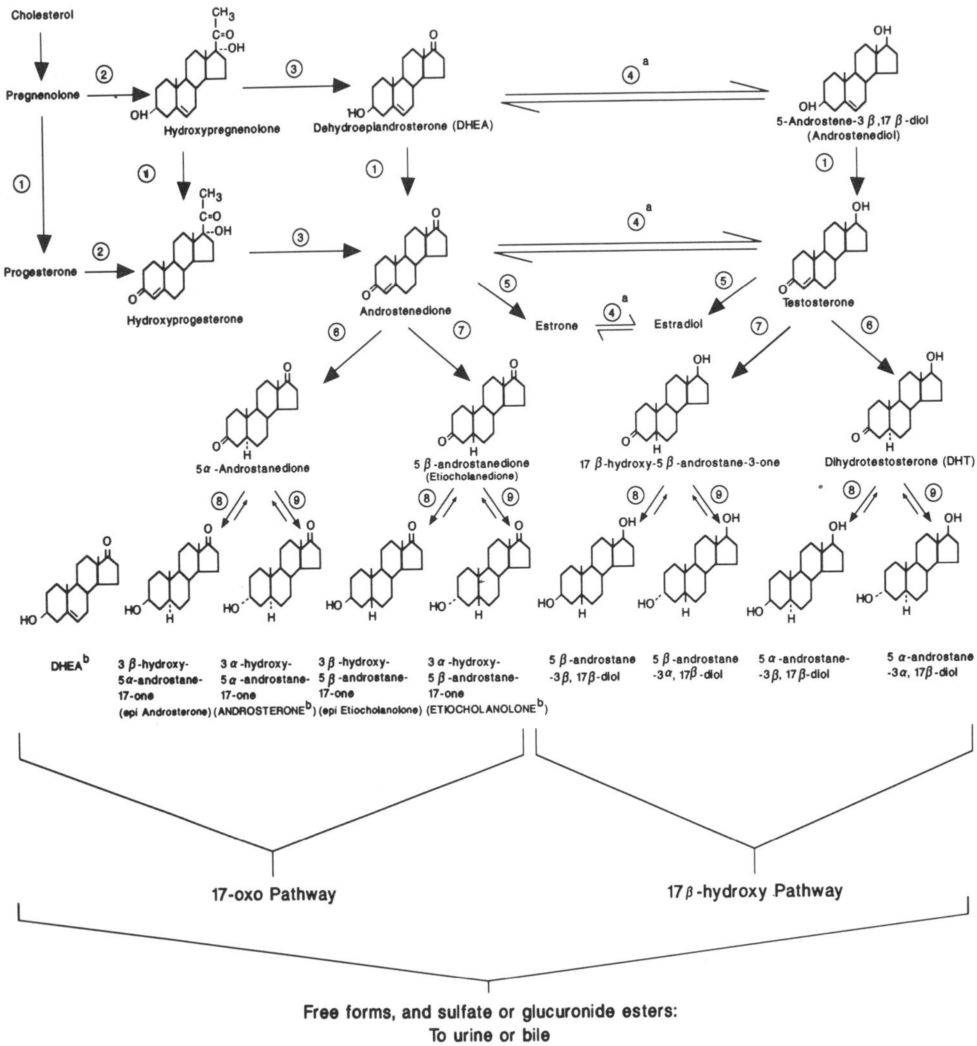

FIG. 1. Principal pathways of androgen synthesis and catabolism. Enzymes: (1) 3β-hydroxysteroid dehydrogenase; (2) 17β-hydroxylase; (3) 17,20-desmolase; (4) 17β-hydroxysteroid dehydrogenase; (5) aromatase; (6) 5α-reductase; (7) 5β-reductase; (8) 3β-oxoreductase; (9) 3α-reductase. [a]In the gonads, the 17β-hydroxysteroid dehydrogenase activity predominantly yields 17β-dehydrogenated products (androstenediol and testosterone), whereas the reverse is true in peripheral tissues. [b]Aldosterone, etiocholanolone, and DHEA are the principal urinary metabolites of androgens. (From ref. 13, with permission.)

(2–4). Although DHEAS is the most abundant androgen in circulation, in a concentration approximately 8,000–10,000 times that of T, these three steroids are very weak androgens compared to T and DHT, and under normal circumstances have a very limited androgenic effect.

T and DHT circulate tightly bound to a hepatic α-globulin called sex steroid binding globulin (TeBG or SHBG) and, to lesser extent, to albumin. Androstenedione is only weakly bound, while DHA and DHEAS circulate mostly unbound (5,6). Since only free (unbound) steroid is able to act on the androgen receptor, the action of T and DHT is greatly influenced by the circulating SHBG level. If the SHBG level is low, the free fractions of T and DHT are going to be higher and their effect greater (7). In addition, the SHBG level influences the clearance of T and DHT from circulation (8), since only free androgen can be metabolized by the liver and peripheral tissues. The circulating SHBG level is decreased by androgens and increased by estrogens (9–12). Thus, if the circulating level of androgens increases, the SHBG concentration will drop resulting in a higher T and DHT clearance. The final result may be that while the total T level remains relatively normal, T production and its free (active or unbound) fraction are increased (7).

Androgen production and clearance are affected by various physiologic states. In obesity androgen production and clearance are accelerated (13). The increased clearance is, in part, due to an obesity-related decrease in SHBG, which leads to higher levels of rapidly metabolizable free T and DHT. In addition, because steroids are fat soluble, the increased amount of adipose tissue in obese women tends to "trap" androgens, increasing their extravascular pool. In obesity a greater percentage of the androgens are metabolized to estrogens, through the action of aromatase, present in the stroma of adipose tissue. Since androgen levels in obese women are generally normal or only slightly decreased, their production rate must be increased to compensate for their higher clearance. The exact mechanism(s) by which androgen production increases is not clear. One-possibility is that obesity leads to subtle increases in adrenal androgen production. Komindr and colleagues observed a greater "responsivity" of DHA and a higher "sensitivity" of A to incremental doses of adrenocorticotropin (ACTH), in obese eumenorrheic women (14). Alternatively, we have been unable to demonstrate any gross abnormalities in the adrenocortical response to acute ACTH stimulation in obese women, with the exception of a slight, but significant increase in the net increment of A (Fig. 2).

ADRENARCHE AND ANDROGEN DEVELOPMENT THROUGHOUT PUBERTY

It is important to understand the changes in serum androgen levels and adrenal function that take place at puberty, in order to clearly diagnose syndromes of androgen excess during this period of time. Total T levels in prepubertal boys and girls are approximately equal, increasing four-fold in girls to reach a mean of 38 ng/dL (range, 20–85 ng/dL) in Tanner stage V (15–19). In comparison, boys in Tanner stage V have T levels ranging from 200 to 1,000 ng/dL (Fig. 3) (15,16). Dihydrotestosterone concentrations increase similarly in normal girls from a mean of 6 ng/dL in Tanner stage I to 17 ng/dL at the completion of puberty (19). Free T also increases during this period of time from a mean of 3.8 pg/ml (range, 2–6 pg/ml) to 8.8 pg/ml (range, 5–13 pg/ml) (18). The SHBG concentration during female puberty changes little (18), although some investigators have reported a minimal decrease (20). It is speculated that the increase in androgen levels during female puberty offsets any positive effect that the increase in estrogens may have on circulating SHBG levels. However Cunningham and colleagues noted a decrease in SHBG levels with chronologic age, regardless of androgen status, in four normal men and their two 46XY androgen insensitive siblings, suggesting that the decrease in SHBG in the puberty is independent of androgen activity and may be under the regulation of other factors (21). Androstenedione levels increase throughout puberty in a similar fashion in both boys and girls, from a mean of 35 ng/dL (range, 10–100 ng/dL) to approximately 141 ng/dL (range, 58–224 ng/dL) in Tanner stage V (15,22,23). The pubertal increases in T and A throughout pu-

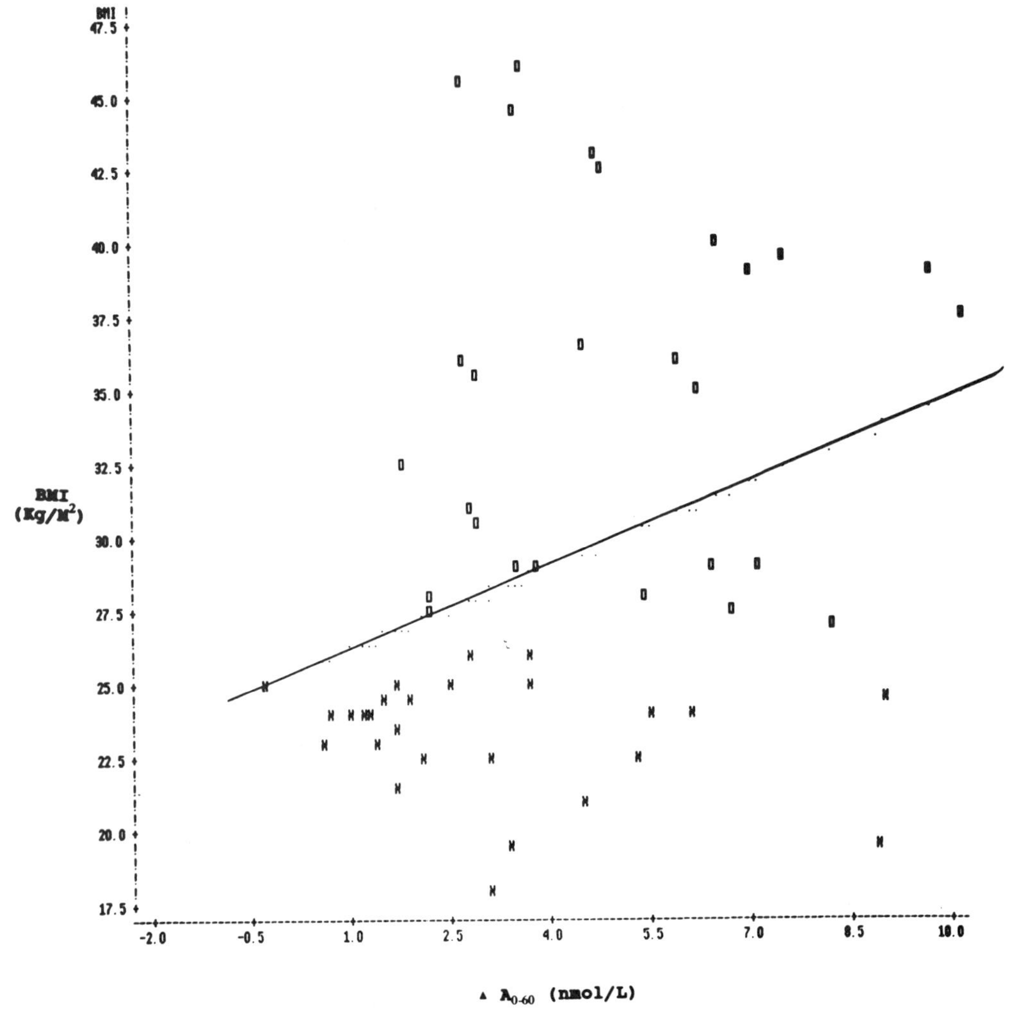

FIG. 2. In normal eumenorrheic nonhirsute women, the increment in androstenedione secretion ($\blacktriangle A_{0-60}$) following acute 1–24 ACTH stimulation appears to be positively correlated with the body mass index (BMI); $r = 0.32$, $p < 0.02$. The difference in mean $\blacktriangle A_{0-60}$ between obese (>120% ideal body weight) and normal weight women was significant; 5.0 ± 2.3 vs. 2.9 ± 2.3 nmol/L ($p < 0.001$), respectively (From reference 179, with permission).

berty appear to be mostly of ovarian origin. In Turner's Syndrome patients the increase in serum T and A are minimal, and at the age of 15 years the concentrations of these androgens were 50% and 60%, respectively, for the corresponding levels in normal girls of the same age (17).

A marked increase in serum DHA and DHEAS concentrations is noted beginning at about the age of five years and continuing throughout puberty (Fig. 3) (16,17,22, 23–27). The levels of these adrenal steroids rise similarly in both boys and girls, from a mean of 133 ng/dL (range, 19–300 ng/dL) to 741 ng/dL (range, 389–1,093 ng/dL) for DHA, and from 43 μg/dL (range 24–86 μg/dL) to 120 μg/dL (range, 78–163 μg/dL) for DHEAS. In patients with Turner's Syndrome after 13 years of age, the mean serum DHA concentration was slightly, but

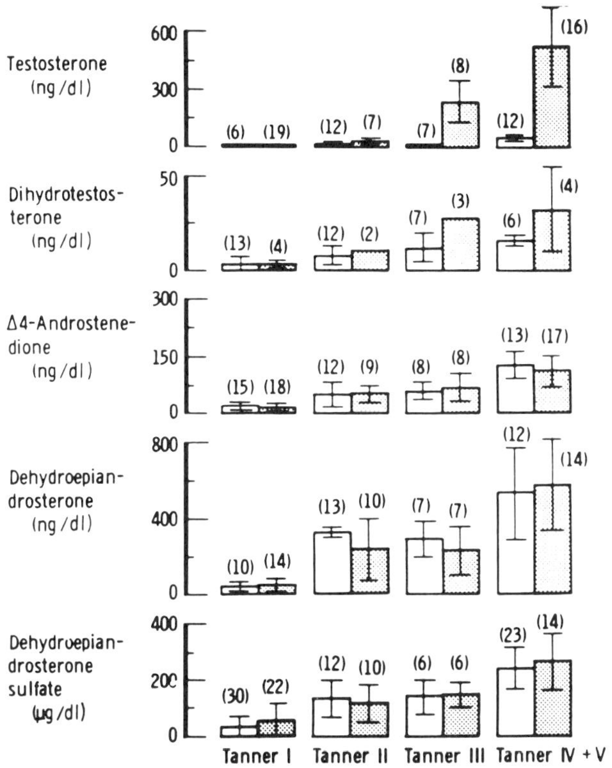

FIG. 3. Mean (± SD) serum concentrations of testosterone, dihydrotestosterone, ▲4-androstenedione, dehydroepiandrosterone, and dehydroepiandrosterone sulfate in normal boys and girls according to pubarchal development (Tanner I, II, III, and IV+V). Testosterone was higher in boys in stages II, III, and IV+V ($p < 0.001$). Dihydrotestosterone was higher in boys in stages III and IV+V ($p < 0.01$). In both sexes, differences between stages I and II are significant for all steroids ($p < 0.001$). Differences between stages II and III are significant in boys for testosterone ($p < 0.001$). Differences between stages III and IV+V are significant for all steroids (except DHA) in girls. (From ref. 16, with permission.)

significantly, lower (20–30%) than that of normal girls of the same age, suggesting that this steroid is produced in part by the ovary (17). The increased adrenal secretion of androgens and estrogens begins 2–3 years before the onset of puberty and is termed pubarche or adrenarche. Histopathologically adrenarche correlates with the appearance of a continuous reticularis zone in the adrenal cortex. Focal development of the reticularis begins at about the age of 5 years and by 8 years of age it is usually present as a continuous zone (28). The measurement of urinary or serum androgens and their metabolites (29), the steroid response to adrenal stimulation (30), and in vitro studies of adrenal microsomal activity (31) suggest that the relative efficiency (activity) of 3β-hydroxysteroid dehydrogenase (3β-HSD) activity decreases and that of 17,20-desmolase (17,20-D) and to a lesser extent 17-hydroxylase increases during adrenarche. Some investigators have also noted a doubling in 21-hydroxylase (21-OH) activity in vitro (31) and a fall in 11β-hydroxylase (11-OH) activities by measurement of urinary steroid metabolites (29). It should be noted that these alterations do not lead to a change in circulating cortisol levels, which remain stable throughout puberty (27).

The mechanisms responsible for initiating and controlling adrenarche are not clear. Adrenarche appears to occur independently of gonadal maturation (32). Some investigators have proposed that the development of the continuous reticularis and the changes adrenocortical biosynthesis are under the control of both ACTH and as yet an unidentified pituitary regulatory factor, the adrenal androgen stimulating hormone (AASH) or cortical androgen stimulating hormone (CASH) (33,34). Experimental evidence for such a substance rests on the observation that bovine and human pituitary extracts stimulate a greater secretion of DHA relative to cortisol, from dog and human adrenals *in vitro* and *in vivo* (34). More recently, the sequence of this peptide has been proposed to be identical to a portion of the joining peptide of the pro-opiomelanocortin (POMC) molecule (35), although this remains to be confirmed. Clinical evidence for the presence of a non-ACTH pituitary factor controlling adrenal maturation and androgen production include the following (36): (a) The pattern of plasma androgens in premature adrenarche is different from that seen in children after protracted ACTH stimulation. (b) Circulating levels of androgens do not exert a negative feed-back on the pituitary secretion of ACTH. (c) There is no difference in ACTH release following metyrapone administration between adults and children. (d) There are numerous instances of a divergence in the secretion of cortisol and adrenal androgens, including alternative day glucocorticoid administration (37), and surgical trauma or severe burns (38,39).

Alternatively, other investigators have suggested that much, if not all, of the changes in adrenal androgen production at puberty can be explained by alterations in the intrinsic adrenocortical hormonal milieu and the progressive development of the reticularis. Rich et al. (30) have suggested that the increase in DHA levels noted at adrenarche results from a combination of changes in the response of the adrenal cortex to ACTH (30). More of the precursor 17-pregnenolone is available and the percentage of this steroid converted to DHA increases as the result of an apparent improvement in 17,20-D activity, whereas DHA is less efficiently converted to A because of an apparent decrease in 3β-HSD activity. These authors noted that the resultant increase in DHA after ACTH stimulation, together with acquisition of sulfokinase activity by the adrenal, was sufficient to explain the adrenarchal rise in DHEAS. Furthermore, Pang et al. (40) noted, in two children with hypopituitarism, that prolonged administration of ACTH resulted in normal DHA responses to a 6-hr ACTH stimulation test. In this same report, corticotropin releasing hormone (CRH) administration to four ACTH-deficient patients caused a rise in DHA and cortisol in those patients who had previously demonstrated a normal response to ACTH, while those with a poor ACTH response had a lesser rise in DHA and cortisol. That ACTH is one of the principle hormones regulating adrenal androgen secretion in prepubertal and pubertal girls was also noted by Pintor et al. (23), who reported that in these children short-term dexamethasone administration decreased the circulating levels of cortisol, pregnenolone, DHA, progesterone, 17-hydroxyprogesterone (17-HP), A, T, and estradiol (E_2). Alternatively, Kreitzer et al. (41) were not able to suppress the circulating DHEAS level in pre-adrenarchal children, although high doses of prednisone for one week were able to reduce circulating DHEAS levels by 70% in postadrenarchal children. This data suggested that there may be two distinct regulatory pathways leading to DHEAS production, one of which is independent of ACTH. Dickerman et al. (42) observed that the shift in the relative activities of 3β-HSD and 17,20-D at adrenarche were associated with changes in the steroidal microenvironment of the adrenal cortex, and that the age-related changes in adrenal size are accompanied by significant changes in intraadrenal steroid concentrations of sufficient magnitude to influence steroidogenesis. These investigators suggested that the developmental changes in adrenal androgen secretion could be explained in terms of shifts in relative enzyme activities induced solely by the necessity to maintain a stable cortisol secretion in face of continued adrenal growth, without the need to invoke the action of a pituitary androgen stimulating hormone. Also using an in vitro model, Hornsby and Aldern noted that cultured human fetal definitive zone cells in serum-free conditions produced cortisol and DHEAS (via DHA) about equally from 17-hydroxypregnenolone following ACTH administration (43). When compared to bovine adrenocortical cells (which secrete only minimal amounts of DHEAS), the difference in DHEAS production between species was felt to be secondary to differences in the intrinsic activity of 3β-HSD and not the presence of an extrinsic adrenal androgen stimulating factor(s). Overall it still remains unclear to what extent is adrenarche and adrenal androgen secretion the result of changes in intra-adrenal hormonal milieu and adrenal response to ACTH, or a result of the secretion of a specific androgen stimulating pituitary hormone.

HIRSUTISM

Hair follicles cover the entire body with the exception of the soles of the feet, the palms of the hands, and the lips. Most hair follicles are present at birth with very few new ones formed thereafter (44). Hair follicles are lost in a generalized fashion beginning in the mid to late 40s leading to the thinning of hair noted thereafter. Although there are racial and ethnic differences in follicle numbers, there are no differences between sexes within each race/ethnic group. The visible differences between men and women do not relate to the number of hair follicles, but rather to the type of hair arising from these follicles. White Caucasians have a higher density of hair follicles than blacks, who in turn have more follicles than orientals.

In general there are three types of hair. Lanugo is the soft unmedullated hair covering the surface of the fetus, which is shed sometime in late gestation or the early postpartum period. Vellus hairs are short (2–5 mm), soft, fine, unmedullated, and usually nonpigmented, and cover the apparently "hairless" areas of the body. Terminal hairs are long, coarse and medullated, making up the eyebrows, the eyelashes, and the scalp, pubic and axillary hair. Although in women many of the hair follicles produce vellus hairs, in men these same follicles produce terminal hairs leading to the appearance of visible facial, chest and abdominal hair. The hair growth cycle can be divided into three phases (44). The hair grows actively during the *anagen phase,* associated with downward progression of the dermal papilla (Fig. 4). During the *catagen phase* the hair follicle involutes, followed by the *telogen phase* in which the hair is eventually shed. Although in many animal species the growth cycles of all hair follicles are in synchrony, in humans this is not the case, which accounts for the impression that hair continuously grows. Occasionally a greater number of hair follicles shift into synchrony, as in pregnancy, menopause or following delivery, or when starting or stopping oral contraceptive medications, which leads to the temporary shedding of excessive numbers of hairs, without an actual reduction in the number of hair follicles. This is a temporary situation which eventually reverts to normal.

There are a number of hormones that control hair growth. Thyroid and growth hormone produce a generalized growth in hair. Hyperthyroidism yields a fine friable hair which is easily lost, while hypothyroidism produces a coarse brittle hair which is also easily lost. Of the reproductive hormones progesterone has a minimal effect, while estrogens basically oppose the effect of androgens, most importantly by increasing circulating SHBG leading to a decrease in free T and DHT. Androgens, in turn, are the most important determinant of the type and distribution of hairs throughout the body.

Circulating androgens, particularly T, are converted in the hair follicle to DHT, through the action of 5α-reductase. DHT then acts on the dermal papilla and sebaceous gland (which compose the pilosebaceous unit) to increase the growth rate and thickness of terminal hairs and increase sebum production. Androgens also transform vellus-producing follicles to terminal hair-producing follicle, an irreversible process.

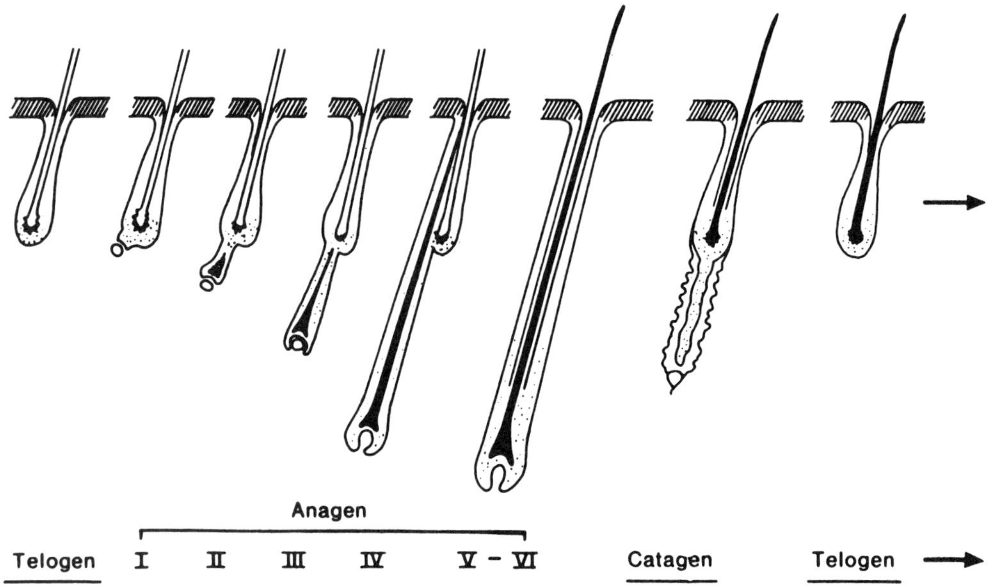

FIG. 4. Diagram of the growth cycle of a hair follicle. Depicted are a club hair (in white) in old telogen, early anagen (I–IV) follicles, and a new hair (in black) in late anagen (V–VI). (From ref. 44, with permission.)

The effect of androgens on the hair follicle will be specific to the area of skin in which it is located (44). Some skin areas (e.g., eyelashes, eyebrows, lateral and occipital aspects of the scalp) appear to be relatively independent of the effects of androgens, and are designated as *nonsexual skin*. Other areas are very sensitive to the effect of even low levels of androgens, due to their high 5α-reductase activity, and include the lower pubic triangle and the axilla, which are designated as *ambosexual areas*. The hair follicles in these areas develop terminal hairs quite early in puberty, accompanying the minimal increases in adrenal androgens. Other parts of the skin contain lower levels of 5α-reductase and respond only to high concentrations of androgens, including the chest, lower abdomen, lower back, upper thighs, upper arms, chin, face and upper pelvic triangle, and are designated as *sexual areas*. Terminal hair growth in these areas is characteristically masculine and, if present in women, is considered hirsutism.

Excessive growth of coarse hairs of the lower forearms and lower legs alone does *not* constitute hirsutism. However, a woman suffering from hirsutism (i.e., terminal hair growth in areas that are exclusively masculine) may also note an increase in the pigmentation and growth rate of hairs on the lower forearm and leg. While hirsutism is usually obvious, it may be important to standardize the examination for future reference by using a scoring system (Fig. 5). It is also important to remember that not all hyperandrogenic women demonstrate hirsutism (e.g., Oriental women rarely do so) (45), whereas some patients with obvious hirsutism have normal circulating androgen levels (see below).

OTHER SIGNS AND SYMPTOMS OF ANDROGEN EXCESS

In addition to hirsutism, androgen excess in women leads to a number of other problems including acne, oligo- or amenorrhea,

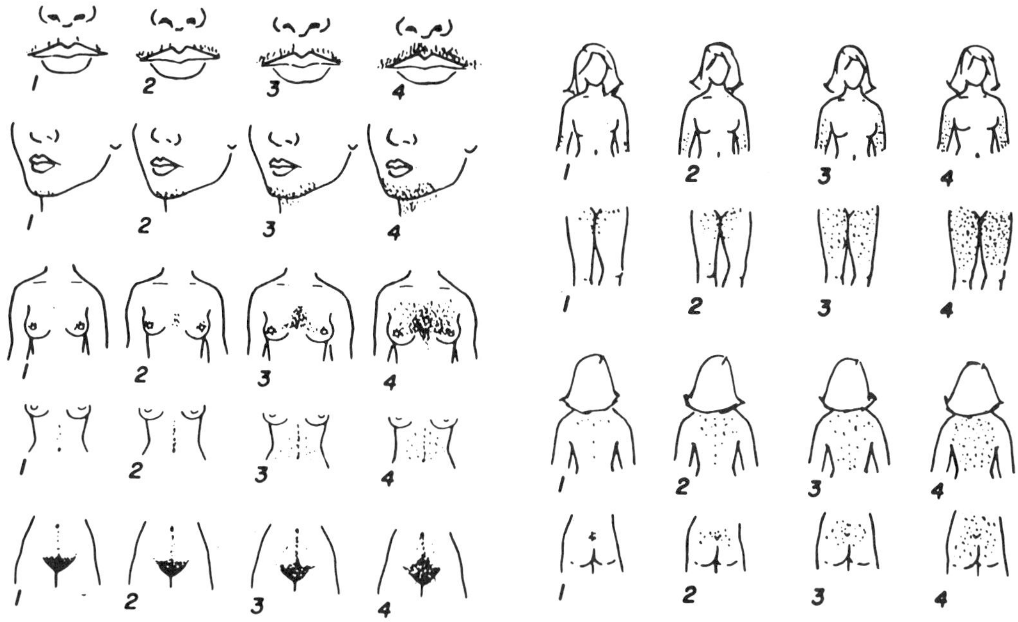

FIG. 5. Hirsutism scoring standard to determine the extent of total body hirsutism. The scores in each area are summed. (From ref. 178, with permission.)

weight gain, and if very severe, virilization/masculinization.

Acne

The pilosebaceous unit, in addition to the hair follicle, also contains a sebaceous gland which produces an oily protective secretion, *sebum,* in response to androgen action. The excessive production of sebum leads to oily skin, clogged hair follicles, folliculitis and subsequent acne. Although all androgens may lead to acne, the sole presence of acne without hirsutism is often associated with excessive levels of the adrenal androgens, DHA and/or DHEAS (46–49). Although these steroids are relatively weak in their stimulation of terminal hair growth, they are relatively effective in increasing sebum production. Elevations in other serum androgen levels have also been noted (50–54), particularly in patients with acne and hirsutism, although not all investigators agree (55–58).

There are conflicting reports as to the incidence in adrenocortical abnormalities following ACTH stimulation in these women (59,60). Some investigators have observed that while serum androgen levels may be relatively normal, the metabolism of such androgens by the affected skin is increased (61–63). It does appear clear, however, that acne frequently improves following treatment with oral contraceptives, glucocorticoid suppression, spironolactone or cyproterone acetate (64–70). Although many teenagers suffer from acne, skin problems that persist into the 20s should raise the suspicion of androgen excess. Empiric treatment with spironolactone, low-dose glucocorticoid or oral contraceptives may be justified in patients without evidence of overt androgen excess.

Oligo- or Anovulation

Very high levels of androgens, in of themselves, can disrupt the hypothalamic-pituitary-ovarian axis with the subsequent development of ovulatory problems. Androgens can also be converted to estrogens in peripheral and hepatic tissue, and the excessive levels of both androgens and estrogens may suppress the hypothalamic-pituitary production of gonadotropins. Furthermore, excessive androgen levels directly inhibit follicular development, which may result in the accumulation of multiple small cysts within the ovarian cortex (the so-called "polycystic" ovary). Adolescent oligomenorrhea is frequently hyperandrogenic in nature (71,72). Approximately one-half of these children will go on to develop persistent hyperandrogenemia, with all its consequences (73).

The appearance of "polycystic" ovaries, either on laparoscopy or more commonly at sonography, is not diagnostic for the so-called polycystic ovarian syndrome (PCOS) (see below) (74–77). Excessive levels of circulating androgens from any source will lead to the disruption of follicular development and the accumulation of many small, atretic follicles in the ovarian cortex, producing a "polycystic" picture. PCOS is a diagnosis of exclusion and should not be established by a sonographic or laparoscopic picture of a "polycystic" ovary. Kim et al. (78) observed ovarian hyperandrogenism in histologically normal and abnormal ovaries, although patients with "polycystic" ovaries appeared to demonstrate a greater degree of androgen excess.

Virilization and/or Masculinization

If the androgen levels are extremely elevated and present prior to puberty the patient's body habitus may become masculinized with amenorrhea, an absence of breast development, an increase in muscle mass, upper body obesity and virilization. Virilization includes temporal and frontal balding, clitoromegaly, reduction in breast size and severe hirsutism. In general, virilization or masculinization should raise the suspicion of an androgen-producing tumor or congenital adrenal hyperplasia. Occasionally girls with severe hyperthecosis, or suffering from the HAIRAN syndrome (see below) may exhibit a moderate degree of virilization.

DIFFERENTIAL DIAGNOSIS OF ANDROGEN EXCESS

Nonandrogenic Causes

Acromegaly

Acromegalic women often demonstrate a generalized increase in hair growth and sebum production, and may present with hirsutism (79). Accompanying the hirsutism will be an enlargement of the hands and feet, and a coarsening of the facial features. This cause of hirsutism is extremely rare, and the diagnosis is based on a determination excessive growth hormone secretion.

Chronic Skin Irritation

Teleologically, hairs protect the skin, and chronic irritation of the skin secondary to depilating agents, environmental toxins, etc., leads to a local increase in hair growth, as well as the increased transformation of vellus to terminal hairs (44).

Anabolic Drugs

Certain anabolic medications cause a generalized growth of many tissues, particularly hair, and include Dilantin, Nilevar, and Anavar. However, these drugs generally lead to hypertrichosis and not hirsutism.

Androgenic Causes

The diagnosis in this category are based on finding elevated circulating androgen levels.

Androgenic Drugs

Rarely will the accidental or deliberate ingestion of danazol, methyltestosterone, stanazol, etc. lead to the development of acne and hirsutism, particularly in young women engaged in body building.

Male Pseudohermaphroditism

The peripubertal onset of hirsutism, breast development and clitoromegaly, accompanied by primary amenorrhea can suggest the presence of incomplete testicular feminization or a Y-bearing dysgenetic gonad (80). If undiagnosed progressive masculinization may result. Upon examination these individuals will demonstrate a blind vaginal pouch and varying degrees of clitoromegaly. These patients may also demonstrate bilateral or unilateral vulvar swelling secondary to the descent of one or both gonads. In some patients with XY gonadal dysgenesis a uterine remnant may be present, invariably accompanied by some degree of genital asymmetry.

Classic Congenital Adrenal Hyperplasia

Also called the adrenogenital syndrome this disorder represents one of the most common autosomal recessive disorders, affecting one of every 5,000–10,000 newborns (81). The disorder results from the inherited deficiency of any enzyme necessary for the adrenocortical biosynthesis of cortisol. In order to maintain normal cortisol levels ACTH levels and adrenocortical activity increases leading to cortical hyperplasia and the excessive accumulation of the enzymatic precursors. The signs and symptoms of these disorders will depend on the severity and location of the enzymatic block. Approximately 90% of children demonstrate a deficiency in 21-OH function (Fig. 6). The accumulation in the bloodstream of precursors to the affected enzyme and the deficiency in steroidal products will result in the signs and symptoms of classic congenital adrenal hyperplasia (CAH). If the defect is extremely severe (as in the total absence of enzymatic activity) cortisol and aldosterone may not be produced in sufficient quantities, with polyuria, dehydration, hypokalemia and seizures ("adrenal crisis") resulting in death if left untreated (81). The accumulation of very high levels of progesterone, 17-HP and particularly A and T leads to severe masculinization of the female genitalia *in utero*. These patients are designated as "salt wasters." Alternatively in "simple virilizing" 21-OH deficient CAH cortisol is produced in amounts sufficient to sustain life, whereas androgens accumulate to lesser degrees, producing a less disfiguring genital abnormalities in girls. Girls with CAH will subsequently develop amenorrhea, acne, hirsutism and virilization. These patients may remain undiagnosed in spite of their progressive masculinization and hirsutism. The diagnosis is usually established by the measurement of basal 17-HP and A levels, with a 17-HP level usually exceeding 10 ng/mL (82).

Other less common causes of congenital virilizing adrenal hyperplasia include 11-OH and 3β-HSD deficiencies. The inherited deficiency of 11-OH will lead to the additional accumulation of deoxycorticosterone (DOC), a potent mineralocorticoid, with the additional symptom of hypertension. Overall, the clinical picture in 11-OH deficient CAH varies significantly (83). The diagnosis can be established by measuring the basal level of 11-deoxycortisol (compound S) which usually exceeds 40 ng/mL (84). Extremely high basal levels of 17-hydroxypregnenolone (above 80 ng/mL) herald 3β-HSD deficient CAH (85,86).

An electrolyte panel and renin activity level should be obtained in all patients suspected of suffering from CAH. Once the diagnosis is established corticosteroid (with prednisone or hydrocortisone) and, if necessary, mineralocorticoid (with fluorocortisone) replacement will suffice. Nevertheless, the hirsutism may not improve

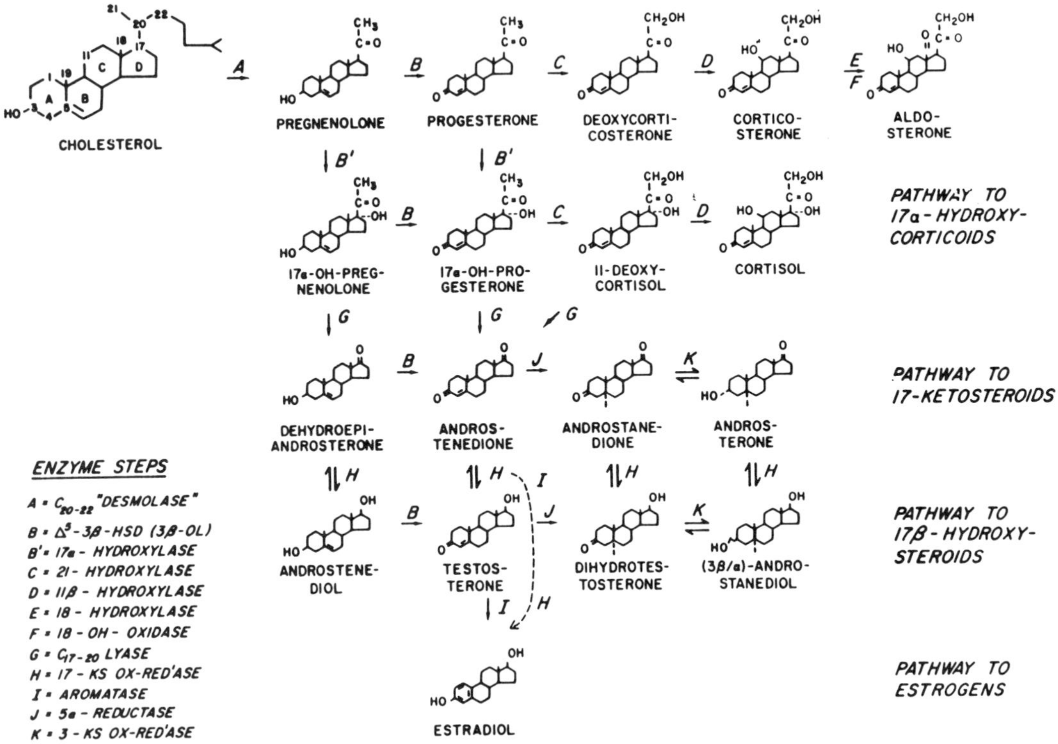

FIG. 6. Major pathways off steroid biosynthesis from cholesterol. The flow of hormonogenesis is usually to the right and downward. C_{17-20} lyase (enzyme step G) is also termed 17,20-desmolase. (From ref. 178, with permission.)

completely, requiring the addition of antiandrogens. Simple virilizing CAH patients may also require low doses of mineralocorticoids in the event their basal renin measurements are elevated (87). Fertility is possible and will depend on the degree of genital virilization (88) (which will determine the overall coital success following reconstructive surgery [89]) and hyperandrogenemia.

Late-Onset Adrenal Hyperplasia

Between 1% and 6% of hyperandrogenic women suffer from 21-OH deficient late-onset adrenal hyperplasia (LOAH) (90). In contrast to CAH, where the enzyme deficiency is so severe that the symptoms of cortisol deficiency and/or androgen excess are present in the newborn or in childhood, patients with LOAH are clinically indistinguishable from other hyperandrogenic patients and usually present peri or postpubertally (90,91).

Serum levels of the exclusive adrenal androgen DHEAS are not any higher than that of other hyperandrogenic women. Although levels of A are higher than in other hyperandrogenic patients, the overlap is sufficient to make the measurement of this steroid useless for screening purposes (Fig. 7). Fortunately, the measurement of a morning 17-HP level in the follicular phase of the menstrual cycle can be used to screen for this disorder (90). If the baseline 17-HP is higher than 2 ng/mL (or 200 ng/dL) then the patient should undergo an ACTH stimulation test to rule-out the disorder (see below). These patients can be easily treated

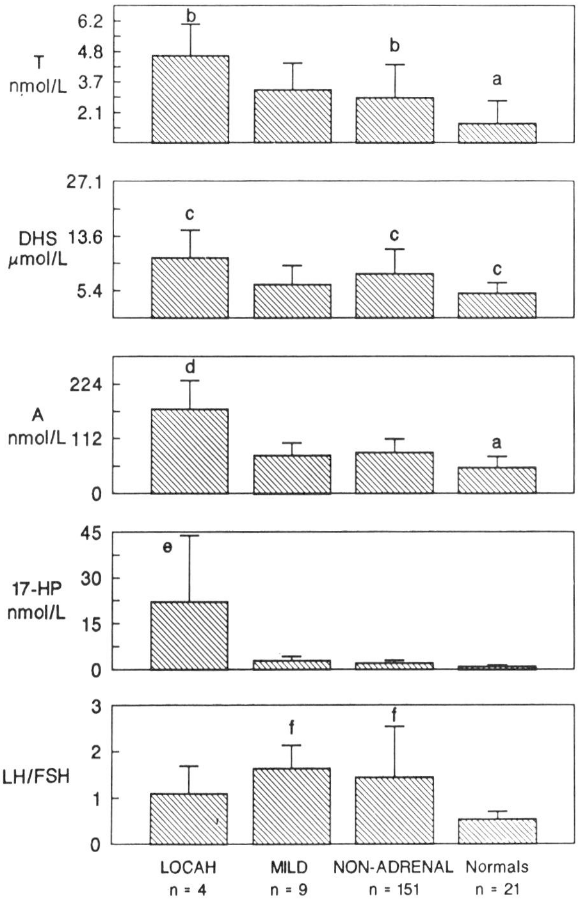

FIG. 7. Mean basal hormone levels in women with 21-OH deficient LOAH (LOCAH), patients with a mild exaggeration in 17-HP response to ACTH (MILD), hyperandrogenic women without an abnormal 17-HP response (NON-ADRENAL), and control subjects (Normals). **A:** Normals lower than all others ($p < 0.02–0.003$). **B:** LOAH higher than NON-ADRENAL patients ($p < 0.01$), but not different from MILD. **C:** LOAH and NON-ADRENAL patients, but not MILD, had higher DHS levels than normal ($p < 0.0005$). **D:** LOAH higher than all others ($p < 0.0001$). **E:** LOAH higher than all others ($p < 0.0001$). **F:** NON-ADRENAL and MILD hyperandrogenic women, but not LOAH, had higher mean LH/FSH ratios than normals ($p < 0.002$). (From ref. 90, with permission.)

with corticosteroid replacement (0.5 mg dexamethasone qday or qod, 5–10 mg prednisone qday, or 20–30 mg hydrocortisone qday). Nevertheless, if long-standing, their hirsutism and ovulatory disorder may not respond solely to corticosteroids, requiring the addition of appropriate medications (92).

Less than one percent of our hyperandrogenic patients, or approximately one-half of the incidence of 21-OH deficient LOAH, consistent with other reports (93), were found to suffer from 11-OH deficient LOAH. Basal measures of 11-deoxycortisol were not found useful as a screening measure. With adrenal stimulation testing, our patients have 11-deoxycortisol levels that exceed three-fold the upper 95th percentile of normal (Fig. 8). One patient demonstrated mild hypertension, whereas the other did not, consistent with the clinical variability already noted for the CAH form. Although 3β-HSD deficient LOAH has been reported its prevalence is unclear (94,95).

Hyperandrogenic-Insulin Resistant-Acanthosis Nigricans Syndrome

Between 1 and 5% of hyperandrogenic women suffer from this disorder. It is characterized by extremely high circulating levels of insulin, generally >80 uU/mL in the fasting state, and >300 uU/mL following an

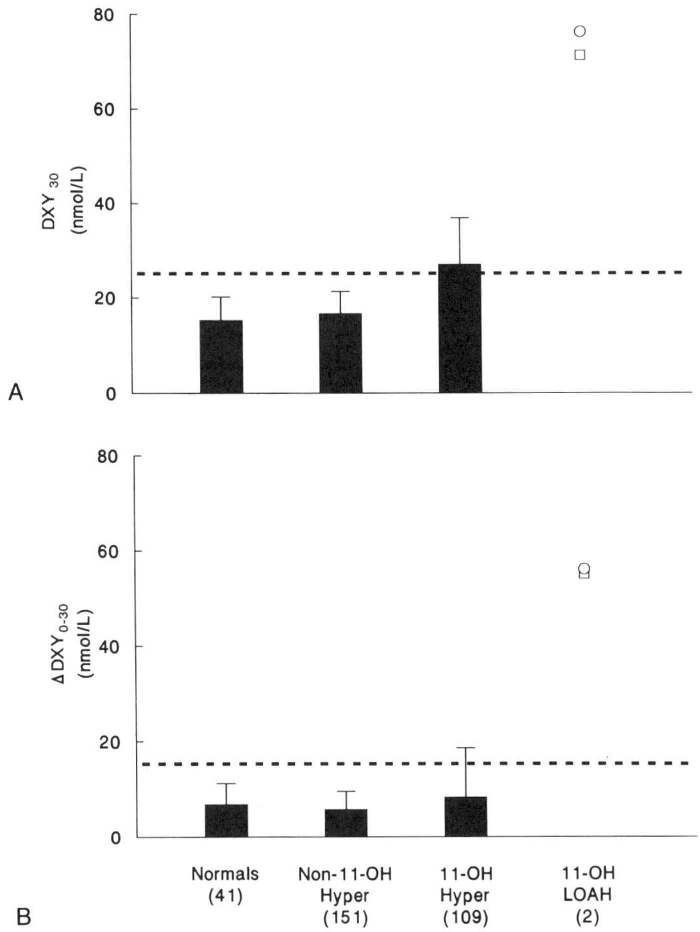

FIG. 8. In a population of 262 hyperandrogenic patients studied consecutively (after excluding all patients with 21-OH deficient LOAH), the increment in 11-deoxycortisol ($\blacktriangle DXY_{0-30}$) and DXY level ($DXY_{30}$) following acute 1–24 ACTH is depicted (mean ± 1 SD) for normal women (Normals), hyperandrogenic women with a normal 11-OH response (Non-11-OH Hyper), and hyperandrogenic patients with a mildly exaggerated DXY response (11-OH Hyper), and in two patients with presumed 11-OH deficient LOAH. The *dashed line* represents the upper 95th percentile of normal. **A:** Higher than control or 11-OH normal hyperandrogenic women ($p < 0.0001$). **B:** Higher than control or 11-OH normal hyperandrogenic women ($p < 0.0007$).

oral glucose tolerance test (96–98). In general, their fasting glucose levels will be relatively normal. The high levels of insulin are usually due to a genetic deficiency in either the number of insulin receptors and/or a postreceptor defect (99–104). Rarely some of these women demonstrate circulating anti-insulin receptor antibodies (105, 106). This syndrome should not be confused with the insulin resistance noted among many patients with PCOS, where the increase in insulin levels are generally mild.

Patients with hyperandrogenic-insulin resistant-acanthosis nigricans (HAIRAN) syndrome demonstrate acanthosis nigricans, a velvety hyperpigmented change of the crease areas of the skin (Fig. 9). These girls are usually severely hyperandrogenic, and can even be virilized or masculinized. A

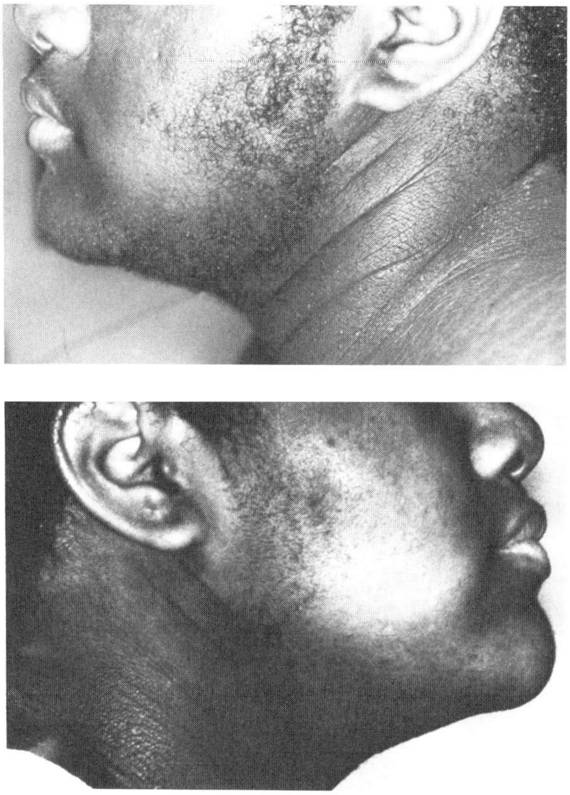

A

B

FIG. 9. Thirteen-year-old patient with HAIRAN syndrome before (**A**) and following 6 months of treatment with leuprolide (**B**). Note acanthosis nigricans and marked improvement in hirsutism following treatment with the long-acting GnRH agonist.

fasting insulin and glucose will serve to diagnose most hyperandrogenic patients with the HAIRAN syndrome. Rarely is an oral glucose tolerance test (measuring both glucose and insulin responses) required.

These patients are relatively difficult to treat, nevertheless standard therapy with antiandrogens and oral contraceptives should be instituted. If no response is noted ketoconazole or long-acting GnRH analogs may be used. Ketoconazole is an antifungal agent that has been found to block androgen synthesis by inhibiting, among others, the cytochrome P450 dependent enzyme 17,20-D. This drug has been successful in the treatment of boys with testoxicosis,or primary testicular hypertestosteronemia, and in a patient with the HAIRAN syndrome (107). Long-acting GnRH analogs inhibit LH-dependent androgen production by reducing circulating gonadotropins to castrate levels. At least 3–6 months of gonadotropin suppression are required to achieve full androgen suppression in HAIRAN syndrome (Fig. 9) (108). If all fails, a bilateral ovarian wedge resection or even oophorectomy may be required.

Cushing's Syndrome

Excessive adrenocortical function, due to either an adrenal neoplasm, an ectopic ACTH-producing tumor, or a pituitary tumor (Cushing's disease) can lead to excessive adrenal androgen secretion and hyperandrogenemia. The incidence of this disorder presenting as hirsutism is rare.

Of approximately 400 hyperandrogenic patients with which this investigator has had contact, only one has been diagnosed with Cushing's disease, by inferior petrosal sinus sampling and CRH stimulation. Most of these patients will present with typical Cushingoid features including "yoke-like" centripetal obesity, thinning and striae of the skin, muscle wasting, glucose intolerance, osteoporosis, etc. However, some patients with ectopic ACTH tumor or adrenal carcinoma may demonstrate few of these signs, presenting malnourished and/or cachectic.

In general, the diagnosis of excessive cortisol production (Cushing's syndrome) can best be established by a 24-hr urine free cortisol. A more simple screening method is the measurement of a morning fasting cortisol following 1 mg of dexamethasone the evening before, although the false positive rate for this test can be as high as 15% among obese women or depressed patients, with a false negative rate of approximately 2%.

Androgenic Tumors

Androgen-producing tumors are relatively rare. They should be suspected when the onset of androgenic symptoms is rapid and sudden, and when virilization and masculinization ensue. Steroid-secreting neoplasms may also be associated with other systemic symptoms including weight loss, anorexia, abdominal bloating, back pain, etc. These tumors are usually of ovarian or adrenal origin. Suppression and stimulation tests (including corticosteroid, oral contraceptive, and human chorionic gonadotropin and ACTH administration) can be misleading and are not encouraged for the screening or diagnosis of these neoplasms (109).

Androgen-producing tumors of the adrenal are relatively rare. These adrenal tumors should be suspected when the serum DHEAS level exceeds 6600 ng/mL, and/or the T level exceeds 200 ng/dL (110). The appearance of Cushingoid features along with hirsutism should also arouse suspicion. The diagnosis is usually established by a CAT scan of the adrenal, with images obtained at 0.5 cm intervals. Adrenal carcinomas are usually associated with Cushingoid features, and are generally large (>6 cm) and irregular on CAT scan. Unfortunately their prognosis is very poor.

Ovarian tumors are somewhat more common. They are usually palpable on pelvic exam and/or are associated with a unilateral ovarian enlargement on ultrasound or computed tomography (CT) scan. They are generally not malignant, and include Sertoli-Leydig cell tumors and lipoid cell tumors. Ovarian tumors should be suspected when the circulating T levels are greater than 200 ng/dL (111). However, it is important to understand that 20–50% of androgen-producing ovarian tumors may have T levels below this value (112), and that the *majority* of women with T levels over 200 ng/dL have either HAIRAN syndrome, hyperthecosis, or PCOS, and *not* an ovarian tumor (113). Adrenal and ovarian vein catheterization, with simultaneous peripheral sampling, to determine the gradient in androgen levels may be used preoperatively when the diagnosis or location of the tumor is in doubt (112,114–116).

Hyperthecosis

These patients are usually severely androgenized and have very high levels of circulating T, often greater than 200 ng/dL (117–120). These girls may be somewhat virilized. The diagnosis is established pathologically after removal or wedge resection of the ovary. Islands of hyperplastic luteinized theca cells are noted throughout the stroma and, in contrast to the ovaries in the PCOS, with relatively few small atretic follicles (121). Circulating LH and FSH levels may be normal to low (4–8 mIU/mL) due to the high circulating levels of T. These patients are particularly difficult to treat, do not respond to conventional therapy (120) and often require an extensive ovarian wedge resection or oophorectomy, although the use of long-acting GnRH agonists appears to be promising (122).

Polycystic Ovarian Syndrome

Although this disorder has been commonly termed the polycystic ovarian syndrome (PCOS), not all patients have "polycystic" appearing ovaries (76,77). A better term would be that of hyperandrogenic chronic anovulatory syndrome (HCAS). These patients comprise between 80% and 90% of all hyperandrogenic women seen (123). The diagnosis is one of exclusion, having eliminated other causes of hyperandrogenemia. Patients with PCOS demonstrate elevated circulating levels of free T and a reduction in SHBG, accompanied by variable increases in total T (7,124,125). Approximately 50% will demonstrate an abnormally high DHEAS level, rarely above 6000 ng/mL (126). Prolactin is usually normal, although up to 17–23% of such patients may demonstrate mild elevations (generally less than 80 ng/mL, depending on the assay) without any other apparent cause (127,128). The LH/FSH ratio is usually 3:1 or greater (129–131), which is observed in approximately 60% of these patients (129). Pathologically, the ovarian cortex contains multiple intermediate and atretic follicles measuring 2–5 mm in diameter, which give the ovary its "polycystic" appearance at sonography or laparoscopy. However, not all HCAS patients demonstrate ovaries that are "polycystic," nor are "polycystic" ovaries diagnostic for PCOS (74–77). Approximately 40% of these patients are obese, 60% are amenorrheic, 15% have regular menses (132). One should note that not all patients with PCOS demonstrate hirsutism (45,132–134). These patients do not generally present with virilization or masculinization. PCOS may result in primary amenorrhea (135,136) and present as early as age 12 years (137).

Idiopathic Hirsutism

The diagnosis of "idiopathic" hirsutism (IH) is reached only when circulating androgen levels appear to be consistently normal, even when assessing the free androgen levels, and the patient is obviously hirsute. Furthermore, these patients usually do not suffer from oligoovulation. Approximately 5–25% of hirsute women will end up with the diagnosis of IH. However, it should be understood that many of these patients simply demonstrate degrees of androgen excess that are not detectable by routine clinical androgen assays, and in fact, may more accurately reflect a nonsensitive laboratory assay (138). However, women with IH may demonstrate excessive 5α-reductase activity of the hair follicle, which leads to hirsutism in face of "normal" circulating androgen levels (139). The measurement of serum 3α-androstanediol-glucuronide (3α-Adiol-G), a metabolite of DHT, may reflect peripheral 5α-reductase activity and may help to confirm the "hyperfunction" of this enzyme (139,140). Measurements of 3α-Adiol-G may also assist in monitoring the efficacy of antiandrogen therapy (141), since it takes at least six months for an improvement in hirsutism to become clinically noticeable and standard serum androgen assays cannot be used to determine the adequacy of gonadal/adrenal suppression in IH. Nevertheless, the diagnosis of IH is usually established by default, when normal free and total circulating androgen levels, after repeated measurements, are encountered in a patient with hirsutism and regular menses.

WORK-UP OF ANDROGEN EXCESS

History

The pace of pubertal development and its relation to the onset of hirsutism, acne and/or obesity should be established. Drug or medication use, exposure or use of skin irritants elicited. Menstrual history, onset and progression of hirsutism and/or acne, change in extremity or head, change in face contour, balding and hair loss, etc., should be noted. A family history of similar signs and symptoms is a powerful clue to the inherited basis of the disorder. The etiology of hirsutism can often be established from the history alone.

Physical Exam

The type and pattern of excessive hair growth and/or acne should be noted and scored. The presence of galactorrhea, virilization, masculinization, clitoromegaly, pelvic and abdominal masses, obesity, Cushoid features, "bluntness" of facial features, thyroid enlargement, or signs of systemic illness, should be sought. If the patient is premenarchal or suffers from primary amenorrhea, the upper/lower body and span/height ratios should be determined. If there has been a delay in epiphyseal closure, due to insufficient sex steroid availability with physiologic growth hormone exposure, the upper/lower body ratio will be decreased (<1) and the span/height ratio increased (>1). Tanner staging of pubertal and breast development should be noted.

It is most important to determine whether hirsutism is truly present and whether it is related to other endocrinologic features. The excessive growth of vellus hairs, producing a "fuzzy" appearance, is called *hypertrichosis* and should not be considered hirsutism. Although a number of medical problems or medications can lead to hypertrichosis, it is more commonly familial, in individuals of Mediterranean origin.

Laboratory Assessment

If the patient demonstrates hirsutism, or any other sign or symptom of androgen excess, initially serum measures of total and free T (which usually includes measures of SHBG activity), DHEAS and 17-HP are ascertained. Optimally these measurements are obtained in the morning (for maximal adrenal output) and in the follicular phase of the menstrual cycle. If the patient is oligoovulatory or amenorrheic a simultaneous measurement of serum progesterone (or urinary pregnanediol using a commercially available kit) can help establish the validity of the 17-HP measurement. If the progesterone level is >5 ng/mL (indicating that the patient is in the luteal phase), the 17-HP level will also be elevated and misleading.

Although A is easily measured it is of limited value in most patients, but should be obtained when the above androgen levels are normal in face of obvious hirsutism. DHA and DHT measurements are rarely used in the clinical setting. Serum 3α-Adiol-G levels may serve to predict the effectiveness of antiandrogen therapy in patients with IH, and should be obtained prior to initiating treatment of any such patient.

If the basal 17-HP level is over 10 ng/mL the patient has a diagnosis of 21-OH deficient adrenal hyperplasia. Whether it is of the classic congenital or late-onset varieties will depend on her clinical characteristics. Alternatively, if the patient demonstrates no signs of virilization and her basal follicular 17-HP level is above 2 ng/mL (200 ng/dL) but below 10 ng/mL, she should undergo an acute adrenal stimulation test to rule-out LOAH. Intravenously 250 μg (1 vial) of Cortrosyn (1-24 ACTH) are administered and blood sampled 60 min afterward. If the poststimulation 17-HP level is >10 ng/mL (or 1,000 ng/dL) the diagnosis of 21-OH deficient LOAH is established (Fig. 10). In order to rule out rarer deficiencies of the adrenal cortex, such as 3β-HSD and 11-OH, the levels of 17-hydroxypregnenolone or 11-deoxycortisol may also be measured, respectively, following adrenal stimulation.

In our laboratory, 11-OH deficient LOAH is presumed (since actual genetic confirmation is not yet available) when the 11-deoxycortisol level exceeds 25 ng/mL (Fig. 8), and 3β-HSD deficient LOAH suspected

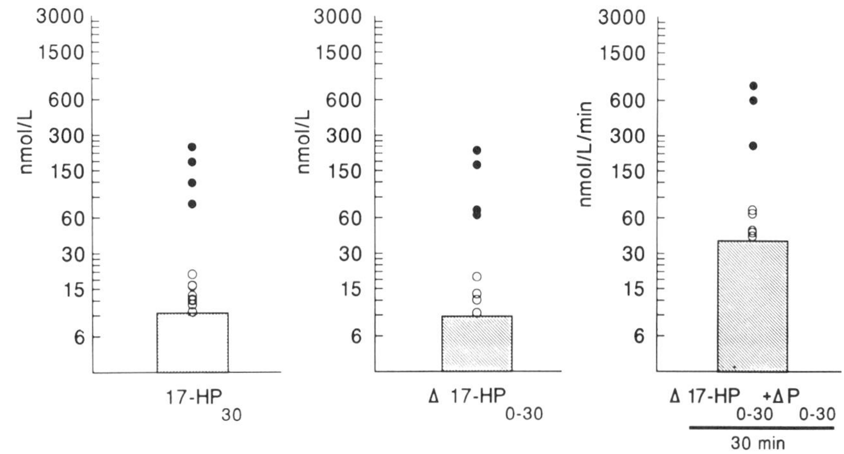

FIG. 10. From a population of 164 hyperandrogenic patients studied consecutively, all women with abnormal 21-OH measures after stimulation with 1–24 ACTH are plotted on a logarithmic scale. Measures include the 17-HP level 30 min. following ACTH administration (17-HP_{30}), the net increment in 17-HP (▲17-HPO-30), and the sum of the increments in 17-HP and progesterone divided by the stimulation time ([▲17-$HP_{0\text{-}30}$ + ▲$P_{0\text{-}30}$]/30 min), yielding the rate of rise of these two steroids. The boxed area represents the control response (up to the 95th percentile of normal). ● LOAH; ● patients with a mild exaggeration in their 17-HP response to ACTH. (From ref. 90, with permission.)

if the 17-hydroxypregnenolone is above 15 ng/mL.

If the patient is also oligoovulatory, an FSH, LH, prolactin, and basal body temperature chart should also be obtained. Although an LH/FSH ratio equal to or greater than three appears to be more common in PCOS patients, it is neither diagnostic nor specific, unless measured repeatedly.

If the patient has signs or symptoms of thyroid disorder (myxedema, tachycardia, hair loss of the lateral eyebrows, goiter, heat/cold intolerance, etc.) a thyroid panel including TSH, T_3RU, and T_4 RIA should be obtained. If available, it may be preferable to obtain a TSH measure using a high sensitivity assay and a free T_4 level. If the patient has features suggestive of acromegaly, a fasting growth hormone (with the patient as unstressed as possible) should be obtained, and normally is <10 ng/mL. If the patient has signs suggestive of Cushing's syndrome a fasting morning cortisol following 1 mg of dexamethasone the evening before, or preferably, a 24-hr urine free cortisol should be obtained. The 24-hr free cortisol should be <100 μg/24 hr, whereas the morning cortisol after overnight dexamethasone should be <5 μg/dL. Obese and depressed individuals may have slightly elevated fasting cortisol levels which will require further testing.

In patients suspected of suffering from male pseudohermaphroditism or XY gonadal dysgenesis, a karyotype should be obtained. In selected women an evaluation of liver function may be necessary, since chronic liver disease (e.g., chronic active hepatitis, congenital causes of biliary cirrhosis, hemochromocytosis, etc.) may result in excessively low SHBG production with a consequent elevation in free T and DHT levels.

TREATMENT OF HIRSUTISM

The treatment of hirsutism should be undertaken *as soon as the diagnosis is established.* Although, in young children or teenagers the degree of hair growth may not be alarming one must remember that these disorders are usually progressive, and the appearance of terminal hairs not reversible. Any terminal hairs remaining after six months of adequate suppression with medical therapy must be removed by electrolysis, which can be very painful, costly and not applicable to large areas of the body. Hirsutism is not only cosmetically disfiguring but can become a significant handicap to a young woman's social life and emotional stability. Furthermore, the treatment of hyperandrogenemia has profound medical implications since the long-term effects of excess androgens include an increased risk of cardiovascular disease (142). Hyperandrogenic oligomenorrhea can also lead to the development of endometrial hyperplasia and subsequent carcinoma at a young age (143–145). Furthermore, 30–50% of adolescents with oligomenorrhea demonstrate hyperandrogenemia which may be persistent in 50% of these girls (71–73).

The hormonal treatment of hirsutism has the prime objective of stopping the development of new terminal hairs. Hormonal therapy also slows the growth, and reduces the diameter and pigmentation of terminal hairs already present. However, it will not reverse the transformation of vellus to terminal hairs. It is important to emphasize that therapy for hirsutism may take up to 6 months before a clinical response is noted.

Mechanical means of hair removal, by themselves, do little to affect the long-term course of hirsutism. However, while awaiting the full effect of hormonal therapy it is best to encourage the patient to shave (either with a blade or a machine) since this causes the least trauma to the skin. Although shaving can lead to a blunt hair end, which may feel "stubble-like," it does not lead to a worsening of hirsutism. It is surprising what satisfactory cosmetic results shaving and the proper application of makeup can produce. Recording the interval between shavings prior to each office visit provides a relatively simple way to monitor the efficacy of treatment. Plucking or waxing should be discouraged since it stimulates the growth of surrounding follicles, and may lead to folliculitis with the subsequent development of ingrown hairs. Depilating agents, particularly on the face, can lead to skin irritation and worsening of hirsutism. Electrolysis is the only method available for the irreversible destruction of hair follicles. It may not be applicable to large areas of the body including sensitive areas, such as the periareolar region. As indicated above, electrolysis should be combined with hormonal therapy, after a clinical response has been observed, for maximum cosmetic benefit.

The mainstay of androgen excess treatment are oral contraceptive pills (OCPs) which, by suppressing the secretion of gonadotropins (LH and FSH), lead to a decrease in ovarian androgen production (146). Full suppression is usually seen within the month. Oral contraceptive pills also decrease adrenal androgen production by a mechanism not yet clear, but may be related to a decrease in circulating ACTH. The progestin in OCPs can also compete for 5α-reductase and the androgen receptor. The estrogen fraction in the OCPs increases circulating SHBG, with a subsequent decrease in free T levels. Since the progestin in the OCPs may in turn decrease SHBG, it is most important to select a pill whose progestin is the least androgenic (e.g., ethynodiol diacetate in Demulen). Birth control pills should be administered in the usual cyclic fashion, and the circulating androgen levels should be checked periodically to assess the adequacy of hormonal suppression.

Retrospective studies of women developing post-pill amenorrhea have observed that between 37% and 63% of these patients had a history of oligomenorrhea (147,148), which appears to be higher than the incidence in the general population, and has lead to the recommendation that OCP administration is contraindicated in oligomenorrheic adolescents. However, the incidence of post-pill amenorrhea appears to be relatively low, less than 0.5% of women taking OCP's (147). Furthermore, the incidence of hyperandrogenemia in adolescent amenorrhea is high (71,72,149) and OCP administration leads to a suppression of their androgen levels (149). Furthermore after cessation of therapy the androgen levels returned to their pretreatment levels (149). Thus, it is very probable that oligomenorrheic patients developing post-pill amenorrhea simply demonstrate a recurrence of their pathology, whereas OCP use actually suppressed the frequently coexisting hyperandrogenemia, with a consequent delay in the appearance of such clinical signs as acne and hirsutism.

Spironolactone (SPA) is an aldosterone antagonist and a mild diuretic. It also is an effective therapy for hirsutism (150–156), competing for the androgen receptor, 5α-reductase, and the binding of T to SHBG (157). Furthermore, SPA blocks the action of various enzymes involved in androgen biosynthesis (157–159). Initially a dose as high as 200 mg a day should be used. If the dose is slowly increased from 25 to 200 mg a day, by 25 mg increments every three days or so, the patient will have minimal side effects. The side effects most commonly associated with SPA use include polyuria, fatigue, headaches, and irregular menses. The incidence of metrorrhagia may be decreased by administering the SPA days 4–21 of the menstrual cycle (160). Hypertensive patients on a potassium-saving diuretic may rarely develop hyperkalemia. Spironolactone is extremely effective for treating hirsutism, in particular IH. Treatment should be continued for at least a year with a subsequent reduction in dose. Since SPA acts through mechanisms different from that of OCPs, it is possible to improve the overall therapeutic effectiveness by combining these medications (161,162). Furthermore, the use of OCPs or estrogen/progestin therapy in combination with SPA minimizes the problems with dysfunctional uterine bleeding or worsening oligomenorrhea often observed in women using SPA alone, while providing adequate contraception (161–163).

Dexamethasone (0.25–0.5 mg every to every other evening) or prednisone (5–10 mg daily) can be used as an adjuvant for the treatment of hirsutism (164–168), particularly in patients with significant adrenal hyperandrogenemia, or for patients suffering from LOAH or CAH. The use of oral estrogen (with a progestin administered in a cyclic fashion when the uterus is present) has been advocated for older women or those not tolerating OCPs. The doses of estrogen needed are higher than that required for regular postmenopausal hormonal therapy. Estrogen therapy increases SHBG, decreases circulating LH and FSH levels, and potentially antagonizes the effect of androgens at the hair follicle. High doses of progestin only (e.g., 20–30 mg of medroxyprogesterone acetate daily) can also be used (169). High doses of progestin increase the clearance of T by the liver and may lead to a decrease in circulating LH. However, this therapy also leads to a decrease in the circulating SHBG concentration which may decrease its therapeutic effectiveness. Furthermore, side effects may become unacceptable and include breakthrough bleeding, liver dysfunction, possibly vascular changes, weight gain, depression and hot flushes. Cyproterone acetate (CPA) is a strong progestin and antiandrogen, and an effective treatment for hirsutism (170). It produces a decrease in circulating T and A levels through a reduction in LH. Furthermore, CPA antagonizes the effect of androgens at the androgen receptor level. Side effects may include adrenal insufficiency and loss of libido. This drug is currently not available in the United States, and it is unlikely that it will become FDA approved since SPA appears to be equally effective. Cimetidine also competes for binding to the androgen receptor, although it does not change circulating levels of T, DHT, and adrenal androgens. Since it is a relatively weak androgen receptor antagonist it has no benefit, but greater side-effects, over SPA use (171).

In the past, ovarian wedge resection has been used with satisfactory results (172, 173). More recently, laparoscopic wedge resection (174) or fulguration of multiple areas of the ovarian cortex has been proposed (175–177), although long term follow-up information is lacking. In general, these destructive procedures should be used as line of last defense, since they almost invariably lead to ovarian adhesions. It is a rare patient who requires a bilateral ovarian wedge resection, with the exception of those suspected of having an ovarian tumor, and some hyperthecotic or HAIRAN syndrome patients. The use of a long-acting GnRH agonist may be a better method of treating these patients (108,122), since it produces a medical "oophorectomy" without the surgical risk or possibility of adnexal adhesions (Fig. 9). Long-acting GnRH agonist treatment should be accompanied by estrogen/progestin replacement in order to reduce the hypoestrogenic side effects (hot flushes, genital dryness, osteoporosis, etc.) and increase circulating SHBG levels. Spironolactone may also be combined for maximum therapeutic effect in these very affected girls. It may take 3–4 months for the full suppressive effects of the agonist to occur. Therapy with ketoconazole may also be considered in these patients (107). Rarely are individuals so affected that a bilateral oophorectomy need be considered, although this may be applicable in some severely affected young girls who have little hope of improvement otherwise (e.g., HAIRAN syndrome). However, these patients are very much the exception. Women who suffer from hirsutism require long-term follow-up, counseling and emotional support, since these disorders are usually life long, and progressive unless adequately treated medically, with electrolysis as an adjuvant.

REFERENCES

1. James VHT, Goodall A. Androgen production in women. In: Jeffcoate SL, ed. *Androgens and anti-androgen therapy*. New York: John Wiley & Sons, 1982;23–40.
2. Rosenfeld RS, Rosenberg BJ, Fukushima DK, Hellman L. 24-Hour secretory pattern of dehydroisoandrosterone and dehydroisoandrosterone sulfate. *J Clin Endocrinol Metab* 1975; 40:850–5.
3. Huq MS, Pfaff M, Jespersen D, Zucker IR, Kirschner MA. Concurrence of aldosterone, androgen and cortisol secretion in adrenal venous effluents. *J Clin Endocrinol Metab* 1976;42: 230–8.
4. Suzuki T. Circadian rhythm of adrenocortical secretory activity. In: *Physiology of adrenocortical secretion*. New York: Karger, 1983: 72–191.
5. Kato T, Horton R. Studies of testosterone binding globulin. *J Clin Endocrinol Metab* 1968; 28:1160–8.
6. Dunn JF, Nisula BC, Rodbard D. Transport of steroid hormones: binding of 21 endogenous steroids to both testosterone-binding globulin and corticosteroid-binding globulin in human plasma. *J Clin Endocrinol Metab* 1981;53:58–68.
7. Rosenfield RL. Plasma testosterone binding globulin and indexes of the concentration of unbound plasma androgens in normal and hirsute subjects. *J Clin Endocrinol Metab* 1971;32: 717–28.
8. Vermeulen A, Verdonck L, Van der Straeten M, Orie N. Capacity of the testosterone-binding globulin in human plasma and influence of specific binding of testosterone on its metabolic clearance rate. *J Clin Endocrinol Metab* 1969; 29:1470–80.
9. Plymate R, Leonard JM, Paulsen CA, Fariss BL, Karpas E. Sex hormone-binding globulin changes with androgen replacement. *J Clin Endocrinol Metab* 1983;57:645–8.
10. Tochimoto S, Olivo J, Southren AL, Gordon GG. Studies of plasma β-globulin: sex difference and effect of ethinyl estradiol and testosterone. *Proc Soc Exp Biol Med* 1970;134: 700–2.
11. Musa BU, Doe RP, Seal US. Serum protein alterations produced in women by synthetic estrogens. *J Clin Endocrinol Metab* 1967;27: 1463–9.
12. Chitkowski RJ, Meldrum DR, Steingold KA, et al. Biologic effects of transdermal estradiol. *N Engl J Med* 1986;314:1615–20.
13. Azziz R. Reproductive endocrinologic alteration in female asymptomatic obesity. *Fertil Steril* 1989;52:703–25.
14. Komindr S, Kurtz BR, Stevens MD, Karas JG, Bittle JB, Givens JR. Relative sensitivity and responsivity of serum cortisol and two adrenal androgens to α-adrenocorticotropin-(1-24) in

normal and obese, nonhirsute, eumenorrheic women. *J Clin Endocrinol Metab* 1986;63: 860–4.
15. Ducharme JR, Collu R. Pubertal development: normal, precocious and delayed. In: Ducharme JR, Collu R, eds. *Clinics in endocrinology and metabolism, vol. 11*. Philadelphia: W.B. Saunders, 1982;57–87.
16. Korth-Schultz S, Levine LS, New MI. Serum androgens in normal prepubertal and pubertal children and in children with precocious adrenarche. *J Clin Endocrinol Metab* 1976;42: 117–24.
17. Apter D, Lenko HL, Perheentupa J, Soderholm A, Vihko R. Subnormal pubertal increases of serum androgens in Turner's Syndrome. *Horm Res* 1982;16:164–73.
18. Moll Jr GW, Rosenfield RL. Plasma free testosterone in the diagnosis of adolescent polycystic ovary syndrome. *J Pediatr* 1983;102:461–4.
19. Apter D, Vihko R. Serum pregnenolone, progesterone, 17-hydroxyprogesterone, testosterone and 5α-dihydrotestosterone during female puberty. *J Clin Endocrinol Metab* 1977;45: 1039–48.
20. Belgorosky A, Rivarola MA. Progressive increase in nonsex hormone-binding globulin-bound testosterone and estradiol from infancy to late prepuberty in girls. *J Clin Endocrinol Metab* 1988;67:234–7.
21. Cunningham SK, Loughlin T, Culliton M, McKenna TJ. Plasma sex hormone-binding globulin levels decrease during the second decade of life irrespective of pubertal status. *J Clin Endocrinol Metab* 1984;58:915–8.
22. Collu R, Ducharme R. Role of adrenal steroids in the initiation of pubertal mechanisms. In: James VHT, Giusti MS, Giusti G, Martini L, eds. *The endocrine function of the human adrenal cortex. Proceedings of the Serono Symposia, vol. 18*. New York: Academic Press, 1978:547–59.
23. Pintor C, Facchinetti F, Puggioni R, et al. Effect of short dexamethasone suppression on plasma steroids in prepubertal and pubertal girls. *J Endocrinol Invest* 1980;3:25–28.
24. De Peretti E, Forest MG. Unconjugated dehydroepiandrosterone plasma levels in normal subjects from birth to adolescence in human: the use of a sensitive radioimmunoassay. *J Clin Endocrinol Metab* 1976;43:982–91.
25. Sizonenko PC, Paunier L. Hormonal changes in puberty III: correlation of plasma dehydroepiandrosterone, testosterone, FSH, and LH with stages of puberty and bone age in normal boys and girls and in patients with Addison's disease or hypogonadism or with premature or late adrenarche. *J Clin Endocrinol Metab* 1975; 41:894–904.
26. Korth-Schutz S, Levine LS, New MI. Dehydroepiandrosterone sulfate (DS) levels, a rapid test for abnormal adrenal androgen secretion. *J Clin Endocrinol Metab* 1976;42:1005–13.
27. Pintor C, Genazzani AR, Carboni G, et al. Adrenal androgens and pubertal development in physiological and pathological conditions. In: Genazzani AR, et al, eds. *Adrenal androgens*. New York: Raven Press, 1980;173–81.
28. Dhom G. The prepuberal and puberal growth of the adrenal (adrenarche). *Beitr Path Bd* 1973; 150:357–77.
29. Kelnar CJH, Brook CGD. A mixed longitudinal study of adrenal steroid excretion in childhood and the mechanism of adrenarche. *Clin Endocrinol (Oxf)* 1983;19:117–29.
30. Rich BH, Rosenfield RL, Lucky AW, Helke JC, Otto P. Adrenarche: changing adrenal response to adrenocorticotropin. *J Clin Endocrinol Metab* 1981;52:1129–36.
31. Schiebinger RJ, Albertson BD, Cassorla FG, Bowyer DW, Geelhoed GW, Cutler Jr GB. The developmental changes in plasma adrenal androgens during infancy and adrenarche are associated with changing activities of adrenal microsomal 17-hydroxylase and 17,20-desmolase. *J Clin Invest* 1981;67:1177–82.
32. Counts DR, Pescovitz OH, Barnes KM, et al. Dissociation of adrenarche and gonadarche in precocious puberty and in isolated hypogonadotropic hypogonadism. *J Clin Endocrinol Metab* 1987;64:1174–8.
33. Grumbach MM, Richards GE, Conte FA, Kaplan SL. Clinical disorders of adrenal function and puberty: an assessment of the role of the adrenal cortex in normal and abnormal puberty in man and evidence for an ACTH-like pituitary adrenal androgen stimulating hormone. In: James VHT, Giusti MS, Giusti G, Martini L, eds. *The endocrine function of the human adrenal cortex. Proceedings of the Serono Symposia, vol. 18*. New York: Academic Press, 1978:583–612.
34. Parker LN, Odell WD. Control of adrenal androgen secretion. *Endocrinol Rev* 1980;1: 392–410.
35. Parker L, Lifrak E, Shively, et al. Human adrenal gland cortical androgen-stimulating hormone (CASH) is identical with a portion of the joining peptide of pituitary proopiomelanocortin (POMC) [Abstract]. Presented at the 71st Endocrine Society Annual Meeting, Seattle, Washington, 1989.
36. Forest MG, de Peretti E, Bertrand J. Developmental patterns of the plasma levels of testosterone, δ^4-androstenedione, 17α-hydroxyprogesterone, dehydroepiandrosterone and its sulfate in normal infants and prepubertal children. In: James VHT, Giusti MS, Giusti G, Martini L, eds. *The endocrine function of the human adrenal cortex. Proceedings of the Serono Symposia, vol. 18*. New York: Academic Press, 1978:561–82.
37. Avgerinos PC, Butler Jr GB, Tsokos GC, et al. Dissociation between cortisol and adrenal androgen secretion in patients receiving alternate day prednisone therapy. *J Clin Endocrinol Metab* 1987;65:24–9.
38. Parker Jr CR, Baxter CR. Divergence in adre-

nal steroid secretory pattern after thermal injury in adult patients. *J Trauma* 1985;25: 508–10.
39. Lephart ED, Baxter CR, Parker Jr CR. Effect of burn trauma on adrenal and testicular steroid hormone production. *J Clin Endocrinol Metab* 1987;64:842–8.
40. Pang S, Legido A, Levine LS, Temeck JW, New MI. Adrenal androgen response to metyrapone, adrenocorticotropin, and corticotropin-releasing hormone stimulation in children with hypopituitarism. *J Clin Endocrinol Metab* 1987; 65:282–9.
41. Kreitzer PM, Blethen SL, Festa RS, Chasalow RI. Dehydroepiandrosterone sulfate levels are not suppressible by glucocorticoids before adrenarche. *J Clin Endocrinol Metab* 1989; 69:1309–11.
42. Dickerman Z, Grant DR, Faiman C, Winter JSD. Intraadrenal steroid concentrations in man: zonal differences and developmental changes. *J Clin Endocrinol Metab* 1984;59: 1031–6.
43. Hornsby PJ, Aldern KA. Steroidogenic enzyme activities in cultured human definitive zone adrenocortical cells: comparison with bovine adrenocortical cells and resultant differences in adrenal androgen synthesis. *J Clin Endocrinol Metab* 1984;58:121–7.
44. Uno H. Biology of hair growth. *Semin Reprod Endocrinol* 1986;4:131–41.
45. McKenna TJ, Loughlin T, Daly L, Smyth PA, Culliton M, Cunningham SK. Variable clinical and hormonal manifestations of hyperandrogenemia. *Metabolism* 1984;33:714–7.
46. Ginsberg GS, Birnbaum MD, Rose LI. Androgen abnormalities in acne vulgaris. *Acta Dermatol Venereol (Stockh)* 1981;61:431–4.
47. Marynick SP, Chakmakjian ZH, McCaffree DL, Herndon Jr JH. Androgen excess in cystic acne. *N Engl J Med* 1983;308:981–1025.
48. Vexiau P, Husson C, Chivot M, et al. Androgen excess in women with acne alone compared with women with acne and/or hirsutism. *J Invest Dermatol* 1990;94:279–83.
49. Pekkarinen A, Sonck CE. Adrenocortical reserves in acne vulgaris. *Acta Dermatol Venereol (Stockh)* 1962;42:200–10.
50. Darley CR, Moore JW, Besser GM, Munro DD, Edwards CRW, Rees LH, Kirby JD. *Clin Exp Dermatol* 1984;9:28–35.
51. Steinberger E, Rodriguez-Rigau LJ, Smith KD, Held B. The menstrual cycle and plasma testosterone levels in women with acne. *J Am Acad Dermatol* 1981;4:54–8.
52. Lucky AW, McGuire J, Rosenfield RL, Lucky PA, Rich BH. Plasma androgens in women with acne vulgaris. *J Invest Dermatol* 1983;81:70–4.
53. Lawrence DM, Katz M, Robinson TWE, Newman MC, McGarrigle HHG, Shaw M, Lachelin GCL. Reduced sex hormone binding globulin and derived free testosterone levels in women with severe acne. *Clin Endocrinol (Oxf)* 1981; 15:87–91.
54. Held BL, Nader S, Rodriguez-Rigau LJ, Smith KD, Steinberger E. Acne and hyperandrogenism. *J Am Acad Dermatol* 1984;10:112–226.
55. van der Meeren HLM, Thijssen JHH. Circulating androgens in male acne. *Br J Dermatol* 1984;110:609–11.
56. Sultan C, Oliel V, Audran F, Meynadier. Free and total plasma testosterone in men and women with acne. *Acta Dermatol Venereol (Stockh)* 1986;66:301–4.
57. Sheehan-Dare RA, Hughes BR, Cunliffe WJ. Clinical markers of androgenicity in acne vulgaris. *Br J Dermatol* 1988;119:723–30.
58. Levell MJ, Cawood ML, Burke B, Cunliffe WJ. Acne is not associated with abnormal plasma androgens. *Br J Dermatol* 1989;120:649–54.
59. Chrousos GP, Peck GL, Gross EG, Cutler GB, Loriaux DL. Adrenal function in women with idiopathic acne. *J Invest Dermatol* 1982;78: 468–71.
60. Lucky AW, Rosenfield RL, McGuire J, Rudy S, Helke J. Adrenal androgen hyperresponsiveness to adrenocorticotropin in women with acne and/or hirsutism: adrenal enzyme defects and exaggerated adrenarche. *J Clin Endocrinol Metab* 1986;62:840–8.
61. Sansone G, Reisner RM. Differential rates of conversion of testosterone to dihydrotestosterone in acne and in normal human skin-a possible pathogenic factor in acne. *J Invest Dermatol* 1971;56:366–72.
62. Lookingbill DP, Horton R, Demers LM, Egan N, Marks JG, Santen RJ. Tissue production of androgens in women with acne. *J Am Acad Dermatol* 1985;12:481–7.
63. Hay JB, Hodgins MB. Metabolism of androgens by human skin in acne. *Br J Dermatol* 1974;91:123–33.
64. Palatsi R, Reinila M, Kivinen S. Pituitary function and DHEA-S in male acne and DHEA-S, prolactin and cortisol before and after oral contraceptive treatment in female acne. *Acta Dermatol Venereol (Stockh)* 1986;66:225–30.
65. Hammerstein J, Moltz L, Schwartz U. Antiandrogens in the treatment of acne and hirsutism. *J Steroid Biochem* 1983;19:591–7.
66. Darley CR, Moore JW, Besser GM, Munro DD, Kirby JD. Low dose prednisolone or oestrogen in the treatment of women with late onset or persistent acne vulgaris. *Br J Dermatol* 1983; 108:345–53.
67. Goodfellow A, Alaghband-Zadeh J, Carter G, et al. Oral spironolactone improves acne vulgaris and reduces sebum excretion. *Br J Dermatol* 1984;2:209–14.
68. Muhlemann MF, Carter GD, Cream JJ, Wise P. Oral spironolactone: an effective treatment for acne vulgaris in women. *Br J Dermatol* 1986; 115:227–32.
69. Nader S, Rodriguez-Rigau LJ, Smith KD, Steinberger E. Acne and hyperandrogenism: impact of lowering androgen levels with glucocorticoid treatment. *J Am Acad Dermatol* 1984;11:256–9.
70. Ettinger B, Goldfield B, Burrill E, von Werder K, Forsham C. Plasma testosterone stimula-

tion-suppression dynamics in hirsute women. *Am J Med* 1973;54:195–200.

71. Siegberg R, Nilsson CG, Stenman UH, Widholm O. Endocrinologic features of oligomenorrheic adolescent girls. *Fertil Steril* 1986;46: 852–7.
72. Emans SJ, Grace E, Goldstein DP. Oligomenorrhea in adolescent girls. *J Pediatr* 1980; 97:815–9.
73. Venturoli S, Porcu E, Fabbri R, et al. Postmenarchal evolution of endocrine pattern and ovarian aspects in adolescents with menstrual irregularities. *Fertil Steril* 1987;48:78–85.
74. Swanson M, Sauerbrei EE, Cooperberg PL. Medical implications of ultrasonically detected polycystic ovaries. *J Clin Ultrasound* 1981;9: 219–22.
75. Polson DW, Wadsworth J, Adams J, Franks S. Polycystic ovaries—a common finding in normal women. *Lancet* 1988;870–2.
76. el Tabbakh GH, Lotfy I, Azab I, Rahman HA, Southren AL, Aleem FA. Correlation of the ultrasonic appearance of the ovaries in polycystic ovarian disease and the clinical, hormonal, and laparoscopic findings. *Am J Obstet Gynecol* 1986;154:892–5.
77. Orsini LF, Venturoli S, Lorusso R, Pluchinotta V, Paradisi R, Bovicelli L. Ultrasonic findings in polycystic ovarian disease. *Fertil Steril* 1985;43:709–14.
78. Kim MH, Rosenfield RL, Hosseinian AH, Schneir HG. Ovarian hyperandrogenism with normal and abnormal histologic findings of the ovaries. *Am J Obstet Gynecol* 1979;134:445–52.
79. Materlik H, Slowko T, Jedrzejczak A. Skin changes in acromegaly. *Pol Med J* 1968;23: 1522–7.
80. Philip J, Trolle D. Familial male hermaphroditism with delayed and partial masculinization. *Am J Obstet Gynecol* 1965;93:1076–83.
81. New MI, Levine LS. *Congenital adrenal hyperplasia*. New York: Springer-Verlag, 1984.
82. Giusti G, Manelli M, Forti G, et al. Plasma steroid values in congenital adrenocortical hyperplasia. In: James VHT, Giusti MS, Giusti G, Martini L, eds. *The endocrine function of the human adrenal cortex, vol. 18*. New York: Academic Press, 1978:271–87.
83. Zachmann M, Tassinari D, Prader A. Clinical and biochemical variability of congenital adrenal hyperplasia due to 11β-hydroxylase deficiency. A study of 25 patients. *J Clin Endocrinol Metab* 1983;56:222–9.
84. Hochberg Z, Schechter J, Benderly A, Leiberman E, Rosler A. Growth and pubertal development in patients with congenital adrenal hyperplasia due to 11β-hydroxylase deficiency. *Am J Dis Child* 1985;139:771–6.
85. Pang S, Levine LS, Stoner E, et al. Nonsalt-losing congenital adrenal hyperplasia due to 3β-hydroxysteroid dehydrogenase deficiency with normal glomerulosa function. *J Clin Endocrinol Metab* 1983;56:808–18.
86. de Peretti E, Forest MG, Feit JP, David M. Endocrine studies in two children with male pseudohermaphroditism due to 3β-hydroxysteroid (3β-HSD) dehydrogenase defect. In: Genazzani AR, Thijssen JHH, Siiteri PK, eds. *Adrenal androgens*. New York: Raven Press, 1980.
87. Griffiths KD, Anderson JM, Rudd BT, Virdi NK, Holder G, Rayer PHW. Plasma renin activity in the management of congenital adrenal hyperplasia. *Arch Dis Child* 1984;59:360–5.
88. Mulaikal RM, Migeon CJ, Rock JA. Fertility rates in female patients with congenital adrenal hyperplasia due to 21-hydroxylase deficiency. *N Engl J Med* 1987;316:178–82.
89. Azziz R, Mulaikal RM, Migeon CJ, Jones Jr HW, Rock JA. Congenital adrenal hyperplasia: long-term results following vaginal reconstruction. *Fertil Steril* 1986;46:1011–4.
90. Azziz R, Zacur HA. 21-Hydroxylase deficiency in female hyperandrogenism: screening and diagnosis. *J Clin Endocrinol Metab* 1989;69: 577–84.
91. Dewailly D, Vantyghem-Haudiquet MC, Sainsard C, et al. Clinical and biological phenotypes in late-onset 21-hydroxylase deficiency. *J Clin Endocrinol Metab* 1986;63:418–23.
92. Spritzer P, Billaud L, Thalabard JC, et al. Cyproterone acetate versus hydrocortisone treatment in late-onset adrenal hyperplasia. *J Clin Endocrinol Metab* 1990;70:642–6.
93. Carmina E, Malizia G, Pagano M, Janni A. Prevalence of late-onset 11β-hydroxylase deficiency in hirsute patients. *J Endocrinol Invest* 1988;11:595.
94. Pang S, Lerner AJ, Stoner E, et al. Late-onset adrenal steroid 3β-hydroxysteroid dehydrogenase deficiency. I. A cause of hirsutism in pubertal and postpubertal women. *J Clin Endocrinol Metab* 1985;60:428–39.
95. Lobo RA, Goebelsmann U. Evidence for reduced 3β-ol-hydroxysteroid dehydrogenase activity in some hirsute women thought to have polycystic ovary syndrome. *J Clin Endocrinol Metab* 1981;53:394–400.
96. Barbieri RL, Ryan KJ. Hyperandrogenism, insulin resistance, and acanthosis nigricans syndrome: a common endocrinopathy with distinct pathophysiologic features. *Am J Obstet Gynecol* 1983;147:90–101.
97. Barth JH, Ng LL, Wojnarowska F, Dawber RPR. Acanthosis nigricans, insulin resistance and cutaneous virilism. *Br J Dermatol* 1988; 118:613–9.
98. Richards GE, Cavallo A, Meyer III WJ, et al. Obesity, acanthosis nigricans, insulin resistance, and hyperandrogenemia: pediatric perspective and natural history. *J Pediatr* 1985;7: 893–7.
99. Kahn CR, Flier JS, Bar RS, et al. The syndromes of insulin resistance and acanthosis nigricans. *N Engl J Med* 1976;14:739–45.
100. Bar RS, Muggeo M, Roth J, Kahn CR, Havrankova J, Imperato-McGinley J. Insulin resistance, acanthosis nigricans, and normal insulin receptors in a young woman: evidence for a postreceptor defect. *J Clin Endocrinol Metab* 1978;47:620–5.

101. Bar RS, Muggeo M, Kahn CR, Gorden P, Roth J. Characterization of insulin receptors in patients with the syndromes of insulin resistance and acanthosis nigricans. *Diabetologia* 1980; 18:209–16.
102. Peters EJ, Stuart CA, Prince MJ. Acanthosis nigricans and obesity: acquired and intrinsic defects in insulin action. *Metabolism* 1986;9: 807–13.
103. Moller DE, Flier JS. Detection of an alteration in the insulin-receptor gene in a patient with insulin resistance, acanthosis nigricans, and the polycystic ovary syndrome (type A insulin resistance). *N Engl J Med* 1988;319:1526–9.
104. Kadowaki T, Bevins CL, Cama A, et al. Two mutant alleles of the insulin receptor gene in a patient with extreme insulin resistance. *Science* 1988;240:787–90.
105. Taylor SI, Dons RF, Hernandez E, Roth J, Gorden P. Insulin resistance associated with androgen excess in women with autoantibodies to the insulin receptor. *Ann Intern Med* 1982; 97:851–5.
106. Kellett HA, Collier A, Raylor R, et al. Hyperandrogenism, insulin resistance, acanthosis nigricans, and systemic lupus erythematosis associated with insulin receptor antibodies. *Metabolism* 1988;7:656–9.
107. Pepper GM, Poretsky L, Gabrilove JL, Ariton MM. Ketoconazole reverses hyperandrogenism in a patient with insulin resistance and acanthosis nigricans. *J Clin Endocrinol Metab* 1987;65:1047–51.
108. Corenblum B, Baylis BW. Medical therapy for the syndrome of familial virilization, insulin resistance, and acanthosis nigricans. *Fertil Steril* 1990;53:421–5.
109. Padilla SL. Androgen-producing tumors in children and adolescents. *Adolesc Pediatr Gynecol* 1989;2:135–42.
110. Yuen BH, Moon YS, Mincey EK, Li D. Adrenal and sex steroid hormone production by a virilizing adrenal adenoma and its diagnosis with computerized tomography. *Am J Obstet Gynecol* 1983;145:164–9.
111. Meldrum DR, Abraham G. Peripheral and ovarian venous concentrations of various steroid hormones in virilizing ovarian tumors. *Obstet Gynecol* 1979;53:36–43.
112. Surrey ES, de Ziegler D, Gambone JC, Judd HL. Preoperative localization of androgen-secreting tumors: clinical, endocrinologic, and radiologic evaluation of ten patients. *Am J Obstet Gynecol* 1988;158:1313–22.
113. Friedman CI, Schmidt GE, Kim MH, Powell J. Serum testosterone concentrations in the evaluation of androgen-producing tumors. *Am J Obstet Gynecol* 1985;153:44–9.
114. Sorensen R, Moltz L, Schwartz U. Technical difficulties of selective venous blood sampling in the differential diagnosis of female hyperandrogenism. *Cardiovasc Intervent Radiol* 1986; 9:75–82.
115. Weiland AJ, Bookstein JJ, Cleary RF, Judd HL. Preoperative localization of virilizing tumors by selective venous sampling. *Am J Obstet Gynecol* 1978;131:797–802.
116. Moltz L, Pickartz H, Sorensen R, Schwartz U, Hammerstein J. Ovarian and adrenal vein steroids in seven patients with androgen-secreting ovarian neoplasms: selective catheterization findings. *Fertil Steril* 1984;42:585–93.
117. Judd HL, Scully RE, Herbst AL, Yen SSC, Ingersol FM, Kliman B. Familial hyperthecosis: comparison of endocrinologic and histologic findings with polycystic ovarian disease. *Am J Obstet Gynecol* 1973;117:976–82.
118. Aiman J, Edman CD, Worley RJ, Vellios F, MacDonald PC. Androgen and estrogen formation in women with ovarian hyperthecosis. *Obstet Gynecol* 1978;51:1–9.
119. Wentz AC, Gutai JP, Jones GS, Migeon CJ. Ovarian hyperthecosis in the adolescent patient. *J Pediatr* 1976;88:488–93.
120. Nagamani M, Lingold JC, Gomez LG, Garza JR. Clinical and hormonal studies in hyperthecosis of the ovaries. *Fertil Steril* 1981;36: 326–32.
121. Scully RE. Correspondence: reply to Dr. Fienberg. *Am J Obstet Gynecol* 1974;119:864–5.
122. Steingold KA, Judd HL, Nieberg RK, Lu JKH, Chang RJ. Treatment of severe androgen excess due to ovarian hyperthecosis with a long-acting gonadotropin-releasing hormone agonist. *Am J Obstet Gynecol* 1986;154:1241–8.
123. Hull MGR. Epidemiology of infertility and polycystic ovarian disease: endocrinological and demographic studies. *Gynecol Endocrinol* 1987;1:235–45.
124. Mathur RS, Moody LO, Landgrebe S, Williamson HO. Plasma androgens and sex hormone-binding globulin in the evaluation of hirsute females. *Fertil Steril* 1981;35:29–35.
125. Vermeulen A, Stoica T, Verdonck L. The apparent free testosterone concentration, an index of androgenicity. *J Clin Endocr* 1971; 33:759–67.
126. Hoffman DI, Klove K, Lobo RA. The prevalence and significance of elevated dehydroepiandrosterone sulfate levels in anovulatory women. *Fertil Steril* 1984;42:76–81.
127. Luciano AA, Chapler FK, Sherman BM. Hyperprolactinemia in polycystic ovary syndrome. *Fertil Steril* 1984;41:719–25.
128. Carmina E, Rosato F, Maggiore M, Gagliano AM, Indovina D, Janni A. Prolactin secretion in polycystic ovary syndrome (PCO): correlation with the steroid pattern. *Acta Endocrinol (Copenh)* 1984;105:99–104.
129. Taymor ML, Barnard R. Leuteinizing hormone excretion in the polycystic ovary syndrome. *Fertil Steril* 1962;13:501–12.
130. Yen SSC, Vela P, Rankin J. Inappropriate secretion of follicle-stimulating hormone and luteinizing hormone in polycystic ovarian disease. *J Clin Endocrinol Metab* 1970;30:435–42.
131. Kazer RR, Kessel B, Yen SSC. Circulating luteinizing hormone pulse frequency in women with polycystic ovary syndrome. *J Clin Endocrinol Metab* 1987;65:233–36.

132. Goldzieher JW, Green JA. The polycystic ovary. I. Clinical and histologic features. *J Clin Endocrinol Metab* 1962;22:325–38.
133. Hosseinian AH, Kim MH, Rosenfield RL. Obesity and oligomenorrhea are associated with hyperandrogenism independent of hirsutism. *J Clin Endocrinol Metab* 1976;42:765–9.
134. Lobo RA, Goebelsmann U, Horton R. Evidence for the importance of peripheral tissue events in the development of hirsutism in polycystic ovary syndrome. *J Clin Endocrinol Metab* 1983;57:393–7.
135. Stanhope R, Adams J, Brook CGD. Evolution of polycystic ovaries in a girl with delayed menarche. *J Reprod Med* 1088;33:482–4.
136. Canales ES, Zarate A, Castelazo-Ayala L. Primary amenorrhea associated with polycystic ovaries. *Obstet Gynecol* 1971;37:205–10.
137. Rao JK, Chihal HJ, Johnson CM. Primary polycystic ovary syndrome in a premenarchal girl. *J Reprod Med* 1985;30:361–5.
138. Kirschner MA, Zucker R, Jespersen D. Idiopathic hirsutism—an ovarian abnormality. *N Engl J Med* 1976;294:637–40.
139. Gompel A, Wright F, Kuttenn, Mauvais-Jarvis P. Contribution of plasma androstenedione to 5α-androstanediol glucuronide in women with idiopathic hirsutism. *J Clin Endocrinol Metab* 1986;62:441–4.
140. Greep N, Hoopes M, Horton R. Androstanediol glucuronide plasma clearance and production rates in normal and hirsute women. *J Clin Endocrinol Metab* 1986;62:22–7.
141. Kirschner MA, Samojlik E, Szmal E. Clinical usefulness of plasma androstanediol glucuronide measurements in women with idiopathic hirsutism. *J Clin Endocrinol Metab* 1987;65:597–601.
142. Wild RA, Painter PC, Coulson PB, Carruth KB, Ranney GB. Lipoprotein lipid concentrations and cardiovascular risk in women with polycystic ovary syndrome. *J Clin Endocrinol Metab* 1985;61:946–51.
143. Jackson RL, Dockerty MB. The Stein-Leventhal syndrome: analysis of 43 cases with special reference to association with endometrial carcinoma. *Am J Obstet Gynecol* 1957;73:161–73.
144. Wood GP, Boronow RC. Endometrial adenocarcinoma and the polycystic ovary syndrome. *Am J Obstet Gynecol* 1976;124:140–2.
145. Farhi DC, Nosanchuk J, Silverberg SG. Endometrial adenocarcinoma in women under 25 years of age. *Obstet Gynecol* 1986;68:741–5.
146. Azziz R, Gay F. The treatment of hyperandrogenism with oral contraceptives. *Semin Reprod Endocrinol* 1989;7:246–54.
147. Steele SJ, Mason B, Brett A. Amenorrhea after discontinuing Oestrogen-progestogen oral contraceptives. *Br Med J* 1973;4:343–5.
148. Buttram VC, Vanderheyden JD, Besch PK, Acosta AA. Post "pill amenorrhea." *Int J Fertil* 1974;19:37–44.
149. Siegberg R, Nilsson CG, Stenman U-H, Widholm O. Sex hormone profiles in oligomenorrheic adolescent girls and the effect of oral contraceptives. *Fertil Steril* 1984;41:888–93.
150. Ober KP, Hennessy JF. Spironolactone therapy for hirsutism in hyperandrogenic women. *Ann Intern Med* 1978;89:643–4.
151. Boisselle A, Tremblay RR. New therapeutic approach to the hirsute patient. *Fertil Steril* 1979;32:276–9.
152. Shapiro G, Evron S. A novel use of spironolactone: treatment of hirsutism. *J Clin Endocrinol Metab* 1980;51:429–32.
153. Cumming DC, Yang JC, Rebar RW, Yen SSC. Treatment of hirsutism with spironolactone. *JAMA* 1982;247:1295–8.
154. Lobo RA, Shoupe D, Serafini P, Brinton D, Horton R. The effects of two doses of spironolactone on serum androgens and anagen hair in hirsute women. *Fertil Steril* 1985;43:200–5.
155. Ylostalo P, Heikkinen J, Kauppila A, Pakarinen A, Jarvinen PA. Low-dose spironolactone in the treatment of female hirsutism. *Int J Fertil* 1987;32:41–5.
156. Barth JH, Cherry CA, Wojnarowska F, Dawber RPR. Spironolactone is an effective and well tolerated systemic antiandrogen therapy for hirsute women. *J Clin Endocrinol Metab* 1989;68:966–70.
157. Taylor A, Pita JC, Santen R. Spironolactone and endocrine dysfunction. *Ann Intern Med* 1976;85:630–6.
158. Young RL, Goldzieher JW, Elkind-Hirsch K. The endocrine effects of spironolactone used as an antiandrogen. *Fertil Steril* 1987;48:223–8.
159. Serafini P, Lobo RA. The effects of spironolactone on adrenal steroidogenesis in hirsute women. *Fertil Steril* 1985;44:595–9.
160. Helfer EL, Miller JL, Rose LI. Side-effects of spironolactone therapy in the hirsute woman. *J Clin Endocrinol Metab* 1988;66:208–11.
161. Pittaway DE, Mazson WS, Wentz AC. Spironolactone in combination drug therapy for unresponsive hirsutism. *Fertil Steril* 1985;43:878–82.
162. Chapman MG, Dowsett M, Dewhurst CJ, Jeffcoate SL. Spironolactone in combination with an oral contraceptive: an alternative treatment for hirsutism. *Br J Obstet Gynecol* 1984;92:983–5.
163. Board JA, Rosenberg SM, Smeltzer JS. Spironolactone and estrogen-progestin therapy for hirsutism. *South Med J* 1987;80:483–6.
164. Emans SJ, Grace E, Woods ER, Mansfield J, Crigler Jr JF. Treatment with dexamethasone of androgen excess in adolescent patients. *J Pediatr* 1988;112:821–6.
165. Ettinger B, Goldfield B, Burrill K, von Werder K, Forsham M. Plasma testosterone stimulation-suppression dynamics in hirsute women. *Am J Med* 1973;54:195–200.
166. Steinberger E, Rodriguez-Rigau LJ, Smith KD. The prognostic value of acute adrenal suppression and stimulation tests in hyperandrogenic women. *Fertil Steril* 1982;37:187–92.
167. Abraham GE, Maroulis GB, Boyers SP, Buster JE, Magyar DM, Elsner WC. Dexamethasone

suppression test in the management of hyperandrogenized patients. *Obstet Gynecol* 1981;57: 158–65.

168. Casey JH, Burger HG, Kent JR, et al. Treatment of hirsutism by adrenal and ovarian suppression. *J Clin Endocrinol Metab* 1966; 26:1370–4.
169. de Oliveira RFC, Novaes LP, Lima MB, et al. A new treatment for hirsutism. *Ann Intern Med* 1975;83:817–9.
170. Belisle S, Love EJ. Clinical efficacy and safety of cyproterone acetate in severe hirsutism: results of a multicentered Canadian study. *Fertil Steril* 1986;46:1015–20.
171. Lissak A, Sorokin Y, Calderon I. Treatment of hirsutism with cimetidine: a prospective randomized controlled trial. *Fertil Steril* 1989; 41:247–50.
172. Adashi EY, Rock RA, Guzick D, Wentz AC, Jones GS, Jones Jr HW. Fertility following bilateral ovarian wedge resection: a critical analysis of 90 consecutive cases of the polycystic ovary syndrome. *Fertil Steril* 1981;36: 320–5.
173. Lunde O. Polycystic ovarian syndrome; a retrospective study of the therapeutic effect of ovarian wedge resection after unsuccessful treatment with clomiphene citrate. *Ann Chir Gynaecol* 1982;71:330–3.
174. Campo S, Garcea N, Caruso A, Siccardi. Effect of celioscopic ovarian resection in patients with polycystic ovaries. *Gynecol Obstet Invest* 1983;15:213–22.
175. Greenblatt E, Casper RF. Endocrine changes after laparoscopic ovarian cautery in polycystic ovarian syndrome. *Am J Obstet Gynecol* 1987;156:279–85.
176. Sumioki H, Utsunomyiya T, Matsuoka K, Korenaga M, Kadota T. The effect of laparoscopic multiple punch resection of the ovary on hypothalamo-pituitary axis in polycystic ovary syndrome. *Fertil Steril* 1988;50:567–72.
177. Sakata M, Tasaka K, Kurachi H, Terakawa N, Miyake A, Tanizawa O. Changes of bioactive luteinizing hormone after laparoscopic ovarian cautery in patients with polycystic ovarian syndrome. *Fertil Steril* 1990;53:610–3.
178. Hatch et al. *Am J Obstet Gynecol* 1981; 140:815–30.
179. Azziz R., Zacur HA, Parker CR, Jr., Bradley EL, Jr., Beets LR. Effect of obesity on the response to acute adreno-corticotropin (ACTH-[1-24]) stimulation in eumenorrheic women. *Fertil Steril* (in press).

Pediatric and Adolescent Gynecology,
edited by S. E. Carpenter and J. A. Rock.
Raven Press, Ltd., New York © 1992.

18

Pelvic Pain in Children and Adolescents

Sergio C. Stone

Department of Obstetrics and Gynecology, University of California–Irvine, Orange, California 92668

Pelvic pain is always a challenge to the gynecologist, especially the chronic, recurrent, intermittent type, that appears unrelated to a specific etiology. Conditions other than gynecological pathology may be involved and emotional or psychological components are difficult to rule out. In the persistent, recurrent or chronic type these conditions may play an important role. Usually, patients become increasingly frustrated and impatient and change doctors frequently.

In children and young adolescents, the challenge is even greater, though with the increased use of pelvic ultrasonography and the early use of diagnostic laparoscopy, a more precise diagnosis is possible in an increasing number of cases. Though in young women, lower abdominal pain is usually attributed to gynecological disorders first, there is a reluctance, on the part of most physicians (including some gynecologists), to obtain gynecological histories and perform gynecological examinations in younger patients, such as adolescents. This compounds the difficulty of dealing with this problem in this group of patients. On the other hand, in prepuberal children and infants, gynecological causes of pelvic or lower abdominal pain are rare, and these young individuals will usually consult pediatricians or emergency room facilities first.

I believe that it is useful and practical to separate acute from chronic pelvic pain when confronted by this complaint in our young patients, and we will review this subject in this manner.

Since the challenge of pelvic pain in young patients is in reaching an adequate diagnosis, we will devote most of this presentation to the diagnostic approach. The therapy becomes more conventional and standard, once the etiological factor of the pain is clear.

ACUTE PELVIC PAIN

Definition

We can arbitrarily define acute pelvic pain, as one that is <1 week old and has characteristics of an urgent or an emergency condition, either due to its intensity, its accompanying symptoms, or to the rapidly progressive nature of its form of presentation. Pain that is insidious in nature, slowly progressive over a prolonged or varied period of time and becomes suddenly acute, fulfills our definition.

Diagnosis

A careful *history* is of invaluable help, so in young patients, a calm and relaxed approach is most rewarding. The physician must have the time and the inclination to deal with such a patient. It is often difficult to relate to infants or young children in acute pain, especially in the presence, in most instances, of an anxious parent or close relative. In infants, parents can usually give an adequate history, though as previously stated, in this age group most cases will be seen first by a pediatrician or a pediatric surgeon.

Young children, can usually give precise information of the circumstances surrounding the onset of acute pain, its location, radiation and its course over the previous few days. The parents or guardian can complete the information and give their consent for further diagnostic and therapeutic steps.

Most cases of acute pain, in this young population consult an emergency service first and when the gynecologist is called, usually some type of initial evaluation has been done and a tentative diagnosis of a gynecological etiology has been made. Nevertheless, it is prudent not to simply rule out other non gynecological conditions, to avoid missing the correct diagnosis. The differential diagnosis especially in pubescent patients must include, besides pathology, the normal physiological events that surround menarche, such as primary dysmenorrhea and ovulatory pain. A differential diagnosis is presented in Table I. Since many of the etiologies of acute pelvic pain may require prompt intervention and even an emergency surgical approach, an adequate and complete work-up in the initial contact is essential. Also, gynecologists may occasionally be consulted during a surgical procedure, if unexpectedly gynecological, pathology is encountered by a pediatric or general surgeon.

In older individuals, especially after puberty, primary consultations with gynecologists become more frequent. If the patient is an adolescent, she may require some measure of confidentiality. It may be difficult to get an adequate gynecological-sexual history, that may give us the clue of the condition, in the presence of parents. Extreme delicate approach is required, and a proper balance, between the adolescent's right to privacy and the parents rights and duties is needed.

As it can be seen in Table 1, there is a long list of both gynecological and non gynecological conditions that can cause acute pelvic pain. The work-up must be directed towards those etiologies that may require acute intervention, and that are more common in each age group. If no clear etiology emerges, consultation is mandatory since, especially in infants, severe conditions are usually masked, are very difficult to diagnose, or may progress rapidly.

A practical evaluation of a patient with acute pelvic pain is presented in Table 2. Not all suggested steps are relevant to all cases. A judicious use of the history and physical examination should allow the physician to order the necessary tests to confirm the initial clinical suspicion. Age, clinical picture and severity of the symptoms should guide the physician to obtain only those tests that are pertinent to the patient's age and symptomatology. After an adequate and complete general *physical exam,* a decision must be made to perform a *gynecological examination.* The gynecological examination must be complete though considerations due to age are necessary. The vulva and perianal area must be inspected. In infants, one of the parents may hold her on his/her lap thus facilitating the exami-

TABLE 1. *Differential diagnosis of acute pelvic pain in children and adolescents*

Gynecological conditions
Physiological causes
1 or 2 dysmenorrhea
Functional follicular cysts
Ovulatory pain
Corpus luteum cyst
Gynecological pathology
Tumors neoplastic/nonneoplastic
True cysts, ruptures
Torsion of adnexa, cyst, tumor
Pregnancy: abortion, ectopic
Acute vaginitis: monilia
Congenital malformations
Pelvic inflammatory disease
Nongynecological pathology
Gastrointestinal
Appendicitis
Gastroenteritis
Crohn's disease
Volvulus
Intestinal obstruction
Urinary
Cystitis, urethritis
Pyelonephritis
Renal calculus
Trauma
Falls, accidents
Sexual molestation
Sports: hip, pelvic fractures, ligamentous-tendinous, musculoskeletal
Malignancies: bone metastasis
Psychological/emotional
Unknown

TABLE 2. *Diagnostic approach to pelvic pain in children and adolescents*

History
General health, allergies, medications
Menstrual, contraceptives, social-sexual
Recent activities
Pain: onset, nature, location, radiation fever, other symptoms related to menses, exercise, food intake
Physical
General exam
Abdominal exam
Pelvic, rectovaginal
Pelvic ultrasound
Laboratory
CBC, urinalysis, KUB, IVP, SMA-18, Sed Rate
Pregnancy test
Cultures: urine
Cervix: gonococcus, chlamydia, chlamydia antibodies (ELISA)
Laparoscopy
Diagnostic
Operative
Laparotomy
Therapeutic

nation. An otoscope can be most useful to visualize the vagina and cervix (1). Normal pelvic organs are usually not palpable in this age group. In older children it is necessary to explain the gynecological instruments and procedures, to obtain her confidence and approval. Preadolescents or adolescents should be given the opportunity to express their preference whether her parents should be present or not. If the patient is alone, a good opportunity arises to ask pertinent questions about sociosexual conduct, menstrual dates etc. An adequate menstrual, social, sexual and contraceptive history is important, especially in older adolescents that are in ever increasing numbers, sexually active at earlier stages of development. It may prove challenging to obtain an accurate history in these young individuals and the presence of her parents may inhibit a candid exchange of information. On the other hand, the presence of one of the parents may be invaluable, especially in the anxious, scared and uncooperative patient. Due to psychological, emotional, or sociocultural reasons, this is the most difficult area to evaluate in young patients with pelvic pain. In other acute etiologies of pain, such as appendicitis or renal calculi the physician does not encounter these especially difficult communication problems.

The laboratory should help to confirm the diagnosis, but in general has less value than an adequate exam and pelvic ultrasonography (Table 2).

Pelvic ultrasonography has become an excellent, reliable, noninvasive, and relatively inexpensive diagnostic tool, and has simplified enormously the diagnosis of pelvic pathology in a large number of conditions (2,3). We may even be close to the time at which ultrasound may replace the routine pelvic exam, except for the need for cultures or tissue sampling. It can certainly diagnose very precisely pelvic masses that are otherwise difficult to assess due to their small size or pain for example. Though we have limited experience on the diagnostic value of pelvic ultrasonography in children and adolescents with pelvic pain, based on our experience in adults, it is a very adequate, accurate, and rewarding method of diagnosis. It is especially useful in cases of ovarian cysts and tumors, tubal pregnancies, hemoperitoneum, torsion of adnexa, inguinal masses, etc. In cases of congenital gynecological abnormalities, such as hydrocolpos, hematocolpos, congenital uterine malformations, etc. it is also most useful. Another advantage is that now pelvic ultrasound is certainly readily available. More and more gynecologists use ultrasound diagnostic technology, either in their offices or in close cooperation with radiologists. Its use will certainly expand enormously over the next few years. In experienced hands, a negative pelvic ultrasound almost always rules out gynecological pathology. CAT scans and magnetic resonance imaging has not been used as widely and access to this technology is more restricted. Its usefulness, and due to cost, its right place in the diagnostic process for pelvic pain remains to be proven. Presently they should be used only as complimentary techniques (4).

If in a patient, all possible etiologies can either be ruled out or considered highly improbable, and the pain persists or becomes progressive, a *diagnostic laparoscopy* is the logical next step. The indications for a diagnostic laparoscopy are presented in Table 3. In very acute, severe difuse pelvic or abdominal pain, renal calculi should be ruled out by a urinalysis, KUB, and an IVP if necessary.

TABLE 3. *Indications for diagnostic laparoscopy in young patients with acute pelvic pain*

Unclear etiology
To rule out early ectopic pregnancy
Unimproved progressive pain after 24–48 hr of treatment
Recurrent acute severe pain
Progressive peritoneal signs, acute abdomen

The benefit/risk ratio favors a diagnostic laparoscopy in all properly indicated cases, even when considering the risk of anesthesia and the surgical cost (Table 3), since the consequences of missing a major diagnosis can be devastating. If the laparoscopy does not help the diagnosis, the exclusion of a gynecological or abdominal condition by itself is worth the admission of the patient to an outpatient surgical facility. Since the procedure may be more than diagnostic and the case may require an extensive surgical procedure, including surgical consultation, it may be best to use the outpatient department within a hospital, so that any major surgical procedure, if necessary can be readily performed.

In acute pelvic pain the laparoscopy can reveal no pathology in up to 30% of the cases, with the most common diagnosis being ovarian cysts and acute pelvic inflammatory disease (PID) (Table 4) (5,6).

It is also possible that in a minority, but still in a good number of patients, the etiology of an acute pelvic pain of short duration may remain unknown, and if no recurrence occurs, no cause will ever be found. Therefore, the gynecologist must prepare the patient and her family for this possible eventuality.

Selected Etiologies

Pelvic inflammatory disease (PID) plays an important etiological role in acute pelvic pain in adolescents and should be suspected in all sexually active patients. A direct relationship between early sexuality and the development of PID has been suggested (7). Since prompt treatment is essential to minimize the severe sequelae, such as chronic pelvic pain and infertility due to pelvic tubal disease, this etiology must be ruled out in all these patients.

After puberty, PID diagnosed by laparos-

TABLE 4. *Laparoscopic findings in adolescents with acute pelvic pain*

Finding	Rate
Ovarian cysts	30–40%
Acute PID	15–30%
Appendicitis	10%
Adnexal torsion	8%
Endometriosis	5%
Ectopic pregnancy	3%
Normal pelvis	15–30%

copy in sexually active adolescents does not seem related to age. It appears as frequent in the 11–13 age group than in the 16–17, (7) with an incidence of 15–20% of all laparoscopies performed for acute pelvic pain. The incidence of PID is related to the percentage of sexually active teens becoming similar to adults in the late teens. Most cases of overt, clear PID may not need a diagnostic laparoscopy, though the clinical diagnosis alone can be wrong in a good number of patients (8,9). If there is any doubt, the laparoscopy must be used to confirm the suspicion, to obtain adequate tubal-pelvic cultures and to initiate treatment.

Another area that requires very judicious approach, is the acute pelvic, vulvar, or vaginal pain associated with trauma (10–11). In all these cases potential physical or sexual abuse must be excluded. Due to the important medicolegal implications and potential liabilities attached to such a suspicion, and the need for reporting, physicians, especially if not adequately trained or experienced, must seek consultation and limit themselves to an accurate, objective, and precise description of the lesions. If sexual abuse is confirmed these patients and their families need adequate psychological support, counselling and long-term follow-up.

Vaginal infections in the very young, especially involving microorganisms known to be sexually transmitted, or the presence of herpes virus or papilloma virus lesions, have also been related to possible sexual abuse (12,13). Adequate cultures to document such type of infection is imperative in all cases. In the older post pubertal patient this type of infections may be related to early sexual activity and experimentation, and not to sexual abuse. The differentiation becomes a real challenge, and requires experience and expert assessment.

Either trauma or infection secondary to abuse may be very difficult to diagnose or differentiate (14). On the other hand, it is of interest to note that it has been estimated that, in up to 30% of sexually abused children, the physical examination detects no abnormalities (15). This underscores the need for referral if the gynecologist is not familiar with this type of situation.

A colposcope is useful to examine young patients with suspected sexual abuse (16). The most common findings are linear lacerations of the hymen, usually posteriorly. Lacerations of the thin vaginal mucosa, local bleeding and hematomas or ecchymosis can also be present. If severe bleeding is encountered injuries to the upper vagina, rectum or intra abdominal organs is possible. General anesthesia may be needed for an adequate diagnosis and surgical repair. Vaginal secretions should be collected for wet preparation to detect sperm or for cultures as needed.

Pregnancy should always be suspected in the sexually active adolescent (post puberal patient) and a pregnancy test is mandatory, even in patients that give a history of normal regular menses without a period of amenorrhea. This is especially true, if the pelvic-lower abdominal pain is accompanied by vaginal bleeding of any type.

Acute, intermittent, cyclic or recurrent pelvic pain can be ovulatory pain, primary dysmenorrhea, or some of the rare cases of congenital malformations, such as imperforate hymen, congenital absence of the cervix, etc. An adequate pelvic examination and an office ultrasound can adequately make the diagnosis, in most cases.

As more and more young females participate in competitive sports, pelvic pain could also be due to acute severe trauma or to repetitive microtrauma. Soft tissue injuries are usually caused by acute strains or due to the repetitive use of muscles and ligaments in this group of skeletally immature individuals. An adequate history and physical examination should direct the physician's attention away from gynecological conditions and to adequate consultation and referral. Referral is important, since some conditions, such as a hip fractures or dislocations, should be considered emergencies and could lead to complications and severe long term sequelae such as avascular necrosis, joint non union or malunion, potentially leading to deformity, and/or functional limitation. Fortunately, these conditions are rare and should be easy to rule out in the initial consultation.

Endometriosis is rare in the young adolescent but is much more frequent than most gynecologists recognize. It has been estimated that about 5% of all cases of endometriosis, occur in adolescents (5). Though most young patients with endometriosis are expected to have chronic symptoms, an occasional patient may well present herself with acute pain secondary to a ruptured or a leaking endometrioma or severe progressive dysmenorrhea.

In children and pre-puberal girls, acute pelvic pain of gynecological origin is rare. Ovarian cysts, adnexal torsion, infections occur only rarely. If an adnexal mass is diagnosed, a true tumor is likely, since other types of functional cysts do not generally develop in the absence of hypothalamic-pituitary maturation. In young children, pelvic ultrasound is especially valuable. Though the normal uterus and adnexa of the pre-puberal child is not palpable, pelvic ultrasound can easily demonstrate its presence and degree of normality. Thus, it can diagnose pelvic pathology, minimizing the limitations of a pelvic-rectal examination.

The torsion of the uterus or adnexa in prepuberal children is very rare and is usually confused with acute appendicitis. Much more frequent is the torsion of an ovarion cyst or tumor. Only about 20% of ovarian enlargement are nonneoplastic and unless there is a torsion, they are mainly asymptomatic until very advanced.

Psychological causes of acute pelvic pain are obviously rare but psychological factors may influence the young patient's perception of her pain or condition. They require adequate evaluation and treatment, especially if the suspected diagnosis is a physiological cause such as primary dysmenorrhea (Table 1). A short, precise but comprehensive explanation may be invaluable in gaining the young patient's attention and confidence. This may be important for her future treatment and subsequent interaction with the physician and the medical profession, as well as her perception of her condition.

Treatment

If an specific etiology is uncovered by our initial evaluation, specific therapy is obviously indicated. Nevertheless, the important number of patients without a clear etiology is a major challenge.

After this initial diagnostic approach, most conditions that can cause acute pelvic pain can be adequately evaluated and proper action can be taken, including surgical referrals for conditions such as acute appendix, bowel obstruction, etc. Most of the other medical or surgical conditions can be treated by the gynecologist, and except for considerations of size and weight, should be treated similarly as in older women. Special mention should be given to benign conditions such as ovarian cysts. If a surgical approach is necessary due to lack of response to medical treatment, the severity of the pain or the progressive nature of it, gynecologists and especially general surgeons, should pay special attention to the potential effects of the surgical procedure in the patient's future fertility. The most conservative surgical procedure is preferable and careful attention should be given to measures to minimize post-operative pelvic adhesions. A cystectomy is better than a oophorectomy; a wedge resection of the contralateral ovary may be unnecessary, "microsurgical" handling of the tissues is best. Laparoscopy is better than laparotomy and is the best choice in most cases. First, it is a diagnostic tool, second, with adequate experience and instruments it is possible to correct most benign gynecological conditions, and third preliminary observations demonstrate considerably less post operative adhesions then those observed after laparotomy. In addition, with the continuous improvement of fibroptics, the development of new micro instruments and lasers and video equipment, operative laparoscopy should allow for the adequate surgical correction of most acute gynecological conditions such as ovarian cysts, endometriosis, tubal pregnancies, etc.

In a few patients, the diagnosis may be questionable and a trial of therapy of the most likely cause with adequate observation is in order. Most authors recommend that in the presence of persistent acute pelvic or lower abdominal pain, a definitive diagnosis, followed by adequate therapy should be initiated within 24–48 hr after the initial consultation. If this is not possible, the case requires additional urgent evaluation and consultation with another specialist.

CHRONIC PELVIC PAIN

Definition

Pain in the lower abdomen and pelvis of 3–6 month duration is considered chronic in nature. Its origin is usually unprecise, and its progression difficult to follow. Patients frequently have a vague idea of pelvic discomfort that becomes increasingly persistent and progressive, requiring consultation.

Diagnosis

As in acute pelvic pain most causes of chronic pelvic pain in infants and children are not of gynecological origin, whereas in adolescents, especially in the older, sexually active individuals, is frequently associated with gynecological disorders. A review of the different etiologies and the relative incidence of each, gives an overall idea of how to organize the work-up based on the most common causes (Table 5).

The diagnostic approach in chronic pelvic pain, must also be organized along the lines presented in Table 2. A careful and detailed history and a complete physical examination, along the lines described above for patients with acute pelvic pain is necessary.

TABLE 5. *Differential diagnosis of chronic pelvic pain in children and adolescents*

- Gynecological conditions
  - Physiologic causes
    - Dysmenorrhea 1 and 2
    - Ovulatory pain
    - Recurrent ovarian cysts: follicular corpus luteum cyst
  - Gynecological pathology
    - Ovarian cyst
    - Ovarian tumor
    - Endometriosis
    - Congenital malformation
    - Pelvic inflammatory disease
    - Pelvic congestion-hyperemia
    - Peritoneal defects
    - Pelvic adhesions
    - Tubal pathology: hydrosalpinx
- Nongynecological pathology
  - Gastrointestinal
    - Constipation
    - Fecaliths
    - Bowel inflammation (crohn's disease), "dysfunction", diverticulitis
    - Dietary allergies
    - Irritable bowel
  - Urinary
    - Chronic urinary tract infection
    - Urinary tract strictures
    - Kidney disease
  - Trauma
    - Chronic injury 2 to sports
  - Orthopedic
    - Cordosis, scoliosis
    - Vertebral pathology
  - Somatic pathology
    - Neurogenic, myofascial
  - Psychological/emotional
    - Sexual abuse
    - Depression
    - Sexual dysfunction
  - Unknown

As in the adult women, the most frustrating feature is the non specific nature of most chronic pains that makes it very difficult to assess it properly. Nevertheless, its characteristics are important to determine its etiology: onset, location, radiation, duration and evolution, relation to bowel movements, voiding or food intake, effect of position and different activities, etc. Precise, detailed, and specific questions about the characteristics of the pain are necessary. In pubertal patients, the pain relation to the menstrual cycle may be important in determining its origin. If the adolescent is sexually active, a detailed sexual history and the relation of the pain to sexual activities is necessary.

The use of pelvic ultrasound is here as useful as in the case of acute pelvic pain. It should be used to rule out a large number of possible etiologies, such as ovarian masses or cysts. Again, if no adequate etiology is uncovered, a diagnostic laparoscopy should be the next step.

Though the literature in this area is scarce, several authors have reported on the laparoscopic findings in children and adolescent with chronic pelvic pain (6,17). It is difficult to compare series due to the differences in age groups and number of patients. Table 6 gives an idea of these findings, based on a review of several authors. The etiology of chronic pelvic pain in adolescents and young women is strikingly similar (18). This fact should certainly assist in the diagnosis of the correct cause of the persistent pain.

TABLE 6. *Laparoscopic findings in adolescents with chronic pelvic pain*

Finding	Rate
Normal pelvis	25–40%
Endometriosis	38–45%
Ovarian cyst	2–5%
Uterine malformations	5–8%
Post operative adhesions	4–13%
Pelvic inflammation	5–15%
Others	2%

Referral to a urologist and orthopedic surgeon is also indicated to rule out pathology related to these areas. Without an adequate, specialized examination, a gynecologist may miss a clear diagnosis in this area.

In long-standing, persistent cases, to explore all possibilities, a multidisciplinary approach may be needed. A comprehensive evaluation may require a team that may include one or more of the following: a gynecologist, an internist, a psychiatrist, an anesthesiologist, a gastroenterologist, a urologist, a orthopedist, and a psychologist. Such a team is usually found in a well established and organized "Pain Center or Clinic." For the diagnosis and management of the most difficult and persistent cases without a clear etiology, consultation or referral may be the right step.

Selected Etiologies

It is interesting to note that in these young individuals, endometriosis as a major finding not only has a high incidence, but that it is similar to that of endometriosis associated with pelvic pain in mature women (Table 6).

The incidence of endometriosis may actually be higher, if we include nontraditional or early lesions, that were not usually recognized as evidence of endometriosis in earlier published series. Most studies report typical endometrial lesions, such as retraction, fibrosis, powder burn lesions or endometriomas. Nevertheless, a careful visual inspection of the pelvic at laparoscopy, may show pigmented, vesicular, pale, cystic or hemorrhagic lesions, that have recently been associated with typical endometrial tissue by pathological examination. Therefore a very careful laparoscopic inspection of the pelvic organs seems well indicated in the absence of other obvious etiological factors. If these lesions are included, a good number of negative laparoscopies could be eliminated and a more pertinent treatment may be started. For all these reasons, a diagnostic laparoscopy is well indicated, despite the surgical and anesthesia risks and the cost involved.

The incidence of PID increases with the age and the sexual behavior of the patient. Furthermore, the incidence of PID appears to double in young women that start their sexual activity before age 16 (7). In the adult woman complaining of pain, PID has been found by laparoscopy in up to 30% of cases (17,18). The observation that, in up to another third, the laparoscopy reveals a normal pelvic, underscores the difficulty in making a clear etiological diagnosis. It also points to the need to look for other etiologies, including psychosocial and emotional.

In young children, gynecological cancers are only 2–3% of all malignancies of this age group and generally preclude chronic symptoms. A total of 70% of all ovarian masses in this age group are neoplastic with the other 30% being nonneoplastic. Germ cell tumors comprise 60% of all neoplastic tumors (19). Ovarian tumors are only 1% of all girl tumors but is the most common gynecological tumor, with 5% of all ovarian tumors occurring in adolescents, especially in the 10–14-year-old group (20).

In women with chronic pelvic pain of undetermined etiology, most reports reveal an alarmingly high rate in the incidence of previous abuse, including sexual abuse as children or adolescents (21,22). Therefore, it is important to explore this possible etiology if no other cause is uncovered. Adequate referral may be in order since most gynecologists are poorly trained to recognize and treat these conditions.

Others (23,24) have also found a high frequency of all types of somatic complaints, including pelvic pain, in victims of previous sexual abuse. Nevertheless, others have reported that the relationship between pelvic pain and previous abuse is stronger for children that have been physically abused only (25).

Rarely, pelvic pain can be caused by a bone malignancy. For instance, 20% of chrondrosarcomas in women 21 years old and younger are located in the pelvic bones (26).

A comprehensive evaluation may uncover a series of somatic or miofascial conditions, and even the effect of chronic injuries secondary to sports, that have precise and adequate treatments (27). Chronic somatic, myofascial, or neurogenic pain is an ill-defined condition, with vague symptoms, associated with menses, coitus, etc. The pain can be poorly localized, constant or intermittent or may be precise, sharp, and triggered by coitus or pelvic examinations. This type of pain is generally not caused by trauma, cysts, acute infection, bleeding, etc. They are due instead to visceral hypersensitivity or referral pain of different sources (27). The correct diagnosis requires careful and systematic examination of the pelvis and abdomen, looking for precise pain locations, trigger points, etc. Even the use of techniques, such as selected anesthetic blocks, may be required.

Dysmenorrhea, primary or secondary is also a common etiology of chronic pelvic pain (28). It is important to differenciate primary from secondary dysmenorrhea since the treatment is quite different. In primary dysmenorrhea, the pain is associated with ovulatory cycles, it's typical of a cramp in the suprapubic or sacral area, and it's short lived, coinciding with menses. In secondary dysmenorrhea, the pain is due to pathology: endometriosis, PID, ovarian cysts or tumors, adenomyosis, vaginal or cervical pathology, uterine polyps or myomas, etc.

Functional symptomatic ovarian cysts are frequent, usually producing mild discomfort or short lived acute pain. Rarely, they can be persistent and recurrent (29). These patients have a history of multiple laparoscopies or laparotomies and chronic ovarian suppression may be needed. After years of frustration and ineffectual treatments, the pain has an important psychological component. We see one or two patients a year in consultation for this type of chronic ovarian condition.

The role of adhesions, secondary to previous infection or surgery in chronic pelvic pain is obscure (30,31). In most cases, adhesions probably do not cause pelvic pain (32,33). Nevertheless, we have all seen cases in which adhesions under tension, pulling pelvic or abdominal organs together, produce very precise and localized pain that improves dramatically after laparoscopic transection.

Chronic pelvic pain has been recognized to have a large psychological component, either as a cause factor or as a consequence of the frustration, anxiety, and tension of a long-standing, poorly defined, and persistent condition. Therefore, an adequate psychological evaluation and a confidential sexual-social history is important. These patients are frequently depressed and depression is frequent in adolescents.

Finally, if no organic disease of any type is documented, and this can occur in up to 25% of all cases, the pain may be psychogenic in origin (34). The diagnosis and treatment is most difficult and adequate referral is best. First, all known causes of somatic pathology must be ruled out and second a multidisciplinary approach is best, including psychological testing. Pain of this type is a complex syndrome, that is related to other symptoms such as depression, sleep disorders, anxiety, hypochondriasis, etc.

Treatment

If our work-up, as detailed, uncovers the etiological factor, direct treatment of the cause of chronic pelvic pain can readily be made. Dysmenorrhea, PID, endometriosis, ovarian cysts, urinary problems, etc. can be managed in a routine manner. It is advisable to spend some time explaining the nature of the condition and reassure and counsel the patient, as needed, to alleviate the psychological component of chronic pelvic pain.

A laparoscopy is most valuable, since besides being diagnostic, as previously stated, it is often therapeutic, given the current advances in operative endoscopy.

It is important to rule out pelvic pathology such as endometriosis, that now can be easily treated at the time of laparoscopy by laser vaporization. Even an uterosacral ablation can be done laparoscopically if indicated and no other obvious disease is encountered, especially in the patient with typical primary dysmenorrhea, that responds poorly to analgesic therapy.

Before suggesting a laparoscopy a trial of treatments with analgesics, antiinflammatory agents, and even oral contraceptives may be indicated for a few months if no obvious pathology is found and the nature of the pain appears benign. Serial ultrasounds can be used to rule out the possible relationship of the pain to follicular cysts, ovulation or the formation of large corpus luteum cysts.

Surgical treatments that are recommended, that may or may not alleviate pelvic pain, are presented in Table 7. Most authors do not recommend surgical treatments unless there is clear organic pelvic pathology, in which case the treatment is usually successful. A good review has recently been published by Slocumb (35).

Non surgical treatment should be directed, if at all possible, to the etiological condition suspected. Avoidance of analgesics is important, since these patients may

TABLE 7. *Suggested surgical treatments for chronic pelvic pain*

Dilatation and curettage
Hysteroscopy-operative: synechiae
Laparoscopy-operative
Polyps
Lysis of adhesions
Ablation of endometriosis
Uterosacral transection ovarian cysts
Myomectomy
Uterine suspension
Closure of laceration of brood ligament
Hysterectomy
Presacral neurectomy

become rapidly addicted and resistant to most, requiring frequent and higher doses, including narcotics.

The treatment of psychogenic chronic pain may require behavior modification, hypnosis, biofeedback, and extensive psychiatric sessions (34). It is important that the patient is not left alone or with the impression that "all is in her head." The usefuless of the comprehensive approach of a well established pain center, is in these cases invaluable.

It is of interest to note that plasma endorphines appear not to be elevated in cases of pelvic pain (35). Therefore, peripheral pain may not be mediated by them, though a role in the central nervous system by some form of endorphines is still possible.

If everything is negative, these patients require careful and close follow-up. Patience and understanding is essential, to gain the patient's confidence and help them during this period of trial and errors. If with adequate counseling and psychological evaluation and treatment, there is no relief, referral to a specialized pain center, that is used to dealing with patients like this, may be the last resort. These centers are specialized in treating unspecific, chronic pain of various and complex etiologies, and can be of real help. The alternative, increasing doses of pain relief medications, not only does not work, but adds potential addiction to an already complex problem.

SUMMARY

Acute pelvic pain of gynecological origin is rare in prepuberal children and it is frequently a finding that requires a gynecological consult on an emergency basis. In adolescents, acute pelvic pain has an incidence similar to that of young women and its etiology is also similar. Conditions such as PID and endometriosis are surprisingly frequent and require early consideration. In sexually active teenagers, pregnancy and its complications, mainly abortion and ectopic pregnancy, must be considered. In chronic pelvic pain, neoplasms, endometriosis, and psychological problems related to prior negative experiences appear prominent in the differential diagnosis. The use of pelvic ultrasound and laparoscopy has helped tremendously in the diagnosis of this condition. The treatment of all etiologies of pelvic pain is similar to that of older women, except for considerations for age, weight and future fertility. In chronic pelvic pain, especially of uncertain etiology adequate consultation and referral is best, after ruling out gynecological pathology.

REFERENCES

1. Emans, SJ, Woods ER, Flagg NT, et al. Genital findings in sexually abused symptomatic and asymptomatic girls. *Pediatrics* 1987;79:778–86.
2. Haller HM. Ultrasonography in pediatrics gynecology. *J Ultrasound Med* 1984;3:509–15.
3. Sanfilippo JS, Lavery JR. The spectrum of ultrasound: antenatal to adolescent years. *Semin Reprod Endocrinol* 1988;6:45–53.
4. Council on Scientific Affairs. Report of the Panel on Magnetic Resonance Imaging. *JAMA* 1989;261:420–33.
5. Goldstein DP. Acute and chronic pelvic pain. *Pediatric Clin North Am* 1989;36:573–80.
6. Vercellini P, Fedele L, Arcaini L, Bianchi S, Rognoni MT, Candiani GB. Laparoscopy in the diagnosis of chronic pelvic pain in adolescent women. *J Reprod Med* 1989;34:827–30.
7. Ledegaard O, Helm P. Pelvic inflammatory disease: the influence of contraceptive, sexual and social life events. *Contraception* 1990;41: 475–83.
8. Allen LA, Schoon MG. Laparoscopic diagnosis of acute pelvic inflammatory disease. *Br J Obstet Gynecol* 1983;90:966–8.
9. Ledger WG. Laparoscopy in the diagnosis of acute pelvic inflammatory disease. *Am J Obstet Gynecol* 1984;148:235–40.
10. Huffman JW, Dewhurst CJ, Capraro VJ. Injuries to the genitalia during childhood. In: Huffman JW, Dewhurst CJ, Capraro VJ, eds. *The gynecology of childhood and adolescence*. Philadelphia: W.B. Saunders, 1981:213–24.
11. Russell DEH. The incidence and prevalence of intrafamiliar and extrafamiliar sexual abuse of female children. *Child Abuse Negl* 1983;7: 133–9.
12. Huffman J. Gynecologic infections during childhood and adolescence. In: Feigian R, ed. *Textbook of pediatric infectious diseases*. Philadelphia: W.B. Saunders, 1981.
13. De John AR, Weiss JC, Brent RL. Condyloma

acuminata in children. *Am J Dis Child* 1982; 136:704–9.
14. Ladson S, Johnson CF, Doty RE. Do physicians recognize sexual abuse? *Am J Dis Child* 1987; 141:411–7.
15. Muran D. Child sex abuse—genital findings in prepubertal girls: II. Comparison of colposcopic and unaided examination. *Am J Obstet Gynecol* 1989;160:333–8.
16. Woodin B, Hegar A. The use of the colposcope in the diagnosis of sexual abuse in the pediatric age group. *Child Abuse Negl* 1989;10:111–7.
17. Goldstein DP, de Cholnoky C, Emans SJ. Laparoscopy in the diagnosis and management of pelvic pain in adolescents. *J Reprod Med* 1980; 24:251–6.
18. Bakary CM, Gorodeski IG. The diagnostic value of laparoscopy in women with chronic pelvic pain. *Am Surgeon* 1987;53:672–4.
19. Golladay E, Mollit D. Ovarian masses in the child and adolescent. *South Med J* 1983;76: 954–61.
20. Kennedy AW. Ovarian neoplasm in childhood and adolescents. *Semin Reprod Endocrinol* 1988; 6:79–91.
21. Harrop-Griffiths J, Katon W, Walker E, Holen L, Russo J, Hickock L. The association between chronic pelvic pain, psychiatric diagnosis and childhood sexual abuse. *Obstet Gynecol* 1988; 71:589–94.
22. Haser J, Roos. Effects of spouse abuse and/ or sexual abuse in the development and maintenance of chronic pelvic pain in women. *Adv Pain Res Ther* 1985;9:889–95.
23. Browne A, Finkelhor D. Impact of child sexual abuse: a review of the research. *Psychol Bull* 1986;99:66–77.
24. Cunningham J, Pearce P. Childhood sexual abuse and medical complaints in adult women. *J Interpers Viol* 1988;3:131–44.
25. Rapkin AJ, Karnes LD, Darke LL, Stampler FM, Naliboff BD. History of physical and sexual abuse in women with chronic pelvic pain. *Obstet Gynecol* 1990;76:92–6.
26. Huuos AG, Marcove RC. Chondrosarcoma in the young. *Am J Surg Pathol* 1987;11:930–42.
27. Slocumb JC. Chronic somatic, myofascial, and neurogenic abdominal pelvic pain. *Clin Obstet Gynecol* 1990;33:145–53.
28. Dawood MY. Dysmenorrhea. *Clin Obstet Gynecol* 1990;33:168–78.
29. Stone SC, Swartz WJ. A syndrome characterized by recurrent symptomatic functional ovarian cysts in young women. *Am J Obstet Gynecol* 1979;134:310–4.
30. Molinak LR. Operative management of pelvic pain. *Clin Obstet Gynecol* 1989;23:191–210.
31. Krisch AJ, Seifer OB, Sacks LB, Barrese I. Laparoscopy in 100 women with chronic pelvic pain. *Obstet Gynecol* 1984;64:672–8.
32. Chan CLK, Wood C. Pelvic adhesiolysis: the assessment of symptom relief by 100 patients. *Aust NZ Obstet Gynecol* 1985;25:295–301.
33. Rapkin AJ. Adhesions and pelvic pain: a retrospective study. *Obstet Gynecol* 1986;68:13–5.
34. Wood DP, Weisner MG, Reiter RC. Psychogenic chronic pelvic pain: diagnosis and management. *Clin Obstet Gynecol* 1990;33:179–95.
35. Slocumb YC. Operative management of chronic abdominal pelvic pain. *Clin Obstet Gynecol* 1990;196–204.
36. Benett TL, Pearson JW, Frederickson RCA. Plasma endorphin-like immunoreactivity in pelvic and abdominal pain. *Pain* 1986;24:41–8.

Pediatric and Adolescent Gynecology, edited by S. E. Carpenter and J. A. Rock. Raven Press, Ltd., New York © 1992.

19

Sexually Transmitted Disease

Jean Anderson

Department of Gynecology and Obstetrics, The Johns Hopkins Hospital, Baltimore, Maryland 21205

The epidemic of sexually transmitted diseases (STDs) currently sweeping the U.S. has special implications for adolescents. Adolescents who are sexually active have the highest age specific rates of STD's (1). Furthermore, the long-term sequelae of certain infections, particularly those involving fertility, are an especially heavy burden in the adolescent female at the beginning of her reproductive life. The increasing occurrence of human immunodeficiency virus (HIV) infection in this population raises the stakes considerably.

PHYSIOLOGIC SUSCEPTIBILITY

Although the clinical manifestations of STD's are similar between adolescents and adults, adolescents have some physiologic characteristics that may make them more susceptible to certain infections if sexually active.

Against the background of earlier sexual maturation, as evidenced by decreasing age of menarche over the past century (2), up to 15% of women are still having anovulatory cycles 6 years after menarche (3). The absence of progesterone with these cycles appears to prolong the time period when cervical mucus is most permeable (4,5); therefore, motile or sperm-born organisms may be more likely to ascend and cause upper tract infection in these women. This may partially explain the fact that a more virulent phenotype of *N. gonorrhea* is more commonly isolated from the cervices of younger women than adults; a less virulent phenotype tends to be found more abundantly in the progesterone-dominant luteal phase in ovulatory cycles (6).

Cervical ectopy is a characteristic of early puberty, with extension of columnar epithelium from the endocervical canal onto the vaginal surface of the cervix. Columnar epithelium is particularly vulnerable to infection with the gonococcus and chlamydia (1). In young adolescent girls, therefore, there is a greater surface area favorable for colonization with these pathogens. With age, metaplastic transformation takes place, and the transformation zone is formed, with less vulnerable multilayered squamous epithelium replacing the fragile single layer of columnar epithelium.

The presence and/or role of age-specific immune mechanisms is currently unknown.

SEXUAL BEHAVIOR

The past two decades have seen an increasing proportion of adolescents who are sexually active and at younger ages. Zelnik and Cantner (7) reported that the percentage of 15–19-year-old women who had been sexually active increased from 30.4% in 1971 to 49.8% in 1979. In 1988, 53% of 15–19-year-old women were sexually experienced. Although black women initiate intercourse an average of 1 year earlier than white women and a greater proportion of black adolescents are sexually active than whites or Hispanics, the greatest rate of increase in sexual activity has been in white teenagers (7,7a,7b) (Fig. 1). The average age at first intercourse is now 16 (8).

Although the frequency of intercourse in adolescent females is significantly lower than in adult women, their sexual partners tend to be males 2–3 years older than themselves. In fact, more than 50% of male sexual partners of adolescent females were at least 20 years old in 1976 (9). Furthermore, 58% of 15–19-year-old sexually active females have had more than one partner (7,7a,7b).

There seem to be two primary patterns of sexual activity in adolescents: (a) serial monogamy—one sexual relationship at a time, often with deep emotional attachments—is the first. However, there is data to suggest that perceptions of the strength of the relationship in heterosexual couples vary dramatically between males and females, with women more likely to perceive the relationship as strong (10). This, coupled with the fact that relationships are initiated at an age when individuals are psychologically unable to make a stable commitment, explains why these relationships are generally short lived. Over one half of adolescent females fit into this pattern of sexual behavior (9).

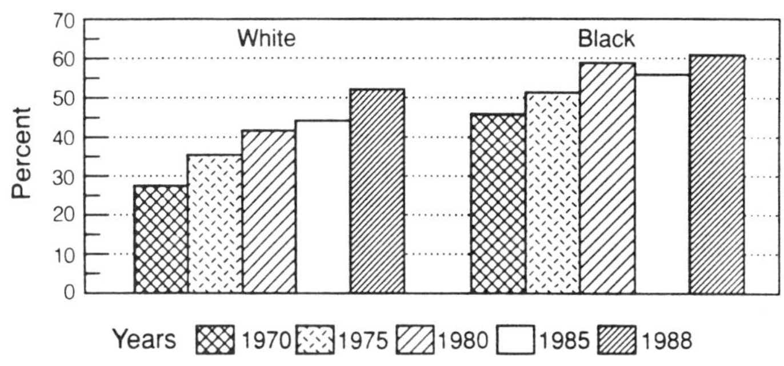

Source: Centers for Disease Control. Premarital sexual experience among adolescent women, United States, 1970-1988. *MMWR* 1991;39:929-932.

FIG. 1. Premarital sexual intercourse among women aged 15–19 years by race in the U.S., 1970–1988.

(b) Sexual adventures—multiple concurrent sexual partners and/or single sexual relationships in rapid sequence—is the second pattern. Approximately 13% of adolescent sexually active women fit into this classification (11).

Contraceptive use also affects risk of infection. In 1982, 15% of sexually active adolescent teens reported that they had never used contraception, and 40% reported inconsistent use. At their last episode of intercourse, 62% reported oral contraceptive use, 22% used condoms, and 6% used the diaphragm (12). In a 1988 survey of 17–19-year-old urban males, condom usage at the most recent intercourse had increased to 58%, most likely reflecting the intensive educational efforts in the wake of the HIV epidemic (12a). However, similar information from 15–19-year-old women that year found that only 17% used condoms (12b). A high pregnancy rate, even among those using contraception, emphasizes the frequency of inconsistent or incorrect usage. It has also been found that the frequency with which contraception is used varies inversely with the level of emotional commitment to the relationship (10). Sexual encounters that are more casual (and with possibly higher risk for transmission of infection) are less likely to be associated with use of contraceptive methods that might be protective against acquisition of infection.

These behaviors are partially explained by the unique place in which adolescents find themselves in terms of both physical and psychosocial development. Adolescence is a time of rapid physical growth and maturation, often outstripping cognitive and social development. Because of the nature of these changes, along with their rapidity and differing time rates, adolescence is a time of marked psychologic stress. During adolescence, there is increasing mobility and independence from parents, and greater identification with peers. Adolescents tend to associate with peers whose values and behavior are similar to what is learned and observed within their own family (13,14). However, peer pressure can be especially significant when the home environment lacks clearly expressed values or exhibits values that are inflexible and authoritarian, or when behavior at home is inconsistent (15). Adolescents also often have a sense of being invulnerable, believing that bad things will not happen to them or will be easily fixed, and thus they may be unable to fully comprehend the consequences of their actions (15). The psychic turmoil of adolescence contributes to frequent discrepancies between beliefs (or attitudes) and behavior. Zabin et al. (10) in a study of 3,500 inner city junior and senior high school students found that 83% of those who had been sexually active cited the best age for first intercourse older than the age at which they themselves initiated intercourse; furthermore, 43% stated a best age for first intercourse older than their current age.

Behavior is also affected by the cultural setting. Geography, ethnicity, and social class all affect behavior. In certain populations, early sexual activity and childbearing are both accepted and expected (16). In cultures where machismo has a strong influence, condom usage is less accepted (17).

Finally, the changes in sexual behavior documented over the past several decades must be seen against the background of increasing urbanization, changing sexual mores, and intensive media bombardment with often explicit sexual content. From 1963 to 1975, the percentage of U.S. adults accepting premarital intercourse increased from approximately 20% to 70% (18). By the time the average American teenager has finished high school, it is estimated that he or she will have spent 15,000 hours watching television and only 12,000 in formal classroom instruction. It is not surprising that teens rank television as first or second as a source of information about sex (19,20).

Incarcerated youths, runaways (many of whom wind up in prostitution), and youths who are victims of sexual assault or abuse stitute groups at particularly high risk for sexually transmitted diseases (15,21).

USE OF AND ACCESS TO HEALTH CARE

A final factor that impacts on the adolescent's risk for a sexually transmitted disease involves issues surrounding use of and access to care. The cost of health care and contraceptives, concerns about confidentiality, spoken or unspoken judgmental attitudes from health care providers, and feelings of embarrassment and shame often conspire to prevent adequate health care delivery to adolescents (15).

A large of survey of Canadian adolescents showed that 70% were interested in discussing STD's; however, discussions actually occurred with physicians only 18% of the time (22). Half of the females suggested that the physician initiate these discussions, since adolescents may be too shy to do so themselves. Education about sexuality, contraception, and STD's necessitates use of easily understood and clearly defined terms, including current slang. Questioning should be direct, sensitive, and nonjudgmental. Confidentiality is a critical issue for adolescents. Parental consent is not required for evaluation and treatment of STD's in any state (23); nevertheless, the goal of the health care provider should be to aid adolescents in communicating with their parents and enlisting the parents' support for the adolescent. The severity of the infection, the need of the teenager for adult assistance to receive adequate medical care, and the developmental maturity of the adolescent all impact on decisions about confidentiality. Once an infection is diagnosed, compliance with prescribed treatment can be poor in adolescents and seems to vary with the nature of the illness and the clinical setting (24). Special considerations regarding metabolism or effectiveness of drugs used to treat STD's in adolescents have not been defined. Single-dose or short-course regimens may be especially desirable in this age group (1).

VIRAL INFECTIONS

HIV

Epidemiology

Adolescents aged 13–21 years currently account for 1.2% of the total number of acquired immune deficiency syndrome (AIDS) cases in the U.S. (25). Not only are the numbers increasing, but there is evolving awareness that the majority of young adults with AIDS were infected as adolescents (26,27). The factors noted at the beginning of this chapter resulting in increased risk for other STD's apply to HIV infection as well. In addition, experimentation with drugs is worse in urban areas hardest hit by HIV disease. In 1986, approximately 10% of high school seniors had used cocaine within the last year, according to a national survey (28). Cocaine may be used intravenously or with other parenteral drugs or alcohol; however, even in the absence of intravenous drug use, there is increased risk for HIV infection in those using cocaine and other drugs of abuse, probably secondary to exchange of sex for money or drugs and disinhibited sexual behavior when "high" (29–31). In large urban areas with the highest HIV prevalence, greater than 50% of the intravenous drug using population may be HIV positive (32). For adolescents involved in drug use, that population may constitute the pool from which the majority of their sexual partners come, forming another link in their chain of risk.

Fourteen percent of adolescents with AIDS are female versus approximately 11% of adult cases (27,33). Forty-six percent of AIDS cases in adolescent females are felt secondary to heterosexual transmission

(27) (Fig. 2). Statistics concerning women who are HIV-infected but not yet necessarily AIDS-defined are even more revealing. In a recent report, Quinn et al. (34) found that almost three-quarters of HIV-positive women under the age of 25 attending the Baltimore City STD Clinics denied recognized risk factors (34). Presumably, a large proportion of these women acquired their infection heterosexually. Ethnic and racial minorities make up 53% of adolescent AIDS cases (35).

The number of adolescents who are infected with HIV but not yet AIDS defined is unknown, but without doubt is much larger than those already carrying a diagnosis of AIDS. Furthermore, the proportion of women seems to be even higher among these HIV-infected adolescents than among those with full-blown AIDS. In Essex, New Jersey, HIV-infected women actually outnumbered men (36). In a study of high-risk homeless and runaway youths at Covenant House in New York City, the HIV seroprevalence was 7% in 1,500 teenagers (37). Prevalence rates are greater than 1% in large urban areas with the greatest numbers of HIV-infected individuals, such as New York, Newark, San Francisco, and Washington, D.C. (37).

Clinical Presentation

Because of the long latency period of HIV, most adolescents will not develop AIDS, and the majority may be asymptomatic. Over 50% of individuals infected with HIV have an acute mononucleosis-like syndrome associated with seroconversion for HIV antibody (38). This acute episode resolves spontaneously, and the individual becomes asymptomatic. The immune system may remain healthy with normal function for many years. Ultimately, however, the majority and perhaps all of those who are HIV infected become progressively immunocompromised and eventually symptomatic. Symptoms and signs at this stage of illness often include lymphadenopathy, chronic and/or recurrent mucocutaneous candidiasis (including vaginal), and recurrent atypical herpetic infection (39). Ultimately, AIDS is diagnosed when the indi-

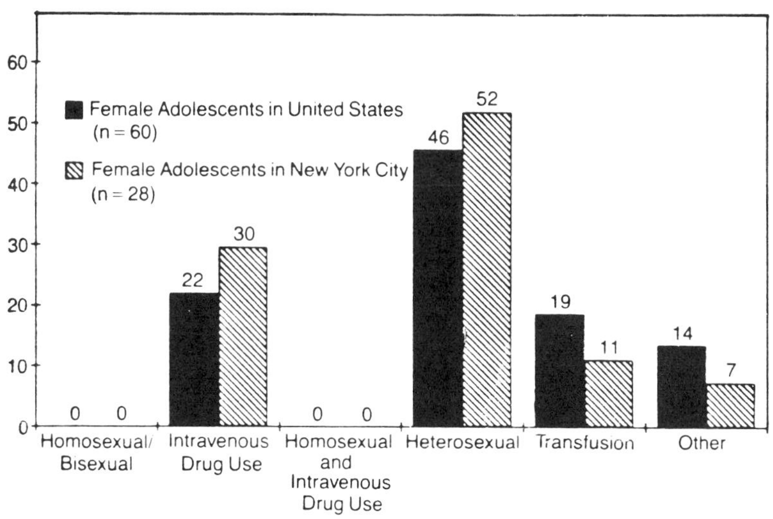

FIG. 2. Transmission profile for female adolescents aged 13–21 years with acquired immunodeficiency syndrome in New York City, and the United States *excluding* New York City.

vidual develops an indicator opportunistic infection or AIDS-associated malignancy. The most common AIDS defining illness is Pneumocystis pneumonia; Kaposi's sarcoma, extremely common in infected male homosexuals, is very rare in HIV-infected women (40).

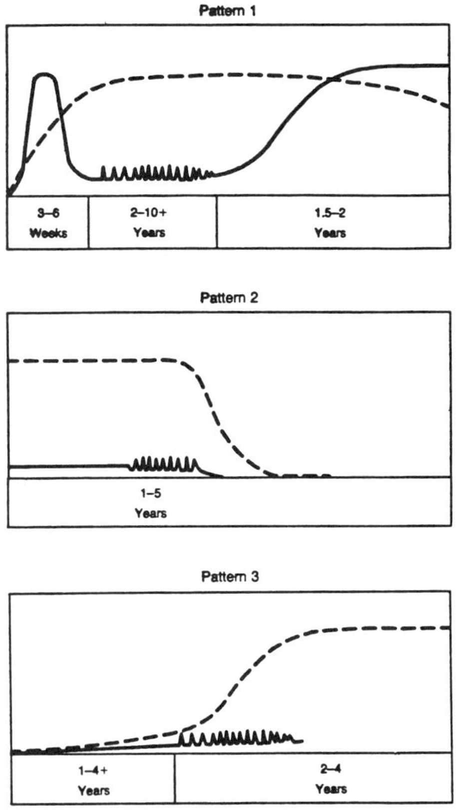

FIG. 3. Three patterns of HIV infection. The unbroken lines denote levels of viral protein (p24), and the broken lines antiviral antibodies. The duration of each phase of the infection is indicated.

Diagnosis

The diagnosis of HIV-1 infection can be made by a variety of serologic and virologic techniques developed during the 1980s. Use of diagnostic tests need to take into consideration the natural course of HIV infection and antibody formation. The characteristic pattern of viremia and antibody response is illustrated in Fig. 3A (41). Two unusual patterns have also been described (Fig. 3B and 3C) (42).

The enzyme-linked immunosorbent assay (ELISA) is the most widely used serologic test for HIV antibody detection. Individuals who are reactive by ELISA should be retested for HIV antibody with a confirmatory assay, most commonly the Western Blot. This assay utilizes essentially the same principle as the ELISA, but has the advantage of identifying antibodies specific for different HIV viral antigens. It yields a profile of viral bands characteristic of HIV when incubated with antibody positive serum. The definition of a "positive" Western Blot is somewhat arbitrary and is not uniform throughout the U.S. Nevertheless, with utilization of this sequence of tests, sensitivity is greater than 99% and specificity is greater than 99.9% (41).

Concern that serologic techniques may miss cases of HIV infection during the period before antibody formation has taken place has led to the development of assays that actually detect the antigens and nucleic acids of the virus. P-24 is an HIV core antigen that is detectable soon after infection. It usually disappears as antibody titers rise and reappears later in the course of the disease as viral antigenemia exceeds antibody production (43). HIV can be cultured from almost all patients with AIDS and from 80–90% of seropositive individuals (43). Culture is not used for routine diagnosis of HIV because of its cost and complexity. The most promising technique in the diagnosis of HIV infection currently is polymerase chain reaction (PCR). PCR amplifies HIV nucleic acid by repetitive DNA synthesis to levels that can be easily detected by DNA hybridization. PCR is positive in almost all seropositive adult patients and can detect HIV infection prior to sero conversion (44–46). This technique has not yet been fully standardized. There have been some reported problems with specificity; furthermore, it is technically complex and demanding. However, it holds much promise and is rapidly becoming much more than a research tool.

Treatment

Follow-up of the HIV-infected individual requires a comprehensive and multidisciplinary approach. Individuals with HIV have a high prevalence of other sexually transmitted infections and should be screened for these regularly if they remain sexually active. Vaginal candidiasis, genital herpes, HPV infection, and squamous intraepithelial lesions all appear to be increased in incidence in this population (47–52). Serial CD-4 cell counts are followed as indicators of immune function and markers of progression. Antiviral therapy with azidothymidine (AZT) is indicated when CD-4 counts drop below 200 and/or in those who are AIDS-defined (39). Recent data suggests that individuals with CD-4 counts between 200 and 500 and who are still asymptomatic also benefit from AZT (53). Persons with HIV infection are also frequently treated with aerosolized Pentamidine or Bactrim to prevent initial or recurrent episodes of Pneumocystis. Median survival once a diagnosis of AIDS is made has been approximately 2 years (54).

Human Papilloma Virus

Epidemiology

Human papilloma virus (HPV) infection of the genital tract is currently the most common viral sexually transmitted disease in the U.S., with an estimated minimum incidence of 1–2 million cases per year (55). Utilizing DNA hybridization techniques for diagnosis, reported prevalence in adolescent populations ranges from 13% to 38% (56,57). Rosenfeld et al. (57) compared 71 teenagers aged 13–18 with multiple lifetime sexual partners and 74 teenagers in the same age group with only lifetime sexual partner using cervicovaginal lavage for cell collection and Southern Blot DNA hybridization; HPV prevalence was 54% and 34%, respectively.

Clinical Presentation

Of the over 60 distinct HPV types that have been identified using DNA hybridization techniques, at least 25 have been found to infect the lower genital tract; these infections may be symptomatic and clinically apparent or, more commonly, asymptomatic and invisible to gross inspection. A recent study indicates that HPV infection is multicentric in over 80% of cases (58). Different sites may be infected with more than one virus type (59). HPV is the etiologic agent for genital warts, or condyloma accuminata (Fig. 4). These are usually asymptomatic unless superinfected but can cause great concern and embarrassment by their presence. Rarely, HPV infection may be transmitted during delivery to a newborn infant resulting in laryngeal papillomatosis.

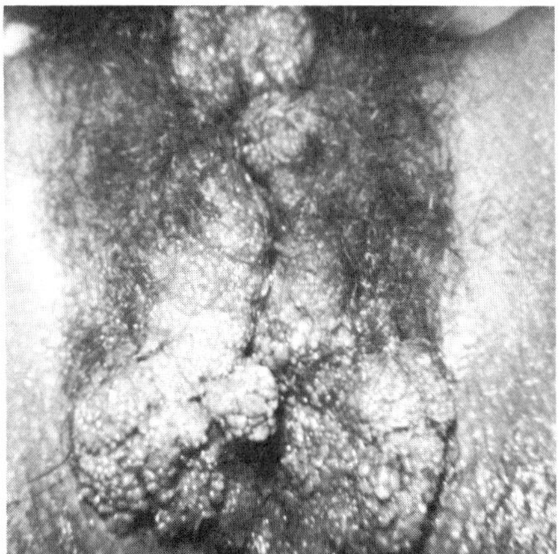

FIG. 4. The condyloma accuminata of human papilloma virus infection.

Natural History

Evidence from prospective follow-up of women infected with HPV and from a correlation of histopathologic evaluation with nucleic acid hybridization data from neoplastic lesions clearly and consistently point to an association, most probably etiologic, between HPV and lower genital tract neoplasia, both intraepithelial and invasive (60,61). Approximately 80–90% of squamous intraepithelial lesions (SIL), as well as invasive cervical cancers, have detectable HPV DNA, and in one recent study, 71% of cases of vulvar neoplasia were associated with HPV (59,62,63). Viral types 16 and 18 have been associated with higher rates of progression or recurrence after treatment, and with more severe disease (59,64–66).

There are few prospective follow-up studies of women with HPV infection. In the largest study, with a mean follow-up of 20 months in 418 women with cervical HPV infection, 24% regressed, 55% persisted, and 21% exhibited progression (67). It is likely that progression of HPV-induced lesions to malignancy requires a cofactor(s). Suggested cofactors thought to possibly influence the natural history of HPV infection include herpes simplex virus or other STDs, cigarette smoking, and immunosuppression (68,69).

Diagnosis

One of the major problems with epidemiologic studies of HPV infection has been the use of relatively insensitive methods for diagnosing the presence of human papilloma virus. Diagnosis of HPV infection may be made on physical examination if the lesion is clinically apparent; however, subclinical infection has been recognized with cytology, colposcopy, histopathology, and more directly and sensitively with DNA hybridization. McNicol (59), in a study of 98 women with cervical intraepithelial neoplasia (CIN), found HPV DNA in 81%, with evidence of HPV infection cytologically and colposcopically in only 31% and 35%, respectively. Southern Blot is considered to be the most sensitive and specific DNA hybridization strategy to detect HPV (70,71). Apart from the use of appropriate diagnostic strategies, adequate cell samples must be obtained in order to draw valid conclusions. In most published studies, cellular material has been collected by ectocervical scrape and an endocervical swab with cotton tip applicator or cytobrush. In recent work reported by Vermund (72), cervicovaginal lavage (CVL) with saline proved superior to cervical scrape/endocervical swab or brush in the amount of cellular material obtained and sensitivity in detecting HPV.

HPV infection and HPV-associated neoplasia of the anogenital tract occur much more frequently in immunodeficient patients—particularly those with defects in cell-mediated immunity—than in the general population. Furthermore, HPV infection and neoplasia in these patients tend to have an accelerated clinical course, are more extensive in area, and recur more frequently, paralleling the severity of immunosuppression (73,74).

Treatment

There is currently no available therapy to affectively eradicate the presence of HPV in the lower genital tract. When grossly visible evidence of the infection is present, the most frequent therapeutic approach is local treatment with chemicals such as Podophyllin and trichloroacetic acid (TCA). Repetitive applications are usually required, and these treatments are generally unsuccessful with bulky disease and in immunocompromised patients. Solutions of 25–85% TCA may be the preferred local treatment, with reapplication recommended three times a week to every 10 days (75). TCA produces less local irritation than Podophyllin, does not need to be washed off, can be used during pregnancy and in highly vascularized tissue, and appears to have greater effectiveness.

Cryotherapy and cautery are effective methods of treating visible warts, with reported cure rates of 63% and 90%, respectively (76). The carbon dioxide laser appears to be the most effective method of treating genital warts, though well-controlled studies are lacking. Reported success rates are as high as 95% (77). The external genitalia, perianal region, vagina, and cervix can be treated concurrently. Urethroscopy and anoscopy, which can be easily performed at the time of laser therapy, is helpful to rule out disease in these areas, especially in patients with extensive lower genital tract involvement. Laser therapy is expensive and usually requires general anesthesia; however, it is the treatment of choice in patients with extensive condylomata or HPV disease that has been refractory to other therapy.

Topical 5-fluorouracil (5-FU) in a 5% cream has been used for the treatment of HPV infections, although it has not been approved by the U.S. Food and Drug Administration for this indication. 5-FU has the theoretical benefit of controlling the reservoir of latent virus. It has been felt to be especially useful in vaginal and urethral condylomata, as prophylaxis in immunocompromised patients, and as an adjunctive measures with surgical treatment. It is contraindicated in pregnancy, and if incorrectly applied may produce an extensive erosive dermatitis. Toxic effects from absorption of 5-FU (i.e., bone marrow suppression or gastrointestinal effects) have not been a clinical problem (75).

Interferon injected intralesionally or intramuscularly has been used for the treatment of HPV infections as part of research protocols for approximately 10 years. An intralesional form is now commercially available. Disadvantages of this form of treatment include flu-like side effects, requirement for multiple injections, and unknown effects on a fetus or on reproductive capacity. It appears to have only moderate efficacy in eliminating genital warts, and its safety has not been established in patients younger than 18 years of age (75).

It should be emphasized that none of the aforementioned methods, despite their frequent efficacy in eliminating gross disease, have been shown to eradicate the presence of HPV. Recurrences are frequent, and the patient should still be considered at increased risk for lower genital tract neoplasia. It is the author's practice to perform colposcopy of the cervix, vagina, and vulva on all patients with physical or cytologic evidence of HPV infection. Colposcopically directed biopsies should be obtained when indicated. Sexual partners should be evaluated as well, and if treatment is given, it should be given to both concurrently. Because of the association with lower genital tract neoplasia, it is appropriate to recommend at least twice yearly pap smears in women with HPV infection who have no cytologic or histologic evidence of SIL. Treatment of HPV infection in the absence of grossly visible disease, other symptomatology, or evidence of intraepithelial neoplasia is probably futile. Patients should be informed about the possibility of transmitting infection to their sexual partners, and condom usage should be encouraged.

Herpes Simplex Virus

Epidemiology

Over the past two decades, genital herpes infections have increased in prevalence in many population groups. In the U.S., there are no nationwide statistics available since genital herpes is not a reportable disease. Various epidemiologic surveys have been performed; however, reported prevalence figures depend on whether clinical, culture, or serologic techniques are used for diagnosis.

Herpes simplex virus (HSV) transmission generally occurs through close contact with an individual shedding virus at a peripheral site or mucosal surface or secretion. The virus is then inoculated on to susceptible mucosal surfaces or through small skin abrasions. At the time of initial infection, the virus ascends peripheral nerves and establishes latency in sensory or autonomatic nerve root ganglia. HSV-II is the most common cause of genital herpes, though 5–15% of first episodes are with HSV-I (78).

Clinical Presentation

Clinical manifestations of genital herpes vary with viral type and host factors such as previous episodes or evidence of past exposure to HSV-I or HSV-II. Retrospective studies suggest that up to 50–70% of HSV-II infections are asymptomatic; more recent prospective studies, however, indicate that most first infections are symptomatic, though often mild (78,79).

Over 50% of women with primary genital HSV-II infection (no serologic evidence of past HSV-I or HSV-II infection) have constitutional symptoms with fever, headache, malaise, and myalgias. These symptoms appear early in the course of disease, peak within 3–4 days after the onset of lesions and gradually recede over a subsequent 3–4 days. The classic hallmark signs of primary herpes are widespread painful lesions on the external genitalia. Beginning as papules or vesicles, these lesions become pustular and then ulcerate, eventually healing with crusting and reepithelization without residual scarring (Fig. 5). Duration of viral shedding is approximately 12 days. Other common local symptoms include itching, dysuria, vaginal or urethral discharge, and tender inguinal adenopathy (78). Concomitant HSV cervicitis occurs in 70–90% of those experiencing primary infection (80,81). Complications of primary genital herpes infection occur more commonly in women and include central nervous system involvement, pharyngitis, and extragenital lesions (78,80).

Patients with first-episode but nonprimary infection with HSV (serologic evidence of past HSV-I or HSV-II infection) are less likely to have systemic symptoms, and tend to have milder and shorter duration of local signs and symptoms than persons with true primary infection.

Recurrent genital herpes is characterized by signs and symptoms localized to the genital region, usually unilaterally. Approximately 50% of persons develop prodromal symptoms before the appearance of lesions (78); these range from mild tingling, to lancinating pains in the buttocks or hips. Symptoms are milder as compared to primary infection, and mean duration of lesions is 9–10 days with viral shedding lasting about 4 days from onset of lesions. Some 10–30% of women have concomitant HSV cervicitis (82). Recurrence rate depends on viral type, severity of initial episode, and host immune response (83,84). Ninety percent of patients recur in the first year after primary episode with HSV-II,

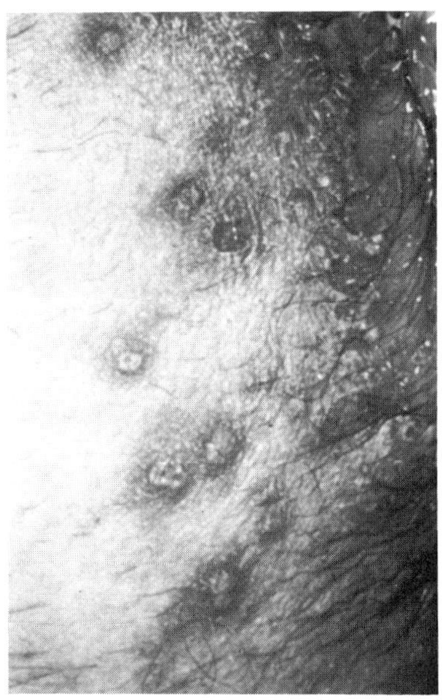

FIG. 5. Vulvar papules and ulcers associated with herpes simplex infection.

versus 60% who have primary HSV-I infection (78,83,80). Patients who develop higher titers of HSV-II neutralizing antibody in convalescent sera are also more likely to recur than those who do not develop neutralizing antibodies (83). Recurrence rate varies between individuals and within a given individual over time.

Immunocompromised individuals, including those with HIV infection, often have more atypical, more frequent, and more prolonged genital herpetic outbreaks. As immune function diminishes, recurrent episodes are likely to have characteristics more similar to primary infection, with systemic symptoms and widespread lesions (49,85). Furthermore, several studies have shown that genital ulcerations, including those secondary to HSV, constitute a risk factor for the acquisition of HIV (86,87).

A major concern in pregnant women with HSV infection is the possibility of transmission to the fetus or neonate. Neonatal herpes, though rare (1 out of 3,000 to 1 out of 20,000 live births) is a disease of high morbidity and mortality (88). Primary genital herpes appears to carry much higher risks (20–50% in several small series) (88,89) of perinatal transmission than recurrent disease (0–8%) (90,91). Greater than 70% of infants with neonatal herpes infections were born to mothers without signs or symptoms at delivery (88,92). Transplacental transmission may occur with primary infection, but most neonatal herpes infection is acquired by contact with the infected maternal genital tract during the intrapartum period. Therefore, women who have clinical evidence of infection or prodromal symptoms at the time of labor should be delivered by Caesarean section. Patients with a history of HSV infection, but without signs or symptoms of HSV at the time of labor, may be allowed to deliver vaginally, although a culture should be obtained from the cervix and vulva to further identify those infants who may be exposed to asymptomatic HSV shedding (93).

Diagnosis

Viral culture is the most sensitive and specific method of documenting a diagnosis of genital herpes. Rapid detection methods, including immunofluorescent, immunoperoxidase, and ELISA techniques for detecting viral antigen and DNA hybridization have sensitivities approaching that of culture when genital lesions are present but reduced sensitivity for asymptomatic viral shedding (94). Cytologic detection has good specificity but poor sensitivity.

Treatment

In primary genital herpes infection, intravenous, oral, and, to a lesser extent, topical therapy with the antiviral agent acyclovir has been shown to markedly reduce duration of symptoms and viral shedding and speed healing (95–98). This has no effect on subsequent natural history of the infection. Patient-initiated therapy with oral acyclovir early in the course of a recurrent episode has some benefit in shortening duration of lesions and viral shedding (99). Several studies have shown that oral acyclovir given daily to patients who have frequent recurrences will prevent recurrences in 65–85% of patients while therapy is continued. This has proven safe and effective for up to 2 years (100–102).

Hepatitis B

Epidemiology

Hepatitis B infects an estimated 300,000 persons each year in the U.S.; most are young adults. Persons having sexual contact with those infected with hepatitis B virus (HBV) or with multiple partners account for 22% of cases of HBV infection in the U.S. (103). In those acquiring infection through heterosexual contact, risk increases with numbers of previous sexual partners (104,105).

Clinical Presentation

After an average incubation period of 120 days, HBV presents insidiously with anorexia, malaise, nausea, vomiting, abdominal pain, and jaundice; skin rash, arthralgies, and arthritis are less common findings. In most cases, infection resolves uneventfully, but approximately 1.4% will die from an acute infection, and 6–10% of adolescents will become chronic carriers of infection. An estimated 25% of carriers develop chronic active hepatitis, often progressing to cirrhosis; furthermore, primary hepatocellular carcinoma is up to 300 times more common in HBV carriers then in the general population (103).

Diagnosis

Specific serologic markers are used to make a diagnosis of HBV infection. Hepatitis B surface antigen (HBsAg) can be identified in serum 1–2 months after exposure to HBV and persist for a variable period of time. Antibody to the core antigen develops in all HBV infections and persists indefinitely. The immunoglobulin M (IgM) antibody fraction is indicative of recent infection. The presence of hepatitis Be antigen (HBeAg) correlates with viral replication and high infectivity. Chronic carrier status is documented by sustained positivity for HBsAG. The appearance of anti-HBs indicates resolution of the infection and is protective against reinfection.

Treatment

There is no specific treatment for acute HBV infection, other than supportive care and monitoring. For postexposure prophylaxis after sexual exposure to an individual who is HBsAG positive, a single dose of hepatitis B immune globulin (HBIG), which contains a high titer of anti-HBs, is 75% effective if given within 2 weeks of sexual exposure (103).

Ongoing sexual contacts of patients with acute or chronic HBV and those with a history of multiple sexual partners in the previous 6 months or who have recently acquired other sexually transmitted diseases should be considered for vaccination. The recommended series of three intramuscular injections of hepatitis B vaccine induces an adequate antibody response in over 95% of adolescents. Universal prenatal screening is now recommended for pregnant women as a means of preventing perinatal transmission (106–108) and universal vaccination of infants and adolescents has been mentioned as a possible strategy for gaining control over this disease. Use of condoms may reduce sexual transmission.

Hepatitis A

Hepatitis A is primarily transmitted by fecal contamination and oral ingestion, but transmission may be facilitated by sexual contact. The average incubation period is 28 days, and greatest infectivity occurs 2 weeks immediately preceeding the onset of jaundice. No chronic carrier state exists with infection by the hepatitis A virus (HAV). Diagnosis of acute infection is made by finding IGM anti-HAV in serum. Immune globulin contains antibodies against HAV and is protective against infection when given preexposure or during the incubation period of the virus. It is recommended for all sexual contacts of persons with hepatitis A (103). The role of sexual transmission in hepatitis C and other forms of non-A–non-B hepatitis is not yet understood.

Cytomegalovirus

Cytomegalovirus (CMV) infection is a prevalent infection spread most commonly by sexual transmission, maternal-fetal transmission, and transfusion-associated transmission. Most infections are asymptomatic, although a mononucleosis-like illness may occur. Congenital CMV infection, however, may be associated with significant morbidity including neurologic abnormalities, jaundice, chorioretinitis, etc. (109). Diagnosis may be made using acute and convalescent antibody titers, or with actual viral isolation. Vaccination holds promise for future preventive efforts.

Molluscum Contagiosum

Molluscum contagiosum is an infection caused by a member of the pox virus family involving the skin and mucus membranes; infection may be spread by both sexual and nonsexual routes of transmission through direct contact with the skin of infected persons or fomites (110,111). After an incubation period averaging 2–3 months, a number of smooth firm papules form with characteristic central umbilications (Fig. 6). Most lesions occur on the thighs, lower abdominal wall, or genital region, and most are asymptomatic. Diagnosis may be made by identifying the characteristic intracytoplasmic molluscum bodies in cytologic or histologic specimens (112).

The infection is benign and self-limited. Treatment usually consists of destruction of lesions with dermal curettage, cryotherapy, or expression of the core of the papule with direct pressure; alternatively, application of a chemical irritant such as Podophyllin or silver nitrate has been utilized but may require more than one treatment (112,113).

BACTERIAL AND CHLAMYDIAL INFECTIONS

Chlamydia

Epidemiology

Chlamydia trachomatis is currently the most common sexually transmitted disease in this country (114). Adolescents have the highest age-related prevalence, with numerous studies showing 8–35% of sexually active adolescents in urban and suburban general health settings to be infected (115–118). Chlamydia is a coexistent pathogen in up to 30–50% of women with gonorrhea (119).

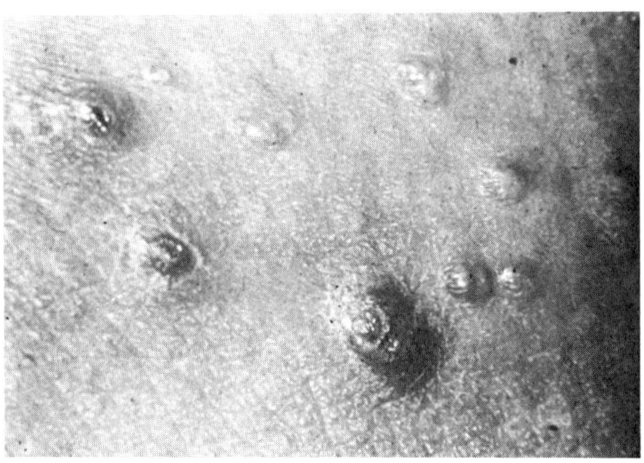

FIG. 6. Characteristic papular lesions of molluscum contagiosum with central umbilications.

Oral contraceptive use has been associated with increased risk of cervical *C. trachomatis* infection, probably because their use tends to increase cervical ectopy (120).

Clinical Presentation

The majority of chlamydial infections are asymptomatic. When symptoms occur, they are likely to include abnormal vaginal discharge, dysuria, frequency, and abnormal vaginal bleeding. On examination, mucopurulent discharge (greater than 10 polymorphonuclear leukocytes, ×1,000 field) (121), cervical edema, erythema, and friability are often found; similarly, the observation of yellow or green cervical discharge on an endocervical swab ("swab test") is associated with the presence of chlamydial infection. Unfortunately, these simple findings do not have sufficient sensitivity or specificity to adequately make a diagnosis of chlamydial infection (117,122).

When women are cultured from both the cervix and urethra, 50% of those with positive culture are positive from both sites and 25% from either site alone (123). Chlamydial urethritis has been implicated as a cause of the urethral syndrome (dysuria, frequency, pyuria with bacteriuria). Histologic evidence of endometritis is present in about 50% of patients with chlamydial cervicitis (124).

Chlamydial infection in pregnancy has been associated with preterm delivery and/or low birth weight and postpartum endometritis. Disease can be transmitted vertically, and result in neonatal conjunctivitis and/or pneumonia (125).

The most common and most serious complication of lower genital tract chlamydial infection is upper genital tract infection or pelvic inflammatory disease (PID), discussed more fully below. Approximately 10–30% of women with cervical chlamydial infection will develop PID (126). Because of the high prevalence of chlamydia in sexually active adolescents, this population should be routinely screened using one of the specific diagnostic techniques outlined below.

Diagnosis

Isolation of *Chlamydia trachomatis* is complicated by the fact that it is an obligate intracellular parasite and has a unique life cycle. It alternates between two morphologically separate forms: the elementary body, relatively resistant to the extracellular environment and responsible for cell-to-cell and host-to-host infection but metabolically inactive; and the reticulate body, requiring an intracellular environment and metabolically active but noninfectious.

Tissue culture is required for isolation and is considered to be the most sensitive and specific diagnostic test available although cost, turn-around time, and fastidious collection transport requirements are real disadvantages. In populations where the prevalence of infection is greater than 10%, newer, more rapid, and less costly diagnostic tests offer satisfactory sensitivity, specificity, and predictive value as compared to culture. The direct immunofluorescent (Microtrak) technique uses monoclonal antibody staining to identify elementary bodies and is somewhat labor intensive. It requires an experienced technician but allows assessment of the adequacy of the sample collected. Chlamydiazyme uses an ELISA with monoclonal or polyclonal antibodies to detect chlamydial antigen; it can be automated and batched allowing performance of a large number of tests and has an objective optical density endpoint. A disadvantage is that specimen quality cannot be monitored. In high-prevalence populations of women, median sensitivity of both of these techniques is 90% or greater, with specificities of 97–98% (127). All diagnostic tests require adequate numbers of cells in collection samples.

Treatment

Treatment of uncomplicated lower genital tract infection with *Chlamydia trachomatis* involves 7 or more days of therapy with Tetracycline or Doxycycline. Erythromycin is the Centers for Disease Control (CDC) recommended alternative, and sulfisoxazole, trimethaprim, and ciprofloxacin have also shown effectiveness (128,129). Single-dose regimens with penicillins or cephalosporins used to treat gonorrhea do not effectively eradicate concomitant chlamydial infection. Sexual partners should also be treated, and women who are sexual partners of men with nongonococcal urethritis should be treated empirically. Because of the high prevalence of chlamydia in adolescents, the sexual behavior patterns in this population, and their increased incidence of noncompliance with therapy, follow-up cultures should be considered approximately 1 month after a course of treatment is completed (130).

Gonorrhea

Epidemiology

The prevalence of *Neisseria gonorrhea* in sexually active adolescent populations studied has ranged from 1.5% to 12% (130,131). Alexander-Rodriguez and Vermund found the prevalence to be 18.3% in girls upon entry into a detention facility in New York City (132). The reported incidence of gonorrhea is almost twice as high for sexually active adolescents 15–19 years old as for sexually active women 20–24 years old (133). Demographic risk factors include low socioeconomic status, urban residence, and nonwhite race. Recent studies in Seattle suggest that approximately 25% of sexually active 16–18-year-old black women living in low socioeconomic urban census tracks acquired gonococcus (GC) each year in 1986 and 1987 (134). It is estimated that 50–90% of women who are sexual consorts of men with GC urethritis will be infected (135,136).

Clinical Presentation

Probably the majority of uncomplicated gonococcal infections in women are asymptomatic, though some studies suggest that gonococcal infections were more apt to be symptomatic then chlamydial infections. Urethritis and cervicitis are the most common clinical syndromes. Urethral colonization is present in 70–90% of infected women(137,138), but is usually accompanied by endocervical infection. Signs and symptoms were the same as those also noted with symptomatic chlamydial infection. Some 35–50% of women with gonococcal cervicitis also have GC isolated from the rectum, although this is usually asymptomatic (134). Most rectal infections in women occur without an acknowledged history of anal intercourse and are felt to be secondary to rectal contamination with infected cervicovaginal secretions. Pharyngeal infection with GC occurs in 10–20% of women but is the sole site of infection in less than 5% (139,140). Over 90% of pharyngeal infections are asymptomatic, and the spontaneous cure rate approaches 100% within 12 weeks of infection (139–141). However, one study noted a possible increased risk of disseminated gonorrhea in persons with pharyngeal GC (139).

Gonorrheal infection occurring during pregnancy may result in septic abortion, preterm delivery, premature rupture of membranes, or prolonged rupture of membranes and chorioamnionitis. Transmission can occur to the newborn with development of ophthalmia neonatorum and, infrequently, gonococcal septicemia (125).

PID is the most common complication of gonorrhea in women and occurs in an estimated 10–20% of those with lower genital tract gonorrhea (142).

Disseminated gonococcal infection is the most common systemic complication of acute gonorrhea and occurs in up to 3% of patients. It is usually manifested clinically as an arthritis/dermatitis syndrome and is more common in women (143).

Diagnosis

Gram-stained smears from the endocervix are highly specific for gonorrhea when typical gram-negative diplococci are seen within polymorphonuclear leukocytes, and such findings facilitate immediate treatment. Their sensitivity is reported to be only 50–70% with uncomplicated gonorrhea. Their predictive value is disappointing in asymptomatic women with normal physical examination (134). Isolation of *N. gonorrhea* is the "gold standard" for diagnosis of gonoccocal infection. Antibiotic-containing selective media are preferred for culturing the endocervix, rectum, and pharynx to suppress other bacteria, which usually outnumber gonorrhea in these locations. Single cultures will detect 80–90% of endocervical infections, and sensitivity may be increased by duplicate cervical cultures or combined cervical and urethral cultures (144). Cultures of areas other than the cervix depend on symptoms and sites exposed. Culture techniques can also identify plasmid-mediated antibiotic-resistant strains to guide therapy.

A rapid detection test for the presence of gonococcal antigen, commercially marketed as Gonozyme, is an enzyme immunoassay. Sensitivity as compared to culture is 73–100% in women, with 88–100% specificity. This test is currently adapted only for cervical and urethral specimens, and cannot be used for determination of antibiotic sensitivity (145,146).

Treatment

Development of antibiotic resistance has been the primary force driving the changing recommendations for adequate gonococcal therapy. Resistance may be of two types: (a) chromosomally mediated resistance requiring incremental increases in dosages of various antibiotics for curative treatment, and (b) plasmid-mediated resistance, usually with production of β-lactamase and resulting in high-level penicillin resistance. These strains were first introduced into the U.S. in 1976 and have increased dramatically since 1985, accounting for over 4% of reported gonorrhea in 1988, and as much as 10% and 33% of strains in New York City and southern Florida, respectively (134,147). Plasmid-mediated tetracycline resistance has now been reported, especially in the northeastern U.S., and sporadic cases of spectinomycin resistance are known (148). Currently CDC-recommended primary and secondary regimens for the treatment of asymptomatic gonorrhea are listed in Table 1 (128).

Pelvic Inflammatory Disease

Epidemiology and Pathogenesis

Teenagers account for 16–20% of the more than 1 million cases of pelvic PID reported each year in this country; although there has been a stabilization of the PID rate for all women, the rate of PID in adolescent women has continued to increase (149). The sexually active 15-year-old has a

TABLE 1. *1989 CDC treatment guidelines—uncomplicated gonorrhea*

First-line
Ceftriaxone 250 mg IM *plus*
Doxycycline 100 mg PO bid × 7 days
Alternative regimens[a]
Spectinomycin 2 gm IM[b]
Ciprofloxacin 500 mg PO
Norfloxacin 800 mg PO
Cefuroxime axetil 1 gm PO + Probenecid 1 gm PO
Cefotaxime 1 gm IM
Ceftizoxime 500 mg IM
Followed by Doxycycline 100 mg PO bid × 7 days

[a]A penicillin should be used only if strain is proven to be penicillin-sensitive.
[b]Preferred.

10 times greater risk for developing active pelvic infection than does a 25-year-old woman (150). Nonwhite adolescents have a PID rate more than twice that of white adolescents, but PID among white teens seems to be increasing at a faster rate (149).

PID, in the absence of recent pregnancy or instrumentation of the genital tract, is generally a polymicrobial sexually transmitted disease. Under certain predisposing circumstances—menses, presence of intrauterine device (IUD) string, presence of motile sperm or trichomonads—the mechanical and immunologic barrier of the cervix is breeched and infecting organisms gain access to the upper genital tract.

It is estimated that approximately 10–19% of females with endocervical gonorrhea and 10–30% with endocervical chlamydia will develop upper tract infection (126). *Mycoplasma hominis* has also been implicated in the development of PID, evenly distributed across age groups; the role of *Ureaplasma urealyticum* is less certain. In addition, endogenous aerobic and anaerobic organisms are usually involved, with or without antecedent infection with a sexually transmitted agent. These commonly include group B streptococci, peptostreptococci, *E. coli, Gardnerella vaginalis,* and bacteroides species. Isolation of these organisms from the upper tract is more common in long-standing and/or in more clinically severe cases and IUD users (151–153).

Microbial etiology and pathogenesis of PID have been very difficult to elucidate, and many points of controversy remain. Existing literature on the subject must be read critically since most studies are based on isolation rates from the cervix, which may not accurately reflect the bacteriologic status of the upper genital tract.

Clinical Presentation and Diagnosis

Clinical diagnosis of PID is hampered by the lack of specificity of traditional signs and symptoms. Only 65% of women diagnosed clinically have PID confirmed when laparoscopy is performed; 23% of women have normal pelvic findings (154). Furthermore, pelvic infection may produce no symptoms at all, or very mild ones. In one series, 6% of patients having PID by laparoscopy had not complained of abdominal pain; only 41% of PID patients have had temperature greater than 38°C (154). Seroepidemiologic studies have confirmed the significant relationship between tubal infertility and the presence of serum antibodies to *Chlamydia trichomatis* and *Neisseria gonorrhea,* even in patients without a history of PID (155–157).

Classic symptoms include lower abdominal/pelvic pain, fever, abnormal vaginal discharge, and abnormal vaginal bleeding. Symptoms with documented chlamydial infection appear to be milder with more indolent onset, whereas infection initiated by GC is associated with more severe symptoms and a more fulminant course. When nausea and vomiting are prominent symptoms, gastrointestinal disease should strongly be considered. In a minority of cases, right upper quadrant pain because of a concomitant perihepatitis (Fitz Hugh Curtis Syndrome) may be the dominating symptom and has been reported as an obscure cause of abdominal pain in adolescents without other symptoms of pelvic infection (158).

On physical examination, fever, pelvic and abdominal tenderness, and abnormal cervical secretions are the hallmark findings associated with PID. This combination of signs, however, was found by Jacobson and Westrom (154) in only 20% of laparoscopically confirmed cases of PID and in 14% of women with a clinical diagnosis of PID but normal tubes at laparoscopy. A palpable adnexal fullness or mass is a common finding and correlates with severity of inflammation as determined by the laparoscope but is also reported not infrequently in women with normal findings on laparoscopy (159). Because of the ascending pathogenesis of PID, women with this diagnosis should also have objective evidence of lower genital tract infection, and the presence of normal cervical secretions essentially rules out the diagnosis of PID. Approximately two-thirds of patients with acute PID have peripheral white blood cell counts over 10,000/ml and three quarters have an erythrocyte sedimentation rate (ESR) of greater than or equal to 15 mm/hr (154). Increased acute phase reactants, such as C-reactive protein, and decreased genital isoamylases are also commonly found in PID, but all of these laboratory tests are relatively nonspecific and discriminate poorly between upper genital tract infection and lower genital tract infection alone (160). Laboratory evaluation should include a serum HCG measurement to exclude the possibility of ectopic pregnancy. Evidence of lower genital tract infection should be a prerequisite for a diagnosis of PID. Evidence of mucopurulent cervicitis on exam and endocervical gram stain helps support a diagnosis of PID. Testing for endocervical gonorrhea and chlamydia should also be performed.

Ultrasound cannot reliably confirm or exclude PID as a diagnosis. It is an important adjunct, however, in identifying the presence of tuboovarian abscess, which occurs in 7–16% of females with acute PID (161). Because of the insensitivity of physical examination, I utilize sonography routinely to identify more severe infection and cases in which anaerobic coverage should be optimal.

More invasive techniques may be useful in making the diagnosis. Culdocentesis productive of purulent material or endometrial biopsy with histologic findings consistent with endometritis are suggestive of PID, but may require sedation in the adolescent. Laparoscopy is currently considered the "gold standard" for the diagnosis of PID. It should be used liberally when a diagnosis is in question or when the patient fails to respond appropriately to treatment. A laparoscopic grading system for severity of infection (Table 2) is helpful in determination of prognosis and predicting rapidity of response to treatment (162). Inaccurate diagnosis of pelvic pain may prevent early treatment for other conditions such as appendicitis or endometriosis; furthermore, once a diagnosis of PID is given, future episodes of pelvic or lower abdominal pain are likely to be labeled—perhaps inappropriately—as recurrent PID.

Treatment

The ultimate objectives of treatment are to preserve fertility, and prevent the complications and long-term sequelae resulting from PID.

There is evidence that early appropriate treatment will reduce damage to the fallopian tubes and, therefore, may decrease the incidence of post-PID infertility and other sequelae (163).

Hospitalization for inpatient treatment should be strongly considered in all adolescents because of the greater number of reproductive years at risk and because of issues of compliance. Appropriate antibiotic therapy must take into account the polymicrobial nature of PID and, in adolescents, the prevalence of nongonococcal agents such as *Chlamydia trachomatis*.

Currently CDC-recommended regimens

TABLE 2. *PID—severity of disease by laparoscopic examination*

Degree	Findings
Mild	Erythema, edema, no spontaneous purulent exudate, tubes freely moveable
Moderate	Gross purulent material evident; more marked erythema and edema; tubes may not be freely moveable and/or patent
Severe	Pyosalpinx or inflammatory complex, abscess (size should be measured)

From ref. 162.

TABLE 3. *1989 CDC treatment guidelines—PID*

Ambulatory treatment
  Cefoxitin 2 gm IM plus Probenecid 1 gm PO
    or
  Ceftriaxone 250 mg IM
    plus
  Doxycycline 100 mg PO bid × 10–14 days
Inpatient treatment
  A. Cefoxitin 2 gm IV q 6 hr or
    Cefotetan 2 gm IV q 12 hr
      plus
    Doxycycline 100 mg IV or PO q 12 hr
  B. Clindamycin 900 mg IV q 8 hr
      plus
    Gentamicin loading dose 2.0 mg/kg
      plus
    Maintenance 1.5 mg/kg IV q 8 hr
The above regimens are given for at least 48 hr after the patient improves. After discharge, continue Doxycycline 100 mg PO bid × 10–14 days total

for inpatient treatment of acute PID are listed in Table 3 (128). It should be kept in mind that these recommendations are not based on well-designed controlled clinical trials, but rather on coverage of organisms isolated in studies of the microbial etiology of PID, along with knowledge of their sensitivity patterns. Antibiotic therapy should be continued until signs and symptoms of inflammation have essentially resolved and for a minimum of 10–14 days. Examination of endocervical secretions may help confirm a satisfactory response to therapy. The patient should be clinically reevaluated at the end of treatment and 1–2 weeks later when repeat cultures from the lower genital tract should be obtained.

An essential adjunct to effective treatment of PID is evaluation and treatment of the woman's sexual partners. In one study, up to 71% of male partners of women with PID who were located had GC or nongonococcal urethritis (164). Furthermore, 20–92% of patients with GC or chlamydial urethritis are asymptomatic (165–168). It is important to treat these male partners with a regimen effective against both organisms, regardless of culture results.

Surgical treatment in PID is indicated when rupture of a pelvic abscess occurs or when medical therapy fails. When surgery is necessary, it should be as conservative as possible. Rarely is hysterectomy and removal of bilateral adnexi indicated; removal of unilateral adnexae or abscess drainage with copious irrigation at laparotomy or laparoscopy is usually sufficient and allows the possibility of future pregnancy.

Complications and Sequelae

The most common long-term complications of PID include recurrent infection, chronic pelvic/abdominal pain, ectopic pregnancy, and infertility. Approximately one quarter of all women with their first episode of PID eventually develop one or more further infections, and women below the age of 20 are reinfected twice as frequently as are older women (169).

Almost one-fifth of patients eventually have chronic abdominal/pelvic pain of more than 6 months duration; this has been correlated with pelvic adhesive disease and with infertility (169,170).

The incidence of ectopic pregnancy has increased almost 400% in the past 20 years, paralleling the increase in PID (171). Ectopic pregnancy occurs in 1 of 24 women after an episode of PID as compared to 1 of 147 control women (170). In two studies, antichlamydial antibodies were more prevalent and of higher titer in women with ectopic pregnancy than age-matched controls with intrauterine pregnancies (172,173). The second leading cause of maternal mortality in the U.S. is ectopic gestation, and women 15–19 years of age have the highest mortality rates in this group (174).

PID has long been recognized as a major cause of infertility. Although infertility rates are significantly lower in women having their first episode of PID before the age of 24, chances of infertility increase at all ages with severity of disease and number of episodes. For adolescents having one episode of severe PID, 27.3% will subsequently be unable to conceive; after three or more episodes, over one half will be infertile (175).

Bacterial Vaginosis

Epidemiology

Bacterial vaginosis (BV) previously known as nonspecific vaginitis, gardnerella vaginitis, or hemophilus vaginitis, is currently the most prevalent vaginitis, accounting for approximately one-third of all cases in women of childbearing age.

In BV, the normal equilibrium of the vaginal microenvironment is disturbed and there is an overgrowth of both aerobic and anaerobic organisms, most notably *Gardnerella vaginalis, Mycoplasma hominis,* and bacteroides and mobiluncus species. The concentration of gardnerella and anaerobes in vaginal secretions is 100–1,000 times greater in this syndrome than in control women without evidence of vaginal infection (176). The role of sexual transmission is unclear, but BV should not be considered an exclusively sexually transmitted disease. Bump and Buesching (177) found no significant difference in prevalence of bacterial vaginosis between virginal and sexually active adolescent females. On the other hand, male partners of women with BV have been found to have an increased rate of *G. vaginalis* and anaerobic isolation from the urethra (178,179).

Clinical Presentation

Up to 50% of women with BV may be asymptomatic (177). Abnormal vaginal discharge and malodor are the most common complaints; irritative symptoms are usually absent or minimal.

Diagnosis

Diagnosis of BV is generally made on the basis of a composite of three of the following four clinical criteria (180): (a) homogenous thin vaginal discharge; (b) vaginal ph greater than 4.5; (c) clue cells on wet mount representing greater than 20% of vaginal epithelial cells; and (d) fishy odor on alkalization of vaginal secretions. In addition, gram stain of vaginal secretions showing a predominance of mixed bacterial types with absent or small numbers of lactobacillus morphotypes is highly correlated with this syndrome (181). Several methods based on detection of the metabolic products of the various microorganisms found in BV have been described but are primarily research tools at the present time.

Treatment

Oral metronidazole, 500 mg. bid for 7 days, is currently considered the treatment of choice. However, treatment with intravaginal metronidazole tablets or sponges, or systemic or topical clindamycin offers promising and attractive alternatives (182,183). To date, routine treatment of male partners of infected women has not been shown to decrease rates of recurrence (184). It is unclear whether asymptomatic women should be routinely treated if BV is diagnosed. There is some evidence that the syndrome often spontaneously resolves, even in the absence of treatment (177). However, recent studies linking BV to complications in pregnant women such as preterm premature rupture of membranes (PROM) (185), preterm labor (185,186), chorioamnionitis (187), and puerperal infectious morbidity (189), as well as polymicrobial upper genital tract infection (189) in nonpregnant women have increased concerns about the implications and possible sequelae of this infection. This may lead to more stringent recommendations as better data become available.

Lymphogranuloma Venereum

Lymphogranuloma venereum (LGV) is an infection caused by certain serovars of *Chlamydia trachomatis;* although it is considered a "minor" STD in North America, it is endemic in much of the developing world (190). The primary lesion is a small papular ulcer, which is relatively asymptomatic and often unnoticed. The secondary stage is characterized by either inflammation and swelling of inguinal lymph nodes (inguinal syndrome) or—more commonly in women—acute proctocolitis with fever, rectal pain, and tenesmus (anogenital rectal syndrome) (191). Even without treatment, most infections resolve after this stage; in a small minority of patients, however, a chronic inflammatory response leads to the development of genital ulcers, genital elephantiasis, and rectal strictures (192,193).

Correct diagnosis is suggested by the clinical picture but may be confirmed by chlamydial isolation from infected tissue or appropriate serologic tests. Currently, recommended treatment is with tetracycline 2 gm daily for 2–4 weeks (128).

Chancroid

Chancroid is a sexually transmitted genital ulcerative disease associated with infection by *Hemophilus ducreyi*. Much more prevalent in men than women, this infection has dramatically increased in incidence in the U.S. over the past decade (194).

The incubation period is usually between 4 and 7 days, with the initial clinical manifestation being a tender papule, which over the course of 1–2 days becomes pustular and then ulcerative. The ulcer classically has ragged undermined edges, is well demarcated, and is without induration (Fig. 7). The base of the ulcer is friable and covered with necrotic purulent debris. Depending on the site of the ulcer, symptoms in women may include pain with urination or defecation, vaginal discharge, dyspareunia, and rectal bleeding. Symptoms in women are often more subclinical than in men. Also a characteristic feature of chancroid, but less commonly seen in women, is painful unilateral inguinal lymphadenitis (195).

Laboratory confirmation of this diagnosis depends on isolation of *H. ducreyi* from a genital ulcer or inguinal node. Gram stain of exudate from the ulcer base shows typical gram negative bacilli in a "school of fish" pattern and may aid in diagnosis. Recommended treatment consists of erythromycin 500 mg qid or trimethoprim-sulfamethoxazole ds bid for 7 days. Ceftriaxone 250 mg. im or ciprofloxacin 500 mg po bid for 1–3 days appear to be effective alternatives (196). Sexual partners should be treated simultaneously and abstinence encouraged until lesions have healed.

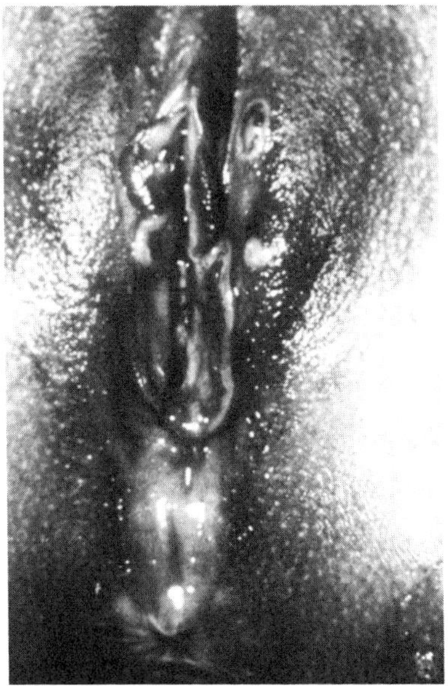

FIG. 7. Ulcerated lesion of the vulva caused by chancroid.

Granuloma Inguinale

Granuloma inguinale, also known as Donovanosis, is a chronic and progressively destructive infection of the genital region caused by the bacterium *Calymmatobacterium granulomatis*. Most common in tropical and subtropical environments, granuloma inguinale has been described in adolescents in the U.S. (197). The role of sexual transmission is controversial (198). There is some evidence that the causative organism may be a normal inhabitant of the intestinal tract and may be autoinoculated into the vagina. Clinical disease then occurs after sexual or nonsexual trauma of sites harboring *C. granulomatis* (199).

The incubation period is not well defined, but appears to be in the range of 8–80 days. The initial lesion is a small subcutaneous nodule(s), which erodes to the skin and forms a painless, beefy red, hypertrophic well-defined ulcerative lesion, which bleeds on contact. Lesions slowly enlarge and often coalesce. In women, most lesions are found on the labia but also have been described in the vagina or on the cervix. Fibrosis and lymphedema of surrounding tissue occur with progressive disease, and the clinical picture has not infrequently been confused with carcinoma (197).

Diagnosis is easily confirmed by stained crushed preparation from the lesion with demonstration of Donovan bodies, deep-staining clusters of organisms with a "safety pin" appearance in the cytoplasm of large mononuclear cells. First-line treatment consists of tetracycline 500 mg qid until lesions have completely healed, for a minimum of 3 weeks. Chloramphenicol and gentamicin are alternative therapies (197).

SPIROCHETE INFECTION

Syphilis

Epidemiology

The incidence of syphilis in the U.S. stands at its highest rate in almost 20 years. In 1989, the rate for diagnosis of all stages of syphilis was 45.1 cases per 100,000 population. The age specific case rate for primary and secondary syphilis among teenaged women 15–19 years of age was 30.9 per 100,000 in 1989, but showed dramatic racial differences; 4.2 per 100,000 for whites, 17.5 per 100,000 for Hispanics, and 166.9 per 100,000 for black teens (200). A study of 285 adolescent girls upon entry into a detention facility in New York City found a 2.5% prevalence of syphilis (132). Rates for syphilis are highest in geographic areas and among populations with the highest prevalence of AIDS.

Clinical Presentation

Approximately 30% of women who have sexual contact with a partner who has early syphilis will themselves become infected (201). The lesion of primary syphilis, the chancre, occurs at the portal of entry of the treponeme an average of 3 weeks after exposure (Fig. 8). It is typically single, indurated, and painless, and is usually associated with regional adenopathy. It heals within a few weeks with or without treatment.

With widespread hematogenous and lymphatic dissemination of *T. pallidum,* a variable systemic illness develops weeks to months after the disappearance of the chancre. A flu-like illness, with low-grade fever, malaise, headache, sore throat, myalgias, and adenopathy, is common. The presence of a papular rash involving the palms and soles should heighten suspicion for secondary syphilis. Condylomatalata are moist confluent papular lesions of secondary syphilis in intertriginous areas and contain large numbers of spirochetes (Fig. 9).

Again, with or without treatment, the manifestations of secondary syphilis resolve and the patient enters the latent stage. During this time, although there is serologic evidence of infection, there are no clinical manifestations. Because transmission re-

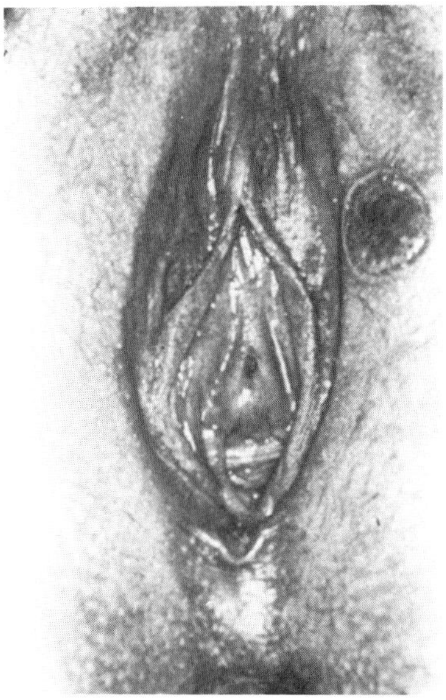

FIG. 8. Chancre of primary syphilis.

quires exposure to mucosal or cutaneous lesions, latency is somewhat arbitrarily divided into early latency (less than 1 year from onset of infection) and late latency on the basis of the time when untreated patients are most likely to develop spontaneous mucocutaneous infectious relapses.

Occurring at times up to 30 years after onset of infection, the signs and symptoms of tertiary syphilis involve the bones, soft tissues, various visceral organs, cardiovascular system (aneurysm, aortic insufficiency), and central nervous system (paresis, tabes dorsalis, etc.). These account for the major morbidity and mortality of the disease.

At each stage of syphilis, the clinical presentation is extremely variable, and "atypical" manifestations are common. This is especially true of patients who are coinfected with HIV (202).

Diagnosis

Dark-field microscopic examination of exudate from the surface of a chancre, aspirate from an involved lymph node, or material from the surface of papules or condylomata can provide the earliest and most direct means of diagnosis of early syphilis. False negative tests may occur when there are too few organisms to identify, the lesion is healing, or topical or systemic treatment has been initiated.

In situations where dark-field exam is not available or appropriate, serologic tests are used to provide indirect evidence of syphilis. Generally, a nontreponemal test such as the VDRL, RPR, or STS is utilized initially to screen for syphilis by detecting reagin, a heterogenous group of substances elevated in syphilis. If this is reactive, a test (FTA-ABS, MHA-TP) detecting specific antibodies to *T. pallidum* confirms the diagnosis. The sensitivity of these tests approaches 100% in secondary syphilis (203–205). Biologic false positives occasionally occur with immunizations, intravenous drug use, febrile illness, or collagen vascular disease, but are usually of low titer (206,207).

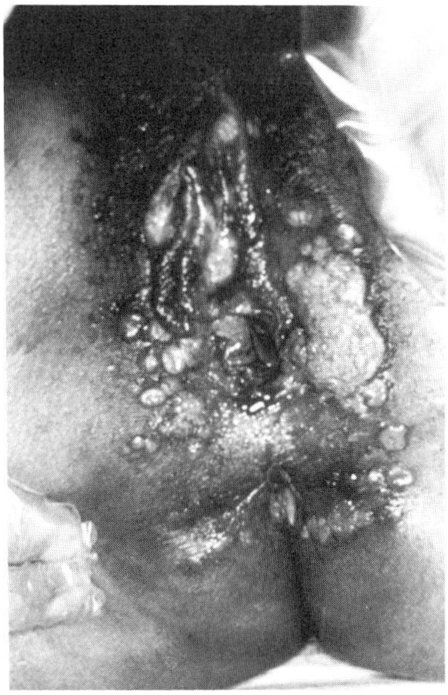

FIG. 9. Condylamatalata of secondary syphilis.

TABLE 4. *CDC treatment guidelines—syphilis*

Early syphilis: Primary, secondary, latent syphilis <1 year
Benzathine penicillin G 2.4 million units IM
Alternative
Doxycycline 100 mg PO bid × 2 weeks
or
Tetracycline 500 mg PO qid × 2 weeks
Late syphilis: Latent syphilis >1 year, tertiary (excluding neurosyphilis)
Benzathine penicillin G 2.4 million units IM given 1 week apart × 3 consecutive weeks.
Alternative
Doxycycline 100 mg PO bid × 4 weeks
or
Tetracycline 500 mg PO qid × 4 weeks

Treatment

The treatment of choice for all stages of syphilis remains intramuscular penicillin in patients who are not allergic. Specific treatment schedules and alternatives recommended by the CDC are noted in Table 4 (128).

After treatment, the patient should be followed with examination and RPR, or other nontreponemal test at 3, 6, 9, 12, and 24 months to detect treatment failure or reinfection. In primary syphilis, the VDRL should become nonreactive approximately 1 year after treatment, and in secondary syphilis it is nonreactive 2 years posttreatment. If clinical signs persist or recur, or if the titer rises, remains high, or fails to decline appropriately, retreatment is indicated (128). For patients with primary syphilis, all sexual partners within the previous 3 months and in patients with secondary syphilis all partners within the proceeding 6–12 months should be located and treated.

ECTOPARASITES

Pediculosis Pubis (Pubic Lice)

Epidemiology

Phthrus pubis, the crab louse, is an ectoparasite that generally infests the pubic area. Sexual contact is the most common, but not the only, means of transmission. Incidence of pubic lice infestation is highest in single persons 15–25 years of age (208).

Clinical Presentation

The louse is dependent on human blood, and symptoms occur largely with sensitization after bites. The primary symptom is itching; scratching leads to erythema with further irritation and inflammation. Small blue spots may be seen in the skin occasionally as a result of bites. After many bites over a short period of time, the individual may have mild fever, malaise, and irritability.

Diagnosis

Diagnosis depends on identification of the adult lice (1 mm long) or their nits (eggs, 0.8 mm long) with the naked eye or microscope. At first glance, pubic lice may appear as scabs over papular areas of irritation.

Treatment

Treatment involves administration topically of a medication that will kill both the adult lice and their eggs. Permethrin 1% creme rinse applied to the affected area and washed off after 10 minutes or Lindane 1% shampoo applied for 4 minutes and washed off appear equally effective, although failure rates as high as 40% have been reported and require retreatment for definitive cure (209). Sexual contacts should be treated similarly, and the patient's clothing and other fomites should be disinfected by laundering in hot water or dry cleaning. A mild antipruritic/antiinflammatory cream may be helpful for treating pruritus, which often persists after treatment of the infestation itself because of residual irritation or allergic reaction (208).

Scabies

Epidemiology

Scabies, a cutaneous infestation caused by the mite *Sarcoptes scabiei,* has been a common disease for at least 3,000 years and occurs in small local outbreaks, as well as large epidemics. In most areas of the world, the highest incidence has been found in children and young adults. Transmission of the mites requires close bodily contact, including but not limited to sexual contact.

Clinical Presentation

Clinical symptoms are generally caused when the mites burrow into the skin to lay eggs. Several weeks later, with sensitization, an erythematous papular rash usually develops, and itching, often exacerbated at night or after a hot bath, is intense and persistent. The mite is quite mobile and likes to gravitate to some favorite places; typical burrows are most commonly found on the hands and wrists. The burrow appears as a short, wavy, "dirty" line that often crosses skin lines.

Diagnosis

Definitive diagnosis requires identification of one of the following: classic burrows, the mite at any stage of development, or its eggs or fecal pellets (210). One technique in wide use involves application of mineral oil to lesions followed by vigorous scraping with a sterile scalpel blade to remove the top of the burrow or papule. The oil and scraped material are then transferred to a glass slide for microscopic exam.

Treatment

The recommended treatment regimen for adolescents is application of 1% Lindane (1 oz of lotion or 30 gm of cream) thinly to all areas of the body from the neck down. This should be washed off thoroughly after 8 hr. This medication is potentially neurotoxic, and to avoid excess absorption, it should not be used after a hot bath or shower and should not be reapplied less than 8 days apart. Permethrin 5% cream has recently been noted to be as effective and safer than Lindane. Both household and sexual partners should be treated simultaneously, and clothes and bed linens disinfected.

FUNGAL INFECTIONS

Vulvovaginal Candidiasis

Epidemiology

It is estimated that three quarters of all women in the U.S. will have at least one episode of vulvovaginal candidiasis. A total of 80–90% of infections are due to *Candida albicans,* but the remainder result from other candidal species that may be more resistant to conventional therapy (211).

Up to 50% of women have asymptomatic vaginal colonization with candida (212). It is unclear just what factors play a role in the development of symptomatic infection, though it has been noted that germination enhances both colonization and tissue invasion (213). It has also been shown that candidal species undergo high-frequency genetic switching, which may provide the capacity to invade different sides of the body or change patterns of resistance to antifungal medications (214).

Predisposing factors for vulvovaginal candidiasis include pregnancy (215), oral contraceptive use (216), broad-spectrum antibiotics (217), allergic or hypersensitivity responses to local irritants (douches, spermicides, etc. . . .) (218), tight, occlusive, or poorly ventilated clothing (219), and immunosuppression [HIV infection (220), diabetes, steroid use].

The role of sexual transmission in the development of vaginal candidiasis is controversial. In a 1987 study, Horowitz (221) evaluated 33 women with recurrent vulvovaginal candidiasis (greater than three culture positive episodes per year) and their sexual partners. He found a high correlation between partners with positive cultures involving the same candidal strains. The oral cavity was the site most often colonized, and 15% of ejaculates were also positive for candidal species. Recurrent vaginal infections were eliminated with systemic antifungal treatment, oral clotrimazole troches, and restriction of oral-genital contact between partners.

Clinical Presentation

Pruritus is the most common clinical symptom, present in approximately 90% of women (222). Other irritative symptoms frequently seen include dyspareunia and vulvar dysuria, often with reflex urgency and frequency. The discharge is classically white and curdy, and may be adherent to the vaginal walls. Vaginal and vulvar erythema are not uncommonly found.

Diagnosis

In patients with candidiasis, vaginal ph is usually within the normal range. Both wet mount and examination of vaginal secretions in 10–20% KOH reveal spores and pseudohyphae with *C. albicans*, lactobacillus predominance, and a relative paucity of white blood cells. Culture with Sabouraud or Nickerson media may be needed to document the diagnosis in vaginitis of unsure etiology or for species identification in chronically recurrent candidiasis.

Treatment

Recommended first-line treatment for vulvovaginal candidiasis is with a topical imidazole compound for 3–7 days. Terconazole, a more recently developed antifungal agent characterized as a triazole compound, appears to have equal or superior efficacy as compared to miconazole and clotrimazole, as well as a more rapid onset of action (223). Short-course therapy is more advantageous in ensuring compliance.

Oral treatment with ketoconazole appears to be highly effective, but it is more expensive and associated with potential hepatotoxicity, making it perhaps a better choice for chronically recurrent or refractory cases (224). The new antifungal agent, Fluconazole, though not yet FDA approved for the treatment of vaginal candidiasis, shows promise as an effective and safe antifungal when administered in a single oral dose (225).

Treatment of male sexual partners is not indicated for the routine management of vulvovaginal candidiasis, but should be considered with chronically recurrent, or refractory cases.

PROTOZOAN INFECTIONS

Trichomonas

Epidemiology

Trichomonas vaginalis is a flagellated protozoan that infects at least 6 million women and their sexual partners each year in the U.S. The highest incidence is found in teenagers with multiple sexual partners (226). Transmission is by sexual contact; nonsexual transmission is theoretically possible, but in reality is thought to be a rare event. Seventy percent of men are found to harbor the organism when examined within 48 hr after sexual contact with an infected woman (227).

Clinical Presentation

Up to 50% of women are asymptomatic, but one-third of these will develop symptoms within 6 months if untreated (226). Abnormal vaginal discharge is the most common symptom and is classically described as profuse, purulent, frothy, and foul smelling, though this composite description is found in a minority of women. Irritative symptoms are common, including pruritus, burning, dyspareunia, and vulvar dysuria. Punctate hemorrhagic lesions of the vagina or cervix ("strawberry spots") are another classic, but infrequent finding (228). Vulvar and vaginal erythema may also be seen (229).

Diagnosis

Vaginal pH is usually elevated greater than 4.5 with vaginal trichomoniasis. The most common way to confirm the diagnosis is with direct observation of motile organisms on wet mount. A significant inflammatory component is usual, manifested by excess numbers of white blood cells. Culture on Kupferberg medium or Diamond medium modified is considered the most sensitive means of making the diagnosis but requires 2–7 days for results. Recent staining methods using monoclonal antibody technology offer promise as rapid, sensitive, and specific alternatives to culture (230).

Treatment

Vaginal trichomoniasis is treated with oral metronidazole given to both partners. Both the single 2-gm dose and more extended 5- and 7-day regimens of 250 mg tid or 500 mg bid have been effective (231). Single-dose treatment, though not as efficacious as extended therapy, is preferred in adolescents because of compliance issues. Trichomoniasis should alert the health care provider to the possible presence of other STDs.

PREVENTION

The topic of prevention could alone fill several chapters. However, a few brief comments must suffice. All adolescents should have access to care that is safe, nonjudgmental, confidential, and inexpensive. A sexual history should be elicited from every adolescent in a sensitive and thorough fashion. Each exposure of the individual to the health care system should be seen as an opportunity to discuss sexual issues, including STDs. This should include education about warning signals, complications of STDs, and means of prevention, including alteration of sexual behavior to minimize the number of sexual partners and the use of barrier methods of contraception. Because of the link among drug use, sexual behavior, and sexually transmitted diseases, each adolescent's education should include information about drug use, abuse, and resources available for aid.

Although each interaction with an adolescent should be considered confidential, a major thrust of the health care provider should be to enlist the parents' support for the adolescent. This may provide the impetus for better understanding and closer interaction in the future.

REFERENCES

1. Bell TA, Hein K. Adolescents and sexually transmitted diseases. In: Holmes KK, Mardh P-A, Sparling PF, Wiesner PJ, eds. *Sexually transmitted diseases*. New York: McGraw-Hill, 1984:73.
2. Tanner JM. *Foetus into man: physical growth from conception to maturation*. Cambridge, MA: Harvard University Press, 1978:152.
3. Vihko R, Apter D. The role of androgens in

adolescent cycles. *J Steroid Biochem* 1980; 12:369.
4. Lee WI, Blandau RJ. Laser light scattering study of the effect of progesterone on sperm mobility. *Fertil Steril* 1979;32:320.
5. Enhorning G, Huldt L, Melen B. Ability of cervical mucus to act as a barrier against bacteria. *Am J Obstet Gynecol* 1970;108:532.
6. James JF, Swanson J. Color/opacity colonial variants of Neisseria gonorrhoeae and their relationship to the menstrual cycle. In: Brooks GF, et al., eds. *Immunobiology of Neisseria gonorrhoeae*. Washington, DC: American Society for Microbiology, 1978: 339.
7. Zelnik M, Kantner JF. Sexual activity, contraceptive use and pregnancy among metropolitan-area teenagers: 1971–1979. *Fam Plann Perspect* 1980;12:230.
7a. Forrest JD, Singh S. The sexual and reproductive behavior of American women, 1982–1988. *Fam Plann Perspect* 1990;22:206.
7b. Centers for Disease Control. Premarital sexual experience among adolescent women, United States, 1970–1988. *MMWR* 1991;39:929.
8. Pratt WF, Mosher WD, Bachrach CA, Horn MC. Understanding U.S. fertility: findings from the national survey of family growth, cycle III. *Popul Bull* 1984;39.
9. Zelnik M, Kantner JF. Sexual and contraceptive experience of young unmarried women in the United States, 1976 and 1971. *Fam Plann Prospect* 1977;9:55.
10. Zabin LS, Hirsch MB, Smith EA, Hardy JB. Adolescent sexual attitudes and behavior: are they consistent? *Fam Plann Perspect* 1984; 16:181.
11. Sorensen RE. *Adolescent sexuality in contemporary America: personal values and sexual behavior, ages thirteen to nineteen*. New York: World Publishing, 1973:122.
12. Hayes C. *Risking the future: Adolescent sexuality, pregnancy and childbearing. Vol. I.* Washington, DC: National Academy Press, 1987.
12a. Sonenstein FL, Pleck JH, Ku LC. Sexual activity, condom use and AIDS awareness among adolescent males. *Fam Plann Perspect* 1989; 21:152.
12b. Mosher WD. Contraceptive practice in the United States, 1982–1988. *Fam Plann Perspect* 1990;22:198.
13. Shah F, Zelnik M. Parent and peer influence on sexual behavior, contraceptive use, and pregnancy experience of young women. *J Marr Fam* 1981;43:339.
14. Nathanson CA, Becker MH. Family and peer influence on obtaining a method of contraception. *J Marr Fam* 1986;48:513.
15. Brookman RH. Adolescent sexual behavior. In: Holmes KK, Mardh P-A, Sparling PF, Wiesner PJ, eds. *Sexually transmitted diseases*. New York: McGraw-Hill, 1990:77.
16. Smith EA, Udry JR. Coital and non-coital sexual behaviors of white and black adolescents. *Am J Public Health* 1985;75:1200.
17. Darrow WW. Attitudes towards condom use and the acceptance of venereal disease prophylactics. In: Redford MH, et al., eds. *The condom: increasing utilization in the United States*. San Francisco, CA: San Francisco Press, 1974:173.
18. Reiss IL. Human sexuality in sociological perspective. In: Holmes KK, Mardh P-A, Sparling PF, Wiesner PJ, eds. *Sexually transmitted diseases*. New York: McGraw-Hill, 1984:39.
19. Strasberger VC, ed. Sex, drugs, rock n' roll—understanding common teenage behavior. *Pediatrics* 1985;76(suppl):659.
20. Strasburger VC. Television and adolescents. *Pediatr Ann* 1985;14:814.
21. Deisher R, Remafedi G. *Adolescent sexuality*. 337.
22. Malus M, LaChance PA, Lamy L, et al. Priorities in adolescent health care: The teenager's viewpoint. *J Fam Pract* 1987;25:159.
23. Holder AR. Minor's rights to consent to medical care. *JAMA* 1987;257:3400.
24. Lih IF, Cuskey WR. Compliance with medical regimens during adolescence *Pediatr Clin North Am* 1980;27:3.
25. Centers for Disease Control. *AIDS Weekly Surveillance Report, United States*. Atlanta, GA: CDC AIDS Program, July 5, 1988.
26. Munoz A, Wang M, Bass S, et al. Acquired immunodeficiency syndrome (AIDS) free time after human immunodeficiency virus type I seroconversion in homosexual men. *Am J Epidemiol* 1989;130:530.
27. Vermund SH, Heim K, Gayle HD, et al. Acquired immunodeficiency syndrome among adolescents: case surveillance profiles in New York City and the rest of the United States. *Am J Dis Child* 1989;143:1220.
28. Johnston LD, Bachman JG, O'Malley PM. *Drug use among American high school students, college and other young adults: national trends through 1986*. Rockville, MD: National Institute on Drug Abuse, 1987.
29. Sande M. HIV infection and AIDS—editorial overview. *Curr Opin Infect Dis* 1990;3:67.
30. Centers for Disease Controls. Continuous increase in infectious syphilis—United States. *MMWR* 1988;37:35.
31. Sterk C. Cocaine and HIV seropositivity. *Lancet* 1988;2:2052.
32. Booth W. AIDS and drug abuse: no quick fix. *Science* 1988;239:717.
33. Centers for Disease Control. AIDS in women—United States. *MMWR* 1990;39:845.
34. Quinn T, Glasses D, Cannon R, et al. Human immunodeficiency virus infection among patients attending clinics for sexually transmitted diseases. *N Engl J Med* 1988;318:197.
35. Brooks-Gunn J, Boyer CB, Heim K. Preventing HIV infection and AIDS in children and adolescents—behavioral research and intervention strategies. *Am Psychologist* 1988;43:958.
36. Burke DS, Brundage JF, Herbold JR, et al. Human immunodeficiency virus infections among civilian applicants for United States military

service, October 1985 to March 1986. *N Engl J Med* 1987;317:131.
37. Interest heightens in defining, preventing AIDS in high-risk adolescent population. *JAMA* 1989; 262:2197.
38. Koenig S, Fauci AS. Immunology of HIV infection. In: Holmes KK, Mardh P-A, Sparling PF, Wiesner PJ, eds. *Sexually transmitted diseases*. New York: McGraw-Hill, 1990:317.
39. Hirsch MS. Clinical manifestations of HIV infection in adults in industrialized countries. In: Holmes KK, Mardh P-A, Sparling PF, Wiesner PJ, eds. *Sexually transmitted diseases*. New York: McGraw-Hill, 1990:331.
40. Volberding P. AIDS-related malignancies. In: Holmes KK, Mardh P-A, Sparling PF, Wiesner PJ, eds. *Sexually transmitted diseases*. New York: McGraw-Hill, 1990:685.
41. Goldstein L. Immunodiagnosis of human immunodeficiency virus infections. In: Holmes KK, Mardh P-A, Sparling PF, Wiesner PJ, eds. *Sexually transmitted diseases*. New York: McGraw Hill, 1990:961.
42. Haseltine. *N Engl J Med* 1989;320:1487.
43. Jackson JB, Balfour HH. Practical diagnostic testing for human immunodeficiency virus. *Clin Microbiol Rev* 1988;1:124.
44. Ou C-Y, Kwok S, Mitchell SW, et al. DNA amplification for direct detection of HIV-1 in DNA of peripheral blood mononuclear cells. *Science* 1988;239:295.
45. Kwok S, Mack DH, Mullis KB, et al. Identification of human immunodeficiency virus sequences by using *in vitro* enzymatic amplification and oligomer cleavage detection. *J Virol* 1987;61:1690.
46. Loche M, Mach B. Identification of HIV-infected seronegative individuals by a direct diagnostic test based on hybridisation to amplified viral DNA. *Lancet* 1988;2:418.
47. Rhoads J, Wright C, Redfield R, Burke D. Chronic vaginal candidiasis in women with human immunodeficiency virus infection. *JAMA* 1987;257:3105.
48. Imam N, Carpenter CC, Mayer KH, et al. Hierarchical pattern of mucosal candida infections in HIV-seropositive women. *Am J Med* 1990;89:142.
49. Maier J, Bergman A, Rose M. Acquired immunodeficiency syndrome manifested by chronic primary genital herpes. *Am J Obstet Gynecol* 1986;155:756.
50. Feingold A, Vermund S, Burk R, et al. Cervical cytologic abnormalities and human immunodeficiency virus. *J Acquir Immune Defic Syndr* 1990;3:896.
51. Vermund S, Kelley K, Burk R, et al. Risk of human papillomavirus and cervical squamous intraepithelial lesions highest among women with advanced HIV disease [Abstract]. Presented at the VI International Conference on AIDS, San Francisco, 1990.
52. Maiman M, Fruchter, Serar E, et al. Human immunodeficiency virus infection and cervical neoplasia. *Gynecol Oncol* 1990;38:377.
53. National Institute of Allergy and Infectious Diseases. State-of-the art conference on azidothymidine therapy for early HIV infection. *Am J Med* 1990;89:335.
54. Berkelman RL, Heyward WL, Stehr-Green JK, Curran JW. Epidemiology of human immunodeficiency virus infection and acquired immunodeficiency syndrome. *Am J Med* 1989; 86:761.
55. Steinberg BM. Papillomavirus—effects upon mother and child. *Ann NY Acad Sci* 1988; 549:118.
56. Martinez J, Smith R, Farmer M, et al. High prevalence of genital tract papillomavirus infection in female adolescents. *Pediatrics* 1988; 82:604.
57. Rosenfeld WD, Vermund SH, Wentz SJ, Burk RD. High prevalence of human papillomavirus infection and association with abnormal Papanicolaou smears in sexually active adolescents. *Am J Dis Child* 1989;143:1443.
58. Spitzer M, Krumholz B, Scltzer V. Multicentric nature of disease related to human papillomavirus infection of the female lower genital tract. *Obstet Gynecol* 1989;73:303.
59. Mcnicol PJ, Guijon FB, Paraskevas M, Brunham RC. Comparison of filter in situ deoxyribonucleic acid hybridization with cytologic, colposcopic, and histopathologic examination for detection of human papillomavirus infection in women with cervical intraepithelial neoplasia. *Am J Obstet Gynecol* 1989;160:265.
60. Broker TR, Botchan M. Papillomaviruses: retrospectives and prospectives. *Cancer Cells* 1986;4:17.
61. Syrjanen KJ. Papillomaviruses and cancer. In: Syrjanen KJ, Gissmann L, Koss L, eds. *Papillomaviruses and human disease*. Berlin: Springer Verlag, 1987:468.
62. Campion MJ, Franklin EW, Stacy CD, et al. Human papillomaviruses and anogenital neoplasia: a fresh look at the association. *South Med J* 1989;82:35.
63. Shah KV, Buscema J. Genital warts, papilloma viruses, and genital malignancies. *Ann Rev Med* 1988;39:371.
64. Kurman RJ, Schiffman MH, Lancaster WD, et al. Analysis of individual human papillomavirus types in cervical neoplasia: a possible role for type 18 in rapid progression. *Am J Obstet Gynecol* 1988;159:293.
65. Reid R, Greenberg M, Jenson AB, et al. Sexually transmitted papillomaviral infections. I. The anatomic distribution and pathologic grade of neoplastic lesions associated with different viral types. *Am J Obstet Gynecol* 1987; 156:212.
66. Gal D, Friedman M, Mitrani-Rosenbaum S. Transmissibility and treatment failures of different types of human papillomavirus. *Obstet Gynecol* 1989;73:308.
67. Syrjanen KJ, Mantyjarvi R, Saarikoski S, et al. Factors associated with progression of cervical human papillomavirus (HPV) infections into carcinoma in situ during a long term prospec-

tive follow-up. *Br J Obstet Gynecol* 1988; 95:1096.

68. Schiffman MH, Haley NJ, Felton JS, et al. Biochemical epidemiology of cervical neoplasia: measuring cigarette smoke constituents in the cervix. *Cancer Res* 1987;47:3886.
69. Vessey MP. Epidemiology of cervical cancer: Role of hormonal factors, cigarette smoking and occupation. In: Peto R, ZurHausen H, eds. *Viral etiology of cervical cancer.* New York: Cold Spring Harbor Laboratory, 1985:29.
70. Ritter DB, Kodish AS, Vermund SH, et al. Detection of human papillomavirus deoxyribonucleic acid in exfoliated cervicovaginal cells as a predictor of cervical neoplasia in a high-risk population. *Am J Obstet Gynecol* 1988; 159;1517.
71. Lorincz AT. Human papillomavirus detection tests. In: Holmes KK, Mardh P-A, Sparling PF, Wiesner PJ, eds. *Sexually transmitted diseases.* New York: McGraw-Hill, 1990:953.
72. Vermund SH, Schiffman MH, Goldberg GL, et al. Molecular diagnosis of genital human papillomavirus infection: Comparison of two methods used to collect exfoliated cervical cells. *Am J Obstet Gynecol* 1989;160:304.
73. Halpert R, Fruchter RG, Sedlis A, et al. Human papillomavirus and lower genital neoplasia in renal transplant patients. *Obstet Gynecol* 1986;68:251.
74. Schneider V, Kay S, Lee LM. Immunosuppression as a high-risk factor in the development of condyloma accuminatum and squamous neoplasia. *Acta Cytol* 1983;27:220.
75. Davis AJ, Emans SJ. Human papilloma virus infection in the pediatric and adolescent patient. *J Pediatr* 1989;115:1.
76. Simmons PD, Langlet F, Thin RNT. Cryotherapy versus electrocautery in the treatment of genital warts. *Br J Venereal Dis* 1981;57:273.
77. Ferenczy A. Treating genital condyloma during pregnancy with the CO_2 laser. *Am J Obstet Gynecol* 1984;148:9.
78. Corey L. Genital herpes. In: Holmes KK, Mardh P-A, Sparling PF, Wiesner PJ, eds. *Sexually transmitted diseases.* New York: McGraw-Hill, 1990:391.
79. Nahmias AJ, Roizman D. Infection with herpes simplex virus 1 and 2. *N Engl J Med* 1973; 29:667.
80. Corey L, Adams HG, Brown ZA, Holmes KK. Genital herpes simplex complications. *Ann Intern Med* 1983;98:958.
81. Barton IG, Kinghorn GR, Walker MJ, et al. Association of HSV1 with cervical infection [Letter]. *Lancet* 1981;2:1108.
82. Koutsky LA. Spectrum of symptomatic and silent genital herpes in women attending an STD clinic. Presented at the International Faculty STD Research, 7th meeting, Atlanta, Georgia, August 2–5, 1987.
83. Reeves WC, Corey L, Adams HG, et al. Risk of recurrence after first episodes of genital herpes: Relation to HSV type and antibody response. *N Engl J Med* 1981;305:315.
84. Zweerink HJ, Corey L. Virus specific antibodies for HSV-2 in sera from patients with genital herpes virus infection. *Infect Immunol* 1982; 37:413.
85. Siegel FP, Lopez C, Hammer GS, et al. Severe acquired immunodeficiency in male homosexuals manifested by chronic perianal ulcerative herpes simplex lesions. *N Engl J Med* 1988; 305:1439.
86. Greenblatt R, Lukehart S, Plummer F, et al. Genital ulceration as a risk factor for human immunodeficiency virus infection in Kenya. *AIDS* 1988;2:47.
87. Stamm W, Handsfield H, Rompalo A, et al. The association between genital ulcer disease and acquisition of HIV infection in homosexual men. *JAMA* 1988;260:1429.
88. Nahmias AJ, et al. Herpes simplex. In: Remington JS, Klein JO, eds. *Infectious diseases of the fetus and newborn infant.* Philadelphia: Saunders, 1983:636.
89. Brown ZA, Vontver LA, Benedetti J, et al. Genital herpes in pregnancy: Risk factors associated with recurrences and asymptomatic shedding. *Am J Obstet Gynecol* 1985;153:24.
90. Arvin AM, Hensleigh PA, Prober CG, et al. Failure of antepartum maternal cultures to predict the infant's risk of exposure to herpes simplex virus at delivery. *N Engl J Med* 1986;315:796.
91. Prober CG, Sullender WM, Yasukawa LL, et al. Low risk of herpes simplex virus infections in neonates exposed to the virus at the time of vaginal delivery to mothers with recurrent genital HSV infections. *N Engl J Med* 1987; 316:240.
92. Whitley RJ, Nahmias AJ, Visintine AM, et al. The natural history of herpes simplex virus infection of mother and newborn. *Pediatrics* 1980;66:489.
93. Gibb RS, Amstey MS, Sweet RL, et al. Management of genital herpes infection in pregnancy. *Obstet Gynecol* 1988;7:779.
94. Corey L, Spear PG. Infections with herpes simplex viruses. *N Engl J Med* 1986;314:749.
95. Corey L, Nahmias AJ, Guinan ME, et al. A trial of topical acyclovir in genital herpes simplex virus infections. *N Engl J Med* 1982; 106:1313.
96. Bryson YJ, Dillon M, Lovett M, et al. Treatment of first episodes of genital herpes simplex virus infection with oral acyclovir: a randomized double blind controlled trial in normal subjects. *N Engl J Med* 1983;308:916.
97. Mertz GJ, Critchlow CW, Benedett JK, et al. Double blind placebo-controlled trial of oral acyclovir in the first episode of genital herpes simplex virus infection. *JAMA* 1984;252:1147.
98. Corey L, Fife KH, Benedett JK, et al. Intravenous acyclovir for the treatment of primary genital herpes. *Ann Intern Med* 1983;98:914.
99. Reichman RC, Badger GJ, Mertz GJ, et al. Treatment of recurrent genital herpes simplex infections with oral acyclovir: a controlled trial. *JAMA* 1984;251:2103.

100. Douglas JM, Critchlow C, Benedetti J, et al. A double blind study of oral acyclovir for suppression of recurrences of genital herpes simplex virus infection. *N Engl J Med* 1984; 310:1551.
101. Strauss SE, Takiff HE, Seidlin M, et al. Suppressing of frequently recurring genital herpes: a placebo-controlled double blind trial of oral acyclovir. *N Engl J Med* 1984;310:1545.
102. Mindel A, Carney O, Freris M, et al. Dosage and safety of long term suppressive therapy for recurrent genital herpes. *Lancet* 1988;1:926.
103. Centers for Disease Control, Immunization Practices Advisory Committee. Protection against viral hepatitis. *MMWR* 1990;39(S-2):1.
104. Aller MJ, Ahtone J, Weisfuse I, et al. Hepatitis B virus transmission between heterosexuals. *JAMA* 1986;256:1307.
105. Szmuness W, Much I, Prince AM, et al. On the role of sexual behavior in the spread of hepatitis B infection. *Ann Intern Med* 1975;83:489.
106. Centers for Disease Control, Immunization Practices Advisory Committee. Prevention of perinatal transmission of hepatitis B virus: prenatal screening of all pregnant women for hepatitis B surface antigen. *MMWR* 1988;37:341.
107. Summers PR, Biswas MK, Pastorek JG, et al. The pregnant heptatis B carrier: evidence favoring comprehensive antepartum screening. *Obstet Gynecol* 1987;69:701.
108. Arevalo JA, Washington AE. Cost-effectiveness of prenatal screening and immunization for hepatitis B virus. *JAMA* 1988;259:365.
109. Weller TH, Hanshaw JB. Virologic and clinical observations on cytomegalic inclusion disease. *N Engl J Med* 1962;266:1233.
110. Wilkin JK. Molluscum contagiosum venereum in a women's outpatient clinic: a venereally transmitted disease. *Am J Obstet Gynecol* 1977;128:531.
111. Postlethwaite R. Molluscum contagiosum: a review. *Arch Environ Health* 1970;21:432.
112. Felman YM, Nikitas JA. Sexually transmitted molluscum contagiosum. *Dermatol Clin* 1983; 1:103.
113. Ginsburg CM. Management of selected skin and soft tissue infections. *Pediatr Infect Dis* 1986;5:735.
114. *Chlamydia trachomatis* infections. Policy guidelines for prevention and control. *MMWR* 1985;
34:535.
115. Fraser JJ, Retting PJ, Kaplan DW. Prevalence of cervical *Chlamydia trachomatis* and *Neisseria gonorrhoeae* in female adolescents. *Pediatrics* 1983;71:333.
116. Blythe MJ, Katz BP, Orr DP, et al. Historical and clinical factors associated with *Chlamydia trachomatis* genitourinary infection in female adolescents. *J Pediatr* 1988;112:1000.
117. Moscicki B, Shafer M, Millstein S, et al. The use and limitations of endocervical Gram stains and mucopurulentcervicitis as predictors for *Chlamydia trachomatis* in female adolescents. *Am J Obstet Gynecol* 1987;157:65.
118. Soren K, Willis E. Chlamydia and the adolescent girl. *Am J Dis Child* 1989;143:51.
119. Barnes RC, Holmes KK. Epidemiology of gonorrhea: current perspectives. *Epidemiol Rev* 1984;6:1.
120. Harrison HR, Constin M, Meder JB, et al. Cervical *Chlamydiatrachomatis* infection in university women: relationship to history, contraception, ectopy and cervicitis. *Am J Obstet Gynecol* 1985;153:244.
121. Brunham RC, Paavonen J, Stevens CE, et al. Mucopurulentcervicitis—the ignored counterpart in women of urethritisin men. *N Engl J Med* 1984;311:1.
122. Lindner LE, Geerling S, Nettum JA, et al. Clinical characteristics of women with chlamydia cervicitis. *J Reprod Med* 1988;33:684.
123. Paavonen J. *Chlamydia trachomatis*–induced urethritis in female partners of men with nongonoccal urethritis. *Sex Trans Dis* 1979;6:69.
124. Paavonen J, Kiviat N, Brunham RC, et al. Prevalence and manifestations of endometritis among women with cervicitis. *Am J Obstet Gynecol* 1985;152:280.
125. Brunham RC, Holmes KK, Embree JE. Sexually transmitted diseases in pregnancy. In: Holmes KK, Mardh PA, Sparling PF, Wiesner PJ, eds. *Sexually transmitted diseases*. New York: McGraw-Hill, 1990:771.
126. Washington AE, Sweet RL, Shafer MA. Pelvic inflammatory disease in the adolescent female and its sequelae. *J Adol Health Care* 1985; 6:298.
127. Stamm WE. Diagnosis of *Chlamydia trachomatis* genitourinary tract infections. *Ann Intern Med* 1988;108:710.
128. Centers for Disease Control. *1989 Sexually transmitted diseases treatment guidelines*. Atlanta, Georgia: 1989.
129. Ahmed-Jushuf IH, Arya OP, Hobson D, et al. Ciprofloxacin treatment of chlamydial infections of urogenital tracts of women. *Genitourin Med* 1988;64:14.
130. Hughes EG, Mowatt J, Spence JH. Endocervical *Chlamydia trachomatis* infection in Canadian adolescents. *Can Med Assoc J* 1989; 140:297.
131. Fraser JJ, Rettig PJ, Kaplan DW. Prevalence of cervical *Chlamydia trachomatis* and *Neisseria gonorrhoeae* in female adolescents. *Pediatrics* 1983;71:333.
132. Alexander-Rodriguez T, Vermund SH. Gonorrhea and syphilis in incarcerated urban adolescents: prevalence and physical signs. *Pediatrics* 1987;80:561.
133. Centers for Disease Control. *Sexually transmitted disease statistics, calendar year 1987, no. 316*. Atlanta: U.S. Public Health Service, 1988:1.
134. Hook EW III, Handsfield HH. Gonococcal infections in the adult. In: Holmes KK, Mardh PA, Sparling PF, Wiesner PJ, eds. *Sexually transmitted diseases*. New York: McGraw-Hill, 1990:771.
135. Holmes KK, Johnson DW, Trostle HJ. An es-

timate of the risk of men acquiring gonorrhea by sexual contact with infected females. *Am J Epidemiol* 1970;91:170.
136. Hooper RR, Reynolds GH, Jones OG, et al. Cohort study of venereal disease: I. The risk of gonorrhea transmission from infected women to men. *Am J Epidemiol* 1978;108:136.
137. Thin RN, Shaw EJ. Diagnosis of gonorrhea in women. *Br J Vener Dis* 1979;55:10.
138. Barlow D, Phillips I. Gonorrhea in women: diagnostic, clinical, and laboratory aspects. *Lancet* 1978;1:761.
139. Wiesner PJ, Tronca E, Bonin P, et al. Clinical spectrum of pharyngeal gonococcal infections. *N Engl J Med* 1973;288:181.
140. Tice W, Rodriguez VL. Pharyngeal gonorrhea. *JAMA* 1981;246:2717.
141. Hutt DM, Judson FN. Epidemiology and treatment of oro-pharyngeal gonorrhea. *Ann Intern Med* 1986;104:655.
142. Holmes KK, Eschenbach DA, Knapp JS. Salpingitis: overview of etiology and epidemiology. *Am J Obstet Gynecol* 1980;138:893.
143. Holmes KK, Counts GW, Beaty HN. Disseminated gonococcal infection. *Ann Intern Med* 1971;74:979.
144. Schink JC, Keith LG. Problems in the culture diagnosis of gonorrhea. *J Reprod Med* 1985; 30(suppl):244.
145. D'Angelo LJ, Mohla C, Sneed J, Woodward K. Diagnosing gonorrhea—a comparison of standard and rapid techniques. *J Adol Health Care* 1987;8:344.
146. Finch CA. Assessment of an enzyme immunoassay for diagnosing gonorrhea. *J Reprod Med* 1985;30(suppl):250.
147. Zenilman JM, Bonner M, Sharp KL, et al. Penicillinase producing *Neisseria gonorrhoeae* in Dade County, Florida: evidence of core-group transmitters and the impact of illicit antibiotics. *Sex Transm Dis* 1988;15:45.
148. Rice RJ, Thompson SE. Treatment of uncomplicated infections due to *Neisseria gonorrhoeaea:* a review of clinical efficacy and in vitro susceptibility studies from 1982 through 1985. *JAMA* 1986;255:1739.
149. Shafer MA, Sweet RL. Pelvic inflammatory disease in adolescent females. *Pediatr Clin North Am* 1989;36:513.
150. Westrom L. Incidence, prevalence, and trends of acute pelvic inflammatory disease and its consequences in industrialized countries. *Am J Obstet Gynecol* 1980;138:880.
151. Mardh P-A. An overview of infectious agents in salpingitis, their biology, and recent advances in methods of detection. *Am J Obstet Gynecol* 1980;138:933.
152. Sweet RL, Draper DL, Hadley WK. Etiology of acute salpingitis: influence of episode number and duration of symptoms. *Obstet Gynecol* 1981;58:62.
153. Persson E, Holmberg K, Dahlbren S, Nilsson L. Actinomycesisraelii in the genital tract of women with and without intrauterine contraceptive devices. *Acta Obstet Gynecol Scand* 1983;62:563.
154. Jacobson L, Westrom L. Objectivized diagnosis of acute pelvic inflammatory disease. *Am J Obstet Gynecol* 1980;138:905.
155. Jones RB, et al. Correlation between serum antichlamydial antibodies and tubal factors as a cause of infertility. *Fertil Steril* 1982;38:553.
156. Brunham RC, Maclean IW, Binns B, Peeling RW. *Chlamydiatrachomatis:* its role in tubal infertility. *J Infect Dis* 1985;152:127.
157. Tjiam KH, Zeilmaker GH, Alberda AT, et al. Prevalence of antibodies to *Chlamydia trachomatis, Neisseria gonorrheae,* and *Mycoplasma hominis* in infertile women. *Genitourin Med* 1985;61:175.
158. Katzman DK, Friedman IM, McDonald CA, Litt IF. *Chlamydiatrachomatis* Fitz-Hugh-Curtis syndrome without salpingitis in female adolescents. *Am J Dis Child* 1988;142:996.
159. Westrom L, Mardh P-A. Acute pelvic inflammatory disease (PID). In: Holmes KK, Mardh P-A, Sparling PF, Weisner PJ, eds. *Sexually transmitted diseases.* New York: McGraw-Hill, 1990:593.
160. Westrom L. *Diagnosis, aetiology, and prognosis of acute salpingitis* [Thesis]. Lund, Sweden: Studentlitteratur, 1976.
161. Landers DV, Sweet RL. Tubo-ovarian abscess. Contemporary approach to management. *Rev Infect Dis* 1983;5:876.
162. Hager WD, Eschenbach PA, Spence MR, Sweet RL. Criteria for diagnosis and grading of salpingitis. *Obstet Gynecol* 1983;61:113.
163. Hedberg E, Anberg A. Gonorrheal salpingitis: views on treatment and prognosis. *Fertil Steril* 1965;16:125.
164. Eschenbach DA. Epidemiology and diagnosis of acute pelvic inflammatory disease. *Obstet Gynecol* 1980;55:1425.
165. Handsfield HH, Lipman TO, Harnisch JP, et al. Asymptomatic gonorrhea in men: diagnosis, natural course, prevalence and significance. *N Engl J Med* 1974;290:117.
166. Schwartz SL, Krauss J. Persistent urethral leukocytosis and asymptomatic chlamydial urethritis. *J Infect Dis* 1979;140:614.
167. Stamm WE, Koutsky LA, Benedetti J, et al. *Chlamydia trachomatis* urethral infections in men. Prevalence, risk factors, and clinical manifestations. *Ann Intern Med* 1984;100: 47.
168. Washington AE, Weisner PJ. The silent clap. *JAMA* 1981;245:609.
169. Westrom L. Effect of pelvic inflammatory disease on fertility. *Am J Obstet Gynecol* 1975;121:707.
170. Kresch AJ, Seifer DB, Sachs LB, Barrese I. Laparoscopy in 100 women with pelvic pain. *Obstet Gynecol* 1984;64:672.
171. Centers for Disease Control. Ectopic pregnancy—United States, 1984–1985. *MMWR* 1988;37:367.
172. Svenson L, Mardh PA, Ahlgren M, Nodrenskjold F. Ectopic pregnancy and antibodies to *Chlamydia trachomatis. Fertil Steril* 1985; 44:313.
173. Brunham RC, Binns B, McDowell J, Paraske-

vas M. *Chlamydiatrachomatis* infection in women with ectopic pregnancy. *Obstet Gynecol* 1986;67:722.
174. Atrash HK, Friede A, Hogue CJR. Ectopic pregnancy mortality in the United States, 1970–1983. *Obstet Gynecol* 1987;70:817.
175. Westrom L. Impact of sexually transmitted diseases on human reproduction: Swedish studies of infertility and ectopic pregnancy. In: *Sexually transmitted diseases, status report, NIAID study group*. Washington, DC: NIH Publications, no. 81-2213, 1980:43.
176. Spiegel CA, Amsel R, Eschenbach DA, et al. Anaerobic bacteria in nonspecific vaginitis. *N Engl J Med* 1980;303:601.
177. Bump RC, Buesching WJ. Bacterial vaginosis in virginal and sexually active adolescent females: evidence against exclusive sexual transmission. *Obstet Gynecol* 1988;158:935.
178. Gardner HL, Dukes CD. *Haemophilus vaginalis* vaginitis. A newly defined specific infection previously classified "non-specific" vaginitis. *Am J Obstet Gynecol* 1955;69:962.
179. Pheifer TA, Forsyth PS, Durfee MA, et al. Non-specific vaginitis. Role of *Haemophilus vaginalis* and treatment with metronidazole. *N Engl J Med* 1978;298:1429.
180. Amsel R, Totten PA, Spiegel CA, et al. Nonspecific vaginitis: diagnostic criteria and microbial and epidemiologic associations. *Am J Med* 1983;74:14.
181. Spiegel CA, Amsel R, Holmes KK. Diagnosis of bacterial vaginosis by direct gram stain of vaginal fluid. *J Clin Microbiol* 1983;18:170.
182. Edelman DA, North BB. Treatment of bacterial vaginosis with intravaginal sponges containing metronidazole. *J Reprod Med* 1989;34:341.
183. Livengood CH, Thomason JL, Hill GB. Bacterial vaginosis: diagnostic and pathogenetic findings during topical clindamycin therapy. *Am J Obstet Gynecol* 1990;163:515.
184. Vejtorp M, Bollerup AC, Vejtorp L, et al. Bacterial vaginosis: a double-blind randomized trial of the effect of treatment of the sexual partner. *Br J Obstet Gynecol* 1988;95:920.
185. Gravett MG, Nelson P, DeRouent, et al. Independent associations of bacterial vaginosis and Chlamydiatrachomatis infection with adverse pregnancy outcome. *JAMA* 1986;256:1899.
186. Martius J, Krohn MJ, Hillier SL, et al. Relationship of vaginal lactobacillus species, cervical *Chlamydiatrachomatis*, and bacterial vaginosis to preterm birth. *Obstet Gynecol* 1988;71:89.
187. Gravett MG, Hummel D, Eschenbach DA, et al. Preterm labor associated with subclinical amniotic fluid infection and with bacterial vaginosis. *Obstet Gynecol* 1986;67:229.
188. Watts DH, Krohn MA, Hillier SL, Eschenbach DA. Bacterial vaginosis as a risk factor for post-Cesarean endometritis. *Obstet Gynecol* 1990;75:52.
189. Eschenbach DA, Hillier S, Critchlow C, et al. Diagnosis and clinical manifestations of bacterial vaginosis.
190. Willcox RR. Importance of the so-called "other" sexually transmitted diseases. *Br J Vener Dis* 1986;5:735.
191. Perine PL, Osoba AO. Lymphogranuloma venereum. In: Holmes KK, Mardh PA, Sparling PF, Weisner PH, eds. *Sexually transmitted diseases*. New York: McGraw-Hill, 1990:195.
192. D'Aunoy R, Von Haam E. Venereal lymphogranuloma. *Arch Pathol* 1939;27:1032.
193. Coutts WE. Lymphogranuloma venereum: a general review. *Bull WHO* 1950;2:545.
194. Schmid GP, Sanders LL, Blount JH, Alexander ER. Chancroid in the United States: re-establishment of an old disease. *JAMA* 1987; 258:3265.
195. Ronald AR, Albritton W. Chancroid and Haemophilus ducrey. In: Holmes KK, Mardh PA, Sparling PF, Weiser PJ, eds. *Sexually transmitted diseases*. New York: McGraw-Hill, 1990: 263.
196. Dangor Y, Ballard RC, Miller SD, Koornhof HJ. Treatment of chancroid. *Antimicrob Agents Chemother* 1990;34:1308.
197. Wysoki RS, Majmudar B, Willis D. Granuloma inguinale (Donavanosis) in women. *J Reprod Med* 1988;33:709.
198. Kuberski TM. Granuloma inguinale (Donavanosis). *Sex Transm Dis* 1980;7:29.
199. Goldberg J. Studies on granuloma inguinale: VIII. Some epidemiological considerations of the disease. *Br J Vener Dis* 1964;40:140.
200. Centers for Disease Control. *Sexually transmitted disease statistics, calendar year 1989, no. 73:2638*. Atlanta: U.S. Public Health Service, 1990.
201. Shroeter AL, Turner RH, Lucas JB, Brown WJ. Therapy for incubating syphilis: effectiveness of gonorrhea treatment. *JAMA* 1971; 218:711.
202. Hook EW III. Syphilis and HIV infection. *J Infect Dis* 1989;160:530.
203. Communicable Disease Center. *Serology and Evaluation and Research Assembly, 1956–1957*. Washington, DC: U.S. Department of Health, Education and Welfare, publication 650.
204. Deacon WE, Lucas JB, Price EV. Fluorescent treponemal antibody-absorption (FIA-ABS) test for syphilis. *JAMA* 1966;198:156.
205. Lesinski J, Krach J, Kadziewicz E. Specificity, sensitivity, and diagnostic value of the TPHA test. *Br J Vener Dis* 1974;50:334.
206. Moore JE, Mohr CF. Biologically false positive serologic tests for syphilis: type, incidence, and cause. *JAMA* 1952;150:467.
207. Tuffanellie DL, Wuepper KD, Bradford LL, Wood RM. Fluorescent treponemal antibody-absorption tests: studies of false positive reactions to tests for syphilis. *N Engl J Med* 1967;276:258.
208. Billstein SA: Human lice. In Holmes KK, Mardh P-A, Sparling PF, Weisner PH, eds. *Sexually transmitted diseases*. New York: McGraw-Hill, 1990:467.
209. Kalter DC, Sparber J, Rosen T, Matarasso S. Treatment of pediculosis pubis. Clinical comparison of efficacy and tolerance of 1% lindane

shampoo vs. 1% permethrin cremerinse. *Arch Dermatol* 1987;123:1315.
210. Green MS. Epidemiology of scabies. *Epidemiol Rev* 1989;11:126.
211. Sobel JD. Pathophysiology of vulvovaginal candidiasis. *J Reprod Med* 1989;34:572.
212. Drake TE, Mailbach HI. Candida and candidiasis: cultural conditions, epidemiology, and pathogenesis. *Postgrad Med* 1973;53:83.
213. Sobel JD, et al. *C.albicans* adherence to vaginal epithelialcells. *J Infect Dis* 1981;143:76.
214. Soll DR. High-frequency switching in *Candida albicans* and its relations to vaginal candidiasis.
215. Morton RS, Rashid S. Candidal vaginitis: natural history, predisposing factors and prevention. *Proc R Soc Med* 1977;70(suppl 4):3.
216. Odds FC. Candida and candidosis. Baltimore: University Park Press, 1979.
217. Oriel JD, Waterworth PM. Effect of minocycline and tetracycline on the vaginal yeast flora. *J Clin Pathol* 1975;28:403.
218. Witkin SS, Jeremias J, Ledger WJ. A localized vaginal allergic response in women with recurrent vaginitis. *J Allergy Clin Immunol* 1988; 81:412.
219. Fleury FJ. Adult vaginitis. *Clin Obstet Gynecol* 1981;24:407.
220. Imam N, Carpenter CC, Mayer KH, et al. Hierarchical pattern of mucosal candida infections in HIV seropositive women. *Am J Med* 1990;89:142.
221. Horowitz BJ, Edelstein SW, Lippman L. Sexual transmission of Candida. *Obstet Gynecol* 1987;69:883.
222. Brown D, Kaufman RH. Vulvovaginitis. In: Glass RH, ed. *Office gynecology*. Baltimore: Williams and Wilkins, 1988.
223. Hirsch HA. Clinical evaluation of terconazole. European experience. *J Reprod Med* 1989; 34:503.
224. Sobel JD. Recurrent vulvovaginal candidiasis. A prospective study of the efficacy of maintenance ketoconazole therapy. *N Engl J Med* 1986;315:1455.
225. Brammer KW, Feczko JM. Single dose oral fluconazole in the treatment of vaginal candidiasis. *Ann NY Acad Sci* 1988;554:561.
226. Thomason JL, Gelbart SM. *Trichomonas vaginalis*. *Obstet Gynecol* 1989;74:539.
227. Weston TET, Nicol CS. Natural history of trichomonal infection in males. *Br J Vener Dis* 1963;39:251.
228. Fouts AC, Kraus SJ. *Trichomonas vaginalis:* re-evaluation of its clinical presentation and laboratory diagnosis. *J Infect Dis* 1980; 141:137.
229. Wolner-Hanssen P, Krieger JN, Stevens CE. Clinical manifestations of vaginal trichomoniasis. *JAMA* 1989;261:571.
230. Krieger JN, Tam MR, Stevens CE, et al. Diagnosis of trichomoniasis: comparison of conventional wet-mount examination with cytologic studies, cultures, and monoclonal antibody staining of direct specimens. *JAMA* 1988; 259:1223.
231. Lossick JG. Treatment of *Trichomonas vaginalis* infections. *Rev Infect Dis* 1982;4 (suppl):801.
232. Centers for Disease Control. Premarital sexual experience among adolescent women, United States, 1970–1988. *MMWR* 1991;39:929–932.

Pediatric and Adolescent Gynecology,
edited by S. E. Carpenter and J. A. Rock.
Raven Press, Ltd., New York © 1992.

20
Uterovaginal Anomalies

Bruce L. Tjaden and *John A. Rock

David Grant USAF Medical Center/SGHO, Travis AFB, California 94535-5300; and
**The Johns Hopkins Hospital, Baltimore, Maryland 21205*

OVARIAN DEVELOPMENT

The gonads develop during the fifth week, initially as a thickening of the medial aspect of the urogenital ridge. This thickening, known as the genital ridge, is produced by a proliferation of coelomic epithelium and the associated underlying mesenchyme. The gonads arise from three sources: primordial germ cells, the previously mentioned mesenchyme, and the coelomic epithelium of the genital ridge (1). The germ cells are extragonadal in origin; arising from the wall of the yolk sac they migrate to the genital ridge where they undergo differentiation and proliferation (1). The germ cells are ultimately incorporated into the gonad by finger-like down growth of the overlying epithelium known as primary sex cords. This stage is known as the indifferent stage of gonadal development (1). The genetic makeup of the embryo will determine further gonadal development. In XY embryos, the inner medulla of the gonad develops and the outer cortex regresses to produce a testis, whereas in embryos with an XX complement the outer cortex develops and the inner medulla regresses to produce an ovary.

GENITAL DUCT DEVELOPMENT

As with ovarian development, there is also an indifferent stage of development of the internal genital duct (1). During this brief time period, it is impossible to differentiate male from female embryos. Two pairs of genital ducts develop in both sexes: the mesonephric ducts and the paramesonephric ducts. The mesonephric ducts drain the mesonephric kidneys which function briefly, if at all, in human embryos. The paramesonephric ducts develop on each side of the urogenital ridge from invagination of coelomic epithelium lateral and ventral to the mesonephric duct. The edges of these invaginations approach each other and fuse to form the paramesonephric ducts. The cranial ends of the ducts open into the abdominal cavity. Migrating caudally, moving lateral and parallel to the mesonephric ducts, each of the mullerian ducts travels to the caudal end of the mesonephros, at which point both paramesonephric ducts turn medially and cross ventral to the mesonephric ducts. The paramesonephric ducts meet and fuse in the midline forming the uterovaginal primordium. This tubular structure projects into the posterior urogenital sinus near the caudal region of the embryo. This elevation is called the Müllerian tubercle. A mesonephric duct enters the urogenital sinus on each side of this tubercle. Paired endodermal invaginations: the sinovaginal bulbs grown from the urogenital sinus into the caudal end of the uterovaginal primordium. The endodermal cells of the bulbs form a solid mass called the vaginal plate, the center of which ultimately degenerates to form the vaginal canal. Distally, the vaginal canal is separated from the urogenital sinus by the hymen until late in fetal life at which time the hymen usually ruptures affording external communication for the vaginal canal.

In embryos with ovaries (or without testes), the mesonephric ducts regress and the paramesonephric ducts develop into the female genital tract (1). The cranial or unfused portions of the ducts become the fallopian tubes. The caudal portion (the fused portion of the ducts forming the uterovaginal primordium), gives rise to the epithelium and the glands of the uterus, whereas the underlying stroma and myometrium are derived from the surrounding mesenchyme (1). The endometrium is derived from epithelium of the mullerian ducts. This epithelium forms the endometrial glands which in turn provoke the development of supporting stroma. The vaginal epithelium is derived from the endoderm of the urogenital sinus while the fibromuscular wall of the vagina develops from the uterovaginal primordium.

The uterus develops from the paired mullerian ducts forming the adult midline unpaired structure. This results from three well defined growth phases: contact of the ducts, fusion of the duct walls, and involution of the dividing septum. Ducts of unequal size or growth rates may result in a unicornuate uterus. A fusion defect may lead to a didelphic or bicornuate uterus while defects in the involution process usually result in a uterine septum.

The cervix is formed about week 20 of embryonic life (2). It is a result of condensation of stromal cells around a specific site of the fused mullerian ducts.

The upper third of the vagina is formed from the mullerian tuberacle while the lower two-thirds develop from the vaginal plate of the urogenital sinus (1). Apparently, Müllerian development and estrogenic stimulation are important for the induction of vaginal development (1). Failure in development of the mullerian ducts at any time from their origin at 5 weeks to their fusion with the urogenial sinus at 8 weeks may lead to partial or complete vaginal agenesis.

The entirely separate origin of the gonads from the gonadal ridges explains the infrequent association of uterovaginal anomalies with ovarian anomalies. Nevertheless, the gonads are important in Müllerian and

Wolffian development. Presence of testicular tissue causes regression of mullerian tissue and promotes development of Wolffian duct structures. Now classic studies by Jost have demonstrated the importance of functional gonadal tissue in the development of Müllerian and Wolffian structures (3).

ASSOCIATION OF RENAL ANOMALIES

The metanephros (the permanent or adult kidney) initially arises as a ureteric bud off the mesonephros (1). Factors affecting the development of the mesonephric duct or the paramesonephric duct may lead to abnormal renal development. Mesonephric duct agenesis would result not only in unilateral agenesis of the wolffian derived genital structures but also unilateral renal agenesis. Thompson and Lynn (4) have reported that 40% of patients with congenital absence of the kidney will be found to have associated genital anomalies.

CLASSIFICATION OF UTEROVAGINAL ANOMALIES

Previously organized on a clinical basis continued research has brought about classification of most uterovaginal anomalies on embryologic grounds. Conversely, the American Fertility Society has devised a classification scheme of mullerian anomalies based upon the degree of failure of normal development (5). The system separates the anomalies into groups with similar clinical manifestation and prognosis for fetal salvage upon treatment. This classification system does not include vaginal anomalies but allows the provider to describe anomalies involving the vagina, tubes or urinary tract as associated malformations.

A modification of the AFS classification system of uterovaginal anomalies based on embryologic considerations has been proposed and is described as follows (J. A. Rock, unpublished observations).

Class I: Dysgenesis of the Müllerian Ducts

Dysgenesis of the Müllerian ducts or agenesis of the uterus and the vagina, the Mayer-Rokitansky-Kuster-Hauser syndrome, is characterized by the absence of the vagina with or without uterine remnants.

Class II: Disorders of Vertical Fusion of the Müllerian Ducts

Disorders of vertical fusion are defects in the fusion between the down growing Müllerian ducts and the upgrowing derivatives of the urogenital sinus. These are usually characterized by patients with an atretic portion of the vagina. This may be a thick segment or a thin membrane and can be further classified as obstructing or nonobstructing. Regardless of the length of the septum of these disorders should be regarded as a transverse vaginal septum. The so-called partial vaginal agenesis with a uterus and cervix present can or should be considered a misnomer as it probably represents a large segment of atretic vagina. The incidence of urinary anomalies are what would be expected with a vertical fusion disorder. Patients with cervical agenesis or dysgenesis are also included in this group.

Class III: Disorders of Lateral Fusion of the Müllerian Ducts

Disorders of lateral fusion of the paramesonephric ducts may be symmetric or asymmetric and may or may not be obstructed. An example of symmetric unobstructed defect would be the double uterus while an example of asymmetric obstructed defect would be unilateral vaginal obstruction or an obstructed uterine horn. Obstructed lesions associated with disorders of lateral fusion are particularly noteworthy in that obstruction is unilateral and almost invariably associated with absence of the ipsilateral kidney. Bilateral obstruction presumably would be associated with bilateral absence of the kidneys not compatible with viability in the developing embryo.

There are two varieties of asymmetric obstruction with ipsilateral renal agenesis: (a) unicornuate uterus with a noncommunicating horn which contains menstruating endometrium or perhaps unilateral obstruction of a cavity of a double uterus and (b) unilateral vaginal obstruction with a double uterus present.

Symmetric unobstructed disorders of lateral fusion include essentially five groups of disorders: (a) didelphic uterus; (b) bicornuate uterus; (c) septate uterus (each a type of double uterus); (d) T-shaped uterus; and (e) unicornuate uterus with or without a rudimentary horn.

The septum within a septate uterus may be complete or partial. When the septum is complete there are inevitably two cervices with a longitudinal vaginal septum, which may be complete (extending to the introitus) or partial (extending partially down with vaginal canal). The bicornuate uterus may also have a partial or near complete separation of the uterine cavities. The term arcuate uterus should be considered a radiologic term referring to a slight septum in the uterine fundus.

The unicornuate uterus may have an attached horn with a cavity which communicates with a unicornuate uterus. Alternatively, there may or may not be a contralateral uterine horn with or without functional endometrium.

Class IV: Unusual Configurations of Vertical/Lateral Fusion Defects

This category includes combinations of uterovaginal anomalies, in other words, combined lateral and vertical fusion defects that do not fit into other categories.

Obstructed defects require immediate attention to remove the obstructing membrane and stop retrograde menstruation. When there is no obstruction, immediate medical attention is not mandated, however, intervention may be ultimately necessary to improve reproductive or coital function.

CLINICAL MANIFESTATIONS OF CLASS I ANOMALIES: DYSGENESIS OF THE MÜLLERIAN DUCTS

Failure of development of the mullerian ducts at any time between their origin and their fusion with the urogenital sinus results in failure of development of the uterus and vagina. The Mayer-Rokitansky-Kuster-Hauser syndrome is the most common clinical example of this anomaly. In approximately 90% of patients, the uterus is present in the form of a rudimentary anlagen with congenital absence of the vagina. Some series have included patients with a uterus and with absence of varying lengths of the vagina, however, these patients are generally not considered to have Rokitansky's syndrome. The latter group of patients are more appropriately considered under the group of defects in vertical fusion. There is a homogeneity and specificity of the Rokitansky syndrome, that is the absence of a vagina and uterus with a high incidence of urinary tract anomalies. Patients with disorders of vertical fusion have a low incidence of urinary tract anomalies.

The incidence of Mayer-Rokitansky-Kuster-Hauser syndrome was reported as one in 4,000 admissions at the Mayo Clinic (6). Evans reported the incidence as one in 10,588 female births in Michigan from 1963 to 1967 (7). As these patients have a 46 XX karyotype and normal ovarian function with normal development of external genitalia and secondary sexual characteristics they usually present with amenorrhea. Ovulation occurs normally, but as these patients lack a uterus and vagina, menstruation does not occur. Abnormal ovarian function as in PCO and gonadal dysgenesis have been reported in patients with Rokitansky's syndrome (8). An exact genetic etiologic diagnosis has not been elucidated. The discordance of monozygotic twins has been reported (9). The occurrence of complete vaginal agenesis in sisters with a 46 XX karyotype suggests an autosomal mode of inheritance at least for these patients (9). Shokeir (10) investigated 13 families with mullerian duct aplasia and found similarly affected females in 10 families, usually on the paternal side. These findings suggest a female limited autosomal dominant inheritance of a mutant gene transmitted by the male relatives. Knab (11) has suggested that the possible etiologic factors of the Rokitansky syndrome are (a) inappropriate production of mullerian regressive factor(s), (b) regional absence of deficiency of estrogen receptors limited to the lower mullerian duct, (c) arrest of mullerian duct development by teratogenic agents, (d) mesenchymal inductive defect, and (e) sporadic gene mutation.

A significant number of patients with mullerian agenesis will have associated anomalies of the upper mullerian duct system as well as anomalies of other organ systems. In the classic form of the mullerian agenesis the uterus is present only in the form of bilateral rudimentary uterine anlagen. These anlagen are located on the lateral pelvic side wall adjacent to the ovaries they are usually connected to the fallopian tubes (Fig. 1). However, they are usually not palpable on bimanual examination. The anlagen may or may not have endometrial tissue, even if the endometrium is functional the cavity of the analagen may not communicate directly with the peritoneal cavity as often there is an obstruction located at the junction of the tube and the uterine bulb. Occasionally anlagen communicate with the peritoneal cavity via the fallopian tubes and active endometrium if present may regurgitate into the peritoneal cavity.

Renal anomalies are perhaps the most well known anomalies associated with Rokitansky syndrome. Fore has (12) reported that 47% of patients in whom evaluation of the urologic tract was performed had associated urologic anomalies. Other studies

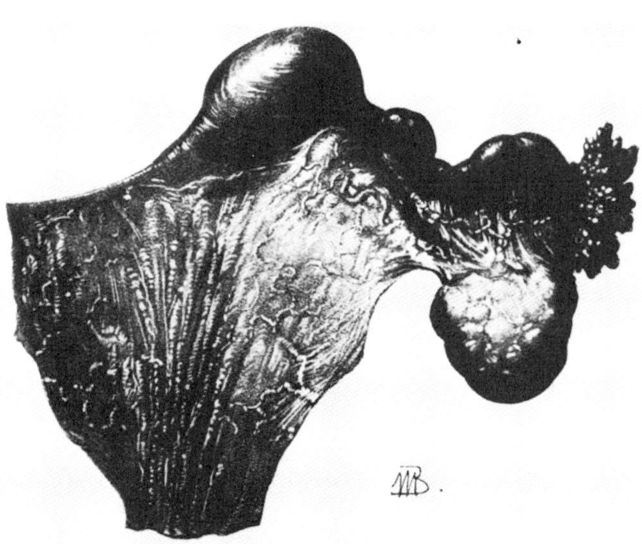

FIG. 1. Left tube and ovary and uterine remnant. The tube and ovary are of normal size. (From ref. 41, with permission.)

have shown approximately 30% of patients with complete vaginal agenesis are found to have significant anomalies.

Griffin (13) found a 12% incidence of skeletal abnormalities in patients with vaginal agenesis. Most of the anomalies involved the vertebral column although abnormalities of the ribs and extremities and digits have been reported.

Laboratory and Diagnostic Testing

Chromosomal analysis to rule out androgen insensitivity or some aberration of the MRKH syndrome should be done. An intravenous pyelogram (IVP) is mandatory to define the excretory system and rule out anomalies. These radiographs can be used to evaluate the lower spine for skeletal anomalies. If symptoms suggest an active uterine anlagen or if a pelvic mass is present appropriate studies such as ultrasonography or MRI can be used to differentiate between hematometria, hematocolpos, endometriomas or other cysts.

Treatment

Preoperative considerations. If functional endometrial tissue is present symptoms from cryptomenorrhea will begin soon after secondary sexual characteristics start to develop. Surgical extripation of the anlagen will afford complete relief of symptoms. Occasionally patients will present with dyspareunia but most commonly patients present around the age of 15 or 16 with primary amenorrhea.

Formerly, it was customary to advise surgical correction until just prior to marriage. More recently the procedure is being performed between the ages of 17–20 when the patient is emotionally mature and intellectually capable of understanding the operative procedure and partaking in her postoperative care which is an extremely important variable in terms of outcome.

Psychological counseling is extremely important in the management of these patients. Evans (14) reported a 15% incidence of psychiatric problems in his patients and has suggested that psychiatric intervention should be initiated prior to surgical intervention. The single most important factor in determining the success of vaginoplasty is the psychological adjustment of the patient to her anomaly.

Methods of Creating a Vagina

Both surgical and nonsurgical methods for creating a vagina have been described and successfully utilized.

Nonsurgical methods utilize dilatation of the vaginal dimple to create a functional vagina. The first method is that described by Robert Frank in 1938 and involves active manipulation by the patient to dilate the neovaginal space (15). Ingram described a technique of creating a new vagina using dilators especially designed for use with a bicycle seat stool (16) (Fig. 2). Ingram reported that 10 of 12 patients with vaginal agenesis and 10 of 14 patients with vaginal stenosis were able to achieve satisfactory vaginal depth and have acceptable coital function (16).

In younger less motivated patients with frank dilatation, technique may prove to be very difficult. At the Johns Hopkins Hospital, we have been encouraged by our results with the Ingram method and we strongly encourage our patients with a vaginal dimple to attempt this method of passive vaginal dilatation as often a major surgical case can be avoided.

There are several described surgical methods of creating a vaginal space. The experience at the Johns Hopkins Hospital has shown us that the McIndoe procedure, or more appropriately the Abbe-Wharton-McIndoe procedure, is superior to all others (17). Under special circumstances, the vulvovaginal pouch of Williams or the sig-

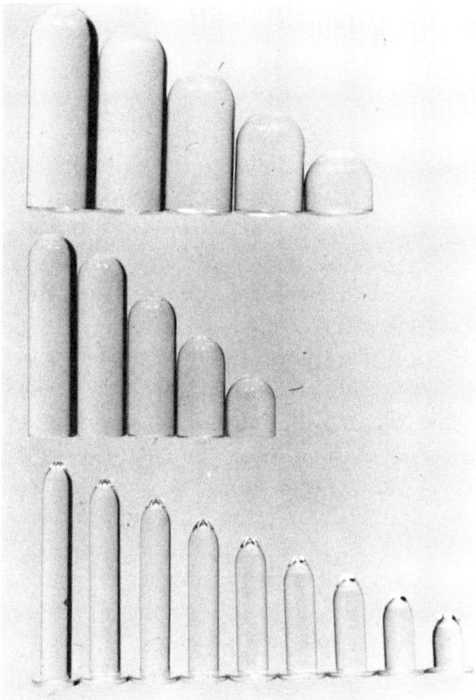

FIG. 2. Series of dilators for passive dilatation.

moid transplant of Pratt may be indicated (18, 19). In essence, a skin graft is taken from the buttock, placed around a vaginal form of foam rubber which is then placed into a surgically created space between the vagina and the rectum.

Serious complications associated with the McIndoe procedure have diminished significantly as techniques and experience have improved. Complications, however, still exist. These include morbidity and mortality from anesthesia, infection, hemorrhage and lack of take of the graft and formation of postoperative granulation tissue. Fistulas from the lower urinary tract or the rectum into the neovagina have been reported to occur in approximately 4% of patients. Malignancies have also been reported to occur in the neovagina (20, 21).

Other surgical procedures have been utilized and may be applicable in special cases, however, the excellent results obtained at the Johns Hopkins Hospital following a modified McIndoe vaginoplasty have prompted us to recommend this operation as the procedure of choice for those women unable to achieve sufficient vaginal length with dilatation or those women with a flat perineum (22).

CLINICAL MANIFESTATIONS OF CLASS II ANOMALIES: LATERAL FUSION DEFECTS

The problems associated with vertical fusion include transverse vaginal septum with or without obstruction. The incidence of transverse vaginal septum have been reported at 1 in 2,100, to 1 in 72,000 (23).

A transverse vaginal septum can develop in any location in the vagina but is more common in the upper vagina at the point of junction between the vaginal plate and the caudal end of the fused mullerian ducts. This defect is thought to be secondary to failure of resorption of the tissue that separates the two embryologic components or by failure of fusion of the two layers.

Septal lengths are variable (Fig. 3). A local abnormality of the vaginal mesoderm or failure of canalization of the epithelial vaginal plate may be the cause. The portion of the vagina originating from the urogenital sinus may at times be considerably more than one-fifth and thus a high transverse vaginal septum may represent the junction of an abnormally long urogenital sinus contribution and a short mullerian portion. Alternatively, there may be a long atretic segment between a small vaginal pouch and a high small segment of vagina.

A septum may be located in the upper, middle or lower portion of the vagina. At The Johns Hopkins Hospital, we have found the incidence to be 46%, 35%, and 19%, respectively (24); while Lodi has reported an incidence of 46%, 40%, and 14%, respectively (25). The thicker septum tend to be located nearer the cervix. In contrast

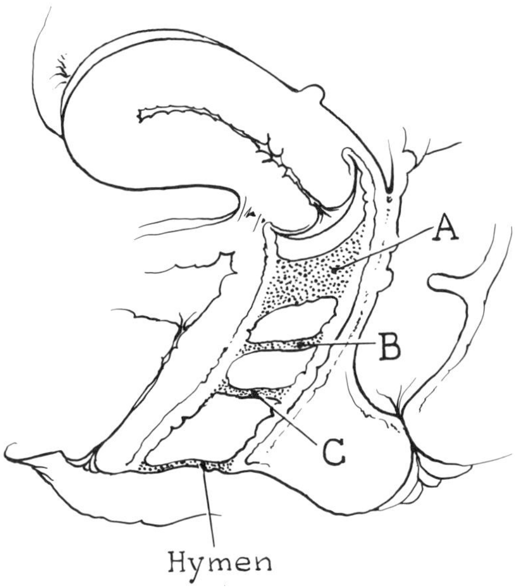

FIG. 3. Positions of septa responsible for complete vaginal obstruction. **A:** High transverse vaginal septum (most commonly thicker than the septum of the middle or lower vagina). **B:** Transverse vaginal septum of the middle third of the vagina. **C:** Transverse vaginal septum of the lower third of the vagina. (From ref. 24, with permission.)

with congenital absence of the mullerian ducts the transverse vaginal septum is associated with few urologic abnormalities. In neonates and young infants, imperforate transverse vaginal septum with obstruction may lead to serious and life threatening problems caused by the compression of surrounding organs by fluid collected above the septum. The fluid is a result of maternal estrogen stimulation of fetal mullerian glandular epithelium. Continued fluid collection in infants even after the first year has been reported. The distended vagina above the septum may create a large mass that can compress abdominal or pelvic organs, vasculature or limit the movement of the diaphragm. Neonatal fatalities have been reported. The hydrocolpos develops along the axis of the upper vagina and therefore may not produce a bulge in the outlet or the perineum even if pressure is applied to the mass. After evaluation of the infant the fluid collection should be drained by incising the septum through a perineal approach.

Vaginal stenosis may develop after the initial procedure, thus close follow-up is required to assure that reaccumulation has not occurred. Vaginal reconstructive surgery may be necessary in later years to allow adequate menstruation and coital function. Symptoms may not develop until the pubertal years at which time a hematocolpos may develop. Patients usually present with cyclic lower abdominal pain, amenorrhea and gradual development of a central pelvic mass. Occasionally, a small tract may allow intermittent passage of menstrual egress. A septum large enough to allow pregnancy may present a problem for the first time as dystocia during labor.

Surgical therapy involves incising a transverse septum but the specific therapy of choice will depend upon the extent and the location of the septum. Therapy for complete obstructing transverse vaginal septum in the lower and middle thirds of the vagina involves excising the septum followed by an anastomosis of the upper and lower vaginal segments (Fig. 4). Others propose a Z-plasty to bridge the gap between the upper and lower portions of the vagina.

The high transverse vaginal septum may pose a difficult surgical problem in that anastomosis of the upper and lower segments may be impossible. In such cases a space is created between the rectum and the bladder to permit identification of the obstructed upper vagina. The mass that has resulted from accumulated menstrual blood must be distinguished from the bladder and the rectum a process that may be facilitated by the mass itself. Laparotomy may be required when it is not possible to delineate the rectum from the bladder or the mass. A sound is passed transfundally through the uterus, through the cervix to tent the vaginal septum where upon the surgeon can make the appropriate incision (Fig. 5). Usu-

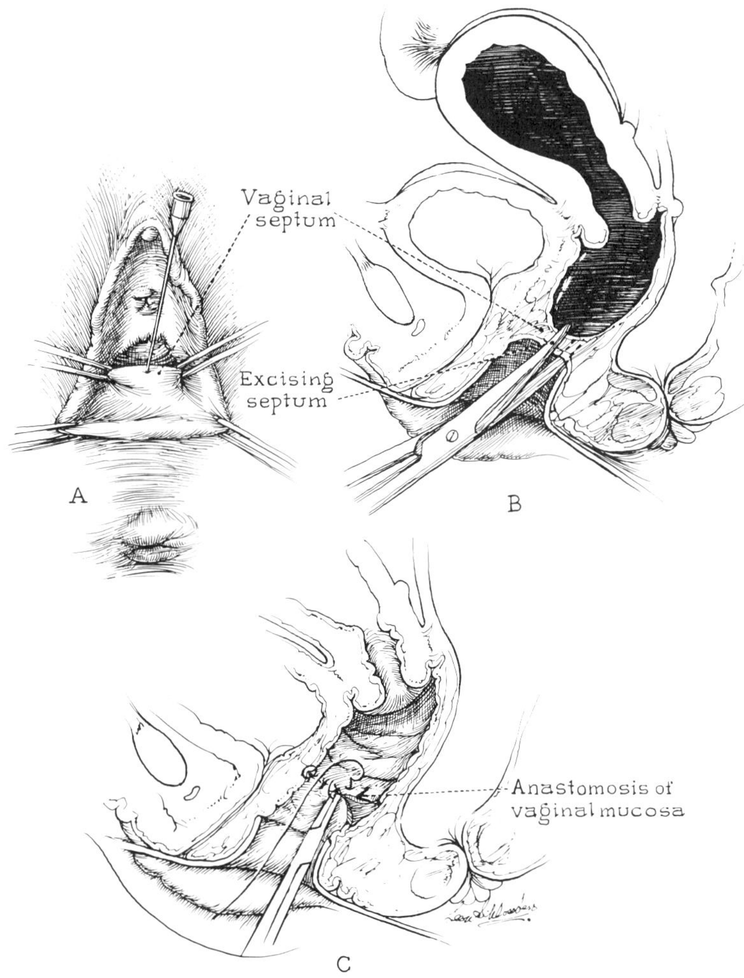

FIG. 4. Transverse vaginal septum of the middle third of the vagina. **A:** The wall of the septum is grasped with Allis clamps. A 14-gauge needle is placed into the vaginal septum, showing the plane of the mass and revealing the trapped accumulated blood. **B:** The septum is then incised with Mayo scissors. The vaginal septum is excised. **C:** The vagina is anastomosed with interrupted sutures of 2–0 chromic catgut (From ref. 26, with permission).

ally, the mass can be readily elucidated with digital exploration. The mass can be probed with an aspirating needle to assure its proper location, over which the septum can be incised with a scapel. Because the distance between the upper and lower segment is frequently too great to permit anastomosis, an indwelling Lucite form consisting of a bulbous end and a channel through which menstrual blood may drain is placed into the vagina. The form can be anchored with a retaining harness. The harness can be removed a few days later after which time the bulbous end of the Lucite form will retain its position in the vagina. The form is left in place for approximately 6 months to be followed by a regular course of vaginal dilatation on a daily basis for another two to four months. The vaginal dilatation is necessary to prevent scarring and stenosis.

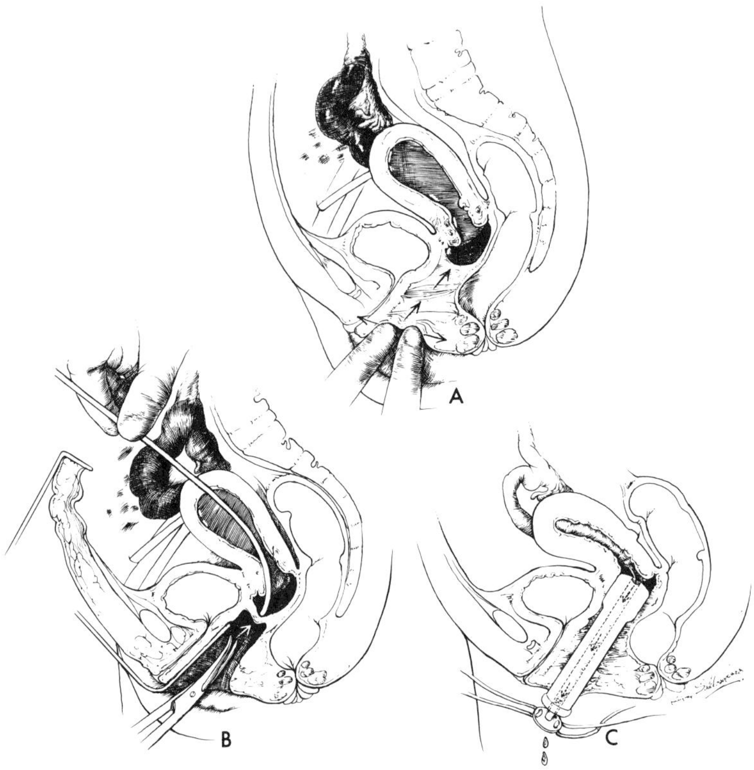

FIG. 5. The surgical management of a high transverse vaginal septum where the upper vagina cannot be safely entered without risk of damage to the bladder or the rectum. **A:** Creation of a neovaginal space. **B:** If unable to enter the vagina from below, a sound may be passed through the uterine fundus to tent the upper vagina. **C:** A Lucite form may be placed in the neovagina, the tip of which occupies the upper vagina space. (From ref. 42, with permission.)

One measure of success of surgical procedures to correct a complete transverse vaginal septum is subsequent pregnancy rates. Location of the vaginal septum is an important determinate of success. The higher the location the lower the success rates (26). In comparing success of corrective procedures the delay between the onset of the symptoms and correction of the defect may directly effect fertility status (Tables 1 and 2). Likewise, patients with an intact vagina obstructed only by an imperforate hymen may be able to accommodate more menstrual blood than the patient with a high transverse septum. The latter case may predispose more to retrograde menstruation and subsequently may lead to endometriosis and the sequelae that follow. Thus, prompt diagnosis and surgical correction to drain the accumulated blood may preserve fertility.

Congenital Absence or Dysgenesis of the Cervix

Agenesis or atresia of the cervix is an uncommon clinical entity. It is often associated with absence or atresia of the vagina. In many cases cyclic abdominal pain and amenorrhea are the presenting symptoms. The diagnosis is difficult to make prior to surgery but the clinician can be aided immensely by radiographic procedures such

TABLE 1. *Pregnancy success following surgical correction of an intact hymen versus correction of a complete transverse vaginal septum*

	Hymen	Transverse septum	Total
Patients	22	26	48
Adequate follow-up	18	22	40
Patients attempting pregnancy	15	19	34
Patients pregnant[a]	13 (86%)	9 (47%)	22 (65%)
Patients with a living child	10 (66%)	7 (36%)	17 (50%)
Total pregnancies	20	18	38
Term	16	8	24
Premature	1	1	2
Abortion	3	9	12

[a]$P < 0.05$ (χ^2 analysis).

as ultrasonography and magnetic resonance imaging (MRI). Making the correct diagnosis prior to surgical intervention offers significant advantages in patient care, the most important of which is preoperative counseling and planning.

Cervical anomalies occur in three forms: (a) aplasia (complete absence of the cervix), (b) absence of the cervix except for small inclusions of endocervical type tissue in a bed of fibrous tissue, and (c) presence of an endocervical stroma, however, there is complete atresia of the endocervical canal.

Treatment of Cervical Agenesis

Many methods have been tried to create a passage through the dense fibrous tissue between the uterine cavity and the vagina. Occasionally, success in maintaining vaginal patency has been reported. Cyclic menstruation and pregnancy have been reported. Vaginal stenosis and constriction are major complications after surgical correction. Other complications include endometriosis along the constructed tract, and recurrent and severe pelvic infections. Many authors have recommended hysterectomy for patients with a functioning corpus with an absence of the cervix. Early hysterectomy will help to preserve ovarian function as the ovaries will not become involved in endometriosis or pelvic infections. Nevertheless, Zarou (27) reported a successful pregnancy in a patient with cervical atresia who had undergone construction of a permanent fistula tract from the uterus to the vagina. Faber reported suc-

TABLE 2. *Pregnancy success following surgical correction of complete transverse vaginal septum*

Site of septum	Lower third	Middle third	Upper third	Total
Patients	5	9	12	26
Adequate follow-up	5	8	9	22 (84%)
Patients attempting pregnancy	4	7	8	19 (73%)
Patients pregnant	4	3	2	9 (47%)
Patients with a living child	4	2	1	7 (36%)
Total pregnancies	6	4	8	18
Term	5	2	1	8
Premature	0	1	0	1
Abortion	1	1	7	9

cessfully maintaining menstrual flow in four patients undergoing similar procedures but pregnancy had not been achieved (28). Cukier et al. (29) have reported a patient with congenital absence of the cervix by construction of aneocervical canal with a split thickness skin graft. In this patient menstruation continued although pregnancy had not been accomplished. More recently attempts to graft the internal portion of the atretic cervix have been successful. Hampton et al. (30) and Thijssen (31) using advanced reproductive technologies report two additional patients delivering a viable pregnancy.

Initially, it may be difficult to distinguish between cervical atresia and high transverse vaginal septum. Dissection begins from below. If it is impossible to enter the mass, laparotomy is performed. If the cervix is atretic a cervicovaginal fistula may be created if cervical stroma is present and if establishment of cyclic menstrual flow is desired. There is general agreement that if the cervix is absent a hysterectomy is advisable (Fig. 6). The ovaries should be preserved so that the patient may consider *in vitro* fertilization with a donor or host uterus.

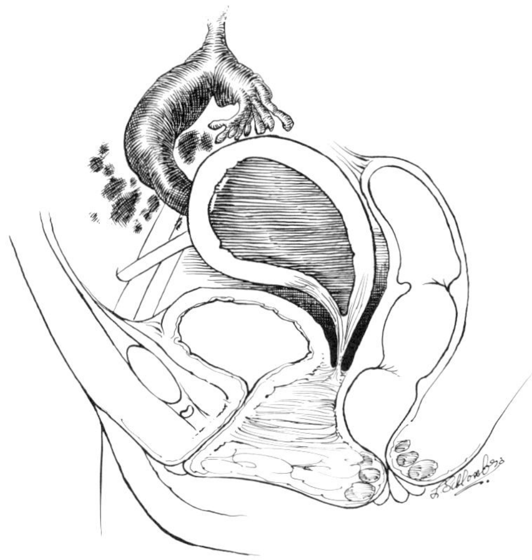

FIG. 6. Congenital absence of uterine cervix with cervical stroma which may contain endocervical glands. (From ref. 43, with permission.)

CLINICAL MANIFESTATIONS OF CLASS III ANOMALIES: LATERAL FUSION DEFECTS

Defects of lateral (midline) fusion can be divided into two groups: (a) those with obstruction and (b) those without obstruction.

Unobstructed lateral fusion disorders include bicornuate, septate or didelphic uterus (Fig. 7). Complete failure of midline fusion may result in two uterine horns, two cervices and two vaginas. Partial failure of fusion may result in a single vagina with two cervices and complete or partial duplication of the uterus. Failure of resorption of the medial junction of the two mullerian ducts may lead to a septate uterus. Each has its own clinical significance. If there is no obstruction, corrective therapy is usually necessary for correction of poor reproductive performance. Classically, the septate uterus is more commonly associated with repeated pregnancy wastage.

Uterine didelphus is most easily recognized, as the patient will have two cervices and most patients will have a longitudinal vaginal septum. The septate or bicornuate uterus may be more difficult to diagnose.

If obstruction is present the diagnosis is usually made shortly after menarche. When obstruction is not present, the diagnosis is most frequently made at the time of hysterosalpingography (HSG) done for evaluation of infertility or repeated pregnancy losses. However, the diagnosis of an anomalous uterus can be suspected by a number of other observations (Table 3). There is no question that uterine anomalies may be associated with normal reproductive history, however, classically Müllerian anomalies are associated with repetitive pregnancy losses, though some forms of double uterus may be related to infertility. The incidence

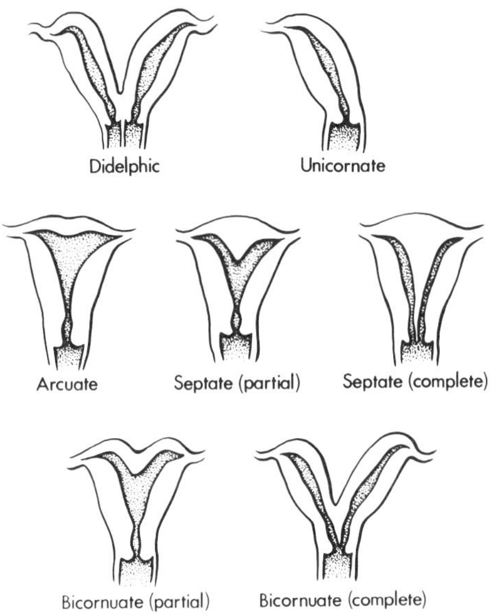

FIG. 7. Seven nonobstructive anomalies of the uterus. This classification is adapted from Jericho, 1946. (From ref. 44, with permission.)

of spontaneous abortion, premature delivery, fetal loss, malpresentation and cesarean section are higher in patients with uterine anomalies. The cause of reproductive failure is unknown though speculation revolves around poor vascularization of the septum. It is difficult to associate cervical incompetence and luteal phase defect with a diminished blood supply to the septum but both have been reported in patients with the double uterus. Likewise, it has been reported that the chance for pregnancy increases with each pregnancy loss; there is no definitive explanation for this observation. Of all patients with repetitive pregnancy losses and premature labor, approximately 10% will have a structural defect on HSG. A thorough and exhaustive search for all etiologic factors should be done on all patients with repetitive losses. Rock and Jones reported seven patients with structural uterine defects who were found to have possibly causative extrauterine factors as an etiology for their repetitive pregnancy losses (32). These patients had a 31% live birth rate prior to therapy, this increased to 71% after therapy for the extrauterine factors. The full-term pregnancy rate for all women with double uterus is not known but is believed to be approximately 25%. For women selected to undergo metroplasty the term pregnancy rate is probably 5–10% prior to the surgical procedure and approximately 80–90% postsurgery. Not all women with uterine anomalies are diagnosed prior to pregnancy, and some are never diagnosed. There is confusion and controversy in the literature about the obstetrical outcome associated with each of the types of uterine defects. The association of other infertility is less strong. Once again, a thorough and exhaustive search for other causes of infertility should be carried out. Considerable differences of opinion exist regarding whether or not metroplasty is indicated for infertility, most authors would resort to metroplasty only as a last resort.

TABLE 3. *Observations leading to diagnosis of an anomalous uterus*

Difficulty using tampons
Difficulty with intercourse
Urinary tract anomaly noted on IVP
Dysmenorrhea
Menorrhagia
Abnormality noted at D&C
Palpable mass
Abnormal ultrasound
Abnormal uterine contour noted during pregnancy
Fetal malpresentation
Pregnancy in spite of an IUD *in situ*

Dysmenorrhea and dysfunctional uterine bleeding have been reported to occur more frequently in the patient with a double uterus. Some reports reveal a favorable response of these symptoms to metroplasty, although this is highly controversial and most authors would not under take metroplasty solely for these reasons.

Hysterosalpingography is best done under fluoroscopy. It is important to remember that the distinction between a septate and bicornuate uterus cannot be established with a hysterosalpingogram. External uterine configuration can only be made by visualizing directly the uterine fundus. An IVP is important to rule out upper tract renal tract anomalies.

Traditionally, the treatment of the double uterus has been a metroplasty performed through the open abdomen using a Jones or a Tompkins procedure (32). More recently, hysteroscopic procedures have received much attention with reports showing success rates comparable with abdominal metroplasty (33–35). Abdominal metroplasty can be used for septate uterus, however, it is the only approach feasible for bicornuate uterus and for didelphic uterus.

Hysteroscopic procedures are performed transcervically utilizing either a scissors or a resectoscope (Fig. 8). These procedures are generally limited to the septate uterus. Even broad septums can be excised, though occasionally a second operative procedure will be required if too little is excised during the first procedure. Usually the procedure is done concomitantly with laparoscopy to lessen the risks of uterine perforation.

Advantages to the hysteroscopic approach include lessened morbidity and less operative time and patients can deliver vaginally versus cesarean section as is usually recommended for patients who have undergone an abdominal metroplasty.

Other symmetric, unobstructed anomalies include the T-shaped uterus and the unicornuate uterus. The T-shaped uterus is classically associated with *in utero* expo-

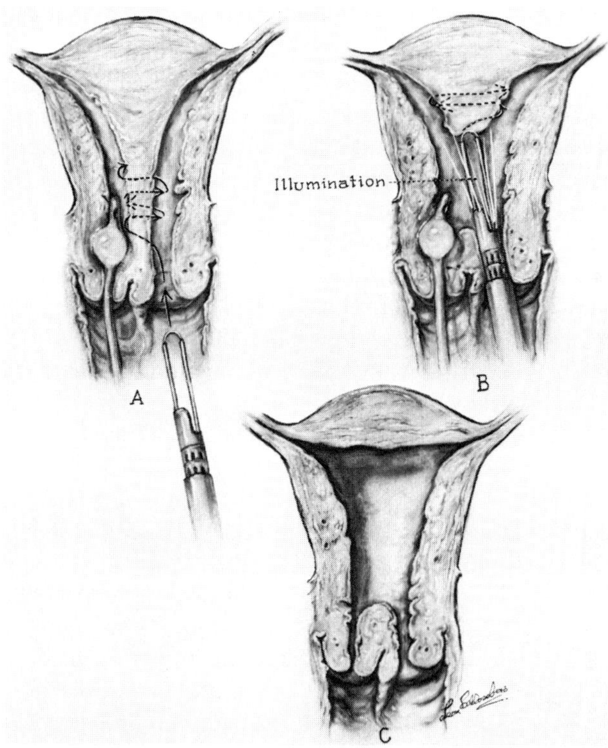

FIG. 8. Transcervical lysis of a uterine septum in a patient with a Class V: Complete septum. **A:** Foley catheter is inserted into the right cervix. The septum is incised until the Foley bulb is identified. **B:** The remaining septum is then cut with electrocautery. **C:** The septum has been cut and the cavities united.

sure to diethylstilbesterol (DES). Poor reproductive performance has likewise been associated with the T-shaped uterus including spontaneous abortion, premature delivery, and ectopic pregnancy. Surgical repair of the uterus is not indicated but patients with a history of DES exposure should be watched for signs and symptoms of premature delivery.

The unicornuate uterus may be present alone or found with a uterine anlagen. The anlagen may or may not contain a cavity with active endometrium. O'Leary and O'Leary (36) reported that 90% of rudimentary horns are noncommunicating. Surgical intervention is not indicated unless the patient is symptomatic from the anlagen at which time a hemihysterectomy is indicated.

Urinary tract anomalies are often associated with a unicornuate uterus. The renal anomaly will arise on the side opposite of the unicornuate uterus. The ovary may be malpositioned most notably high-riding as reported by Rock et al. (37).

Reports suggest that patients with a unicornuate uterus have the poorest fetal survival of all uterine anomalies. The noncommunicating uterine horn found on the contralateral side of most patients with a unicornuate uterus can be a site of an ectopic pregnancy as a result of transperitoneal migration of the sperm or ovum. This rudimentary horn is at risk of rupture should an ectopic pregnancy develop within it.

Failure of medial fusion of the lower mullerian ducts that form the vagina result in longitudinal vaginal septa that maybe partial or complete. Such septa may be entirely asymptomatic and may be identified only at the time of a routine examination. On the other hand, patients may present with dyspareunia or difficulty in using tampons. Generally, it is recommended that the septum be removed. This can usually be accomplished easily by a skilled gynecologic surgeon.

Asymmetric Obstruction: Lateral Fusion Defects

Asymmetric obstruction of the uterus such as unicornuate uterus with a noncommunicating uterine anlagen with active endometrium or unilateral obstruction of a cavity of a double uterus (obstructed horn) are rare and may present a diagnostic dilemma (Fig. 9). Dysmenorrhea or cyclic abdominal pain from cryptomenorrhea may be the only symptoms. Endometriosis from retrograde menstruation or a tender mass may be present. Removal of the obstructed horn is the procedure of choice and should alleviate the symptoms.

Another rarely seen entity is the double uterus with an obstructed hemivagina and ipsilateral renal agenesis. These patients

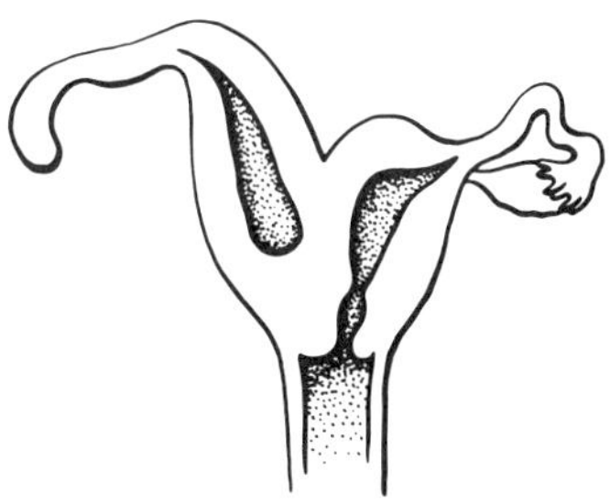

A

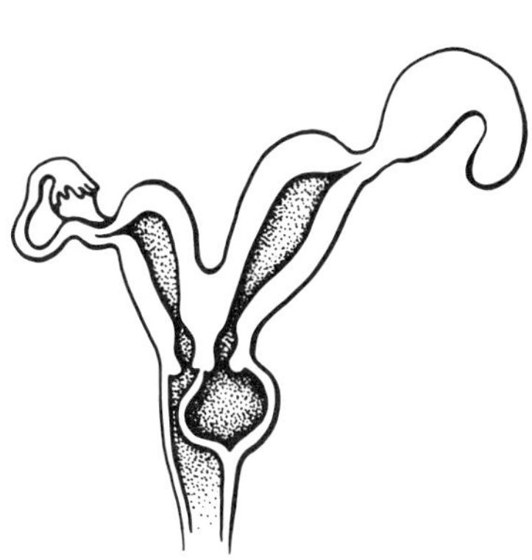

B

FIG. 9. A: Unilateral obstruction of a horn. **B:** Vagina. (From ref. 44, with permission.)

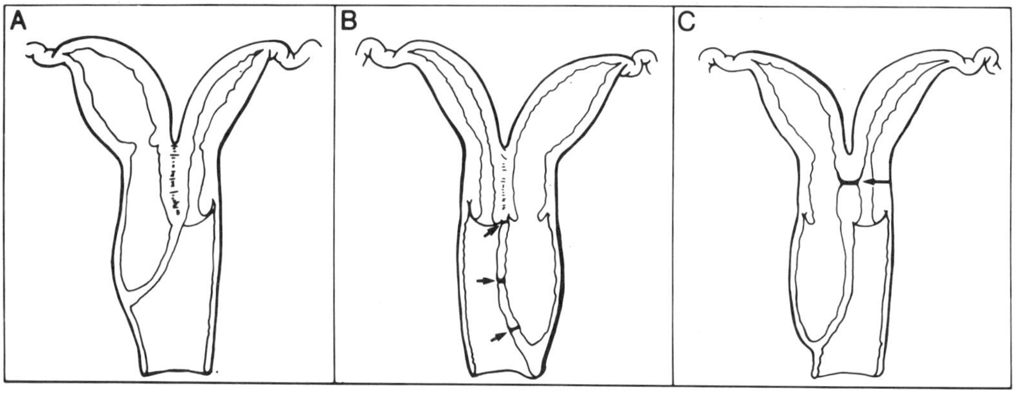

FIG. 10. Double uterus, complete or incomplete vaginal obstruction, and ipsilateral renal agenesis. **A:** Complete vaginal obstruction. **B:** Incomplete vaginal obstruction. **C:** Complete vaginal obstruction with a lateral communicating double uterus. (From ref. 45, with permission.)

have a double uterus, obstruction of the vagina (unilateral, partial or complete) and ipsilateral renal aplasia. These patients can be divided into three diagnostic groups: (a) complete unilateral vaginal obstruction with uterine communication, (b) incomplete unilateral vaginal obstruction without uterine communication, and (c) complete vaginal obstruction with lateral uterine communication (Fig. 10). The diagnosis can be difficult to make, however, MRI imaging is an extremely useful tool toward making appropriate diagnosis. A double uterus may be noted associated absence of the kidney on the side of vaginal obstruction (Fig. 11). Treatment consists of surgical excision of the vaginal septum which may be quite thick, making the surgery challenging. Generally, abdominal exploration is unnecessary and uterine reconstruction is not indicated. Reproductive performance is related to the type of double uterus unless a delay in diagnosis has resulted in endometriosis or has destroyed tubal function.

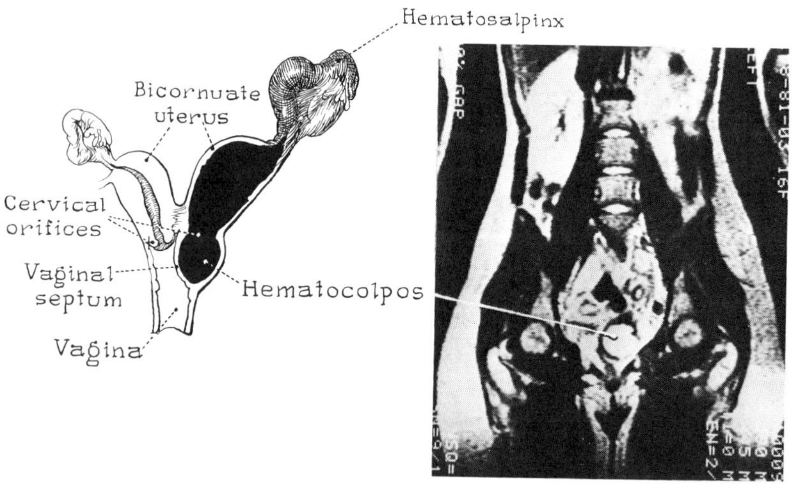

FIG. 11. Magnetic resonance imaging (MRI) demonstrates absence of kidney on the side of the vaginal obstruction. A double uterus is noted. (From ref. 46, with permission.)

CLINICAL MANIFESTATIONS OF CLASS IV ANOMALIES: UNUSUAL DEFECTS OF LATERAL AND VERTICAL FUSION

Müllerian duct anomalies that do not fit into any of the other well defined categories are unusual. These anomalies may occur with a variety of other problems. Jones and Stanton (38,39) independently reported mullerian anomalies in patients with bladder exstrophy. Stanton (39) noted that 43% of the 70 patients with bladder exstrophy had mullerian anomalies including vaginal agenesis and all forms of double uterus. Operative techniques for repair of the genital anomalies associated with bladder exstrophy were reported by Jones (40). A large number of vaginal and perineal anomalies are seen in patients with uterine anomalies. Hendren and Donahoe (40) reported on the surgical correction of these rare combinations in the pediatric age group.

SUMMARY

A sound embryologic foundation is necessary to fully comprehend, evaluate and treat patients with mullerian anomalies. Embryologic development of the generative tract is complex and may require frequent review of the subject matter. An embryologic perspective will remind the physician of other anatomic defects frequently associated with mullrian anomalies, i.e., renal anomalies associated with the Mayer-Rokitansky-Kuster-Hauser syndrome. A thorough evaluation is imperative to definitively identify the exact nature of the mullerian anomaly so as to provide appropriate counselling and the appropriate therapy. Recently reported successes of nonsurgical approaches to the creation of the vagina mandate consideration of this approach in nearly every patient with congenital absence of the vagina. In those cases where surgical creation of a vagina is necessary, an experienced surgeon is an absolute must. Endoscopic treatment of uterine septa is providing similar success rates to the traditional laparotomy and significantly decreasing the morbidity associated with the latter. Likewise, recently reported successes of aggressively conservative approaches to cervical agenesis rather than the traditionally recommended hysterectomy would mandate this as an option for the patient though not necessarily the appropriate choice for all patients.

Radiologic imaging is invaluable in assisting the gynecologist in making the diagnosis and providing care. It is important that the gynecologist remember that mullerian defects can be complex and confusing and the history and physical examination remain an important part of the evaluation.

REFERENCES

1. Moore KL. The urogenital system. In: *The developing human: clinical orientated embryology*. Philadelphia: WB Saunders, 1977:229.
2. Mattingly RF, ed. *TeLinde's operative gynecology*. 6th ed. Philadelphia: JB Lippincott, 1977: 347.
3. Jost A. Development of sexual characteristics. *Science J* 1970;6:67.
4. Thompson DP, Lynn HB. Genital anomalies associated with solitary kidney. *Mayo Clin Proc* 1966;41:538.
5. American Fertility Society Classification of Mullerian Anomalies. *Fertil Steril* 1988;49:952.
6. Counsellor VS. Congenital absence of the vagina. *Surg Clin North Am* 1957;37:1107.
7. Evans TN. The artificial vagina. *Am J Obstet Gynecol* 1967;99:944.
8. Mattingly RF, ed. The vermiform appendix in relation to gynecology. In: *TeLinde's operative gynecology*. 5th ed. Philadelphia: JB Lippincott, 1977:350.
9. In: Mattingly RF, ed. *TeLinde's operative gynecology*. 5th ed. Philadelphia: JB Lippincott, 1977:347.
10. Shokeir JP. Aplasia of the mullerian system: evidence for probably sex-limited autosomal dominant inheritance. *Birth Defects* 1978;14:147.
11. Knab DR. Mullerian agenesis: a review. Department of Gynecology and Obstetrics, Uniformed Services University School of Medicine and Naval Hospital, Bethesda, MD, 1983.
12. Fore SR, Hammond CB, Parker RT. Urologic and genital anomalies in patients with congenital absence of the vagina. *Obstet Gynecol* 1973; 46:410.

13. Griffin JE, Edwards C, Madden JD. Congenital absence of the vagina. *Ann Intern Med* 1976; 85:224.
14. Evans TN, Poland ML, Boving RL. Vaginal malformations. *Am J Obstet Gynecol* 1981;141: 910.
15. Frank RT. The formation of an artificial vagina without operation. *Am J Obstet Gynecol* 1938;35: 1035.
16. Ingram JM. The bicycle seat stool in the treatment of vaginal agenesis and stenosis: a preliminary report. *Am J Obstet Gynecol* 1981;140: 867.
17. Abbe R. New method of creating a vagina in a case of congenital absence. *Med Rec* 1898; 54:836.
18. Pratt JH. Vaginal atresia corrected by use of small and large bowel. *Clin Obstet Gynecol* 1972; 15:639.
19. Williams EA. Congenital absence of the vagina, a simple operation for its relief. *J Obstet Gynecol Br Comm* 1964;71:511.
20. Gallup DG, Castle CA, Stock RJ. Recurrent carcinoma *in situ* of the vagina following split thickness skin graft vaginoplasty. *Gynecol Oncol* 1987;26:98.
21. Rotmensch J, Rpsensein NB, Dillon M. Carcinoma arising in the neovagina: case report and review of the literature. *Obstet Gynecol* 1983;61:534.
22. Rock JA, Jones HW Jr. Construction of a neovagina for patients with a flat perineum. *Am J Obstet Gynecol* 1989;160:845.
23. Mattingly RF, ed. *TeLinde's operative gynecology*. 6th ed. Philadelphia: JB Lippincott, 1977:347.
24. Rock JA, Zacur HA, Dlugi AM. Pregnancy success following surgical correction of imperforate hymen and complete transverse vaginal septum. *Gynecology* 1982;59:448.
25. Lodi A. Contributo clinico stastico sulle malformazioni della vagina osservate mella. Clinica Obstetricia e Ginecologica di Milano dal 1906 al 1950. *Ann Obstet Gynecol Med Perinatol* 1951;73:1246.
26. Rock JA. Anomalous development of the vagina. *Semin Reprod Endocrinol* 1986;4:1.
27. Zarou GS, Esposito JM, Zaroeu DM. Pregnancy following the surgical correction of congenital atresia of the cervix. *Mt J Gynecol Obstet* 1973;11:143.
28. Farber M, Marchant DJ. Reconstructive surgery for congenital atresia of the uterine cervix. *Fertil Steril* 1976;27:1277.
29. Cukier J, Batzofin JH. Conners JS, Franklin RP. Genital tract reconstruction in a patient with congenital absence of a vagina and hypoplasia of the cervix. *Obstet Gynecol* 1986;68:325.
30. Hampton HL, Meeks RG, Bates W, Wiser WL. Pregnancy after successful vaginoplasty and cervical stenting for partial atresia of the cervix. *Obstet Gynecol* 1990;76:900.
31. Thijssen RFA, Hollanders JMG, Williemsen WNP, Van der Heyden PMF, Van Dongen PWJ, Rollard R. Successful pregnancy after ZIFT in a patient with congenital cervical atresia. *Obstet Gynecol* 1990;76:902.
32. Rock JA, Jones HW Jr, eds. *Reparative and constructive surgery of the female generative tract*. Baltimore: Williams & Wilkins, 1983.
33. Fayex JA. Comparison between abdominal and hysteroscopic metroplasty. *Obstet Gynecol* 1986;68:399.
34. DeCherney A, Polan ML. Hysteroscopy management of intrauterine lesions and intractable bleeding. *Obstet Gynecol* 1983;61:392.
35. Daly DC, Witten CA, Soto-Albors CE, Riddick DH. Hysteroscopic metroplasty: surgical technique and obstetrics outcome. *Fertil Steril* 1983;39:623.
36. O'Leary JL, O'Leary JA. Rudimentary horn pregnancy. *Obstet Gynecol* 1963;22:371.
37. Rock JA, Parmley T, Murphy AA, Jones HW. Malposition of the ovary associated with uterine anomalies. *Fertil Steril* 1986;45:561.
38. Jones HW. An anomaly of the external genitalia in female patients with exstrophy of the bladder. *Am J Obstet Gynecol* 1981;117:49.
39. Stanton SL. Gynecologic complications of epispadios and bladder exstrophy. *Am J Obstet Gynecol* 1974;119:749.
40. Hendren WH, Donahoe PK. Correction of congenital abnormalities of the vagina and perineum. *J Pediatr Surg* 1980;15:751.
41. Kelly H. Operations on the vagina: congenital affections. In: *Operative gynecology, vol. 1*. New York: D Appleton & Co., 1868.
42. Rock JA. Surgical correction of uterovaginal anomalies. In: Sciarra J, ed. *Gynecology and obstetrics, vol. I*. 49th revision. Philadelphia: Harper & Row, 1984.
43. Rock JA, Schlaff WD, Zacur HA, et al. The clinical management of congenital absence of the uterine cervix. *Int J Gynaecol Obstet* 1984; 22:233.
44. Rock JA. Diagnosing and repairing uterine anomalies. *Contemp Obstet Gynecol* 1981;17:44.
45. Rock JA, Jones HW Jr. The double uterus associated with an obstructed hemivagina and ipsilateral renal agenesis. *Am J Obstet Gynecol* 1980;138:340.
46. Rock JA. Mullerian anomalies. In: Mattingly RF, Rock JA, eds. *TeLinde's operative gynecology*. 7th ed. Philadelphia: JB Lippincott, 1991.
47. Rock JA et al. Resectoscopic techniques for lysis of a class V: Complete uterine septum. *Fertil Steril* 1987;48:496.

Pediatric and Adolescent Gynecology,
edited by S. E. Carpenter and J. A. Rock.
Raven Press, Ltd., New York © 1992.

21
Adolescent Sexuality

Melinda B. Stein and Peter J. Fagan

Francis Scott Key Medical Center, Baltimore, Maryland 21224; and Sexual Behaviors Consultation Unit, Baltimore, Maryland 21205

Adolescent sexual development is the basis for further adult sexuality (1,2). How the adolescent sexually changes, adapts and matures will provide him/her with the foundation of future intimate relationships (1,3). Adolescent sexuality evolves through the interface of biological, familiar, social, academic and cognitive issues (4). In this chapter, we discuss the various emotional and behavioral changes, phases, and risks during adolescent sexual development.

ADOLESCENT DEVELOPMENT: IDENTITY AND INTIMACY

Erikson (1) theorized that the adolescent is faced with the development of identity in which a stable sense of self is achieved. This is followed by the young adult task of developing intimacy which allows for openness, sharing, mutual trust, self-abandon, and commitment to another. Although this step-wise developmental progression has been challenged by Gilligan (5) who suggests that identity development in adolescent girls involves relationship components. In any case, it is likely that the developing identity in both genders involves some attempts to develop intimate relationships.

As a result of physical, cognitive and social changes (6), adolescents experiment with sexual relationships and explore sexual roles in their dating and social interaction. Their affectionate and sexual involvement in relationships helps to consolidate sexual identity (7). It is in the managing of the conflict between sexual drives and the emotional, interpersonal and biological results of sexual behavior that the adolescent struggles to achieve adult sexual maturity (8).

SEXUAL DEVELOPMENTAL TASKS

Sexual identity is established on the foundation of gender identity. Gender identity is the sense of maleness or femaleness that the individual predicates to his or her self, e.g., "I am a man" or "I am a woman." It is a profound psychological development typically achieved in the first 2 years of life, detectable in an infant before the end of the first year. In adolescence, gender identity becomes firmly established as sexuality is experienced and integrated into the adolescent's identity.

Sexual identity/role is awareness of self as a sexual person who can be sexually in relationship to persons of the same gender, opposite gender, or both. In one sense, it is the eroticization of gender identity, i.e., the erotic expression self as a young man or young woman.

Biological and psychosocial factors are involved in the initiation of sexual activity for both male and female adolescents. However, for males, interpersonal sexual activity appears to be facilitated primarily by the release of free testosterone in males (9), whereas for females it is the influence of peer groups that is related to sexual activity with others (10).

The age-specific sexual behavior of early adolescence is masturbation; of older adolescence it is sexual experimentation (including intercourse) with another (2). In masturbation, the adolescent learns to integrate sexual pleasure with the fantasy of relatedness with another. Both somatic autoeroticism (self-pleasuring) and cognitive alloeroticism (erotic relatedness to other) processes are developing in tandem. The central or core masturbatory fantasy of the adolescent is often indicative of the main themes, e.g., object and conflicts, of the individual's sexual relatedness (11). The masturbatory fantasy may not be expressed autoerotically in some adolescents but the cognitive aspects nevertheless can develop, e.g., in hero-worship of sport or performing arts figures.

The autoeroticism of masturbation develops into the sex play with another in the developing adolescents as the central fantasy seeks alloerotic expression. The adolescent "practices" his/her sexual identity in sexual roles which are significantly determined by social and peer group factors (12). The 1988 National Survey of Family Growth reported that 27% of 15-year-old and half of 17-year-old women has had intercourse (13).

COGNITION AND MORAL DEVELOPMENT

Sexuality and its meaning to the adolescent seems contingent upon the interaction between adolescents and the world around them (14). Turmoil or conflicts are necessary for working through adolescent tasks including the task of figuring out what should or should not be done sexually. The cognitive development of formal operations (abstract thinking) characteristic of most 11–12-year-olds (15) indicate that when the adolescent begins to move from concrete to more abstract thought processes, he/she is able to engage in responsible sexual decision making. Concrete thinking does not allow for complete understanding of the risks involved in sexual behavior (15). Concrete thought processes are marked by undimensional and unilateral problem solving. A "relationship" is an abstract concept which requires logical, systematic and deductive decision making in order to deal with myriad of possibilities and consequences. Although abstract reasoning ability does not insure appropriate problem solving, it will afford an individual the capacity for responsible sexual judgments.

Transition from elementary to middle school is a difficult time for most youngsters. Lower academic performance, as well as lower educational aspirations correlates with premature adolescent sexual involvement (16). Many youngsters may not reach formal operations or abstract thinking until later adolescence making these transitions more difficult.

Sexual intimacy includes a blending of sensuality, abstract thinking emotional closeness, mutual caring, commitment, and trust. Adolescents who have sex prior to achieving intimacy in their relationships are at risk for undesirable consequences of their sexual actions. Moreover, an adolescent's level of intimacy and cognitive development may influence his/her determination of appropriate sexual initiation, sexually transmitted disease (STD) protection, and contraceptive practices (17,18).

More intelligent adolescents are less reliant on external moral values for directing sexual decision making (14). Further, more religious adolescents are more oriented towards societal sexual norms. An internal focus of control or self identity also influences better practical judgment for males in sexual relationships (14).

Sexual behavior is highly influenced by social forces as indicated by the variety of sexual mores reported in different cultures as well as the differences between generations in the same culture. Although sexuality is at base a biologically motivated behavior, the meaning attributed to sexual expression is largely a social construction. Ethical debates about sexual behavior usually concern whether the meaning of sexual behavior is totally constructed by the situation and the participants, e.g. mutual consenting partners, or whether there is a predetermined meaning in sexual behavior, e.g., for procreation and love in marriage.

FAMILY INFLUENCES

Adolescence marks the transition from dependence on the family to establishing an independent identity. Sexual development is affected by parents' attitude in the home environment (16,18–20). Permissive maternal attitudes reflect adolescents who are more sexually active (21). Adolescents who had a close relationship with their mothers were more likely to share their mother's sexual attitudes and behavior (22). Further, parental supervision and single parent households seem to influence the onset of intercourse (23). Parents who hold permissive attitudes toward sexual behavior have adolescents who are more sexually active and more likely to use contraception (24). Adolescents whose mothers remarry have more permissive attitudes than mothers who are divorced but do not remarry. Maternal sexual attitudes strongly influence adolescent attitudes.

SEXUAL ABUSE

Adolescents with histories of sexual abuse may have more difficulty with identity formation and establishing and maintaining healthy relationships with others (1,2). The abused adolescent may engage in premature sexual behavior in an attempt to achieve pseudointimacy. The latter may temporarily recapitulate or derive for the adolescent feelings of nuturance and gratification of unmet dependency needs, which he/she wishes from their family (2). For example, a male or female adolescent may become sexually involved with an older or female individual in order to attain an adequate parent figure. Depressive, Personality, and Conduct Disorders are frequently associated with disturbed identity and sexual development (2,4).

Sexually abused children and adolescents are frequently overstimulated and seek immediate release of sexual tension. These youngsters are vulnerable to promiscuity, highly suggestible and act without sufficient thought or deliberations. Hence, they are at high risk for pregnancy and STD.

CONTRACEPTION

The United States exceeds the level of teen pregnancies over most other industrialized nations (25). The latter is in part due to poor contraceptive practices among American teenagers. Younger adolescents are poor users of contraception (25,4). It appears that knowledge alone does not determine effective contraceptive use (4).

Positive sexual self-concept is associated with frequent contraceptive use during intercourse (26). Further, sexual self-concept seems to improve with age. Parental support increases contraceptive use (27). Contraceptive use was negatively associated with lower social-economic status, low educational achievement, low self-esteem, and poor family relationships (28,29).

PREGNANCY

Pregnancy can compromise an adolescent's ability to lead a productive and healthy life (17). A pregnant female adolescent is characteristically under 16 years old and from a divorced, single parent home where the mother conceived out of wedlock (30). Adolescent birth lowers a female's likelihood of economic success and increases the likelihood of having a large family (31). Pregnant females are at risk to jeopardize their academic success, by dropping out of school (31).

Zabin et al. (32) studied 360 adolescents seeking pregnancy tests. A 2-year follow-up revealed that the adolescents who aborted their pregnancies were more likely to graduate high school and were generally economically more secure. Additionally, the adolescents who obtained abortions had a lower occurrence of another pregnancy within the 2-year follow-up period. The abortion group also showed a more positive psychological profile, including lower anxiety, higher self-esteem, and internal control. The postponement of childbearing appears to improve the social, psychological, academic, and economic outcome of an adolescent's life.

PROBLEMS IN GENDER AND SEXUAL IDENTITY/ROLE

Problems of gender identity in a female adolescent present as rejection of menarche and secondary sexual characteristics. She may also resent the loss of buddy relationships with young male adolescents. Gender dysphoric female adolescents are typically homosexual in sexual orientation. Among male adolescents cross-dressing is one of the manifestations of a potential gender dysphoria in later years. During preadolescence, both genders tend to engage in cross-gender behavior, e.g., tomboy play for girls, effeminacy for boys (33,34). Female family members, e.g. older sisters, mother, grandmother, frequently played an etiological role in the cross-dressing behaviors of male adolescents by having dressed them as girls (even if only "in play") when younger.

Problems of sexual identity/role in adolescents tend to group around the extremes of near total repression of sexuality or health/life threatening promiscuity (35). Repression of sexuality may be present under the guise of religious, political, academic, or other ideological rationale in the mind of the adolescent. It is marked by severe emotional discomfort with sexual pleasure and the avoidance of situations in which sexual role behavior might be appropriate, e.g., school dances, parties. In some cases, it is part of a psychiatric disorder such as anorexia nervosa or major affective illness. When the sexual dysphoria is part of a psychiatric disorder, referral should be made to a mental health professional who has an expertise in treating adolescents with the psychiatric disorder in question.

Care must be taken to ensure that the label "sexual promiscuity" is not simply the imposition of an older generation's mores upon the younger or applied differentially to each gender, e.g., girls are "promiscuous," whereas boys are "sowing their oats." If, however, the frequency and variety of sexual partners risks physical or psychological health, then the sexual behavior in question is usually an indication of poor integration of sexual identity/role in the adolescent. The adolescent is using promiscuous sexual behavior for purposes which sexual behavior by itself is ill-suited, e.g., security in gender and sexual identity/role, acceptance by others, status in the peer group. It does little good to criticize the promiscuous sexual behavior of the adolescent without first addressing the psychosexual and psychosocial conflicts which the behavior is an attempt to mollify.

PRECOCIOUS AND DELAYED PUBERTY

John Money's longitudinal research and case studies of children with hormonal disorders has provided important data on the effects of precocious or delayed puberty on the sexual behavior of the adolescent. He concludes (36), "Pubertally precocious children do not become erotosexually wild and delinquent (37,38), and pubertally delayed teenagers are not inevitably erotosexually inert, though they tend to be neglected by their pubertally developed agemates, except in nonromantic comradeships (39,40,41)." This conclusion has been supported in a study (42) of female adolescents who experienced idiopathic precocious puberty (IPP). The subjects experienced sexual milestones (first holding hands to first intercourse) about one year prior to their controls. First masturbation occurred approximately 5 years earlier (9.2 years). Later adolescent sexual behavior was not different between the IPP adolescents and their controls.

While a review of the question of general psychological reaction to delayed or precocious puberty is beyond scope of this chapter, a recent study (43) found that among a sample of more normally developing adolescents self-esteem did not vary significantly with pubertal development (measured with Tanner stage-like self-reports) in either males or females. There was a modest correlation between self-esteem and the timing of pubertal events in males but not in females. Thus, adolescent boys experienced increased self-esteem with an early (but not precocious) puberty. For adolescent girls, pubertal development was but one of many unspecified factors affecting self-esteem.

Pubertal development may be arrested by environmental stressors or by an intrapsychic condition such as an eating disorder in both female and male adolescents. In the former, intervention should be directed at alleviating the cause of the stress (44). Although the etiology of eating disorders is typically multifactorial, one of the possible factors in both genders is difficulty in integrating the sexual identity role of a young adult (45). Amenorrhea, loss of secondary sex characteristics and lowered testosterone, remove the eating disordered adolescent from some of the normal stress of assuming responsibility for sexual desire and behaviors. It would be a mistake, however, to consider eating disordered adolescents as being sexually naive. Preliminary studies have shown that general sexual attitudes and behaviors of eating disordered females are not significantly different from standardized norms (46). Male eating disordered adolescents in an inpatient setting have been reported to have a 25% incidence of homosexual orientation—approximately twice that of the general population (45).

SEXUAL ORIENTATION

For the majority of adolescents, sexual fantasies and sexual activity with others are exclusively heterosexual (with the possible exception of some same-sex play in early adolescence). The heterosexual orientation of sexual identity and sexual role is taken for granted by themselves, by their parents and by their peers. There may be occasional distress that he or she is not as ideal a sexual young man or young woman as the culture demands ("Will I get invited to the prom? How will I do when I do IT for the first time?"), but there is no distress that one is qualitatively different from the ideal.

The same cannot be said for the adolescent who is primarily attracted to others of the same sex. For the homosexual adolescent, the clash between erotic fantasies and behaviors on one hand and the cultural expectation of heterosexuality on the other frequently make for notable distress. As the sense of homosexual orientation emerges during adolescence both for the young men or women (47), the primary developmental task for the homosexual adolescent is adjustment to a socially stigmatized sexual role (48).

The etiology of homosexual orientation is highly controverted (49–53). At this point in our knowledge, the question of causality might best be framed as an inquiry into the etiologies of homosexualities. There may be genetic, physiological, and environmental determinants which converge in a multifactorial fashion in the individual. Hypothetically, these may affect the degrees of homosexual and heterosexual orientation in the individual adolescent.

When a clinician is asked about sexual orientation by an adolescent or her parents the question is usually a dichotomous one: "Am I lesbian? Is he homosexual?" It is not a question that often lends itself to a simple categorical answer. Sexual orientation, especially in a developing adolescent is a far more subtle and complex reality. As so aptly stated by Kinsey et al. (54):

> The world is not divided into sheep and goats. Not all are black nor all things white. It is a fundamental of taxonomy that nature rarely deals with discrete categories and tries to force facts into separated pigeon holes. The living world is a continuum in each and every one of its aspects. The sooner we learn this concerning human sexual behavior the sooner we shall reach a sounder understanding of the realities of sex.

To measure the continuous degrees of both homosexuality and heterosexuality in an individual the Kinsey researchers utilized sexual fantasy and sexual behavior as the two determining factors (54) upon which subjects would be rated 0 to 6. Exclusive heterosexuality was represented by 0, and exclusive homosexuality by 6. Today, most who write about the assessment of sexual orientation add to erotic fantasy and sexual behavior other determinants involving sexual identity and sexual social role.

Additional determinants of sexual orientation are sexual attraction, sexual behavior, sexual fantasies, emotional preference, social preference, self-identification, and hetero/gay lifestyle (55–57). The Klein Sexual Orientation Grid (KSOG) employs the Kinsey 7-point ratings on past, present, and ideal dimensions of these seven determinants of sexual orientation (57). The resultant dimensional profiles can provide a description of the variations in the sexual orientation of the subjects. For the clinician choosing not to utilize such an instrument, the KSOG offers a temporal and topical structure which can be utilized in the exploration of sexual orientation with the adolescent.

It is typically the mental health professional who has the professional time and expertise to assist the adolescent who is conflicted or ambiguous about his or her sexual orientation. As a lengthy review of the literature (58) concludes, attempts to change the homosexual adult's sexual orientation have a poor prognosis. The work of therapy with such an adolescent whose sexual identity/role is still developing involves primarily a nonjudgmental exploration into the adolescent's experience of his/her sexual identity/role. Anxiety will be patent as bisexual attractions are dealt with. Premature closure by "deciding" on one orientation simply to bind the anxiety should be avoided. Encouragement to explore the desired sexual orientation will be evident in the therapist by her willingness to process the reactions of the adolescent to this exploration.

If the work of therapy or the self-awareness of the adolescent indicates that there is a clearly homosexual orientation, then the adolescent should be assisted to integrate this sexual orientation into his/her sexual identity/role. Therapy will address not only the negative reactions of family members to an emerging homosexual orientation in their child but also the negative self-judgments which the adolescent has internalized as a member of a culture which is predominantly homophobic. This is facilitated if suitable role models are available to the adolescent in a therapeutic setting, e.g., group therapy, or identified to the youth as public persons who are homosexual.

Parents and Friends of Lesbians and Gays (PFLAG) is a nation-wide organization whose purpose is to assist parents of homosexual children through information and group support. The national address is: Federation PFLAG, P.O. Box 27605, Washington, DC. 20038. Nearby university or college student services might also be contacted for the local chapter's meeting place and time.

TALKING ABOUT SEX

Sexually active adolescents have described themselves as being quite ready to receive information on pregnancy and the prevention of venereal disease (58). The importance of talking about sexuality with adolescents and taking a careful sexual history have obviously increased since the pandemic of AIDS. To the previous aims of reproduction education (59) and the diagnosis and treatment of STDs (60) is added the protection of life itself. It is not merely the homosexual male and the IV drug user that is at risk for HIV transmission. For example, a recent national survey of 5514 first year Canadian college students (mean age, 19.7 years) reported a distressing incidence of high risk STD-HIV behavior among this population (61). Of the 74% of the men sexually active, 14% had participated in anal intercourse and only 25% always used a condom. In the 69% of the sexually active women, 19% had participated in anal intercourse and a mere 16% always used a condom. Nearly 6% of both genders reported a previous STD.

MacDonald et al. (61) suggested three components in effective STD/HIV risk reduction education which should guide clinical conversation about sex with the adolescent. First, the adolescents must be given relevant information which allows them to make an accurate assessment of the risks which they are taking in their sexual practices. With this information, they can determine the changes that they can take to reduce risks in their particular social and sexual environment. This requires inquiry into the number of partners, the incidence of oral-anal, oral-genital, anal and vaginal intercourse, and the use of condoms. Concurrent use of alcohol and drugs should also be seen as an increased risk factor.

The second component involves assisting the adolescents to develop successful techniques for practicing safer sex. This is largely the young person's development of interpersonal skills, e.g. how to abstain from intercourse, how to be assertive enough to demand the use of a condom from a partner. The third component is assisting adolescents to be sufficiently motivated to act upon their knowledge of STD/HIV risk behavior with interpersonal effectiveness even when this is counter to prevailing social norms. The later two components suggested by MacDonald et al. (61) will generally entail public health programs beyond the clinical interview and sexual history.

A competent sexual history will occur in the atmosphere of supportive and nonjudgmental rapport with the adolescent. The clinician's first task is thus to create an environment which is permissive for the adolescent to discuss sexual matters. Sexual orientation should never be presumed because the adolescent appears to conform to sexual stereotypes. The confidentiality of the doctor-patient relationship needs to be conveyed especially relative to any limitations which may be mandated by law, e.g., parental notification of abortion. To discuss embarrassing or emotionally conflicted sexual issues the adolescent must be able to trust that what is said will remain confidential.

When a clinician takes a sexual history, she is not merely obtaining quantitative data about behavior, attitudes and medical conditions. She is also immersing herself in the cultural milieu of the adolescent. At times the prejudices of the clinician may affect the interaction. For example, physicians assessing abdominal pain in an emergency room setting asked black and Hispanic girls about sexual history more frequently than white girls (62).

Taking the sexual history of homosexual males who are sexually active requires a comprehensive evaluation of the risk factors for possible HIV transmission. A 1986 survey (63) of nonclinical male homosexual teenagers found that the average number of sex partners was seven; the partners averaged seven years older; two-thirds of the initial encounters originated in bars or public places; one-third exchanged no personal identification information; nearly half had a history of STD and the majority met criteria for substance abuse. Sexually active gay adolescents should be periodically evaluated for STD with special attention given to disorders of the urethra, pharynx, proctorectal region and skin (60).

Lastly, the more comfortable the clinician is talking about sex, the more at ease will the respondent be. There is no easy way to learn how to talk seriously about sex with another adult. With adolescents generational and cultural differences make it more difficult. Psychodynamic theory suggests that the adult's own repressed adolescent sexuality issues are brought into (pre)–consciousness when talking about sex with an adolescent. This can make conversation about sex emotionally difficult for the adult and secondarily for the adolescent. Desensitization is usually necessary by repeated exposure to the anxiety-provoking stimulus in the *in vivo* situation. The only way to be at ease talking about sex with adolescents is to do it—repeatedly.

CONCLUSION

Adolescent sexual development is a multifaceted process. It includes the interface of biological, familiar, psychological, cognitive, economic and academic determinates. As sexual identity, orientation and intimacy develop, the adolescent is faced with a myriad of choices and decisions. Pregnancy and STD are major challenges and pitfalls for the adolescent. Clinicians can provide a supportive, sensitive, and instructive environment to assist adolescents through their sexual development.

REFERENCES

1. Erikson EH. *Identity, youth and crisis.* New York: Norton, 1968.
2. Scharff DE. *The sexual relationship: an object relations view of sex and the family.* Boston: Routledge & Kegan Paul, 1982.
3. Sullivan HS. *The interpersonal theory of psychology.* New York: Norton, 1953.
4. Brooks-Gunn J, Furstenberg F. Adolescent sexual behavior. *Am Psychol* 1989;44:249–57.
5. Gilligan C. *In a different voice: psychological theory and women's development.* Cambridge, MA: Harvard University Press, 1982.
6. Berndt T. The features and effects of friendship in early adolescence. *Child Dev* 1982;53:1447–60.
7. McCabe MP. Toward a theory of adolescent dating. *Adolescence* 1984;19:160–9.
8. Steinberg L. *Adolescence.* New York: Knopf, 1985.
9. Udry JR, Billy JO, Morris NM, Groff TR, Raj MH. Serum androgenic hormones motivate sexual behavior in adolescent boys. *Fertil Steril* 1985;43:90–4.
10. Udry JR, Talbert L, Morris NM. Biosocial foundations for adolescent female sexuality. *Demography* 1986;23:217–29.
11. Laufer M, Laufer ME. *Adolescence and developmental breakdown: a psychoanalytic view,* New Haven: Yale University, 1984.
12. Gagnon JH, Simon W. *Sexual conduct: the social sources of human sexuality,* Chicago: Aldine, 1973.
13. Barringer F. What is youth coming to? *NY Times* 1990; August 19:E1,E5.

14. Juhasz A, Schneider M. Adolescent sexuality: values, morality and decision making. *Adolescence* 1987;87:579–89.
15. Piaget J. Intellectual evolution from adolescence to adulthood. *Hum Dev* 1972;15:1.
16. Hayes CD, ed. *Risking the future: adolescent sexuality, pregnancy and childbearing (Vol. I)*. Washington DC: National Academy Press, 1987.
17. Grant LM, Demetriou E. Adolescent sexuality. *Pediatr Clin North Am* 1988;35(6):1271–1289.
18. Sarrel LJ, Sarrel PM. Sexual unfolding. *J Adolesc Health Care* 1981;2:93.
19. Furstenberg FF Jr. Implicating the family: teenage parenthood and kinship involvement. *Teenage pregnancy in a family context*. Philadelphia: Temple University Press, 1981.
20. Hercez-Baron R, Furstenberg FF Jr. Adolescent contraception use: The impact of family support systems. *The childbearing decision: fertility attitudes and behavior.* Beverly Hills: Sage, 1982.
21. Thornton A, Camburn D. The influence of the family on premarital sexual attiudes and behavior. *Demography* 1987;24:323–40.
22. Weinstein M, Thornton A. Mother-child relation and adolescent sexual attitude and behavior. *Demography* 1989;26:563–77.
23. Newcome S, Udley JR. Parental mental status effects on adolescent sexual behavior. *J Marriage Family* 1987;49:235–40.
24. Baker SA, Thalberg SP, Morrison OM. Parents' behavioral norms as predictors of adolescent sexual activity and contraceptive use. *Adolescence* 1988;23:265–81.
25. Jones E, Forrest JD, Goldman N, et al. Teenage pregnancy in developed countries, Determinants and policy implications. *Family Planning Perspectives* 1985;17:53–63.
26. Winter L. The role of sexual self-concept in the use of contraceptives. *Family Planning Perspectives* 1988;20:123–7.
27. Jay MS, DuRant RH, Lih IF. Female adolescents' compliance with contraceptive regimens. *Pediatr Clin North Am* 1989;36:731–45.
28. Chilman CS. Some psychosocial aspects of adolescent sexual and contraceptive behavior in a changing American Society. In: Lancaster JB, Hamburg BA, eds. *School-age pregnancy and parenthood biosocial dimensions*. New York: Aldine De Gruyter, 1986:191–217.
29. Morrison DM. Adolescent contraceptive behavior, a review. *Psychol Bull* 1985;98:538–68.
30. Curtis HA, Lanerence CJ, Tripp JH. Teenage sexual intercourse and pregnancy. *Arch Dis Child* 1988;63:373–9.
31. Furstenberg FF Jr, Brooks-Gunn J, Morgan SP. Adolescent mothers and their children in later life. *Fam Plann Perspect* 1987;19:142–51.
32. Zabin L, Hirsch M, Emerson M. When urban adolescents choose abortion: effects on education, psychological status and subsequent pregnancy. *Fam Plann Perspect* 1989;21:248–55.
33. Green R. *The "sissy boy syndrome" and the development of homosexuality*. New Haven: Yale University, 1987.
34. Steiner BW, ed. *Gender dysphoria: development, research and management*. New York: Plenum, 1985.
35. Fagan PJ, Meyer JK, Schmidt CW Jr. Sexual dysfunction within an adult developmental perspective. *J Sex Marital Therapy* 1986;12:1–12.
36. Money J. *Venuses penuses: sexology, sexosophy and exigency theory*. Buffalo: Prometheus Books, 1986.
37. Money J, Alexander D. Psychosexual development and absence of homosexuality in males with precocious puberty: review of 18 cases. *J Nerv Ment Dis*, 1969;148:111–23.
38. Money J, Walker P. Psychosexual development, maternalism, nonpromiscuity and body image in 15 females with precocious puberty. *Arch Sex Behav* 1971;1:45–60.
39. Money J, Clopper R. Postpubertal psychosexual function in postsurgical male hypopituitarism. *J Sex Res* 1975;11:25–38.
40. Clopper R, Adelson JM, Money J. Postpubertal psychosexual function in male hypopituitarism without hypogonadotropinism after growth hormone therapy. *J Sex Res* 1976;12:14–32.
41. Money J, Clopper R, Menefee J. Psychosexual development in postpubertal males with idiopathic panhypopituitarism. *J Sex Res* 1980;16: 212–25.
42. Ehrhardt AA, Meyer-Bahlburg HF. Idiopathic precocious puberty in girls: long-term effects on adolescent behavior. *Acta Endocrinol [Suppl]* 1986;279:247–53.
43. Brack CJ, Orr DP, Ingersoll S. Pubertal maturation and self-esteem. *J Adolesc Health Care* 1988;9:280–5.
44. Eisenstein TD, Gerson MJ. Psychosocial growth retardation in adolescence. A reversible condition secondary to severe stress, *J Adolesc Health Care* 1988;9:436–40.
45. Fagan PJ, Andersen AE. Sexuality and eating disorders in adolescence. In: Sugar M, ed. *Atypical adolescence and sexuality*. New York: W.W. Norton (in press).
46. Rothschild BS, Fagan PJ, Woodall C, Andersen AE. Sexual functioning of female eating disordered patients [Abstract]. Presented at the International Conference for Eating Disorders. New York, April 1990.
47. Chapman BE, Brannock JC. Proposed model of lesbian identity development: an empirical examination. *J Homosex* 1987;14:69–80.
48. Hetrick ES, Martin AD. Developmental issues and their resolution for gay and lesbian adolescents. *J Homosex* 1987;14:25–43.
49. DeCecco JP. Homosexuality's brief recovery: from sickness to health and back again. *J Sex Res* 1987;23:106–14.
50. DeCecco JP. The two views of Meyer-Bahlburg: a rejoinder. *J Sex Res* 1987;23:123–27.
51. Meyer-Bahlburg HF. Psychoendocrine research and the societal status of homosexuals: a reply to DeCecco. *J Sex Res* 1987;23:114–20.
52. Gagnon JH. Science and the politics of pathology. *J Sex Res* 1987;23:120–3.

53. Perper T. Enough is enough: reflections on the views of DeCecco and Meyer-Bahlburg. *J Sex Res* 1987;23:127–9.
54. Kinsey AC, Pomeroy WB, Martin CE. *Sexual behavior in the human male*. Philadelphia: Saunders, 1948.
55. Klein F. *The bisexual option*. New York: Arbor House, 1978.
56. Klein F. Are you sure you're heterosexual? or homosexual? or bisexual? *Forum Magazine* 1980 December:41–5.
57. Klein F, Sepekoff B, Wolf TJ. Sexual orientation: a multivariate dynamic process. *J Homosex* 1985;9:35–49.
58. Acosta FX. Etiology and treatment of homosexuality: a review. *Arch Sex Behav* 1975;4:9–29.
59. Amann-Gainotti M. Sexual socialization during early adolescence: the menarche. *Adolescence* 1986;21:703–10.
60. Zenilman J. Sexually transmitted diseases in homosexual adolescents. *J Adolesc Health Care* 1988;9:129–38.
61. MacDonald NE, Wells GA, Fisher WA, et al. High-risk STD/HIV behavior among college students. *JAMA* 1990;263:3155–9.
62. Hunt AD, Litt IF, Loebner M. Obtaining a sexual history from adolescent girls. *J Adolesc Health Care* 1988;9:52–4.
63. Ramefedi GJ. Adolescent homosexuality; psychosocial and medical implications. *Pediatrics* 1987;79:331–7.

Pediatric and Adolescent Gynecology,
edited by S. E. Carpenter and J. A. Rock.
Raven Press, Ltd., New York © 1992.

22
Adolescent Contraception

Vanessa Elaine Cullins and George R. Huggins

Department of Obstetrics and Gynecology, The Francis Scott Key Medical Center, 4940 Eastern Avenue, Baltimore, Maryland 21224

U.S. adolescent pregnancies number over 1 million per year. Since the late 1970s, approximately 47% of conceptions have resulted in live births and 38 to 40% have been terminated through legal abortion (1). The average age of first intercourse, 16.2 for U.S. females and 15.7 for U.S. males (2), is comparable to the age of coital initiation in industrialized countries such as Canada, Great Britain, France, the Netherlands, and Sweden, yet the birth, pregnancy, and abortion rates are significantly higher among U.S. adolescents (3). The categorical distinction between U.S. teens and teens of other nations is contraceptive use. U.S. teens, like older U.S. women, are poor contraceptors when compared to women of similarly industrialized countries (4).

Early adolescent coitus is a well documented phenomenon. Age at first intercourse has decreased steadily since the 1960s sexual revolution. Factors responsible for this explosion of early coital experiences include a decline of institutional influences such as church and family, and the surge of media exploitation of sex, sex appeal, and sex without consequences. The consequences of unprotected adolescent intercourse reverberate through U.S. society in the form of rising maternal/perinatal morbidity, rising sexually transmitted disease rates, increased private and public expenditures, and the oft arrested educational and financial growth of the affected teen, her consort, and her immediate/extended family.

The cultural diversity found within the United States contributes to this nation's inability to develop a cohesive strategy to combat teen childbearing. Regardless of personal convictions, any health professional caring for adolescents must be prepared to discuss all aspects of sexual responsibility including abstinence, contraception, and prevention of sexually transmitted diseases.

APPROACH TO THE ADOLESCENT

Constant change is the only invariable feature of adolescence. During this transition from childhood to adulthood, all teens experience varying degrees of physiologic, psychologic, and behavioral growth. This time is punctuated by adolescent attempts towards independent behavior often contrary to childhood upbringing and parental advice. If proper rapport is developed, the obstetrician/gynecologist is in a unique position to provide sensitive guidance to teens during this often confusing, transitional time. The tone of dialogue with teens must be nonjudgmental. The setting must be private. Confidentiality is a must. The goal is to help the teen develop her own set of values; to provide her with the tools to live according to values which she may modify as she grows older. In order to approach the sensitive and anxiety provoking subject of adolescent sexuality, the clinician must first determine the adolescent's behavior, attitudes, and concerns relating to sexuality. This may be approached by asking the young woman:

1. How she feels about teenagers having sex?
2. Are any of her friends engaging in sexual intercourse?
3. Has she had sexual intercourse?
4. How does she feel about her sexual behavior?

Once the above information is gained, the physician will know whether to emphasize abstinence or contraceptive counselling. Throughout the conversation the adolescent should be treated as an independent decision maker. She must be helped to see the long term commitment of raising a child. Often teens define sexual activity in terms of frequency. They often equate infrequent sex with no risk of pregnancy. The adolescent patient must be helped to acknowledge that one voluntary sexual act makes her a sexually active individual. With sexual activity comes responsibility to self, i.e., protection against pregnancy and sexually transmitted diseases. She must also come to understand that taking charge of her sexuality and life does not preclude love and spontaneity. Help her understand the nature of relationships—that they are dynamic and often short lived. The role of the physician is one of motivator/re-enforcer of all positive aspects of the teens life, including postponement of intercourse and/or maintenance of sexual health. As the motivator, reenforcer, the physician should offer additional perspectives to the teen's life experiences. This can often be done by listening to and exploring the patient's motivations.

Abrahamse et al. (5) found that teens most likely to consider single parenthood tend to exhibit problem behaviors such as school disciplinary problems and nonconforming behavior. They found adolescents with the most to lose educationally, economically, and socially are least likely to consider early childbearing. One overriding goal in professional dialogue is to emphasize the educational, economic, and social costs of early childbearing. This can be accomplished by incorporating a discussion of each teen's future aspirations and by developing a general plan for the accomplishment of these goals. This translates into an active discussion of abstinence for the virgin and of contraception for the sexually active teen. This position can be reinforced in subsequent visits by reference to progress towards previously mentioned educational, social, and economic goals.

CONTRACEPTIVE METHODS

As the word implies, contraception is designed to prevent conception. For adolescents and adults who practice any mode of interpersonal sexuality excepting lifetime monogamy, contraception must perform the dual role of preventing conception and preventing sexually transmitted disease.

ORAL CONTRACEPTION

The mainstay of adolescent contraception continues to be oral contraception. Today's low dose combined oral contraceptives (OCs) are highly effective (99%) (6–8) when used correctly. Low dose pills prevent pregnancy by (a) preventing ovulation, (b) thickening cervical mucus, (c) atrophy of the endometrium, and (d) altering tubal motility. The increase in cervical mucus viscosity also decreases the risk of upper genital tract sexually transmitted disease (9).

Combined oral contraceptives containing less than 50 μg of estrogen have a low incidence of serious side effects such as venous and arterial thromboembolism. The original data on the relationship between OCs and pulmonary emboli relate only to older high dose pills. Rates of pulmonary embolus, heart attack and stroke are much lower for low dose pills (10,11).

Low dose oral contraceptive pills continue to be associated with such nuisance side effects as nausea, breast tenderness, mood changes, and breakthrough bleeding. The adolescent should be warned of these side effects. She should be reassured that these side effects will usually subside within the first 3 months of use. Assure her that her pill formulation can be changed if she has persistent problems after approximately 3 cycles of continuous use and ask that she contact her clinician with her concerns. Too often, adolescent patients discontinue contraception in response to relatively minor or transient symptoms without seeking medical advice. The non contraceptive benefits of oral contraceptives should be stressed. These include a decreased risk of ovarian cancer, anemia, menorrhagia, dysmenorrhea, functional ovarian cysts, benign breast disease, and pelvic inflammatory disease. For adolescents with a history of acne or hirsutism, the salutary effect of low dose pills on SHBG and free testosterone will be a benefit. No clinically significant weight gain is associated with current low dose formulations. If the teen has a family history of carbohydrate intolerance or hyperlipidemia, a pill containing norethindrone may be chosen (12); a monophasic pill should be prescribed if the adolescent occasionally misses pills (13,14) or if she suffers significant dysmenorrhea (15). An important advantage of the combined oral contraceptive is that it is not a coitally related method.

Disadvantages for the adolescent are that the pill must be taken every day, preferably at the same time each day, and generally requires a pelvic exam prior to its initiation. The cost of the pills can be prohibitive to teen unless she is covered by a prescription plan, has a substantial source of income, or is a patient in a federally subsidized family planning program.

For teens, it is prudent to prescribe a 28-day rather than a 21-day pill. Taking a pill every day tends to encourage pill compliance and prevent extension of the hormone-free interval beyond the recommended 7 days.

The progestin only "mini-pill" is generally reserved for patients that are unable to take estrogen. Very few teens will be medically unable to take estrogen. In addition to decreased effectiveness, progestin only pills have the disadvantage of more frequent and persistent, irregular bleeding episodes. The pregnancy rate associated with missed pills among mini pill users is quite high. Because of the high incidence or irregular bleeding and higher pregnancy rates, mini pills are not well suited for teens.

BARRIER METHODS

Barrier methods available in the United States include spermicidal foams, jellies, creams, suppositories, male condom, female condom, diaphragm, cervical cap, and contraceptive sponge. These methods vary in effectiveness, with pregnancy rates of 4–30% in the first year of contraceptive use (8.16–19). For barrier methods, both the theoretical effective rate and use effective rate is best for the male condom. For the male condom, both the theoretical failure rate and use effective failure rate approach 2% in older, highly motivated couples

(16,17). For all the barrier methods, use effectiveness tends to increase with increasing age. The older and more motivated the user, the more consistent the barrier method use and the lower the failure rate. Theoretically, barrier contraception, especially the male condom, is an ideal method for teens because barrier methods provide excellent dual protection against pregnancy and sexually transmitted diseases, when used correctly. Barrier method failure rates, however, are high in teens. Even when used correctly, barrier method continuation rates are low in younger patients. One year continuation rates for adolescents range from approximately 20 to 80% (18–20).

The major disadvantage of barrier methods is that they are coital related, and require comfort/familiarity with the patient's own genitalia; or in the case of the male condom, comfort with the partner's genitalia. Self assurance is needed to purchase condoms over the counter. Adolescents tend to be intolerant of the inconvenience of preparation required for barrier methods. The cost of barrier methods can be prohibitive unless the teen gives the need for the method a high priority, i.e., considers barrier method cost as a necessary expense, just as a new article of clothing may be considered necessary for the next date.

A barrier method may be a good choice for adolescents who engage in infrequent intercourse, or are poor pill takers. The condom is a must for teens with multiple sexual partners, or who engage in frequent serial monogamy, or who are intimate with partners who have multiple partners, for preventing sexually transmitted diseases, including AIDS.

Comfort with tampon insertion is a good initial indicator of whether a teen is a good candidate for a female barrier method. A teen who is not comfortable inserting or removing a tampon cannot be expected to effectively use a barrier method. As alluded to before, the teen's acknowledgment of sexuality and assertiveness should be gauged prior recommending a barrier method.

As with any contraceptive method, the adolescent should be given detailed instructions on the contraceptive's use. The teen must know exactly what to buy, how to use it, and how to care for any multiple use device.

Male Condom

The major advantage of the male latex condom is superior protection against sexually transmitted diseases. Latex condoms have been shown to prevent the transmission of chlamydia, trichomonas, gonorrhea, herpes, human immunodeficiency virus, cytomegalovirus, hepatitis B virus, and probably human papilloma virus (21–27). In the well motivated couple, condoms also are an effective safeguard against pregnancy. The first year failure rate for the condom can be as low as 1 to 4% (28). Among typical users, failure rates are 10–20% (6,8). Adolescents should be instructed on both the type and correct use of the condom. As natural membrane condoms do not afford effective protection against sexually transmitted diseases, a latex condom should always be used. A new condom should be used with each sexual act. The condom should be placed on the erect penis and rolled from the glans to the base. If a condom without a reservoir tip is used, room must be left at the tip to collect semen and prevent breakage. The rim of the condom must be held when the penis is withdrawn from the vagina. Only a water-based lubricant should be used. The teen should be advised that the most effective protection against sexually transmitted disease transmission is the combination of condom and spermicidal agent. Suggest that in place of a lubricant, a spermicide can be used.

Diaphragm, Cervical Cap, Contraceptive Sponge, and Spermicides

Diaphragm

Diaphragms are shallow, flexible domes of rubber that are placed high in the vagina to cover the cervix. There are three types of diaphragms based on the type of spring located in the rim—the arcing spring, coil spring, and flat spring diaphragm. Adolescent patients tend to fare best with either an arcing or coil spring diaphragm. Both the coil and arcing spring diaphragms are easier to compress and correctly insert than the flat spring. The arcing spring diaphragm forms an arc when compressed. This enables the diaphragm to be inserted easily and correctly in patients with marked ante- or retroversion. The coil spring diaphragm is fitted easily in women with normal pelvic anatomy without marked uterine ante- or retroversion. All three diaphragm types, are produced in a range of sizes 50–105 mm in diameter. In order to receive the proper size and type of diaphragm, the patient must be fitted by a knowledgeable health professional. The diaphragm is used with a spermicidal jelly or cream and can be inserted up to 6 hours prior to intercourse. It must be left in place for at least 6 hours after the last act of intercourse. For continued efficacy, additional spermicide must be inserted for each repeat coital act. The diaphragm pregnancy rate can be as low as 1.1 per 100 women per year for a highly motivated couple. Typical pregnancy rates are 10–20% (6,8,17). Failure rates and discontinuation rates are much higher for new users, and younger women (16,30). For adolescents, the one year continuation rate may be as low as 23% (20).

Side effects from the diaphragm include potential allergy to the spermicide and/or rubber, and an increased risk of urinary tract infections (31–33). Disadvantages of the diaphragm include that it is a coital related method, and therefore interferes with the spontaneity of sex; preparation and insertion is sometimes messy; insertion of additional spermicide is often inconvenient; it must be fitted and prescribed by a health professional.

When fitted for a diaphragm, the patient should receive extensive instruction on its use. In the office, she should both remove and replace the diaphragm. She should be seen back in 1–2 weeks for a recheck of her placement and removal. In addition to routine instructions on use, she should be warned that she will experience a greater chance of diaphragm displacement in female superior positions. She must also be instructed that the diaphragm will need to be refitted after pregnancy. Instruct her on inspection of the diaphragm for holes or tears and on the soap and water cleansing after each diaphragm use. She must be instructed to never leave the diaphragm in more than 24 hr in order to avoid toxic shock syndrome (34–35).

Cervical Cap

The cervical cap is a thimble shaped dome of rubber which is used with a spermicide and is applied over the cervix. Fitting the cap to the cervix is more difficult than the fitting of a diaphragm. Caps available in the United States are manufactured in four different sizes. Because of the limitation in sizes, approximately 6% of women cannot be fitted (36). The cervical cap is considered as efficacious as the diaphragm (19). Although considered less messy than a diaphragm, its insertion and removal tends to be more difficult. It is, however, not necessary to use additional spermicide if repeat intercourse occurs less than 6 hr after the placement of the first application of intracap spermicide. If intercourse occurs longer than 6 hr after initial placement of the cap, additional spermicide should be placed intravaginally. An advantage of the cap is that it may be left in place for up to

48 hr. Cleaning and storage is analogous to diaphragm cleaning and storage. In general, the cervical cap is not a good method for adolescents because of the difficulty involved in placement and removal (36).

Vaginal Contraceptive Sponge

The vaginal contraceptive sponge is a spermicide containing polyurethane foam barrier designed to fit over the cervical os. This single use device, which contains 1 gr of nonoxynol 9, is available in one size, and is purchased over the counter. It is moistened with water prior to insertion, and can be inserted anytime up to 24 hr prior to intercourse. Contraceptive action lasts for 24 hr. The sponge may be left in place for a total of 30 hr. No additional spermicide is needed for additional acts of intercourse within the 24-hr period. For the nulliparous, the first year failure rate of the sponge is similar to that of the diaphragm. The failure rate can be up to 28% for women with children (8,37). As with the diaphragm and cervical cap, adolescents need to be given detailed instructions on sponge use. They should be warned of potential for dislodgement. Although the incidence of toxic shock syndrome is rare, the adolescent should be made aware of the relationship between prolonged sponge exposure and this illness. It is prudent to instruct the adolescent on sponge usage as one would instruct for the diaphragm or cervical cap, i.e., have the adolescent insert and remove the sponge in the office.

Spermicides

Spermicides (jellies, creams, foams, suppositories, tablets and films) may be used independently or in conjunction with the condom, cervical cap or diaphragm. The active ingredient found in spermicides available in the United States is either nonoxynol-9 or octoxynol. Contraceptive efficacy is a result of the surfactant's action on sperm. Additionally, these spermicides are bactericidal and inactivate viruses (9,38–42). Because it is a compliance dependent method, the failure rate of spermicides used independently of other barrier methods is approximately 21% during the first year of use. This contrasts to the theoretical failure rate of 3% (8,17). As with other barrier methods, spermicides are perceived by adolescents as messy and inconvenient. Not only must the spermicide be introduced intravaginally prior to intercourse, but repeat applications should be inserted prior to additional coital acts. Compared with other barrier methods, adolescents may achieve better compliance with spermicidal agents delivered through tubular vaginal applicators, as the insertion mechanism is similar to that of a tampon or medicinal vaginal cream. Even though applicator inserted spermicides are potentially easier and quicker to use than other barrier methods, consistent use and continuation rates are low.

Norplant

Approved by the Federal Drug Administration (FDA) in December, 1990, Norplant is the most exciting contraceptive method to be offered to U.S. women since oral contraceptives. Norplant is a long acting, levonorgestrel containing contraceptive designed to be implanted subdermally in the upper arm of the woman. Each of the six matchstick sized capsules is 34 mm long and 2.4 mm in diameter. Each capsule contains 36 mg of levonorgestrel. Once steady state serum levels are obtained, approximately 30 mcg of levonorgestrel are released a day (43). The failure rate is 0.04% in the first year of use, which is less than any other form of reversible contraception (8). If inserted within the first 5 days of menses, Norplant is effective within hours of insertion; contraceptive efficacy lasts for 5 years (43,44).

Serum levonorgestrel concentrations vary

according to body weight and individual clearance rate. Earlier studies found that the lowest failure rates occurred in patients weighing less than 50 kg. The 5-year cumulative failure rate for patients weighing less than 50 kg was 0.2 per 100 users. This failure rate rose to 8.5 for patients greater than or equal to 70 kg (45). It should be noted however, that a 5-year cumulative pregnancy rate of 8.5 per 100 users is still less than the cumulative 5-year pregnancy rate for typical users of oral contraceptives.

The Norplant capsule used in the U.S. is a modification of original Silastic capsules used in early testing. Current data show that these new capsules may be equally effective in women weighing over 50 kg.

Norplant primarily prevents pregnancy through thickening of the cervical mucus and atrophic effects on the endometrical lining (46). Because serum levels of levonorgestrel are low, ovulation is inconsistently inhibited. The steady, low levels of levonorgestrel also result in this method's primary side effect, irregular bleeding. Menstrual irregularities may include prolonged bleeding during the first months of use, unexpected bleeding, spotting between periods, or amenorrhea. It should be noted, that although frequency of bleeding may be increased, blood loss is usually less than normal menses (43). Other side effects of this method include side effects common to progestin containing compounds including headache, nervousness, nausea, dizziness, acne, change in appetite, weight gain, mastalgia, hirsutism, or hair loss. Although not medically serious, these side effects may account for a substantial percentage of discontinuations. There has been no evidence of adverse cardiovascular, respiratory, or central nervous system disorders as a result of Norplant (43). Return to fertility, once the implant system is removed, is quite rapid and is comparable to rates seen following discontinuation of barrier methods. The resumption of fertility is somewhat faster than that seen after patients have discontinued oral contraceptives (43,45).

This method should prove to be extremely valuable in the prevention of adolescent pregnancy. Because of the cervical mucus effect, a modicum of protection against upper genital tract sexually transmitted diseases is expected. This protection, similar to that seen with oral contraceptives, is incomplete, and adolescents should be advised to use condoms along with the Norplant.

To assure continued use of this method, the adolescent should be counselled in depth about the irregular bleeding patterns. She should be reassured that the irregular bleeding and amenorrhea seen with this method are a normal occurrence and does not indicate an abnormal condition. Management of this irregular bleeding is very different from management of irregular bleeding or amenorrhea associated with birth control pills. For patients on birth control pills, it is very common to stop the method, change pills, or add additional estrogen in an attempt to regularize the cycle. This is an inappropriate response with the Norplant. Most practitioners with extensive Norplant experience recommend that the irregular bleeding and amenorrhea be managed with repetitive patient reassurance as opposed to hormonal manipulations.

Depo-Provera

Depo-medroxyprogesterone acetate—Depo-Provera—is a first generation, long acting, injectable, progestin contraceptive. One hundred and fifty milligrams of Depo-Provera via deep intramuscular injection provides contraceptive efficacy for 3 months. The failure rate of Depo-Provera is less than 1 per 100 women years of use (46). Although an approved FDA medication, Depo-Provera has not been approved by the FDA for contraceptive use. It is currently used as a contraceptive by approximately 4 million women worldwide (44). United States FDA approval of Depo-Provera has been stalemated by political activism influenced by findings of breast cancer in beagles and endometrial cancer in monkeys—findings that have been unsubstantiated in humans (47,48). With the availability of Norplant, it is wise to refrain from prescribing Depo-Provera, except in situations where Depo-Provera is the only rational alternative—for example, the adolescent who does not tolerate or is not compliant with other forms of contraception, and who will not tolerate or allow insertion/removal of the implants.

The most common side effect of Depo-Provera is menstrual irregularities. As with Norplant, this bleeding is unpredictable and may eventually lead to amenorrhea. With Depo-Provera, approximately 50% of users are amenorrhic at the end of the first year of use (47). Other side effects include those related to any progestin containing compound—headache, dizziness, abdominal bloating, mood changes, nervousness, nausea, acne, mastalgia, hirsutism, or hair loss.

FUTURE CONTRACEPTIVE METHODS

The future is most promising for long acting, hormonal, contraceptive methods. Methods in development include: Norplant II, biodegradable implants, injectable microspheres and microcapsules, and vaginal rings. Norplant II is a two capsule levonorgestrel system designed for 3 years of use. Biodegradable implants have the advantage of no need for removal when the contraceptive efficacy wanes. There are two biodegradable implants currently in development: (a) Capronor, a single capsule containing levonorgestrel, designed for 18 months of protection and (b) Norethrindone pellets that provide protection for 12 months. Injectable microspheres and microcapsules can prevent pregnancy for 1, 3, or 6 months. The microspheres or microcapsules contain either estrogen and progestin, progestin, or natural progesterone. Vaginal rings containing levonorgestrel or natural progesterone may remain in the vagina for up to 3 months. Combined estrogen-progestin rings remain in the vagina for 3 weeks and are removed for 1 week out of the month to allow menses.

A new barrier method which will soon be available is the vaginal or female condom. It consists of a loose, 15 cm, soft, polyurethane sheath with flexible polyurethane rings at each end. The inner ring is placed as high as possible in the vagina. The outer ring covers the perineum and thus provides protection against perineal contact with sexually transmitted diseases. The female condom is used in conjunction with a spermicide. It is designed for one time use, and will be available in one size and sold over the counter. Although comparative data is lacking, it is felt the vaginal condom will be as efficacious as the male condom for pregnancy and sexually transmitted disease prevention.

CONTRACEPTIVE METHODS NOT SUITABLE FOR ADOLESCENTS

The two methods least suitable for adolescents include sterilization and the IUD. Because of the increased risk of pelvic inflammatory disease, the IUD is an inappropriate device for adolescents. Tubal sterilization should not be considered a reversible procedure, and thus should not be performed in teens. Because of their tendency towards irregular menses, anovulatory cycles, poor motivation and discomfort with methods that require extensive genital manipulation, most teens are poor candidates for natural family planning methods, i.e., rhythm, basal body temperature method, mucus method, or symptothermal method.

PREGNANT ADOLESCENTS

One of the most disconcerting situations a gynecologic health professional faces is the pregnant adolescent. Pregnant teens need to be advised of all options: (a) childbearing with raising the infant, (b) childbearing with adoption, and (c) abortion. The teen should be referred to appropriate counselling and service facilities, pending the chosen option. As much as possible, she should be made to understand the implications of her decision for her and her family's future.

ABORTION

Approximately one and one half million legal abortions are performed each year in the United States. Since 1981, abortions among women younger than 20 have comprised approximately 27% of all abortion procedures. The percentage of pregnancies terminated by abortions is approximately 45% among adolescents less than age 15 and 40% among adolescents aged 15–19 (49). In 1987, the latest year of the Center for Disease Control (CDC) Abortion Surveillance report, approximately one-half of all abortions were performed before the eighth week of pregnancy and more than 85% were performed during the first trimester of pregnancy (50).

Recriminalization of abortion would have a tremendous impact on adolescent childbearing. Joyce and Mocan (51), using statistical modelling, estimate that if legal abortion was banned in New York City, adolescent births would rise by 18.7% among blacks and 14.0% in whites.

Most laws restricting adolescent access to fertility control services are levied from the state level. It is, therefore, important to know the laws of the state in which the clinician practices. Thirty states have laws requiring parental consent or notification prior to performance of an abortion in a minor[1] (52).

In twenty-one states, a woman is required to wait a designated amount of time between consent for the abortion and performance of the procedure[2] (52).

First Trimester Abortion

Abortion continues to be much safer than childbirth, overall. The risk of death from an abortion is approximately 0.6 per 100,000 cases (52). The safest abortions are those done in the first trimester. The death rate from an abortion performed at 8 weeks gestation or less is 0.2 deaths per 100,000 procedures. This rate increases to 0.6 at 11 or 12 weeks gestation (52).

First trimester abortions are performed by suction curettage (synonymous with vacuum curettage and vacuum aspiration) The cervix is dilated and the uterine contents are evacuated using vacuum aspiration. For nulliparous patients greater than 10 weeks gestational age, initial cervical dilatation is accomplished using a hydroscopic cervical dilator such as laminaria tents or Dilapan. The use of these hydroscopic devices minimizes the incidence of cervical trauma possible during rapid operative dilatation. Almost all first trimester procedures use local anesthesia rather than general anesthesia. The incidence of uterine perforation, intraabdominal hemorrhage, and cervical trauma is less in women receiving local anesthesia (53).

The complication rate for first trimester abortion is low. Complications include hemorrhage (transfusion rate of 0.6 per 100 abortions) (53), hematometra (0.2 to 1 per 100 abortions) (54,55), coagulopathy (8 per 100,000 cases) (56), perforation of the uterus (0.2 per 100 procedures) (53,57), cervical injury (0.18–0.96 per 100 abortions) (53,57), retained products of conception (0.61 cases per 100 abortions) (53), and in-

---

[1]Alabama, Arizona, Arkansas, California, Florida, Georgia, Idaho, Illinois, Indiana, Kentucky, Louisiana, Maine, Maryland, Massachusetts, Michigan, Minnesota, Missouri, Montana, Nebraska, Nevada, North Dakota, Ohio, Pennsylvania, Rhode Island, South Carolina, South Dakota, Tennessee, Utah, West Virginia, Wyoming.

[2]Arizona, Arkansas, Delaware, Idaho, Illinois, Indiana, Kentucky, Louisiana, Maine, Massachusetts, Minnesota, Nebraska, Nevada, North Dakota, Ohio, Pennsylvania, Rhode Island, South Dakota, Tennessee, West Virginia and Wyoming.

fection (0.75 per 100 procedures) (53). The risk of fatal pulmonary embolus is low for first trimester abortions (56).

U.S. studies have not shown a decrease in fertility in patients who have undergone first trimester abortion (58). Chung et al. (59) did not find an increase in frequency of fetal wastage among women with prior legal abortions. Results have varied as to whether induced abortion results in increased risk of premature deliveries (60).

Second Trimester Abortion

In 1987, the latest year for which abortion surveillance data is available, approximately 25% of abortions performed in adolescents less than age 15 and approximately 16% of abortions among those aged 15–19 were second trimester abortions. Second trimester abortions comprised approximately 11% of the total abortions performed in the United States (50). Second trimester abortions are attended by higher mortality and morbidity than first trimester abortions. The risk of major complications is between .5 and 1.8% (52). This complication rate is significantly lower than the childbirth complication rate (52). Adolescents are not at increased risk for developing major complications (52).

There are many different methods of performing second trimester abortions. The two major types of second trimester abortions are (a) dilatation and evacuation and (b) labor induction methods. Dilatation and evacuation is the appropriate technique for gestations between 13 and 16 weeks. Between 16 and 20 weeks, dilatation and evacuation or a labor induction method may be used. Labor induction is generally the preferred method for pregnancies greater than 20 weeks. Both of these two major methods of pregnancy termination require hydroscopic cervical dilators such as laminaria or Dilapan. In dilatation and evacuation, a large suction cannula is used to drain the amniotic fluid and remove remaining placental tissue and clot after most of the uterine contents have been evacuated with long, heavy forceps. There are many different methods and variations of methods for second trimester labor induction. Intravaginal PGE_2, intramuscular 15 methyl PGF_2 alpha, high dose pitocin, hypertonic saline, intraamniotic urea, or a combination of prostaglandins and intraamniotic methods may be used. Complications associated with second trimester abortions include hemorrhage, infection, uterine rupture, disseminated intravascular coagulopathy (hypertonic saline, intraamniotic urea, dilatation and evacuation) and cervical laceration. Fortunately, the major complications are rare (52,61).

As stated previously, adolescents undergoing abortion need extensive counselling. The psychological impact of abortion will vary per individual. In 1989, the Surgeon General, C. Everett Koop concluded, after review of over two hundred and fifty studies, that abortion is not detrimental to a woman's mental health (62). Zabin et al. (63) found that adolescents who terminated their pregnancies were more likely to have graduated from high school or still be in school at the appropriate grade level, than teens who decided to carry their pregnancy to term.

ADOLESCENT SEXUAL RESPONSIBILITY

Promotion of sexual responsibility must be the charge of all health professionals dealing with adolescents. The framework of sexual responsibility includes prevention of pregnancy, sexually transmitted diseases, and early childbearing. The integration of an effective method with the desires and maturational state of the adolescent is often difficult. Method or compliance failure must, therefore, be backed up with childbearing or childraising alternatives.

REFERENCES

1. Henshaw SK, Kenney AM, Somberg D, Van Vort J. *Teenage pregnancy in the United States. The scope of the problem and state responses.* New York: The Alan Guttmacher Institute, 1989.
2. Center for Population Options. *The facts: teenage sexuality, pregnancy and parenthood.* Washington, DC: April 1987.
3. Jones EF, Forrest JD, Goldman N, et al. Teenage pregnancy in developed countries: determinants and policy implications. *Fam Plann Perspect* 1985;17:53.
4. Jones EF, Forrest JD, Henshaw SK, Silverman J, Torres A. Unintended pregnancy, contraceptive practice and family planning services in developed countries. *Fam Plann Perspect* 1988; 20:53.
5. Abrahamse AF, Morrison PA, Waite LJ. Teenagers willing to consider single parenthood: who is at greatest risk? *Fam Plann Perspect* 1988; 20:13.
6. Liskin L, Kak N, Rutledge MS, Smit LC, Stewart S. *Youth in the 1980's: social and health concerns. Population information program. The Johns Hopkins University Population Reports. Series M. No. 9.* November-December 1985.
7. Foster DC. Low dose monophasic and multiphasic oral contraceptives: a review of potency, efficacy and side effects. *Semin Reprod Endocrinol* 1989;7:205.
8. Trussell J, Hatcher RA, Cates W, Stewart FH, Kost K. Contraceptive failure in the United States: an update. *Stud Fam Plann.* 1990;21:51.
9. Grimes DA, Cates W Jr. Family planning and sexually transmitted diseases. In: *Sexually transmitted diseases.* New York: McGraw-Hill, 1990:1087.
10. Mann JI. Progestogens in cardiovascular disease. An introduction to the epidemiologic data. *Am J Obstet Gynecol* 1982;142:752.
11. Meade TW, Greenberg G, Thompson SG. Progestogens and cardiovascular reactions associated with oral contraceptives and a comparison of the safety of 50 and 30 microgram oestrogen preparations. *Br Med J* 1980;280:1157.
12. Godsland IF, Crook D, Simpson R, Proudler T, Felton C, et al. The effects of different formulations of oral contraceptive agents on lipid and carbohydrate metabolism. *N Engl J Med* 1990; 323:1375.
13. Grimes DA, ed. *The contraception report. Vol. I, no. 4. OC compliance and contraceptive failure.* Morris Plains, NJ: Emron, 1990:3–6.
14. Chowdhury V, Joshi UM, Gopalkrishna K, et al. "Escape" ovulation in women due to the missing of low dose combination oral contraceptive pills. *Contraception* 1980;22:241.
15. Nabrink M, Birgersson L, Colling-Jaltin, Solum T. Modern oral contraceptives and dysmenorrhea. *Contraception* 1990;42:275.
16. Ory HW, Forrest JD, Lincoln R. *Making choices—evaluating the health risks and benefits of birth control methods.* New York: The Alan Guttmacher Institute, 1983.
17. Grimes DA, ed. *The contraceptive report. Vol. I, no. 4. Which patients may benefit from alternative contraceptive methods?* Morris Plains, NJ: Emron, 1990:7–12.
18. Goldman JA, Dicker D, Feldberg D, et al. Barrier contraception in the teenager: a comparison of four methods in adolescent girls.*Pediatr Adolesc Gynecol* 1985;3:59.
19. Kulig JW. Adolescent contraception: non-hormonal methods. *Adolesc Gynecol* 1989;36:717.
20. Lane ME, Arceo R, Sobero AJ. Successful use of the diaphragm and jelly by a young population: report of a clinical study. *Fam Plann Perspect* 1976;8:81.
21. Stone KM, Grimes DA, Magder LS. Personal protection against sexually transmitted diseases. *Am J Obstet Gynecol* 1986;155:180.
22. Conant MA, Spicer DW, Smith CD: Herpes simplex virus transmission: condom studies. *Sex Transm Dis* 1984;11:94.
23. Katznelson S, Drew WL, Mintz L. Efficacy of the condom as a barrier to the transmission of cytomegalovirus. *J Infect Dis* 1984;150:155.
24. Conant M, Hardy D, Sernatinger J, Spicer D, Levy JA. Condoms prevent transmission of AID-associated retrovirus. *JAMA* 1986;255: 1706.
25. Rietmeijer CA, Krebs JW, Feorino PM, et al. Condoms as physical and chemical barriers against human immunodeficiency virus. *JAMA* 1988;259:1851.
26. Connell EB. Barrier contraceptives. *Clin Obstet Gynecol* 1989;32:377.
27. Richardson AC, Lyon JB. The effect of condom use on squamous cell cervical intraepithelial neoplasia. *Am J Obstet Gynecol* 1981;140:909.
28. Schirm AL, Trussell J, Menken J, Grady WR. Contraceptive failure in the United States: the impact of social, economic and demographic factors. *Fam Plann Perspect* 1982;14:68.
29. Vessey M, Lawless M, Yeates D. Efficacy of different contraceptive methods. *Lancet* 1982; 1:841.
30. Mishell DR. Contraception. *N Engl J Med* 1989;320:777.
31. Gillespie L. The diaphragm: an accomplice in recurrent urinary tract infections. *Urology* 1984; 24:25.
32. Fihn SD, Latham RH, Roberts P, Running K, Stamm WE. Association between diaphragm use and urinary tract infection. *JAMA* 1985;254:240.
33. Foxman B, Frerichs R. Epidemiology of urinary tract infection: I. Diaphragm use and sexual intercourse. *Am J Public Health* 1985;75:1308.
34. Jaffe R. Toxic shock syndrome associated with diaphragm use [Letter to the editor]. *New Engl J Med* 1981;305:1585.
35. Baehler EA, Dillon WP, Cumbo TJ, et al: Prolonged use of a diaphragm and toxic shock syndrome. *Fert Steril* 1982;38:248.
36. Klitsch M. FDA approval ends cervical cap's marathon. *Fam Plann Perspect* 1988;20:137.
37. McIntyre SL, Higgins JE. Parity and use-effec-

tiveness with the contraceptive sponge. *Am J Obstet Gynecol* 1986;155:796.

38. Bolch OH Jr, Warren JC. In vitro effects of emko on neisseria gonorrhoeae and trichmonas vaginalis. *Am J Obstet Gynecol* 1973;115:1145.
39. Stone KM, Grimes DA, Magder LS. Personal protection against sexually transmitted diseases. *Am J Obstet Gynecol* 1986;155:180.
40. Cutler JC, Singh B, Carpenter U, et al. Vaginal contraceptives as prophylaxis against gonorrhea and other sexually transmissible disease. *Adv Plann Parenthood* 1977;12:45.
41. Hicks DR, Martin LS, Getchell JP, et al. Inactivation of HTLV III/LAV infected cultures of normal human lymphocytes by nonoxynol-9 in vitro. *Lancet* 1985;2:1422.
42. Austin H, Louv WC, Alexander WJ. A case-control study of spermicides and gonorrhea. *JAMA* 1984;251:2822.
43. *Norplant fact sheet.* New York: The Population Council, April 1989.
44. *Long-acting steroid contraceptive technology—a status report. Health and sexuality. Vol 2, no. 1.* Washington, DC: Association of Reproductive Health Professionals, Winter 1991.
45. *Norplant System (levonorgestrel implants) prescribing information. Product literature.* Philadelphia: Wyeth Laboratories, December 1990.
46. Liskin L, Blackburn R, Ghani R. *Hormonal contraception: new long acting methods. Population Information Program. The Johns Hopkins University Population Reports. Injectables and Implants. Series K. no 3.* March–April 1987.
47. Rosenfield A. Injectable contraception. In: Carson SL, Derman RJ, Tyrer LB, eds. *Fertility Control.* 1st ed. Boston: Little, Brown, 1985: 187–195.
48. Rosenfield A, Maine D, Rochat R, Shelton J, Hatcher RA. The Food and Drug Administration and medroxyprogesterone acetate. What are the issues? *JAMA* 1983;249:2922.
49. *Table 1. Number and percentage distribution of legal abortions, abortion rate per 1,000 women, and percentage of pregnancies terminated by abortion, by age, United States, 1973–1985.* The Alan Guttmacher Institute. Personal communications, S. K. Henshaw, 1990.
50. Koonin LM, Atrash HK, Smith JC, Ramick M. Abortion surveillance, 1986–1987. *CDC Surveillance Summaries, Vol 39, no. SS-2.* June 1990: 23–56.
51. Joyce TJ, Mocan NH. The impact of legalized abortion on adolescent childbearing in New York City. *Am J Public Health* 1990;80:273.
52. Gold RB. *Abortion and women's health. A turning point for America?* New York: The Alan Guttmacher Institute, 1990.
53. Grimes DA, Schulz KF, Cates W Jr., Tyler CW. Local versus general anesthesia: which is safer for performing suction curettage abortions? *Am J Obstet Gynecol* 1979;135:1030.
54. Sands RX, Burnhill MS, Hakim-Elahi E. Postabortal uterine atony. *Obstet Gynecol* 1974; 43:595.
55. Nathanson BN. The postabortal pain syndrome: a new entity. *Obstet Gynecol* 1973;41:739.
56. Kaunitz AM, Grimes DA. First-trimester abortion technology. In: Corson SL, Derman RJ, Tyrer LB, eds. *Fertility control.* 1st ed. Boston: Little, Brown, 1985:63–76.
57. Bozorg N. Statistical analysis of first trimester pregnancy terminations in an ambulatory surgical center. *Am J Obstet Gynecol* 1977;127:763.
58. Daling JR, Sapdoni LR, Emanuel I. Role of induced abortion in secondary infertility. *Obstet Gynecol* 1981;57:59.
59. Chung CS, Smith RG, Steinhoff PG. Induced abortion and spontaneous fetal loss in subsequent pregnancies. *Am J Public Health* 1982; 72:548.
60. Hogue CJR, Cates W Jr, Tietze C. The effects of induced abortion on subsequent reproduction. *Epidemiol Rev* 1982;4:66.
61. Stubblefield PG. Induced abortion in the midtrimester. In: Corson SL, Derman RJ, Tyrer LB, eds. *Fertility control.* 1st ed. Boston: Little, Brown, 1985:77–87.
62. *Congressional Record.* March 21, 1989:E908.
63. Zabin LS, Hirsch MB. Emerson MR. When urban adolescents choose abortion: effects on education, psychological status and subsequent pregnancy. *Fam Plann Perspect* 1989;21:248.

Pediatric and Adolescent Gynecology,
edited by S. E. Carpenter and J. A. Rock.
Raven Press, Ltd., New York © 1992.

23
Tumors of the Vulva

*Robert A. Ambros and †Robert J. Kurman

*Departments of *·†Pathology and †Gynecology and Obstetrics, Johns Hopkins Hospital, Baltimore, Maryland 21205*

Tumors of the vulva are very uncommon in the pediatric age group. The relative frequent occurrence of vulvar neoplasms in adult women compared to children and adolescents is most likely related to the accumulated influence of environmental factors including exposure to sexually transmitted diseases such as human papillomaviruses. Most vulvar growths in children and adolescents do not represent neoplastic growths and require little treatment. Due perhaps to their rarity, when true benign and malignant neoplasms do occur, they can be confused with other conditions such as congenital adrenal hyperplasia and abuse leading to delays in diagnosis and appropriate treatment. Conversely, neoplasms and other vulvar growths in infancy and childhood can also signal other problems such as child abuse or genetic syndromes, underscoring the need for careful evaluation of all vulvar lesions in this age group.

BENIGN TUMORS

Hymenal Tags

Hymenal tags are relatively common and represent small nonneoplastic nodules of fibroconnective tissue at the margin of the hymen. Excision is recommended if the tags are large and cause discomfort, or if there is any doubt as to their nature.

Simple Cysts in the Neonate

Several types of simple cysts can occur in the neonate all of which are fairly uncommon. They may be lined by cuboidal, columnar, or squamous epithelium and most frequently occur near the urethral meatus and hymen.

Hymenal Cysts

These lesions must be differentiated from an imperforate membrane with hydrocolpos (1). Hymenal cysts have an opening and usually regress spontaneously. They may also be treated by incision and drainage. Simple puncture without anesthesia has also been successfully performed (2).

Paraurethral Cysts

These cysts are lined by squamous epithelium and are thought to arise from remnants of the wolffian duct by some (3) and as invaginations from the vagina mucosa by others (4). They either rupture spontaneously or are treated by marsupialization. These cysts can closely simulate ureteroceles and conversely, a significant percentage of ectopic ureteroceles present initially as paraurethral cysts (5). For this reason, complete urologic examination is necessary after discovery of any neonatal paraurethral cyst (4).

Simple Cysts in Childhood and Adolescence

Epithelial Inclusion Cysts

Epithelial inclusion cysts are uncommon but may occur in the adolescent age group. They develop by invagination of the surface epithelium into the underlying dermis. Histologically, they are lined by squamous epithelium with keratinaceous material filling the lumen. Treatment is simple excision.

Mucous Cysts

Mucous cysts lined by mucus producing columnar epithelium may occur in the vulvar vestibule. They are more common in adults but have been reported in adolescents (6). They are usually small but can become symptomatic by obstructing the urethra. They most likely arise by the obstruction of small mucinous glands, which are normal constituents of the vulvar vestibule (6,7).

Hydroceles

Hydroceles, also known as cysts of the Canal of Nuck, represent swellings of the blind remnant of the "processus vaginalis" (8). Normally, this remnant regresses, but a cyst develops if the peritoneal protrusion that extends into the labium majus fills with fluid and persists. Like scrotal hydroceles, vulvar hydroceles must be distinguished from true inguinal hernias. The latter can contain bowel or adnexal structures and are usually reducible. Hydroceles are treated by surgical excision.

Urethral Prolapse

Urethral prolapse of the urethral mucosa may produce a painless vulvar mass. In a report of 12 cases by Capraro et al (9), the mean age was 5 years, with patients presenting either with a vulvar mass or bleeding. Redundancy of the urethral mucosa, increased abdominal pressure, and lack of estrogen have been proposed as predisposing factors. Treatment is simple excision.

Bartholin's Gland Cysts

Bartholin's gland cysts have been reported in adolescents (10). They may develop as a result of occlusion of a main duct or small ductule of Bartholin's gland. They are lined by transitional or mucinous epithelium depending on their derivation from the main duct or ductule respectively. Cysts may present as a mass or become secondarily infected to form a painful Bartholin's gland abscess. Bartholin's gland cysts are treated by excision or marsupialization.

Squamous Papillomas and Condylomas

Squamous Papillomas

These (skin tags, acrochordons) are polypoid growths that usually involve the outer aspects of the labia. Microscopically, the lesion is characterized by squamous epithelium overlying a fibroconnective tissue core. Complexity, arborization of the papillae and koilocytosis as seen in a condyloma acuminatum does not occur in a papilloma.

Condylomata Acuminata

Condylomata acuminata result from infection by a specific type of the human papillomavirus (HPV), most frequently types 6 and 11 (11). Although uncommon, the frequency of genital HPV infection in children is believed to be increasing (18). Transmission is by direct contact. In the pediatric patient, this suggests either transmission during childbirth or sexual abuse. Since the incubation period can be up to 3 months (12), the development of condylomas after this time period is suggestive of sexual abuse. Patients range in age from 10 months to adolescence (13–21). In many of the reported cases of vulvar condylomas, sexual abuse was either not admitted or suspected by the parents and the mode of transmission could not be established. Parents sought medical attention because of the observation of a vulvar mass or bleeding following minor trauma. Condylomas are similar to squamous papillomas on gross and microscopic examination but show a more highly arborized pattern of the papillary fronds and often display koilocytosis, a feature pathognomonic of HPV infection. This finding is characterized by nuclear enlargement and wrinkling of the nuclear membrane, and formation of a perinuclear halo (Fig. 1). A diagnosis of vulvar condylomata acuminata mandates the search for other venereally transmitted infections since these may also coexist in these pa-

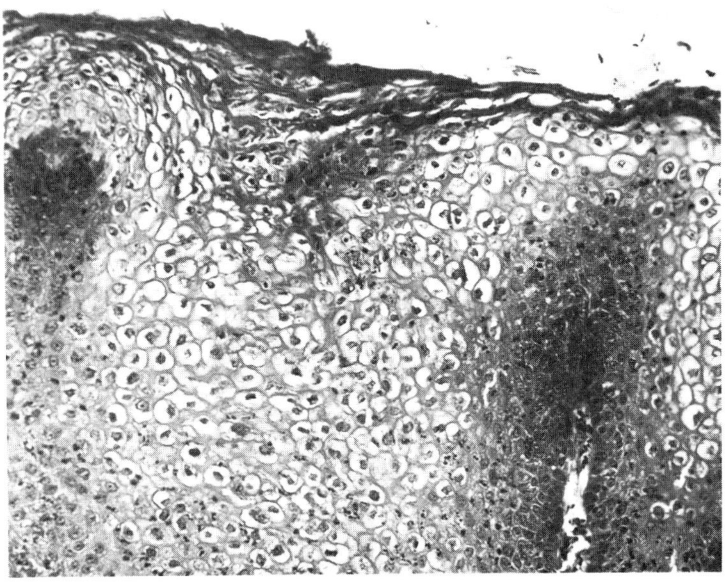

FIG. 1. Condyloma in a 16-year-old girl characterized by koilocytotic cells with enlarged nuclei, wrinkled nuclear membranes, and perinuclear halos.

tients (20). In sexually active adolescents, a cervicovaginal smear should be obtained. Treatment includes the application of trichloroacetic acid, podophyllin, surgical excision, electrocoagulation, and laser vaporization. Laser therapy is widely believed to produce the least scarring and has been advocated particularly for periurethral lesions (18).

Vascular Lesions

Hemangiomas

Hemangiomas are the most common vascular lesions and are divided into two groups based on their gross and microscopic appearance; capillary and cavernous. Although their appearance is usually characteristic, hemangiomas of the vulva can be confused with other conditions. For example, ulcerations of hemangiomas have been confused with burns secondary to child abuse and clitoral hemangiomas have been confused with phallic structures (22, 23). Rarely, vulvar hemangiomas may occur as a component of a syndrome such as vulvar congenital dysplastic angiopathy (Klippel-Trenaunay syndrome) (24). The protean manifestations of vulvar hemangiomas emphasize the need for histologic examination of vulvar growths.

Capillary Hemangiomas

Capillary hemangiomas (strawberry nevi) are flat or slightly elevated neoplasms composed of small blood vessels. On microscopic examination, they are composed of aggregations of thin-walled capillaries in the dermis that may extend with finger-like projections into deeper tissue resembling a malignant tumor.

Cavernous Hemangiomas

Cavernous hemangiomas are composed of large thin-walled vessels and can be more deeply located than capillary hemangiomas. Cutaneous vascular tumors in the infant can be mixed and show both capillary and cavernous areas. They may be present at birth but commonly develop during the first two months. After a period of rapid growth, lasting from several months to several years, the vast majority regress and complete regression by age 5 years is seen in approximately 80% of the patients (25). The percentage of vulvar lesions undergoing spontaneous regression is probably smaller. Treatment is reserved for lesions which fail to regress, are associated with psychologic trauma or develop complications such as bleeding or ulceration (22, 26,27). Ulceration is particularly prone to occur in hemangiomas having a cavernous component. Treatment may be sclerotherapy, cryotherapy, laser therapy, or surgical excision. Radiotherapy is no longer used (28) due to the potential adverse effects on the ovary (27).

Port Wine Nevus

Port wine nevus (nevus flammeus, birthmark) is present from birth and does not represent a true neoplasm. It must be distinguished from a capillary or cavernous nevus. The port wine nevus is variable in size, and is pink to purple in color. The lesion is rarely limited to the vulva. Microscopically, it is composed of dilated vessels in the dermis. It may occasionally be associated with the Sturge-Weber syndrome and Klippel-Trenaunay-Weber syndrome. Port wine nevi at other sites have been treated for cosmetic purposes but are rarely treated on the vulva.

Angiokeratoma

Angiokeratoma is a form of cavernous hemangioma in which the blood vessels are intimately associated with the overlying epidermis that typically displays acanthosis and hyperkeratosis (29) (Fig. 2). The le-

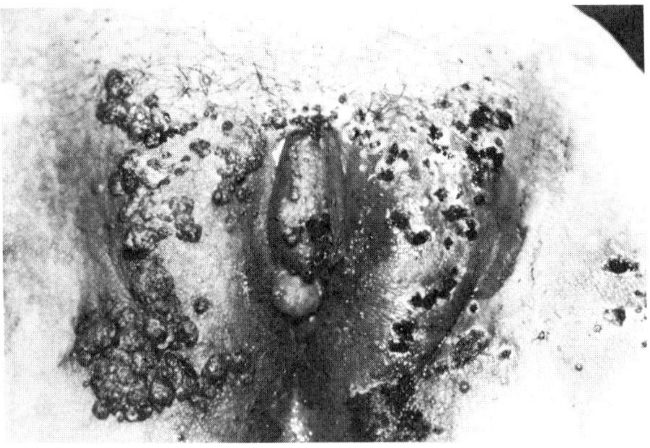

FIG. 2. Vulvar angiokeratoma involving the clitoral hood, labia majora, and inner thighs. (From ref. 30, with permission.)

sions appear as dark red elevations ranging in size from 1 to 10 mm. Angiokeratomas can be localized to the vulva or widely distributed in other sites. In the latter form, they tend to occur on the fingers, toes, and scrotum/vulva (30). Rarely, they are manifestations of a metabolic disorder and may be associated with renal and central nervous system dysfunction, i.e., Fabry's disease (31). Angiokeratomas most frequently occur in adult women but have been reported in adolescents (29,32). They are frequently asymptomatic but can cause discomfort, irritation, and bleeding (30). Treatment which currently is with the argon laser is reserved for symptomatic lesions.

Lymphangiomas

Lymphangioma of the vulva are rare but have been reported in women with congenital lymphedema of the lower extremities (33). More commonly, lymphatic lesions in the vulva are acquired and represent dilatations of existing lymphatic vessels due to disruption of more proximal channels. Lymphangiectasis is a more appropriate term for the latter, as they do not represent true neoplasms. Vulvar lymphangiectasis has been reported in adult women following radiation therapy for cervical carcinoma. A single case has been reported in a six year old child, four years after pelvic exenteration for a malignant bladder tumor (34) (Fig. 3).

Soft Tissue Tumors

Soft tissue tumors other than vascular lesions are rare but include lipomas and leiomyomas (1,35) (Fig. 4).

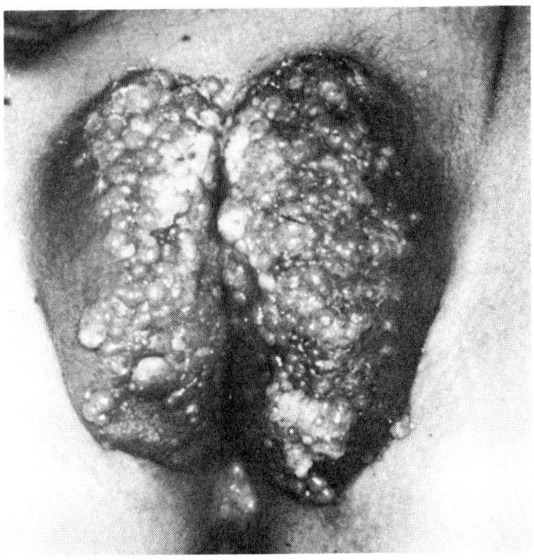

FIG. 3. Acquired vulvar lymphangiectasis 6½ years after radical therapy for rhabdomyosarcoma of the bladder. (From ref. 34, with permission.)

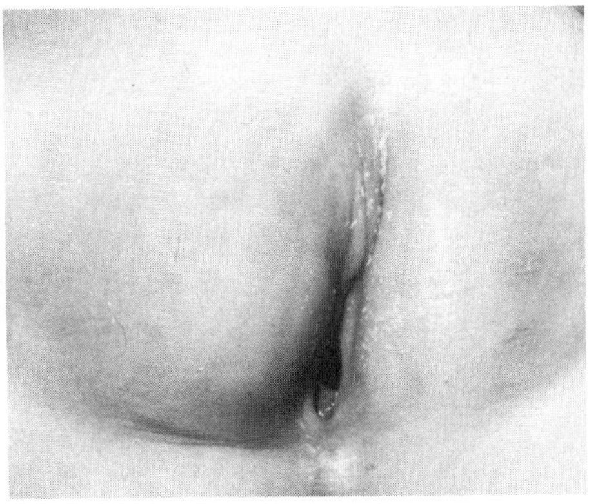

FIG. 4. Lipoma of the vulva involving the right labium majus in a young girl. (Courtesy of Dr. C.J. Dewhurst.)

Neurogenic Tumors

Neurofibromas

Vulvar neurofibromas are very uncommon in children but can occasionally represent the earliest clinical manifestation of neurofibromatosis. Neurofibromatosis is transmitted as a Mendelian dominant disease with variability in gene expression. The origin of this disease has recently been traced to a specific gene region on chromosome 17 (36). Approximately 50% of patients have a family history of the disorder. The lesions in the remainder are believed to arise from new mutations. The disorder is usually manifested in young children by the presence of multiple cafe-au-lait spots. More than six spots are considered to be pathognomonic of the disease. Neurofibromas may appear in late childhood and adolescence. Other manifestations include bone overgrowth, congenital bowing and pseudoarthrosis of bone and soft tissue, kyphoscoliosis, focal gigantism, and megalencephaly (37,38). In addition, approximately 10% of children have mild to moderate mental retardation. The diagnosis is currently based on physical findings but in the near future will probably be based on molecular genetic analysis. Neurofibromas are well circumscribed tumors arising from Schwann cells (Fig. 5). Histologically, they are composed of elongated spindle cells forming interlacing bands admixed with nerve fibers. The frequency of malignant neurogenic tumors in patients with neurofibromatosis is higher than in the general population with rates varying from 5% to 30% (39,40). Malignant transformation, however, is rare in children. Presentation as a solitary vulvar neurofibroma is very unusual but can occur and be confused with other conditions. Usually, the neurofibroma is confused with a phallus leading to a diagnosis of pseudohermaphroditism (41–44). The diagnosis should be suspected in a child with multiple cafe-au-lait spots. Physical examination and cystoscopy may reveal additional neurofibromas in the vagina and bladder (37).

Granular Cell Tumor

This is a benign neoplasm occurring in the breast and tongue and less commonly in

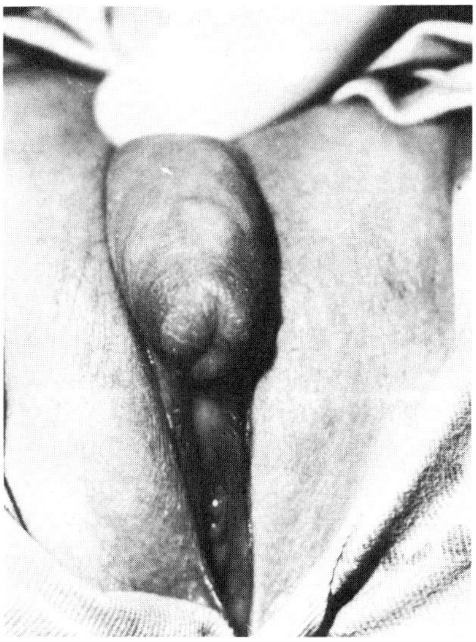

FIG. 5. Neurofibroma of the clitoris presenting as phallus-like structure. (From ref. 44, with permission.)

the vulva. Several vulvar lesions have been reported in the pediatric age group (45,46). Based on electron microscopic and immunohistochemical studies, a Schwann cell origin of this neoplasm has been proposed (47). Excision is curative.

Melanocytic Lesions

Nevi

Vulvar nevi are uncommon in the pediatric age group. In a 14-year review of patients with pigmented vulvar lesions at The Johns Hopkins Hospital, only two of 59 nevi occurred in patients under the age of 20 (48). In the same review, the frequency of dysplasia was not higher in the vulva compared to nevi in other locations. Vulvar lesions did, however, show greater tendency to display variability in the size and shape of melanocytic nests. Both junctional and intradermal nevi have been described.

MALIGNANT NEOPLASMS

Malignant tumors of the vulva are rare in the pediatric age group but have been sporadically reported since the latter part of the 19th century. Our review of the world literature since 1871 revealed 38 cases (49–55). Although it is difficult to determine histologic type in many of these cases, it appears that squamous cell carcinomas, embryonal rhabdomyosarcomas, and endodermal sinus tumors are the most common. The rarity of squamous cell carcinomas in this age group underscores the role of environmental factors in the development of these tumors in adults. Conversely, the occurrence of sarcomas and endodermal sinus tumors in this age group and their virtual absence in the adult population suggests a role of congenital genetic factors in the development of these neoplasms.

Squamous Cell Carcincomas

Although rare, squamous cell carcinomas of the vulva have been reported in adolescents and some have proved to be fatal (49,56). As in other sites, squamous carcinoma presents as a raised lesion which can be ulcerated and confused with an infectious process (56) (Figs. 6 and 7). Biopsy reveals nests of malignant squamous cells in a desmoplastic stroma. Patients have been treated by radical vulvectomy with inguinal node dissection or by radiation therapy. Although precursor lesions have not been well studied in this age group, atypias of the vulvar epithelium have been reported (57,58). The relationship of these lesions to HPV infection has not been studied in these patients.

Sarcoma Botryoides

Sarcoma botryoides (embryonal rhabdomyosarcoma) of the vulva are rare. Almost all patients have been infants who pre-

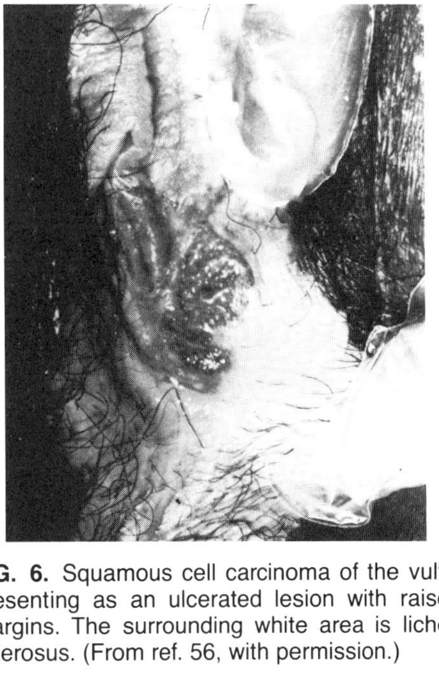

FIG. 6. Squamous cell carcinoma of the vulva presenting as an ulcerated lesion with raised margins. The surrounding white area is lichen sclerosus. (From ref. 56, with permission.)

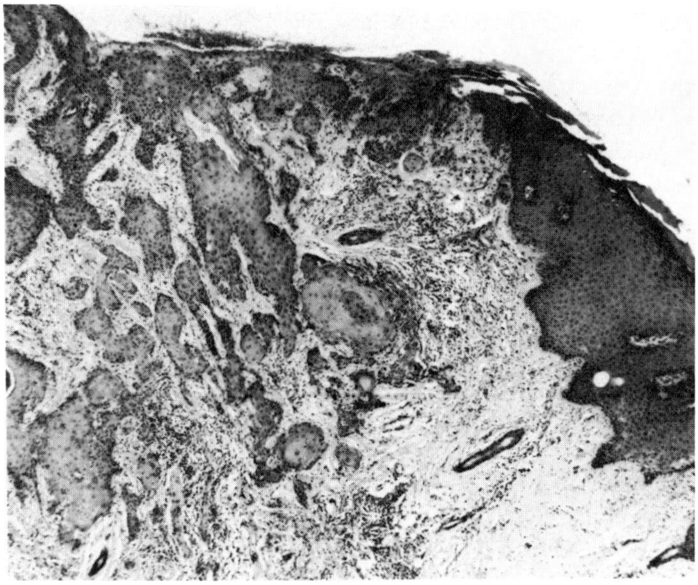

FIG. 7. Well-differentiated squamous carcinoma characterized by irregular nests of squamous epithelial infiltrates underlying the stroma. The adjacent epithelium shows squamous hyperplasia but no evidence of carcinoma *in situ* (hematoxylin and eosin). (From ref. 56, with permission.)

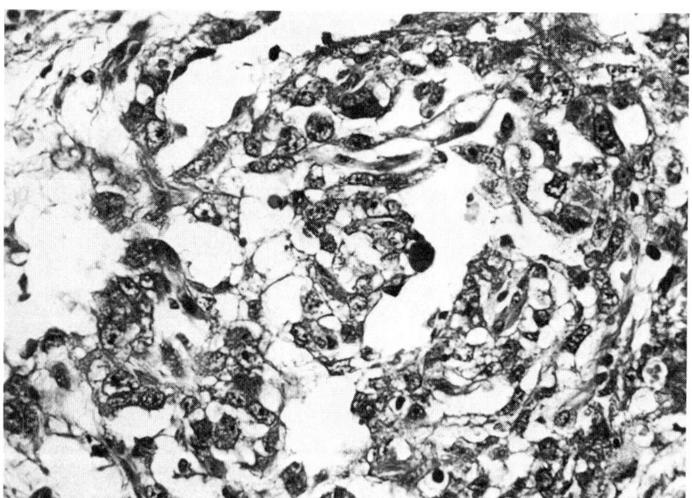

FIG. 8. Endodermal sinus tumor of the vulva characterized by a reticular pattern (hematoxylin and eosin). (From ref. 68, with permission.)

sented with a vulvar mass (59–64). Large lesions may involve both vulva and vagina. Microscopically, the tumor is composed of immature rhabdomyoblasts showing varying degree of differentiation towards skeletal muscle. A condensation of primitive cells designated the "cambium layer" is frequently seen immediately beneath the epithelium and aids in the histologic diagnosis. The stroma is frequently myxoid and on gross examination results in the appearance of a "bunch of grapes" accounting for the term "sarcoma botryoides." Although these tumors are highly aggressive and have a tendency to recur locally (59,61,62), the multimodality approach utilizing surgery, radiation therapy, and chemotherapy has increased survival in genitourinary rhabdomyosarcomas from 18% to 75% (65). A similar aggressive approach has resulted in long term survival in the patients with vulvar sarcoma botryoides (60).

Endodermal Sinus Tumor

Three pediatric cases of endodermal sinus tumor have been reported involving the vulva (66–68). Two were young children younger than 3 years of age at presentation, and the third was an adolescent. Histologically, the tumor is composed of nests of primitive cells in a reticular pattern identical to its counterpart in the ovary. Intracytoplasmic inclusions containing alpha-fetoprotein were common (Figs. 8 and 9). Serum alpha-fetoprotein levels have not been elevated. One of the three cases showed areas of embryonal carcinoma in addition to the endodermal component. These tumors have been highly malignant with two of the three patients dying of tumor despite radical surgery and adjuvant chemotherapy.

Malignant Melanoma

Only three vulvar cases in the pediatric age group have been reported to our knowledge. All three patients were adolescents (51,52,69). The 5-year survival for malignant melanoma of the vulva in the adult age group is approximately 75% for lesions confined to the vulva when treated by radial vulvectomy and lymph node dissection (70).

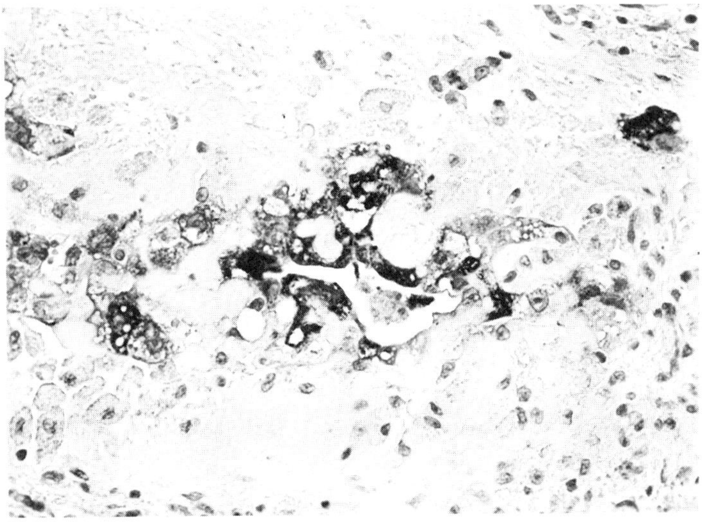

FIG. 9. Immunohistochemical positivity for intracytoplasmic alpha-fetoprotein in an endodermal sinus tumor of the vulva (same case as in Fig. 8). (From ref. 68, with permission.)

REFERENCES

1. Dewhurst CJ. Tumors of the genital tract in childhood and adolescence. *Clin Obstet Gynecol* 1977;20:595–606.
2. Lottmann H, Cendron J, Baviera E, Eyssautier C. Kystes vulvaires a revelation neonatale. *Ann Urol* 1985;19:259–62.
3. Cohen HJ, Klein MD, Laver MB. Cysts of the vagina in the newborn infant. *Am J Dis Child* 1957;94:322.
4. Blaivas JG, Pais VM, Retik AB. Paraurethral cysts in female neonate. *Urology* 1976;7:504–7.
5. Williams DI. Problems in the management of ectopic ureteroceles. *J Urol* 1964;92:635.
6. Friedrich EG, Wilkinson EJ. Mucous cysts of the vulvar vestibule. *Obstet Gynecol* 1972;42:407.
7. Robboy SJ, Ross JS, Prat J, et al. Urogenital sinus origin of mucinous and ciliated cysts of the vulva. *Obstet Gynecol* 1978;51:347.
8. Huffman JW. Tumors of the vulva and vagina during childhood. In: *The gynecology of childhood and adolescence*. Philadelphia: W. B. Saunders Company, 1981:225–59.
9. Capraro VJ, Bayonet-Rivera NP, Magoss I. Vulvar tumor in children due to prolapse of urethral mucosa. *Ame J Obstet Gynecol* 1970;108:572–5.
10. Lee YH, Rankin JS, Alpert S, Daly AK, McCormack WM. Microbiological investigation of Bartholin's gland abscesses and cysts. *Am J Obstet Gynecol* 1977;129:150–3.
11. Reid R, Greenberg M, Jenson AB, et al. Sexually transmitted papillomaviral infection. *Am J Obstet Gynecol* 1987;156:212–22.
12. Powell LC. Condyloma acuminatum: recent advances in development, carcinomgenesis and treatment. *Clin Obstet Gynecol* 1978;21:1061–79.
13. McCoy CR, Applebaum H, Besser AS. Condyloma acuminata: an unusual presentation of child abuse. *J Pediatr Surg* 1982;17:505–7.
14. Seidel J, Zonana J, Totten E. Condylomata acuminata as a sign of sexual abuse in children. *J Pediatr* 1979;95:553–4.
15. DeJong AR, Weiss JC, Brent RL. Condyloma acuminata in children. *Am J Dis Child* 1982;136:704–6.
16. Sadan O, Koller AB, Adno A, Beale PG. Massive vulvar condyloma acuminata in a 10 month old child with suspected sexual abuse [Case report]. *Br J Obstet Gynecol* 1985;92:1201–3.
17. Stumpf PG. Increasing occurrence of condylomata acuminata in premenarchal children. *Obstet Gynecol* 1980;56:262–4.
18. Randrup ER, Sangisetty KV. Condyloma acuminatum in children. *Urology* 1985;26:176–7.
19. Grace DA, Ochsner JA, McLain CR, Smith JP. Vulvar condylomata acuminata in prepubertal females. *JAMA* 1967;201:151–2.
20. Goldman L, Clarke GE. Infectious papilloma (so called condyloma acuminatum) with genital, perineal, and lip lesions in a 3 year old girl. *Urol Cutan Rev* 1940;44:677–8.
21. Eftaiha MS, Amshel AL, Shonberg IL. Condyloma acuminata in an infant and mother: report of a case. *Dis Colon Rectum* 1978;21:369–71.
22. Levin AV, Selbst SM. Vulvar hemangioma simulating child abuse. *Clin Pedatr* 1988;27:213–5.
23. Kaufman-Friedman K. Hemangioma of the clitoris confused with adrenogenital syndrome. *Plast Reconstr Surg* 1978;62:452–4.
24. Tjaden BL, Buscema J, Haller JA, Rock JA. Vulvar congenital dysplastic angiopathy. *Obstet Gynecol* 1990;75:552–4.
25. MacColum DW, Martin LW. Hemangioma in infancy and childhood. A report based on 6479 cases. *Surg Clin North Am* 1957;36:1947.
26. Bellone F, Gloria M, Diani F. Considerazioni cliniche sugli emangiomi della vulva in eta infantile. *Minerva Ginecologia* 1985;37:747–50.
27. Urbanowisz W. Naczyniaki sromu u dziewczynek. *Ginekol Pol* 1973;44:687–91.
28. Mobius VW, Krause W. Das Vulvahamagiom biem Saugling und Kleinkind und seine Behandlung. *Zbl Gynak* 1974;96:280–6.
29. Cohen PR, Young AW, Tovell MM. Angiokeratoma of the vulva: diagnosis and review of the literature. *Obstet Gynecol Surg* 1989;44:339–46.
30. Dotters DJ, Fowler WC, Powers SK, McCune BK. Argon laser therapy of vulvar angiokeratoma. *Obstet Gynecol* 1986;68:56S–9S.
31. Robbins SL, Cotran RS, Kumar V. *Pathologic basis of disease*. Philadelphia: W.B. Saunders, 1984:152–3.
32. Imperial R, Helwig EB. Angiokeratoma of the vulva. *Obstet Gynecol* 1967;29:307–12.
33. Wilkinson EJ. *Pathology of the vulva and vagina*. New York: Churchill Livingston, New York, 1987:211.
34. Rabinowitz R, Churchill BM, Alexis ME, Boxall L. Acquired vulvar lymphangiectasis in a child. *Urology* 1977;10:459–60.
35. Tavassoli FA, Norris HJ. Smooth muscle tumors of the vulva. *Obstet Gynecol* 1979;53:213–7.
36. Diehl SR, Boehnke M, Erickson RP, Ploughman CM, et al. A refined genetic map of the region of chromosome 17 surrounding the von Recklinghausen neurofibromatosis (NF1) gene. *Am J Hum Genet* 1987;44:33–7.
37. Rink RC, Mitchell ME. Genitourinary neurofibromatosis in childhood. *J Urol* 1983;130:1176–9.
38. Vaughan V, McKay RJ, Behrman RE. *Nelson textbook of pediatrics*. Philadelphia: W.B. Saunders Company, 1979;1765,1865–72.
39. D'Agostina AN, Soule EH, Miller RH. Sarcomas of the peripheral nerves and somatic soft tissues associated with multiple neurofibromatosis (von Recklinghausen's disease). *Cancer* 1963;16:1015.
40. Das Gupta TK, Brasfield RD. Von Recklinghausen's disease. *Cancer* 1971;21:174.
41. Labardini MM, Kallet HA, Cerny JC. Urogenital neurofibromatosis simulating an intersex problem. *J Urol* 1968;98:627–32.
42. Ogawa A, Watanabe K. Genitourinary neurofibromatosis in a child presenting with an enlarged penis and scrotum. *J Urol* 1986;135:755–7.
43. Schepel SJ, Tolhurst DE. Neurofibromata of cli-

toris and labium majus simulating a penis and testicle. *Br J Plast Surg* 1981;221–3.
44. Kaneti J, Liebrman E, Moshe P, Carmi R. A case of ambiguous genitalia owing to neurofibromatosis-review of the literature. *J Urol* 1988; 140:584–5.
45. Brooks GG. Granular cell myoblastoma of the vulva in a 6 year old girl. *Am J Obstet Gynecol* 1985;153:897–8.
46. Hashem M. The pathology and histogenesis of the granular cell myoblastoma. *J Egypt Med Assoc* 1959;42:239–60.
47. Coates JB, Hales JS. Granular cell myoblastoma of the vulva. *Obstet Gynecol* 1973;41:796.
48. Christensen WN, Friedman KJ, Woodruff JD, Hood AF. Histologic characteristics of vulvar nevocellular nevi. *J Cutan Pathol* 1987;14: 87–91.
49. Mesrogli M, Lelle RJ. Vulvakarzinom bei einem 13ahrigen Madchen. *Geburtsh u. Frauenheilk* 1986;46:754–6.
50. Addison A. Adenocarcinoma of Bartholin's gland in a 14 year old girl: report of a case. *Am J Obstet Gynecol* 1977;127:214–5.
51. Pack GT, Oropeza R. A comparative study of melanomas and epidermoid carcinomas of the vulva: a review of 44 melanomas and 58 epidermoid carcinomas (1930–1965). *Rev Surg* 1967;5: 305–24.
52. Chung AF, Woodruff JM, Lewis JL. Malignant melanoma of the vulva: a report of 44 cases. *Obstet Gynecol* 1975;45:638–46.
53. Lister UM, Akinla O. Carcinoma of the vulva in childhood. *J Obstet Gynaecol Br Commonwealth* 1972;79:470–3.
54. Elaraby II, Dent PB, Hunter JDW, Miniella JA. Histiocytosis X: late manifestations in a long-term survivor of Letterer-Siwe disease. *J Pediat* 1976;89:961–2.
55. Egwuatu VE, Ejeckam GC, Okaqro JM. Burkitt's lymphoma of the vulva. Case report. *Br J Obstet Gynaecol* 1980;87:827–30.
56. Cario GM, House MJ, Paradinas FJ. Squamous cell carcinoma of the vulva in association with mixed vulvar dystrophy in an 18 year old girl. Case report. *Br J Obstet Gynaecol* 1984;91: 87–90.
57. Friedrich EG. Reversible vulvar atypia: a case report. *Obstet Gynecol* 1972;39:173–81.
58. Shafi MI, Luesley DM, Byrne P, et al. Vulval intraepithelial neoplasia-management and outcome. *Br J Obstet Gynaecol* 1989;96:1339–44.
59. Moonen WA, Jankneg RA, vdHoek WD. Sarcoma Botryoides: radical treatment by pelvic exenteration with 11 years survival. *Arch Chirur Neerlan* 1970;22:1–6.
60. Piver MS, Rose PG. Long-term follow-up and complications of infants with vulvovaginal embryonal rhabdomyosarcoma treated with surgery, radiation therapy, and chemotherapy. *Obstet Gynecol* 1988;71:435–7.
61. Hildebrand HF, Krivosic I, Grandier-Vazeille X, Tetaert D, Biserte G. Perineal rhabdomyosarcoma in a newborn child: pathological and biochemical studies with emphasis on contractile proteins. *J Clin Pathol* 1980;33:823–9.
62. Talerman A. Sarcoma botryoides presenting as a polyp on the labium jaus. *Cancer* 1973;32: 994–9.
63. James GB, Guthrie W, Buchan A. Embryonic sarcoma of the vulva in an infant. *J Obstet Gynaec Br Commonwealth* 1969;76:458–61.
64. Piver MS, Barlow JJ, Wang JJ, Shah NK. Combined radical surgery, radiation therapy and chemotherapy in infants with vulvovaginal embryonal rhabdomyosarcoma. *Obstet Gynecol* 1973;42:522–6.
65. Ghavimi F, Herr H, Jereb B, et al. Treatment of genitourinary rhabdomyosarcoma in children. *J Urol* 1984;132:313.
66. Castaldo TW, Petrilli ES, Ballon SC, Voet RL, Lagasse LD, Lubens R. Endodermal sinus tumor of the clitoris. *Gynecol Oncol* 1980;9: 376–80.
67. Ungerleider RS, Donaldson SS, Warnke RA, Wilbur JR. Endodermal sinus tumor: The Stanford experience and the first reported case arising in the vulva. *Cancer* 1978;41:1627–34.
68. Dudley AG, Young RH, Lawrence WD, Scully RE. Endodermal sinus tumor of the vulva in an infant. *Obstet Gynecol* 1983;61:76S–9S.
69. Friedman RJ, Knopf AW, Jones WB. Malignant melanoma in association with lichen sclerosus on the vulva of a 14 year old. *Am J Dermatopathol* 1984;6:253–6.
70. Morrow CP, Rutledge FN. Melanoma of the vulva. *Obstet Gynecol* 1972;39:745–52.

Pediatric and Adolescent Gynecology,
edited by S. E. Carpenter and J. A. Rock.
Raven Press, Ltd., New York © 1992.

24

Tumors of the Vagina and Cervix in the Neonate, Child, and Adolescent

Michelle Dudzinski

Department of Gynecology and Obstetrics, The Johns Hopkins Hospital, Baltimore, Maryland 21205

Tumors of the vagina and cervix in the neonate, child, and adolescent are rare. Although in the adult, squamous cell carcinomas are most commonly seen, in the child and adolescent a unique variety of tumors is found, which are discussed in this chapter.

The most common neoplasm of the lower genital tract in infants and adolescents is embryonal rhabdomyosarcoma of the botryoid type, or sarcoma botryoides. Endodermal sinus tumors and a variety of benign masses may also be found in the infant vagina.

Clear cell adenocarcinoma of the vagina and cervix in infants and adolescents was found to increase in incidence in the 1970s and early 1980s. This increase was felt to be due to *in utero* exposure to diethylstilbesterol (DES), which was used in the mid-1940s and 1950s for a variety of indications. Fortunately, the use of DES declined significantly after 1955. Since the oldest reported patient to date with clear cell adenocarcinoma related to DES was 34 years of age (1), the incidence of this neoplasm and other DES sequelae such as adenosis and dysplasia should again be decreasing and should rarely be found in children and adolescents.

Although squamous cell carcinomas of the vagina and cervix are rare before age 18, dysplastic lesions are often seen in adolescents. Risk for these lesions begins with the onset of sexual activity, which, today, often begins in the teenage and even pre-teen years.

This chapter examines the presentation, diagnosis, and management of each of these neoplastic processes.

SARCOMA BOTRYOIDES

The most common form of soft tissue sarcoma in childhood is the rhabdomyosarcoma, of which approximately 20% involve the genitourinary tract (2,3). The botryoid type, or sarcoma botryoides, accounts for 3–3.5% (2,4) of pediatric rhabdomyosarcomas and usually originates in the vagina or cervix. It is the most common tumor of the vagina and cervix in children younger then 16 years of age (5). The vast majority of cases are found in infants and very young children, with the peak incidence occurring in the first 2 years of life and 90% occurring before age 5 (6). As the child's age increases, lesions tend to originate higher in the genital tract (5), and, indeed, cervical tumors predominate in adolescents, forming a second peak in the bimodal incidence of this disease (7,8).

Children with sarcoma botryoides usually present with vaginal bleeding or bloody discharge. A soft, friable, polypoid mass resembling a bunch of grapes may be found protruding from the vagina (Fig. 1). Other less frequent symptoms may include serous vaginal discharge, the passage of sloughed tissue, fever, or pain (7).

Definitive diagnosis requires biopsy of the lesion, as endodermal sinus tumors (Fig. 2) and some benign polypoid masses (Fig. 3) may have a similar presentation. Biopsy may be accomplished in the office if the tumor is protruding from the vaginal introitus. In children with tumors confined to the cervix or vagina, an examination under anesthesia with biopsy may be necessary. The examination under anesthesia is an invaluable aid to determine extent of disease in all infants and children. Cystoscopy and proctoscopy can also be performed to determine if involvement of the bladder or rectum is present. Although most cases of sarcoma botryoides arise from the anterior vaginal wall and are confined to the pelvis at diagnosis, hematogenous and lymphogenous metastases can occur. The urethra and posterior bladder wall are frequently involved with tumor. Less often, the rectum, vulva, pelvic lymph nodes, lung, liver, and bone can be involved (9). A complete staging work-up should, therefore, be performed, including chest x-ray and abdominal-pelvic CT scan. An intravenous pyelogram and bone scan may also be useful.

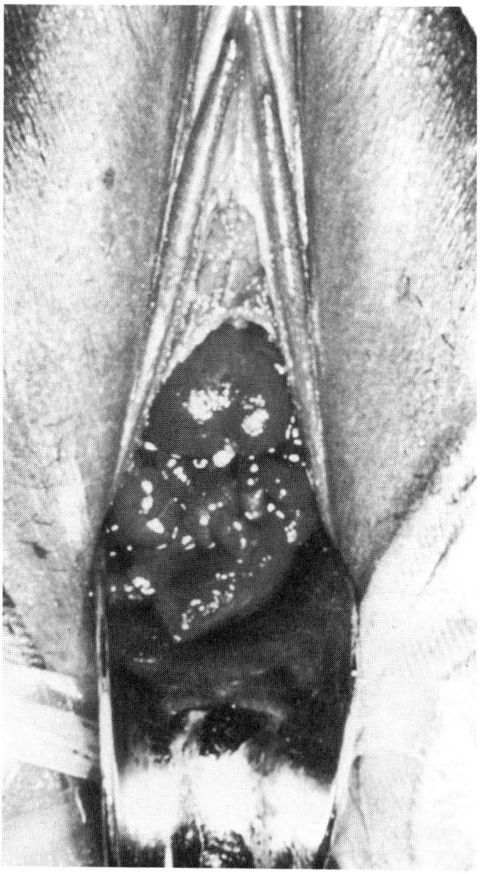

FIG. 1. Sarcoma botryoides protruding from infant vagina.

Sarcoma botryoides is felt to arise from primitive embryonal mesenchyme in the lamina propria (2,5,6). It spreads beneath the mucous membrane of the vaginal wall or other pelvic structures, producing the characteristic polypoid appearance (Fig. 4). Microscopically, the tumor consists of poorly differentiated round or spindle cells (Fig. 5). Striated muscle cells may be present (6).

The therapy of embryonal rhabdomyosarcoma of the female genital tract has changed dramatically over the last 20 years. The evolution of therapy from radical sur-

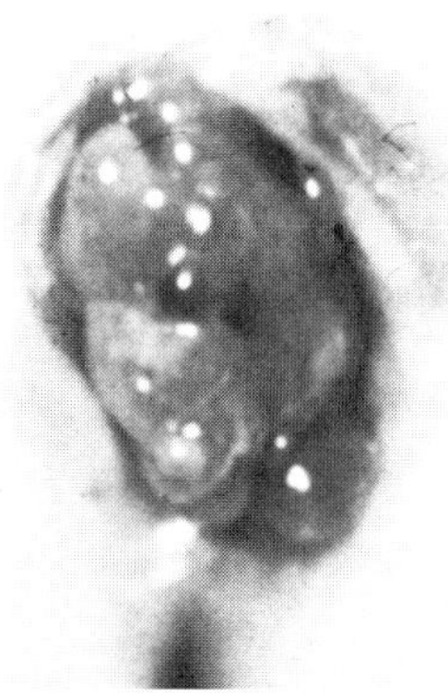

FIG. 2. Endodermal sinus tumor arising in infant vagina.

gery alone to multimodal therapy was described well by Bell et al. (2) and by Hays (10) in their 1986 reviews. Prior to 1960, therapy consisted of palliative radiation, limited excision, or pelvic exenteration, which was introduced by Shackman in 1947 (2) and remained the mainstay of therapy until the 1960s. The prognosis for survival, however, continued to be poor. The introduction of multiagent chemotherapy, particularly vincristine, actinomycin D, and cytoxan (VAC), and its combination with surgery and radiation dramatically improved survival. Indeed, the combination of pelvic exenteration, pelvic radiation, and 2 years of VAC chemotherapy resulted in 90% survival (10).

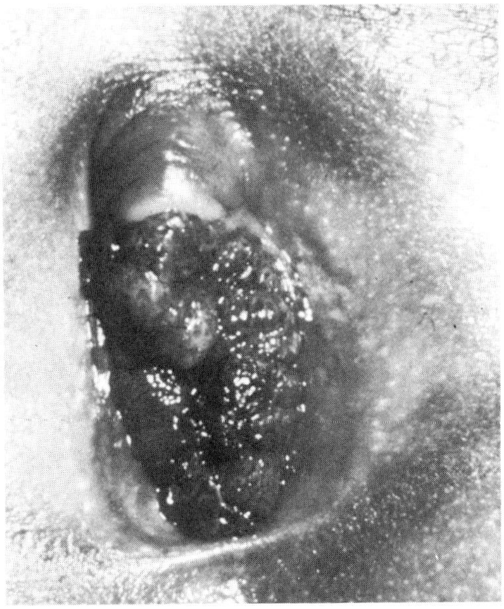

FIG. 3. Benign vaginal condylomata acuminata in an infant.

In an attempt to preserve normal anatomical structure and function in children with sarcoma botryoides, most recent therapeutic approaches have centered on initial use of chemotherapy (3 months) to induce shrinkage of the tumor mass. Surgical excision can then be tailored to the amount and location of residual disease. Radiation therapy can be employed if there is no response to chemotherapy, if there is residual disease after chemotherapy or surgical therapy, or if there is nodal involvement. Adjunctive chemotherapy with VAC should then be continued for a total of 18–24 months. The success of initial therapy in this disease is crucial, as recurrences are rarely cured.

Children who are successfully cured of sarcoma botryoides may develop serious sequelae from the treatment regimen. Radiation complications can include ovarian insufficiency, vaginal stenosis, urethral stenosis, bladder contraction, colorectal stenosis, ureteral stenosis, and vesicovaginal or rectovaginal fistula formation. Ovarian insufficiency can be prevented by transposition of the ovaries prior to initiation of radiation to remove them from the radiation field. In a small series by Piver and Rose (11), there was little effect of pelvic irradiation on eventual height or on intellectual ability.

Flamant et al. (4) recently reported their experience using chemotherapy and local brachytherapy for vulvar and vaginal childhood rhabdomyosarcomas in an attempt to avoid radical pelvic surgery. Two of their patients successfully achieved pregnancy after therapy. Indeed, if complete remission

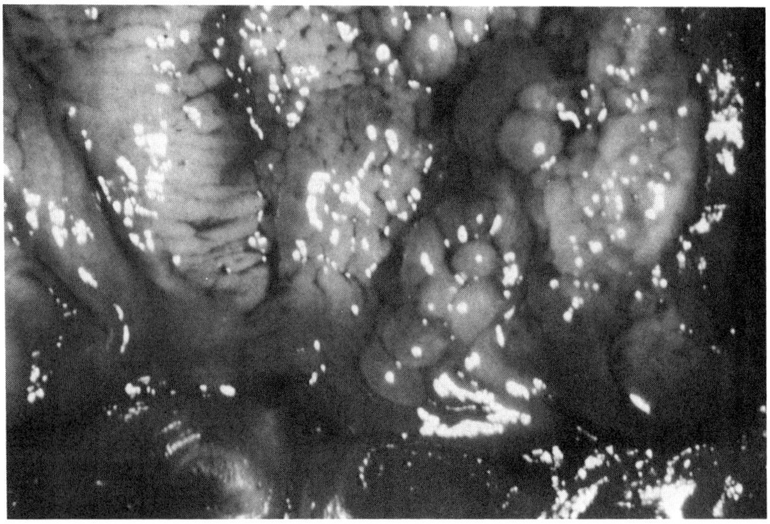

FIG. 4. Gross appearance of polypoid masses arising from vagina in sarcoma botryoides.

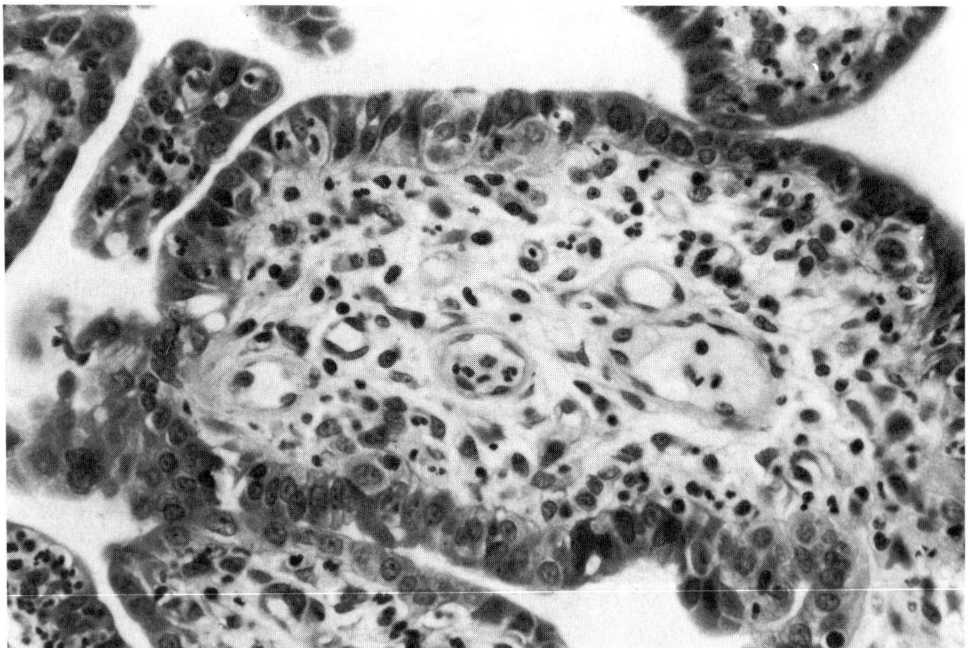

FIG. 5. Microscopic appearance of sarcoma botryoides.

can be achieved by chemotherapy alone, surgery and radiation may be unnecessary.

Several recent reports have examined sarcoma botryoides of the uterine cervix without vaginal involvement (7,8,12). As stated previously, cervical primaries tend to predominate in late childhood and adolescence. As with vaginal primaries, the initial presentation is usually vaginal bleeding. Occasionally, the mass will protrude from the vagina, or fragments of tissue may be passed. Average age of presentation is approximately 18 years. Biopsy and staging work-up should be performed as with vaginal disease. Clinical staging may be classified according to the criteria of the Intergroup Rhabdomyosarcoma Study (13) (Table 1).

The therapy of cervical sarcoma botryoides has undergone a similar evolution to that of its vaginal counterpart. Radical pelvic surgery with loss of reproductive function has been replaced by local surgery combined with chemotherapy for early stage disease. Indeed, Daya (8) successfully treated four patients by polypectomy or cervicectomy alone, and Gordon and Montag (12) successfully treated a patient by local excision followed by VAC chemotherapy in an attempt to preserve reproductive function. Overall survival for cervical sarcoma botryoides is approximately 80% (7).

As with vaginal disease, current management of cervical embryonal rhabdomyosarcoma should be tailored to the extent of disease and should take into consideration preservation of bladder, rectal, and reproductive function. Primary therapy should consist of VAC chemotherapy, with subsequent surgical resection tailored to the amount of residual disease. For early disease confined to the cervix, initial local resection followed by chemotherapy may be appropriate. Radiation therapy may be appropriate for more extensive disease or for surgical/chemotherapeutic failures.

TABLE 1. *Clinical staging classification of intergroup rhabdomyosarcoma study*

Group 1.	Localized disease, completely resected A. Tumor confined to muscle or organ of origin B. Infiltration beyond site of origin. Regional nodes not involved
Group 2.	Gross excision with microscopic residual disease or adjacent organ or regional nodes involved A. Microscopic residual disease B. Grossly resected but involves regional nodes or extends into an adjacent organ C. Grossly resected but involves regional nodes and has microscopic residual
Group 3.	Incomplete resection or biopsy showing gross residual disease
Group 4.	Distant metastatic disease present at onset

Data from ref. 13.

ENDODERMAL SINUS TUMOR

Endodermal sinus tumor (EST) of the infant vagina is an extremely rare neoplasm occurring in infants younger than 3 years of age (14). Fewer than 50 cases have been reported in the literature (15). The clinical presentation is similar to that of sarcoma botryoides, with both tumors presenting with vaginal bleeding and polypoid masses protruding from the vagina (Figs. 1 and 2). Definitive diagnosis is, therefore, made by biopsy.

Histopathologically, EST of the infant vagina is identical to EST of the ovary and may have a tubuloacinar, reticular, or solid pattern. Schiller-Duvall bodies, PAS-positive globules, and positive staining for α-fetoprotein (aFP) should be present. The serum aFP level that can be measured by radioimmunoassay may be used both for diagnostic purposes and also to follow the status of the disease throughout therapy.

Clinical evaluation of extent of disease and definitive diagnosis by biopsy may necessitate examination under anesthesia, as with sarcoma botryoides. Staging procedures are also similar.

The evolution of therapy that occurred

with sarcoma botryoides has also occurred with EST. Prior to 1965, the mainstay of therapy was radical surgery and radiation (9). Survival was poor. With the introduction of the use of chemotherapy by Vawter in 1965 (16), the ability to treat this disease and survival have increased dramatically. In recent years, many reports have been published outlining excellent therapeutic results with multiagent chemotherapy followed by surgery and even chemotherapy alone (9,14,15,17,18). The role of radiation therapy is unclear but is probably limited.

In 1989, Collins et al. (15) reported a 5-month-old girl treated exclusively with chemotherapy. The tumor originally extended to the right pelvic sidewall, and after five courses of vinblastine, bleomycin, and cisplatinum chemotherapy the tumor had completely resolved by CT scan evaluation and clinical assessment. The patient was then begun on maintenance chemotherapy with vincristine, actinomycin D, and cyclophosphamide. The child was without evidence of disease 45 months later, and all pelvic organs were preserved. Andersen et al. (17) also reported a case of a 13-month-old girl treated by primary VAC chemotherapy with subsequent limited surgical resection and preservation of all pelvic organs.

The sensitivity of this tumor to various chemotherapeutic drugs, listed in Table 2, may allow for successful therapy with multiagent chemotherapy alone, as illustrated in these most recent reports. If complete regression does not occur, surgical resection of the residual disease can be performed. As there is no standard therapy for this rare disease, treatment plans must continue to be individualized.

TABLE 2. *Chemotherapeutic agents useful in the therapy of endodermal sinus tumor*

Vincristine
Vinblastine
Actinomycin D
Adriamycin
Cyclophosphamide
Bleomycin
Cisplatinum
Etoposide (VP-16)

The success of initial therapy for EST is crucial, as it is for sarcoma botryoides, as recurrences have rarely been cured. Children with this disease should be followed closely, and aFP should be measured routinely as it may become elevated before clinical evidence of disease can be detected.

BENIGN DISORDERS

Occasionally, benign disorders in infants and children can simulate more serious tumors, as shown in Fig. 3. Vulvar, vaginal, and cervical condylomata, the manifestation of infection by the human papilloma virus (HPV), are often seen in children and are discussed in the chapter by Woodruff. In order to distinguish condylomata from other tumors, a biopsy of the lesion for pathologic evaluation should be obtained prior to the initiation of therapy. Treatment options for infants and young children, which often must be performed with the aid of anesthesia, include laser vaporization, local excision, and topical therapy such as trichloracetic acid. The method of therapy should be chosen based on the location and extent of disease. In the teenage years, 5-fluorouracil cream may be employed to treat diffuse vaginal condylomata if the patient is judged mature enough to understand and comply with the treatment regimen.

Mesonephric duct cysts arising from the vaginal wall may produce masses in the vagina of varying size. Small cysts can be followed without therapy. Larger cysts can easily be treated by performing a wedge resection of a portion of the overlying vaginal mucosa.

Hemangiomas are a common birth defect and, although rare, can occasionally arise in the vagina or cervix. Many will involute and resolve spontaneously over several years. Persistent hemangiomas may present with vaginal bleeding (19). They can present at any age and have been diagnosed in children and adolescents (19,20).

If the diagnosis of hemangioma is suspected, biopsy of the lesion should be undertaken with extreme caution as severe hemorrhage can result. CT scanning with rapid injection of intravenous contrast or radiolabeled red cell scanning may aid in the diagnosis.

The therapy of hemangiomas is controversial. Small localized lesions may be treated by local excision. Steroid therapy, as described by Cook et al. (19), as well as laser therapy, as described by Bellina et al. (20), have also been utilized.

DIETHYLSTILBESTEROL-RELATED DISORDERS

DES-related disorders in the child and adolescent are rapidly becoming of historical interest only. DES, a nonsteroid estrogen, was originally introduced in 1946 as treatment for a variety of high-risk pregnancy disorders to prevent fetal wastage. Some indications included threatened abortion, recurrent spontaneous abortions, essential hypertension, and a history of prior stillbirths (21,22).

It was used most extensively during 1950 and 1951. The therapeutic benefit of DES was disputed in the literature in 1953, and its use declined significantly after 1955. It was discontinued totally from obstetric use in 1972. There are, therefore, no remaining patients younger than 19 years of age who were exposed to DES *in utero,* and the sequelae of DES should no longer be seen in this patient population.

The consequences of *in utero* exposure to DES included both structural abnormalities, clear cell adenocarcinoma of the lower genital tract, and an increased risk of dysplasia. The most common structural abnormality associated with DES is vaginal adenosis, the presence of endocervical type glands in the vagina (Fig. 6). Originally, the

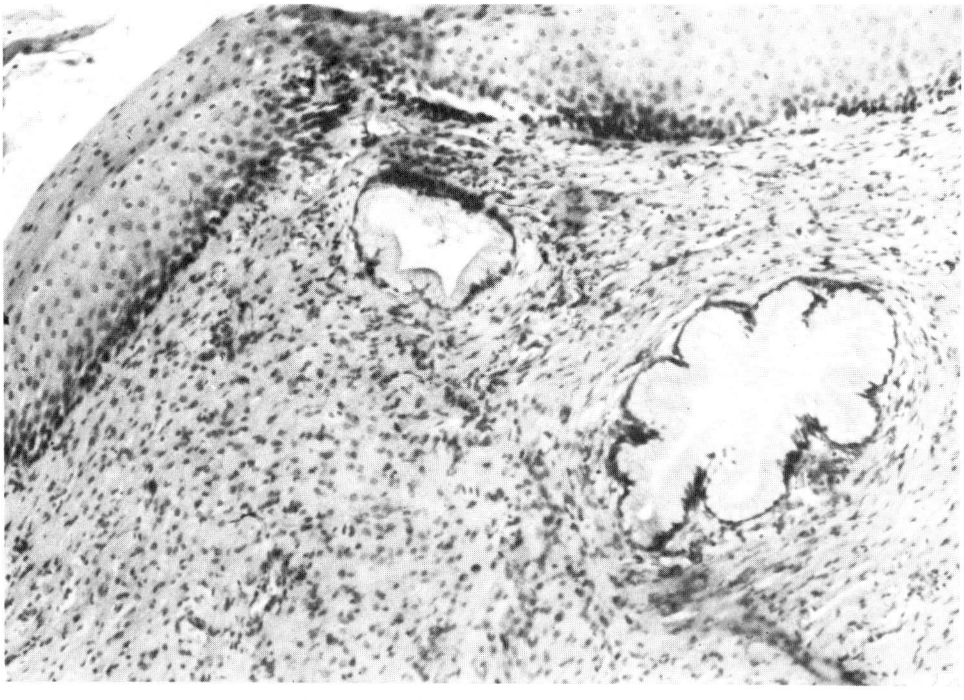

FIG. 6. Vaginal adenosis. Endocervical type glands beneath vaginal squamous epithelium.

glandular epithelium is on the surface of the vagina and can be easily identified by the villous appearing areas of pink/red columnar tissue. Gradually, by the process of squamous metaplasia, the glandular epithelium is covered by squamous epithelium and the columnar tissue is hidden from view. These areas of adenosis may maintain a cystic or nodular configuration that is visible (Fig. 7) and palpable beneath the vaginal mucosa. Patients who manifest this abnormality must be followed closely, as clear cell adenocarcinomas have been reported to arise even while the patient is under observation (23).

Other structural abnormalities include a wide cervical eversion with columnar epithelium covering portions of the exocervix (Fig. 8), cervical hoods, and cockscomb deformities of the cervix (Fig. 9). Cervical hypoplasia may also occur. As with vaginal adenosis, cervical eversions are gradually covered by squamous epithelium, often forming Nabothian cysts. Both vaginal adenosis and wide cervical eversions can occur in patients not exposed to *in utero* DES; however, the incidence is much less frequent. Structural abnormalities of the uterus after DES exposure include a T-shaped endometrial cavity and uterine hypoplasia.

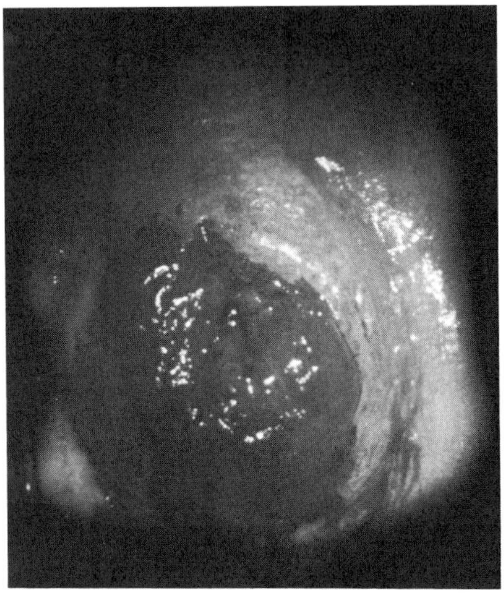

FIG. 8. Cervical eversion with darker columnar epithelium extending onto exocervix.

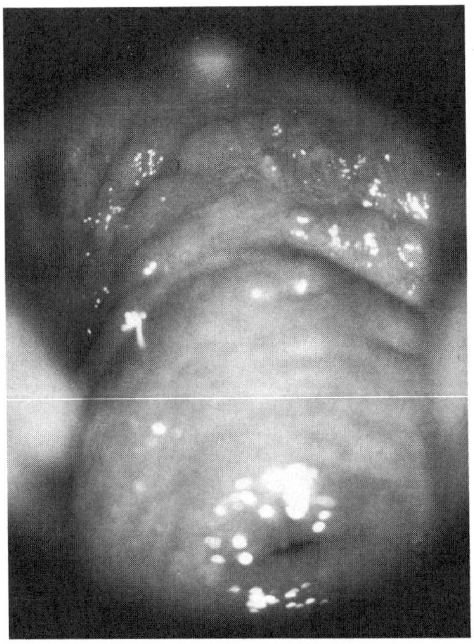

FIG. 7. Anterior vaginal wall with manifestations of vaginal adenosis.

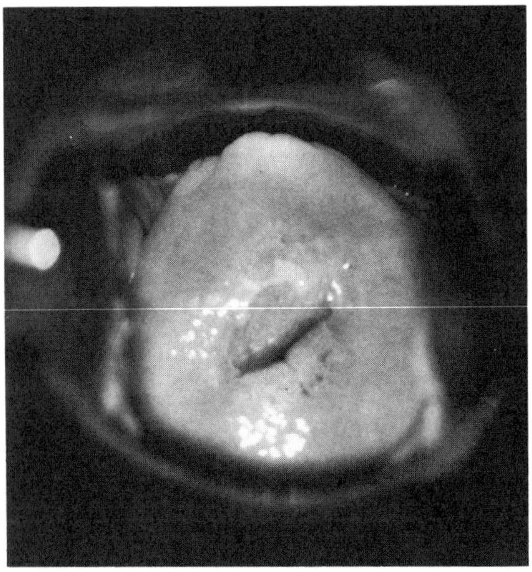

FIG. 9. Cockscomb abnormality of anterior cervix.

Clear Cell Adenocarcinoma

The association of DES exposure and clear cell adenocarcinoma of the female genital tract was first discovered after a report by Herbst and Scully in 1970 detailing seven cases of adenocarcinomas of the vagina in adolescence. Further epidemiological investigation demonstrated that the majority of patients had been exposed to DES *in utero* (25). Since that time, over 500 cases of clear cell adenocarcinoma have been accessioned into an international registry. Two-third of these cases have been positive for DES exposure (26). Certainly, clear cell adenocarcinoma of the female genital tract occurs in the absence of *in utero* DES exposure, with approximately 32% of cervical cases and 14% of vaginal cases having no history of hormone exposure (27). The youngest age on onset was 7 years, and the oldest 34, with a peak frequency at age 19 (27) in patients with a positive history for DES exposure. The reported number of cases has declined steadily since 1975.

The most common symptom of clear cell adenocarcinoma is abnormal vaginal bleeding or discharge, as described by Jones et al. (1). An abnormal Papanicolaou (Pap) smear may lead to the diagnosis, as may an abnormality on routine pelvic examination. Definitive diagnosis is made on biopsy of the lesion, which may arise from any portion of the vagina or cervix, but which, most frequently occurs on the anterior wall or the upper vagina. This also corresponds to the most frequent site of vaginal adenosis, which has universally been found accompanying vaginal clear cell carcinoma (27,28).

Histopathologically, the tumor is most often composed of solid sheets of clear cells or in a tubulocystic pattern, with tubules and cysts lined by the characteristic hobnail cells (28). The tumor most often spreads by local extension but may also metastasize by the hematogenous and lymphogenous routes. Lymph node involvement is relatively common, being present in approximately 16% of stage I and 30% of stage II disease (27).

Therapy for clear cell carcinoma of the vagina and cervix consists of radical pelvic surgery, radiation therapy, or a combination of both modalities, and depends on the stage of disease at diagnosis. Routine staging procedures for cervical or vaginal carcinoma should be performed. These include an examination under anesthesia, chest x-ray, and intravenous pyelogram. An abdominal pelvic CT scan is useful to assess the status of pelvic lymph nodes or disease outside the pelvis. Cystoscopy and proctosigmoidoscopy may be helpful if disease is clinically suspected to involve the bladder or rectum.

If the tumor is confined to the cervix or extends only to the upper vagina, radical hysterectomy, upper vaginectomy, and bilateral pelvic lymphadenectomy is the treatment of choice. The ovaries need not be removed and should be transposed out of the pelvis if the addition of radiation therapy is anticipated. Radiation therapy should be added if the pelvic lymph nodes are positive for metastatic disease. All other stages of more advanced tumor of the vagina or cervix are most appropriately treated by primary radiation therapy, employing 5,000–6,000 rads of whole-pelvis radiation followed by brachytherapy. Pelvic exenteration should be considered for radiation failures.

The therapy for stage IV patients with disease outside the pelvis should be individualized as should therapy of very small, stage I tumors, which have on occasion been treated with local combination therapy with preservation of reproductive function (27). An overall 5-year survival rate of 80% has been reported (27,28).

Although the population of patients exposed to DES is aging and the risk of clear cell adenocarcinoma is decreasing, patients with a history of DES exposure should continue to undergo close follow-up including visualization of the cervix and entire vagina, cervical and vaginal Pap smears, palpation of the vagina, and periodic colposcopy. As the incidence of clear cell carcinoma in patients over 30 is unknown (23), some tumors may still develop in this patient cohort.

Dysplasia

Patients exposed *in utero* to DES have also been shown to have an appropriate twofold higher incidence of cervical and vaginal dysplasia than nonexposed women (21). This may be due to the frequent presence of a large transformation zone in cases with vaginal adenosis or cervical eversions, which results in a larger area susceptible to the neoplastic transformation of carcinogens.

SQUAMOUS CELL LESIONS

Squamous cell carcinoma of the cervix in patients under 18 years of age are essentially unknown. Likewise, vaginal squamous cell carcinoma in this age group is extraordinarily rare, with only five documented cases between ages 11 and 20, as reported by DiDomenico (29). Two of these patients were pregnant at the time of diagnosis. Common symptoms of vaginal squamous carcinoma include vaginal bleeding and/or pelvic pain. Symptoms related to the urinary tract, including hematuria, dysuria, or urgency, may also occur. Diagnosis is confirmed by biopsy of the vaginal lesions. Radiation in the mainstay of therapy, although radical hysterectomy can be performed on lesions confined to the upper vagina.

Dysplasia

More commonly encountered in the adolescent are premalignant squamous lesions of the cervix or dysplasia. Any sexually active female is at risk for the development of dysplasia, and screening should, therefore, begin with the onset of sexual activity or age 20, whichever occurs first. Although the frequency of screening is controversial, most clinicians in the United States continue to screen normal sexually active women at yearly intervals and high-risk women, such as those with a past history of dysplasia, more frequently.

Pathologically, cervical dysplasia consists of a proliferation of undifferentiated basal cells with malignant features and a decrease in superficial cell differentiation. Cervical dysplasia has been divided into three grades (Table 3): cervical intraepithelial neoplasia (CIN) I, or mild dysplasia, CIN II, or moderate dysplasia; and CIN III, or severe dysplasia/carcinoma *in situ* based on the degree of proliferation of the undifferentiated cells. In CIN I, these cells occupy approximately one-third of the epithelium, with the upper two-thirds demonstrating some cytoplasmic differentiation. In CIN II, the lower two-thirds of the epithelium are occupied by undifferentiated cells; in CIN III, full-thickness changes occur. Mitosis and nuclear pleomorphism are common.

The development of cervical dysplasia is felt to be dependent, at least in part, on infection by HPV, and, indeed, manifestations of this infection, such as koilocytosis (cells with eccentric nuclei with perinuclear clearing representing the episomal viral particles), are often seen in early dysplastic lesions (Fig. 10). As the severity of dysplasia increases, the presence of koilocytes often decreases, as the viral DNA becomes integrated into the host genome (Fig. 11).

TABLE 3. *Classification of cervical dysplasia*

	Low grade SIL
CIN I	HPV changes Mild Dysplasia
	High grade SIL
CIN II	Moderate Dysplasia
CIN III	Severe Dysplasia
CIN III	Carcinoma in situ

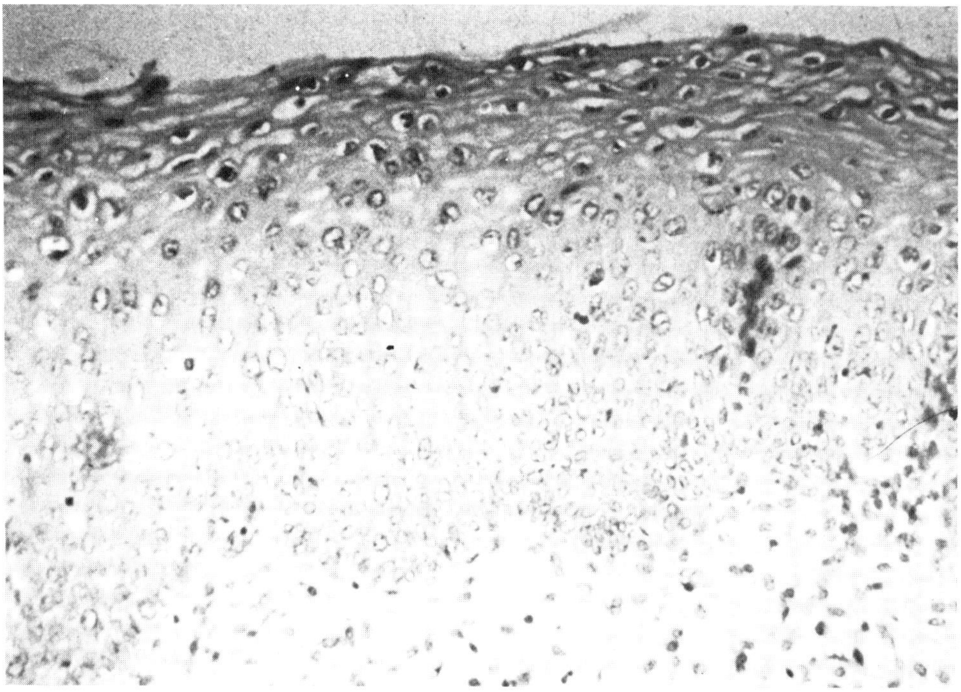

FIG. 10. CIN I with koilocytosis.

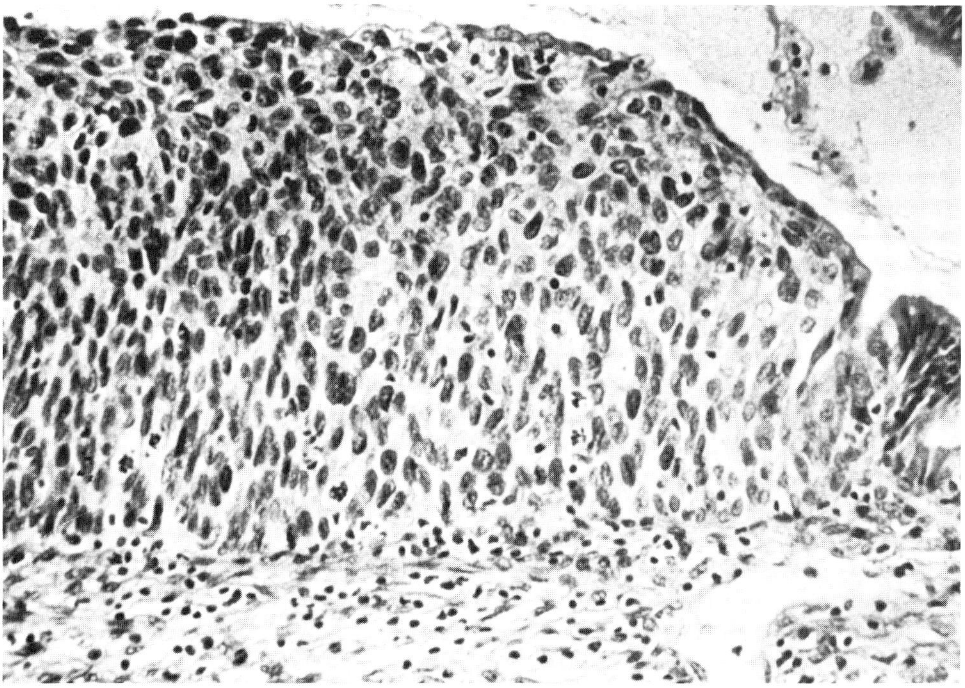

FIG. 11. CIN III. Note absence of koilocytosis.

For a further discussion of HPV, see the chapter by Anderson.

Recently, a new system for classification of cervical dysplasia has been proposed. The Bethesda System (29) divides cervical dysplasia into low-grade squamous intraepithelial lesions (SIL), including HPV changes and CIN I, and high-grade SIL, including CIN II and CIN III. This two-tiered system had not been universally accepted, as the natural history and therapeutic management plan for the categories within each group may differ significantly.

Evaluation of dysplasia in the adolescent is identical to the evaluation performed in an adult. A complete discussion of the evaluation and therapy of dysplasia is beyond the scope of this chapter, and the interested reader is referred to one of the many texts on gynecologic oncology or colposcopy. A synopsis of the diagnosis and management of CIN will be presented.

The diagnosis of cervical dysplasia begins with the abnormal Pap smear. In order to obtain the highest yield and the lowest false negative rate, the Pap smear must be performed correctly. Most dysplasia originates in the transformation zone or at the squamocolumnar junction. This area must, therefore, be sampled with the exocervical scrape. In adolescents, a wide eversion may be present, necessitating sampling away from the endocervical canal and near the vaginal fornices. An endocervical sample should also be obtained. The sample should be smeared on the slide uniformly thin and should be fixed immediately in order to avoid air-drying artifact. Performance of the Pap smear during heavy vaginal bleeding should be avoided, as the blood may obscure the epithelial cells and make evaluation difficult. A small amount of bleeding usually presents no difficulty.

All abnormal Pap smears should be evaluated with colposcopy and biopsy, if indicated (Table 4). This includes Pap smears with persistent atypia that is not of inflammatory origin, glandular atypia, HPV, squamous dysplasia of any degree, or any indication of carcinoma.

TABLE 4. *Indications for colposcopy*

- persistent squamous atypia (non-inflammatory)
- glandular atypia
- HPV changes
- squamous dysplasia
- suspicion of carcinoma

Colposcopic evaluation of the cervix is performed after the application of 3% acetic acid. The acetic acid not only serves to remove cervical mucous but also dehydrates the cells, turning those cells with larger nuclei a bright white due to greater reflection of light. The magnification of the colposcope and the use of the green filter, which accentuates vascular patterns, allows the identification of abnormal dysplastic tissue. The main patterns seen with dysplasia are white epithelium (Fig. 12), mosaicism (Fig. 13), and punctation. When squamous metaplasia is present, it appears

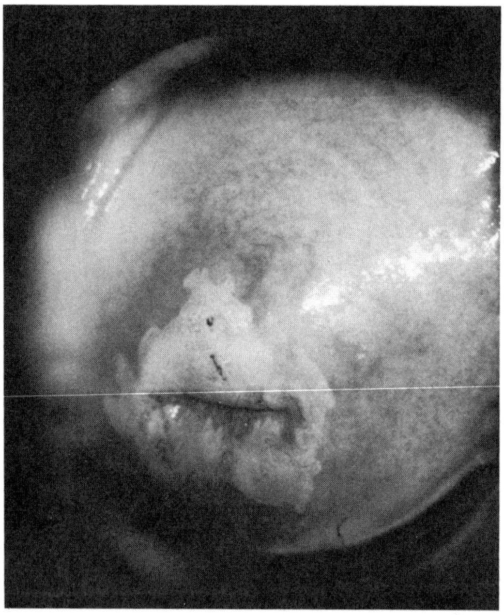

FIG. 12. CIN III. Colposcopic view with white epithelium and mosaic pattern at 12 o'clock.

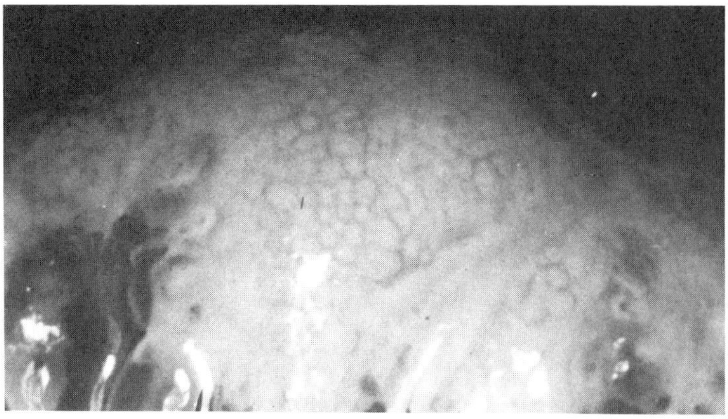

FIG. 13. Mosaicism. High-power view.

as a thin white covering over glandular epithelium, which can often be peeled away by a cotton swab. The hallmark of invasive cervical cancer is the presence of abnormal vessels. Abnormal vessels are characterized by their abnormal branching pattern and not by their size, as enlarged but normally branching vessels can be seen overlying Nabothian cysts and in inflammatory processes. Any colposcopic abnormality should be biopsied to obtain a definitive diagnosis. Any gross lesion of the cervix should also be biopsied regardless of the Pap smear result.

During the colposcopic procedure, a decision must be made regarding the adequacy of the study. An adequate colposcopy is one in which the entire lesion and the entire squamocolumnar junction can be visualized. If the lesion extends into the canal beyond visualization capability, even after the use of an endocervical speculum, or if the entire squamocolumnar junction cannot be seen, further diagnostic procedures such as a cervical conization may be necessary.

Although the routine sampling of the endocervix at the time of colposcopy is somewhat controversial, many colposcopists feel that this important step should never be omitted. Endocervical curettage not only allows the detection of squamous lesions in the endocervical canal that may be missed on colposcopic visualization of the cervix, but also aids in the detection of adenocarcinoma of the endocervix, which is often difficult to detect on Pap smear. Certainly, it is absolutely necessary in any patient being evaluated for glandular atypia on Pap smear, which is often the only indication of adenocarcinoma. Endocervical curettage should not be performed during pregnancy.

Therapy

After the cervical biopsy is performed, the pathology must be correlated with the Pap smear result (Table 5). If the biopsy is equal to or more abnormal than the Pap smear (with one degree of latitude), and the colposcopy is adequate, then definitive therapy may be performed. If the biopsy is less abnormal than the Pap smear, if the colposcopy is inadequate, or if the ECC is positive, then a cervical conization should be performed. If frankly invasive cervical carcinoma is found, definitive therapy may be planned. However, the finding of microinvasive carcinoma without vascular or lymphatic invasion on biopsy necessitates cone biopsy prior to definitive treatment planning.

When cervical conization is not required

TABLE 5. *Management of the abnormal Pap smear*

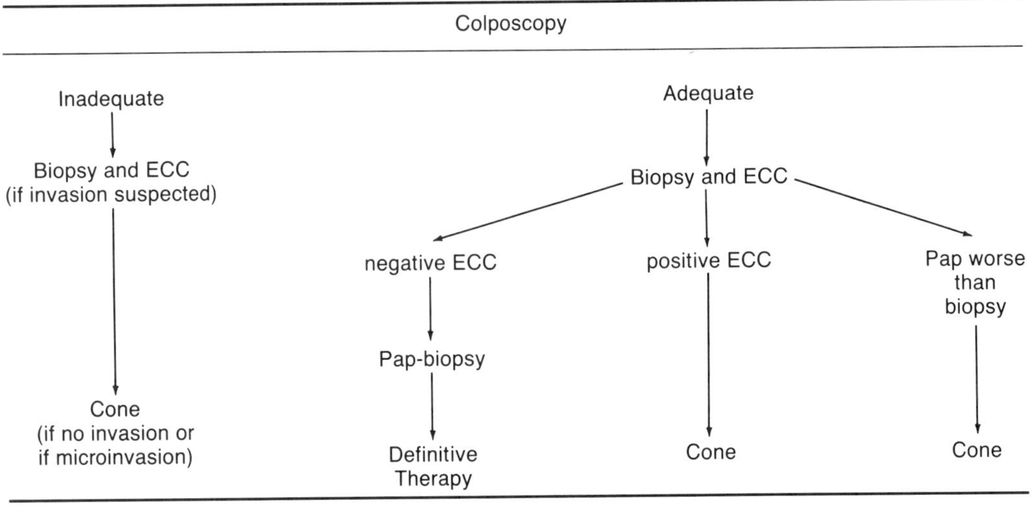

for further evaluation, there are several options for the therapy of CIN I, II, and III that have been adequately evaluated and correlated (Table 6). These include observation, cryotherapy, laser ablation, loop excision of the transformation zone, conization, or hysterectomy.

Observation alone may be utilized in patients with subclinical HPV infection only and no evidence of dysplasia. It may also be elected in highly motivated patients with mild dysplasia, as up to 62% (30) of untreated mild dysplasia may regress to normal without therapy. Observation should never be chosen in patients who are noncompliant, and therapy should be instituted immediately if progression of the dysplasia is noted at follow-up visits, which should be performed every 3–4 months. Observation alone has some distinct advantages in adolescents whose low-grade dysplasia may purely be a manifestation of infection with the HPV virus. The initiation of ablative therapies at a young age may result in increasingly difficult cervical evaluation should the process recur. This may lead to repetitive and increasingly aggressive procedures for this low-grade abnormality.

TABLE 6. *Available therapies for cervical dysplasia*

- Observation
- Cryotherapy
- Laser Vaporization
- Laser Conization
- Cold Knife Conization
- Loop Excision
- Hysterectomy

Cryotherapy, laser ablation, or loop excision are appropriate therapies for CIN I, II, and small CIN III lesions. Cryotherapy has the advantage of being inexpensive, easily and quickly performed, and readily available. Although few serious side effects are noted from cryotherapy, patients do note a thin watery discharge for approximately 14 days, and the procedure may cause the squamocolumnar junction to migrate into the endocervical canal, making further colposcopic evaluation difficult. Laser ablation is more costly, is more difficult and time consuming to perform, and may cause pain and bleeding. Healing after laser therapy, however, is more rapid and the position of the squamocolumnar junction on the exocervix can often be preserved, thus facilitating future colposcopic evaluation. The cure rates for cryotherapy and laser therapy for CIN I, II, and small CIN III lesions are identical. Large CIN III lesions have a higher failure rate and are often treated by cervical conization. An approximate 2% incidence of invasive disease is present when cervical conization is performed (31).

Loop excision of the transformation zone is a new procedure that has tremendous potential in the therapy of all grades of CIN (32,33). This technique has the advantage of being fast, easy, and well tolerated. It has few side effects and provides a tissue specimen for definitive pathological evaluation. Indeed, the diathermy loop may be used to perform cone biopsies in an office setting (34). The major disadvantage of loop excision is the necessity for injection of local anesthesia with a vasoconstrictor into the cervix for anesthesia and the prevention of bleeding. When performed properly, the incidence of bleeding is minimal and healing rapid. The location of the squamocolumnar junction is usually preserved on the exocervix. Although a large body of data has not yet been collected on loop excision of the transformation zone, it seems a very promising new technique.

Hysterectomy as a therapy for cervical dysplasia has a limited role and should be reserved for those patients with CIN III who have no further childbearing in mind.

Follow-up after therapy for cervical dysplasia should be performed 4 months after therapy and every 3–4 months thereafter. If Pap smears remain normal for 1 year, the patient may then be seen at 6-month intervals. Any recurrence of abnormality on Pap smear should reinitiate the entire evaluation and therapeutic process.

ACKNOWLEDGMENT

The author is grateful to J. Donald Woodruff, M.D., for providing the photographs for Figs. 1–5.

REFERENCES

1. Jones WB, Koulos JP, Saigo PE, et al. Clear-cell adenocarcinoma of the lower genital tract: Memorial Hospital 1974–1984. *Obstet Gynecol* 1987;70:573–7.
2. Bell J, Averette H, Davis J, et al. Genital rhabdomyosarcoma: current management and review of the literature. *Obst Gyn Survey* 1986;41: 257–63.
3. Fleming ID, Etcubanas E, Patterson R, et al. The role of surgical resection when combined with chemotherapy and radiation in the management of pelvic rhabdomyosarcoma. *Ann Surg* 1984;199:509–14.
4. Flamant F, Gerbaulet C, Nihoul-Fekete C, et al. Long-term sequelae of conservative treatment by surgery, brachytherapy, and chemotherapy for vulvar and vaginal rhabdomyosarcoma in children. *J Clin Oncol* 1990;8:1847–53.
5. Copeland LJ, Gershenson DM, Saul PB, et al. Sarcoma botryoides of the female genital tract. *Obstet Gynecol* 1985;66:262–6.
6. Blaustein A, Sedlis A. Diseases of the vagina. In: Blaustein A, ed. *Pathology of the female genital tract*. 2nd ed. New York: Springer-Verlag, 1982:59–98.
7. Brand E, Berek JS, Nieberg R, et al. Rhabdomyosarcoma of the uterine cervix—sarcoma botryoides. *Cancer* 1987;60:1552–60.
8. Daya DA, Scully RE. Sarcoma botryoides of the uterine cervix in young women: a clinicopathological study of 13 cases. *Gynecol Oncol* 1988;29:290–304.
9. McHenry CR, Reynolds M, Raffensperger JG. Vaginal neoplasms in infancy: the combined role of chemotherapy and conservative surgical resection. *J Pediatr Surg* 1988;23:842–5.
10. Hays DM. Rhabdomyosarcoma: management in children and young adults. *Current Concepts in Oncology* 1986; Winter.
11. Piver MS, Rose PG. Long-term follow-up and complications of infants with vulvovaginal embryonal rhabdomyosarcoma treated with surgery, radiation therapy, and chemotherapy. *Obstet Gynecol* 1988;71:435–7.
12. Gordon AN, Montag TW. Sarcoma botryoides of the cervix: excision followed by adjuvant chemotherapy for preservation of reproductive function. *Gynecol Oncol* 1990;36:119–24.
13. Maurer HM. The Intergroup Rhabdomyosarcoma Study (NIH): objectives and clinical staging classification. *J Pediatr Surg* 1975;10:977–8.
14. Copeland LJ, Sneige N, Ordonez NG, et al. Endodermal sinus tumor of the vagina and cervix. *Cancer* 1985;55:2558–65.
15. Collins HS, Burke TW, Heller PB, et al. Endodermal sinus tumor of the infant vagina treated exclusively by chemotherapy. *Obstet Gynecol* 1989;73:507–9.
16. Vawter GF. Carcinoma of the vagina in infancy. *Cancer* 1965;18:1479–84.
17. Andersen WA, Sabio H, Durso N, et al. Endo-

dermal sinus tumor of the vagina—the role of primary chemotherapy. *Cancer* 1985;56:1025–7.

18. Young RH, Scully RE. Endodermal sinus tumor of the vagina: a report of nine cases and review of the literature. *Gynecol Oncol* 1984;18:380–92.
19. Cook CL, Sanfilippo JS, Verdi GD, et al. Capillary hemangioma of the vagina and urethra in a child: response to short-term steroid therapy. *Obstet Gynecol* 1989;73:883–5.
20. Bellina JH, Gyer DR, Voros JI, et al. Capillary hemangioma managed by the CO_2 laser. *Obstet Gynecol* 1980;55:128–31.
21. Bornstein J, Adam E, Adler-Storthz K, et al. Development of cervical and vaginal squamous cell neoplasia as a late consequence of in utero exposure to diethylstilbestrol. *Obstet Gynecol Survey* 1988;1:15–21.
22. Ostergard DR. DES-related vaginal lesions. *Clin Obstet Gynecol* 1981;24:379–94.
23. Carlson JA. Morgan M, Boothby R, et al. Stage II papillary clear cell adenocarcinoma of the vagina during observation in a diethylstilbestrol-exposed daughter. *Gynecol Oncol* 1989;32:86–7.
24. Herbst AL, Scully RE. Adenocarcinoma of the vagina in adolescence—a report of 7 cases including 6 clear-cell carcinomas (so-called mesonephromas). *Cancer* 1970;25:745–57.
25. Herbst AL, Ulfelder H, Poskanzer DC. Adenocarcinoma of the vagina: association of maternal stilbestrol therapy with tumor appearance in young women. *N Engl J Med* 1971;284:878–81.
26. Horwitz RI, Viscoli CM, Merino M, et al. Clear cell adenocarcinoma of the vagina and cervix: incidence, undetected disease, and diethylstilbestrol. *J Clin Epidemiol* 1988;41:593–7.
27. DiSaia PJ, Creasman WT. *Clinical gynecologic oncology*. 3rd ed. St. Louis: The C.V. Mosby Company, 1989.
28. Robboy SJ, Young RH, Herbst AL. Female genital tract changes related to prenatal diethylstilbestrol exposure. In: Blaustein A, ed. *Pathology of the female genital tract*. 2nd ed. New York: Springer-Verlag, 1982;99–118.
29. National Cancer Institute Workshop. The 1988 Bethesda System for reporting cervical/vaginal cytologic diagnoses. *JAMA* 1989;262:931–4.
30. Nasiell K, Roger V, Nasiell M. Behavior of mild cervical dysplasia during long-term followup. *Obstet Gynecol* 1986;67:665–9.
31. McIndoe GA, Robson MS, Tidy JA, et al. Laser excision rather than vaporization: the treatment of choice for cervical intraepithelial neoplasia. *Obstet Gynecol* 1989;74:165.
32. Prendiville W, Cullimore J, Norman S. Large loop excision of the transformation zone (LLETZ). A new method of management for women with cervical intraepithelial neoplasia. *Br J Obstet Gynecol* 1989;96:1054–60.
33. Whiteley PF, Olah KS. Treatment of cervical intraepithelial neoplasia: Experience with the low-voltage diathermy loop. *Am J Obstet Gynecol* 1990;162:1272–7.
34. Mor-Yosef S, Lopes A, Pearson S, et al. Loop diathermy cone biopsy. *Obstet Gynecol* 1990;75:884–6.

Pediatric and Adolescent Gynecology,
edited by S. E. Carpenter and J. A. Rock.
Raven Press, Ltd., New York © 1992.

25

Tumors of the Uterine Corpus and Gestational Trophoblastic Disease

Janet S. Rader

Department of Gynecology and Obstetrics, The Johns Hopkins Hospital, Baltimore, Maryland 21205

UTERINE CORPUS

Uterine tumors rarely develop in early life. However, when tumors of the uterus are found in children and adolescents, they are likely to be malignant. The clinical presentation of most uterine tumors is vaginal bleeding. Therefore, the possibility of a neoplasm of the genitalia must be seriously considered and explored, whenever vaginal bleeding occurs in a child younger than 9 years old or in any child without secondary sexual development.

Difficulties in treatment of genital neoplasms in children frequently arise because of delayed diagnosis. Often, neoplasms are detected only after the tumor has reached an advanced stage or large size. Further difficulties arise in the surgical management of children because of delicate tissues, undeveloped genital organs, and small pelvis size.

The patient's subsequent sexual and somatic development and future child bearing should be considered in choosing treatment options. Chemotherapeutic treatments that preserve ovarian function rather than radiation or surgical removal of the uterus and ovaries should be selected when possible.

Endometrial Hyperplasia and Cancer

Endometrial adenocarcinoma, the most common malignancy of the adult female genital tract, is the least common malignancy in children. Endometrial cancer is predominately a neoplasm of obese postmenopausal women. Only a few cases of endometrial cancer have been reported in children or teenagers. The clinical presentation of the adolescents included; a rapidly growing tumor, vaginal bleeding, and no signs of sexual precocity. Most of the patients died within 6 months even with aggressive treatment due to the advanced stage of the disease at diagnosis (1,2).

The predisposing factor for this malignancy and its associated lesion, endometrial hyperplasia, is unopposed estrogen stimulation, either endogenous or exogenous. Unopposed estrogen causes incomplete shedding of the endometrium. The abnormal endometrial proliferations range from various degrees of glandular crowding and cytologic atypia to invasive cancer. Endometrial hyperplasia can be seen in children with Turner's syndrome given unopposed estrogen therapy or women with polycystic ovarian syndrome where extraglandular aromatization of androgens to estrone occurs (3,4).

The diagnosis is usually made by endometrial curettage when the patient presents with vaginal bleeding. Most cases of endometrial hyperplasia do not progress to invasive cancer (5,6). Therefore, young women with endometrial hyperplasia can be treated medically with progestin therapy and monitored with periodic endometrial sampling (Fig. 1). The progestin therapy ensures more complete sloughing of the endometrium, which in turn prevents the continued proliferation. Only when patients are unresponsive to progestin therapy or progress to endometrial carcinoma is hysterectomy necessary. When an adenocarcinoma of the uterus is present, an abdominal hysterectomy with bilateral salpingoophorectomy and intraoperative staging is done. Further radiation therapy can be based on examination of the surgical specimen.

In adolescents who are anovulatory and have irregular bleeding (polycystic ovarian syndrome), progesterone should be given to interrupt the steady estrogen stimulation of

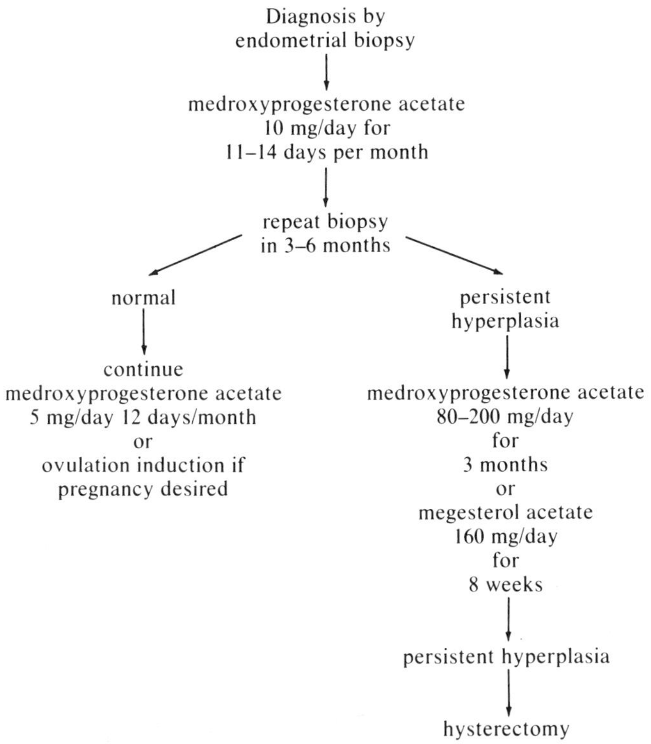

FIG. 1. Management of endometrial hyperplasia.

the uterus. Patients should be given 10 mg medroxyprogesterone acetate for at least 10 days each month to insure complete withdrawal bleeding and to prevent endometrial hyperplasia. If the patient is also in need of contraceptive, a low dose combination oral contraception in the usual cyclic fashion can be given in place of progesterone therapy alone (7). Hormonal therapy should be used until the patient establishes normal ovulation or is ready for ovulation induction and childbearing.

Leiomyomas of the Uterus

Leiomyomas are benign tumors composed mainly of smooth muscle cells and various amounts of fibrous connective tissue. A case of uterine leiomyoma has been reported in a child 10 years old along with a few reported cases in teenagers. Wiscot et al. (8) described the case of a 13-year-old girl who presented with profuse vaginal bleeding and a lower abdominal mass 8 months after beginning menses. Augensen (9) described a 15-year-old who presented with amenorrhea for 8 weeks, urinary retention and a lower abdominal mass. Both patients were treated conservatively with myomectomy and did well postoperatively with resumption of normal menses. Farber et al. (10) presented the case of a myoma developing in a rudimentary muscular bud in a patient with vaginal and uterine agenesis (Rokitansky-Kuster-Hauser syndrome). The patient was treated with excision of the leiomyoma from its attachment to the right myometrial bud. These are rare medical occurrences but should be recognized so patients may be treated conservatively and reassured about future reproductive potential.

Sarcomas of the Uterus

Most of the reported malignancies of the uterine fundus in adolescents have been sarcomas with mixed mesodermal tumors being the most common. Mixed mesodermal tumors is a group of neoplasms that arise from malignant epithelial and mesenchymal stromal elements of the uterus. They are classified according to the nature of the sarcomatous component into homologous (tissue normally found in the uterus) or heterologous (tissue not normally found in the uterus, i.e., striated muscle, cartilage, etc.). The tumors are firm and sessile filling the uterine cavity unlike the grapelike sarcomas of the vagina. This tumor also is usually found in postmenopausal women but several mixed mullerian tumors have been reported in children and adolescents from 4 to 19 years old (1,11–13). Patients usually presented with vaginal bleeding and a pelvic mass. The treatment of the tumors requires early diagnosis and radical surgery followed by radiation and chemotherapy tailored to the patient.

Careful staging of the extent of disease is very important in the treatment and prognosis of children with rhabdomyosarcoma. Pelvic ultrasound and computed tomography can be very useful in evaluating the extent of disease and measuring tumoral regression during chemotherapy (14). Hayes et al. (15) in a large review of 47 children and adolescents with rhabdomyosarcoma of the female genital tract in 1972–1984 had six patients with uterine disease. The patients ranged in age from 4 to 15 years old. Four patients each had a single large polyp protruding from the cervix and two patients had intramural involvement of the uterus. All were treated with vincristine and actinomycin with or without cyclophosphamide and adriamycin. The four patients with polypoid lesions also had local excision performed in three patients and the fourth had a radical hysterectomy. All four patients were disease-free 2.7–6.5 years after treatment. Both patients with intramural corpus involvement had intraperitoneal disease. One patient died of sepsis during chemotherapy and the other patient died of distant disease after radiation and chemotherapy.

Other Tumors

Other reported uterine tumors in children and adolescents include; glioma, peripheral primitive neuroectodermal tumor, hemangioendothelioma, nonHodgkin's lymphoma, and Wilms' tumor (16–21). Corpus uteri cancer in children and adolescents is a rarity, all available information primarily emanates from individual case reports, and treatment has consequently been empirical.

GESTATIONAL TROPHOBLASTIC DISEASE

Gestational trophoblastic diseases are a spectrum of benign and malignant conditions derived from early embryonic tissues of conception. In addition to their malignant potential, molar pregnancies are associated with significant complications including hemorrhage, intrauterine infection, and toxemia. Since these conditions are associated with pregnancy they are a particularly threatening disease in young women. The overall teenage pregnancy rate has increased from 96 to 110 per 1000 women 15–19 years old from 1973 to 1985. In 1985, there were over one million teenage pregnancies in the United States (21).

Gestational trophoblastic diseases are pathologically divided into four distinct forms: (a) Hydatidiform mole is a local degenerative process with histologic features of hydropic villi and trophoblastic hyperplasia. (b) Invasive hydatidiform mole is a tumor that invades the uterine myometrium in addition to the presence of placental villous structures and trophoblastic hyperplasia. (c) Choriocarcinoma is an uncontrolled growth of the cytotrophoblast and syncytiotrophoblast without the presence of villous structures. (d) Placental site trophoblastic tumor is an uncommon tumor composed of infiltrating intermediate trophoblastic cells resembling cells found at the placental implantation site.

Clinically, patients are classified on the basis of high and low risk factors and whether the tumor is metastatic or nonmetastatic (23).

Hydatidiform Mole

Molar pregnancy rates in population-based studies range from 0.2 to 1.2 cases per 1,000 pregnancies or births (24). The incidence of hydatidiform mole in adolescents 15–19 years old in the United States in the 1970s was about 860 per year (25). A woman's age appears to be a risk factor with molar pregnancy rates higher at the extremes of reproductive life. Studies have shown pregnancy in women under 20 and over 35–40 years of age is more likely to result in a molar gestation and persistent trophoblastic disease (25–29). However, several other authors have not shown an increased risk of disease in the adolescent population (30–32).

Grossly, hydatidiform mole is characterized by a mass of vesicles that partially or completely replace the normal placental architecture. The vesicles are individual villi that have become edematous (hydropic degeneration) varying in size from a few millimeters up to 2–3 cm in diameter (Fig. 2). Microscopic examination reveals three major features of hydatidiform mole: (a) edematous swelling of chorionic villi, (b) proliferation of trophoblast, and (c) absence of fetal blood vessels in the villi. As a result of cytogenetic studies, hydatidiform mole is divided into two principal forms: partial and complete (Table 1) (33,34).

Partial moles are characterized by (a) focal hydropic villi with scalloping, (b) focal mild to moderate trophoblastic hyperplasia, and (c) identifiable fetal or embryonic structures. Chromosome analysis reveals a polypoid karyotype, which is most frequently triploid.

Complete moles are characterized by (a) hydropic swelling of all villi, (b) marked hyperplasia and anaplasia of the trophoblast, and (c) complete absence of fetal struc-

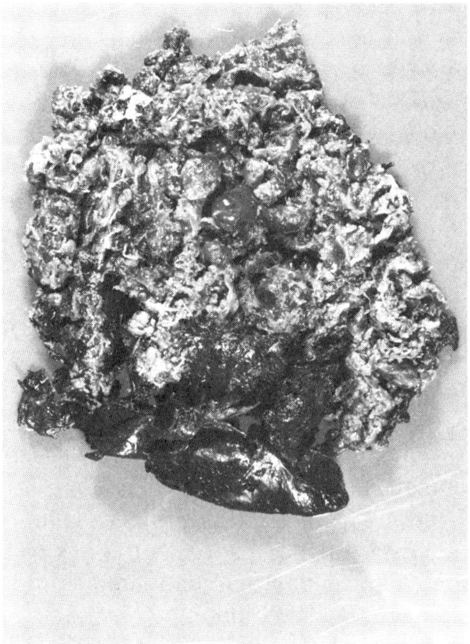

FIG. 2. Hydroponic degeneration of a molar pregnancy showing edematous villi varying in size from a few millimeters to two centimeters in diameter.

tures. The karyotype of the complete mole is 46 XX. Chromosomal banding studies have found that the chromosomal material of complete hydatidiform moles is totally inherited from the paternal contribution (35). Most fertilizations occur with an egg from which the nucleus has been lost or is inactivated by a sperm. The paternal 23 X chromosomes then duplicate to 46 XX (35–37). Jacobs et al. (38), in a study of molar pregnancy in Hawaii, found an excess of women aged <20 years in the group with complete moles when compared to partial moles.

TABLE 1. *Features of complete and partial hydatidiform mole*

	Complete	Partial
Karyotype	46XX, 46XY	Triploid
Fetal or embryonic tissue	Absent	Present
Swelling of chorionic villi	Diffuse	Focal
Trophoblastic hyperplasia	Diffuse	Focal
Percent persistent GTD	20%	5%

About 80% of complete hydatidiform moles will totally resolve after evacuation of the uterus. The remainder of the patients will develop malignant trophoblastic sequelae (invasive mole or choriocarcinoma). About 15% of the persistent disease will be local uterine invasion and 4% distant spread (39). In contrast, patients with a partial molar pregnancy are much less likely to develop persistent trophoblastic disease with a range of 0–6.6% (40–43).

Invasive Mole

Invasive mole is characterized by hydropic chorionic villi and trophoblastic hyperplasia within the myometrium and vascular spaces. The tumor may also metastasis to the vulva, vagina and lung. The frequency of invasive mole is difficult to determine because a uterine curettage is unlikely to yield villi invading the myometrium and therefore, a hysterectomy specimen is necessary for an accurate diagnosis (44). In fact, a pathologic diagnosis is rarely made between invasive mole and choriocarcinoma prior to treatment. This is made possible by the reliability of hCG levels as a tumor marker and the effectiveness of chemotherapeutic agents to kill trophoblastic disease with various histologic types and anatomic locations. Therefore, these tumors are treated under the general clinical terms of "gestational trophoblastic disease," "gestational trophoblastic tumor," and "metastatic trophoblastic tumor" (23).

Choriocarcinoma

Choriocarcinoma is a highly malignant tumor derived from trophoblastic epithelium that lacks chorionic villi. The tumor is extremely vascular and prone to bloodborne metastasis. Microscopic examination shows the abundant growth of both cytotrophoblast and syncytiotrophoblast in anaplastic sheets and columns invading uterine muscle. Hemorrhage and necrosis is usually present (45). As with invasive mole, this tumor is very difficult to diagnose in uterine curettings.

Most cases of choriocarcinoma appear to follow a recognizable gestation. About 50% of choriocarcinomas are preceded by a hydatidiform molar pregnancy, 25% occur following a spontaneous abortion, 22.5% following normal pregnancy, and 2.5% following ectopic pregnancy. About one of every 40 molar gestations is followed by choriocarcinoma (46). There are also reported cases of choriocarcinoma arising from the trophoblast of an otherwise normal placenta (47). Choriocarcinoma usually occurs shortly after the preceding pregnancy. However, very long latency periods of over 10 years have been reported (48,49). Some studies show higher rates of choriocarcinoma for adolescents (50,51), whereas other reports note lower rates for adolescents than women 20–40 years old (52,53).

Abnormal uterine bleeding is the most frequent clinical presentation for choriocarcinoma. Other manifestations of choriocarcinoma usually relates to the location of the metastases. The lungs are the most frequent site of extrauterine spread (54,55), and disease is usually picked up on x-ray examination. In addition, the patient may present with hemoptysis, cough, or dyspnea (56,57). Other sites of metastasis, in the order of decreasing frequency, are vagina, brain, liver, kidneys, small intestine, and spleen. The symptoms usually relate to hemorrhage in these areas (54). Thyrotoxicosis may also occur with choriocarcinoma (58). This tumor was uniformly fatal prior to the advent of chemotherapeutic treatment in 1956.

Classification and Staging

Gestational trophoblastic tumors can be classified according to an anatomical staging or clinical prognostic scoring system. The International Federation of Gynecology and Obstetrics (FIGO) staging system is based on clinical exam and radiologic findings (Table 2) (59). However, most treatment centers in the United States determine therapy according to good and poor prognostic factors other than just the anatomic location of the tumor. These systems take into account additional information regarding antecedent pregnancies, laboratory values, and symptoms. Patients are identified in need of initial aggressive multiagent chemotherapy. The gestational trophoblastic tumors are divided into three groups: nonmetastatic, metastatic low-risk, and metastatic high-risk (Table 3). The high risk patients are those that are not likely to be cured with single agent methotrexate or actinomycin D chemotherapy (23,60,61). Another prognostic scoring system was proposed by Bagshawe based on the patient's age, history of prior chemotherapy, antecedent pregnancy, and number, site and size of metastatis. A weighted score is applied to each variable and the individual scores added. Patients with a final score of 4 or less are considered low risk, those with a score of 5–7 are middle risk, and those with a score of 8 or greater are high risk (Table 4) (23,62,63).

Clinical Management

Clinical suspicion for gestational trophoblastic disease should arise when a pregnancy is accompanied by excessive nausea and vomiting, vaginal bleeding, a uterus large for gestational age, or preeclampsia occurring early in pregnancy.

TABLE 2. *Gestational trophoblastic disease FIGO staging system*

Stage	Disease state
I	Disease confined to the uterus
II	Disease confined to the pelvis
III	Disease confined to pelvis and lungs
IV	Metastatic to any other site

TABLE 3. *Prognostic group classification*

Nonmetastatic
- Persistent hydatidiform mole
- Invasive mole
- Choriocarcinoma

Metastatic
- Low risk, good prognosis
  - Serum hCG, <40,000 mIU/ml
  - Duration of symptoms, <4 months
  - No brain or liver metastasis
  - No prior chemotherapy for GTD
  - Disease after GTD, abortion, or ectopic (not term delivery)
- High risk, poor prognosis
  - Serum hCG, >40,000 mIU/ml
  - Duration of symptoms, >4 months
  - Brain or liver metastasis
  - Prior failed chemotherapy
  - Disease after term delivery
  - Recurrent or metastatic placental site trophoblastic tumor

The method of choice for diagnosing a molar pregnancy is ultrasonography which is an accurate, noninvasive technique. The ultrasonic picture of the mole depends on the gestational age of the patient. In the first trimester, an endometrial cavity filled with an irregular mixed echodense/echospared mass is present similar to that of an incomplete or missed abortion. By the second trimester, the characteristic fluid-filled vesicles are evident. Their size varies from 2 mm at 8.5 weeks gestation to 10 mm or more at 18.5 weeks gestation. The sonographic picture reveals multiple echoes in the uterine cavity which is usually described as a "snow storm" pattern (Fig. 3). This characteristic picture is due to the multiple interfaces between the hydropic chorionic villi (64,65). However, ultrasound can not always differentiate a mole from a first trimester abortion, degenerating fibroids, or even ovarian dysgerminomas (66,67). Taylor et al. (68) have described a technique of assessing blood flow and tissue perfusion of the uterus by duplex Doppler ultrasound. They showed higher systolic and diastolic Doppler shifts in gestational trophoblastic neoplasia when compared to a nongravid uterus, first trimester pregnancy, and incomplete abortion.

When the diagnosis of hydatidiform mole is confirmed, the uterus is emptied as soon as possible by suction and sharp curettage regardless of the uterine size. This allows preservation of fertility in the young patient. Curettage in patients with a uterine size less than 16 weeks has a low complication rate. Patients with a larger uterus are at increased risk of hemorrhage, sepsis, and uterine perforation. Application of oxytocin infusion during evacuation will decrease uterine bleeding and the risk of uterine perforation (69). During evacuation, molar tissue may enter the maternal venous sinuses and invade the lungs. About 2% of

TABLE 4. *Prognostic scoring system*[a]

Prognostic factor	Score 0	1	2	4
Age of patient (years)	≤39	>39		
Preceding pregnancy	Mole	Abortion	Term	
Months since prior pregnancy	<4	4–6	7–12	>12
hCG level (IU/L)	$<10^3$	10^3–10^4	10^4–10^5	$>10^5$
ABO groups (female × male)		O × A A × O	B, AB	
Largest tumor diameter (cm)		3–5	>5	
Site of metastases		Spleen	GI tract	Brain
Number of metastasis		1–4	4–8	>8
Prior chemotherapy			1 drug	≥2 drugs

[a]Total score: ≤4, low risk; 5–7, middle risk; ≥8, high risk. The total score for a patient is obtained by adding the individual prognostic factors.

Modified from ref. 23.

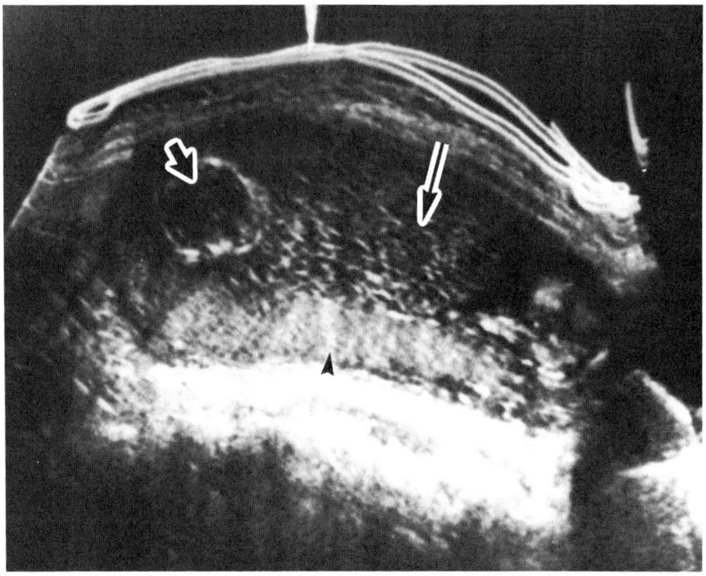

FIG. 3. Ultrasonic picture of a twin pregnancy. → Fetal head twin A; > Normal placenta twin A; ⟶ "Snow storm" Pattern of hydatiform twin B.

patients with molar pregnancy develop pulmonary embolisms and exhibit such symptoms as tachycardia, tachypnea, cyanosis, cough, and chest pain (70).

Preeclampsia has been diagnosed in 27% of patients with complete mole. Toxemia occurs almost exclusively in patients with markedly elevated hCG levels and excessive uterine size. The syndrome is associated with hypertension, proteinuria, and hyperreflexia. Toxemia occurs in the third trimester of pregnancy and the diagnosis of molar pregnancy should be considered in any patient who suffers toxemia early in gestation (71).

Antigenic fetal products may enter the maternal circulation after evacuation of the mole causing sensitization against antigens of the Rh system. These antibodies can be detrimental to an Rh incompatible fetus of a subsequent pregnancy. Therefore, all unsensitized Rh-negative patients should receive human anti D-gamma-globulin (Rhogam). The Rhogam should be given intramuscularly within 72 hr after evacuation of the hydatidiform molar pregnancy (72).

At the time of molar evacuation, a complete physical exam and chest x-ray is done to rule out metastatic disease. If disease is confined to the uterus, patients are then followed with serial β-hCG. The purpose of following hCG levels after evacuation of a hydatidiform mole is to detect continued trophoblastic activity and to begin appropriate chemotherapy. Weekly levels are obtained until three consecutive assays are normal (nondetectable) and then monthly for 1 year. The time for β-hCG levels to return to normal is influenced by the initial pre-evacuation level and the clearance rate. Most patients with spontaneous regression of trophoblastic disease will have normal levels by 12 weeks postevacuation (23,73). However, it is the trend in β-hCG levels that is important and the most specific prognostic indicator (39). Persistent trophoblastic disease requiring treatment is indicated by hCG levels that maintain a plateau over three consecutive weeks or increase at any time. The frequency of persistent trophoblastic disease is increased in pregnancies with large-for-dates uterus, ovarian theca-lutein cysts >5 cm, and post-evacuation uterine bleeding (30,73). Approximately 20–25% of patients with hydatidiform mole will require chemotherapy after evacuation (30,39,74).

Pregnancy prevention for 6 months to 2 years following evacuation of a hydatidiform mole is standard practice. In following the patient, the β-hCG assay is unable to differentiate normal pregnancy from other postmolar sequelae. Oral contraceptives are usually given because of their safety and high effectiveness. Stone et al. (26,75) reported a delay in the fall of hCG after molar evacuation and the need for chemotherapy increased two to three times in patients taking oral contraceptives. However, other studies have not confirmed this and have shown no abnormal hCG regression time after molar evacuation in oral contraceptive users (76–78). If a patient were to become pregnant shortly after evacuation, the β-hCG can be correlated with serial ultrasonography for accurate diagnosis.

Treatment

The prophylactic use of chemotherapy at the time of evacuation of the uterus resulted in a two- to threefold decrease in the development of persistent trophoblastic disease in some studies (79–81). Goldstein (79) used Actinomycin D for 5 consecutive days at the time of evacuation in 100 patients. He had only two cases of persistent disease and no cases of metastatic trophoblastic disease in the treated group compared to 16 cases of persistent disease and four cases of metastatic disease in the untreated group of 100 patients. Kashimura et al. (81) treated patients with 10 mg methotrexate daily for 7 days with a 27% minor complication rate and no severe complications. There was a decrease in persistent trophoblastic disease but not a significant decrease in metastatic disease, choriocarcinoma, or deaths from disease in patients receiving prophylactic chemotherapy. Ayhan et al. (82) showed no difference in the incidence of postmolar gestational trophoblastic disease between prophylactically untreated and treated groups in 233 patients with complete moles. In a randomized, prospective trial, Kim et al. (83) decreased the incidence of trophoblastic tumor from 48% to 14% in a group of patients at high risk of developing postmolar tumors. However, the routine use of prophylactic chemotherapy in all patients with molar pregnancy remains controversial because 80% of patients with hydatidiform mole will experience spontaneous resolution. In addition, if patients are followed closely and treated appropriately nearly all are curable. Therefore, it may only be useful in special situations where the risk of developing a molar pregnancy is very high or where β-hCG levels are unavailable.

Chemotherapy is initiated in trophoblastic disease when either the metastatic lesions are identified or β-hCG titers are plateauing or rising. Once either one of these occurrences is noted, the patient is completely reevaluated with x-ray studies to examine the brain, lungs, liver, and pelvis to determine the extent of disease. A repeat uterine curettage for histologic confirmation is not needed because invasive mole and choriocarcinoma is intramuscular and curettings are often negative.

Patients requiring chemotherapy have a wide spectrum of disease ranging from a few thousand trophoblastic cells remaining in the uterus to large metastatic lesions. The extent of disease greatly affects a patient's future outcome. Therefore, various prognostic factors have been identified to predict long-term survival or bad outcome. This allows patients at high risk of treatment failure to be recognized and given aggressive combination chemotherapy. After complete reevaluation physical exam and radiographic studies, patients are categorized as having nonmetastatic or metastatic gestational trophoblastic disease. Patients with metastatic tumors are further classified as being at high risk based on the presence of one or more of the following: (a) pretreatment serum β-hCG of 40,000 mIU/ml, (b) greater than 4 months from an antecedent pregnancy event to treatment, (c) metastasis to other than the lungs or vagina, (d) antecedent term gestation compared with hydatidiform mole, abortion, or ectopic pregnancy, or (e) prior unsuccessful chemotherapy (Table 3) (23,62,84). Chemotherapy is then given according to a patient's prognostic factors.

Approximately 80% of all patients are in the low-risk metastatic and nonmetastatic group and are treated with single-agent methotrexate or actinomycin D (Table 5). The preferred treatment for the low-risk groups with normal renal and hepatic function is methotrexate followed by folinic acid rescue. Chemotherapy is changed to Actinomycin D if the hCG level plateaus or rises or if toxicity precludes an adequate dose or frequency of treatment.

The methotrexate-folinic acid regimen has been found to be less toxic than methotrexate alone (85). The decreased toxicity on the methotrexate-folinic acid regimen may be due to the alternating day administration of methotrexate. Rotmensch et al. (86) showed that methotrexate at a dose of 1 mg/kg by intramuscular or intravenous administration had plasma levels at 24 hr below the critical threshold dose for toxicity of 2×10^8 at 48 hr (87). Therefore, the dose may be so low as to not require folinic acid rescue at 24 hr.

TABLE 5. *Gestational trophoblastic disease single-agent chemotherapy*

Methotrexate
0.4 mg/kg/day i.m. or i.v. for 5 days every 7–9 days, 14 days
30–50 mg/M^2 i.m. every week
Methotrexate and folinic acid
Methotrexate 1 mg/kg/day i.m. on days 1, 3, 5, and 7
Folinic acid 0.1 mg/kg/day i.m. on days 2, 4, 6, and 8 every 7–10 days
Actinomycin-D
10–12 μg/kg/day for 5 days every 7–9 days, 14 days
1.25 mg/M^2 i.v. every 14 days

All gestational trophoblastic tumors' response to chemotherapy can be accurately monitored in all cases by the tumor marker β-hCG. The patient's response to chemotherapy is described in terms of the fall in hCG which is monitored weekly in patients receiving treatment. A plateau of the hCG level over 2 weeks indicates resistance to the chemotherapy drugs. Once the hCG values are below the limit of detection by serum radioimmunoassay there are fewer than 10^4–10^5 tumor cells (88). Complete remission is diagnosed after three consecutive weekly hCG levels are within normal range and there is no clinical or radiologic evidence of disease. An additional two courses of chemotherapy are usually given after the first normal hCG level to decrease the incidence of relapse (84).

The most common toxic reactions to these drugs are oropharyngeal ulcerations (stomatitis) as well as ulceration of the esophagus, stomach, and small and large bowel. Topical anesthetics combined with antibiotics and systemic analgesics will provide some relief from these complications. A reversible elevation of hepatic enzymes may occur in some patients. Less common toxic reactions are skin rash, nausea and vomiting, significant alopecia, and myelotoxicity (89).

Present studies show a 86–97% initial complete remission in nonmetastatic gestational trophoblastic patients initially treated with single agent chemotherapy (90–92). Patients with low-risk metastatic disease can achieve similar cure rates. About 10–15% of patients will require combination chemotherapy with or without surgery to achieve complete remission. When a young patient with nonmetastatic disease is resistant to single agent chemotherapy, further treatment options include conservative operative treatment, pelvic arterial infusion chemotherapy, or multi-agent chemotherapy. Wilson et al. (93) reported on the local uterine resection of invasive trophoblastic tumors in five patients. All five patients achieved complete sustained remissions with no further treatment, and one patient had two subsequent term pregnancies. Maroulis et al. (94) performed pelvic arterial infusion chemotherapy with methotrexate or actinomycin D in five patients whose disease was resistant to systemic chemotherapy. Two patients were cured. Three others subsequently underwent hysterectomy and entered remission.

Patients with high-risk metastatic disease are initially treated with aggressive combination chemotherapy with or without adjunctive surgery. Present chemotherapy regimens include MAC (methotrexate, actinomycin D, cyclophosphamide) (95) or EMA-CO (etoposide, methotrexate, actinomycin D, cyclophosphamide, oncovin) (Table 6) (63). Studies have shown complete remission rates in high-risk metastatic cancer patients to be 63–83% in those treated initially with combination chemotherapy (63,95). However, high-risk patients treated with single agent therapy followed by combination treatment had about half the cure rate (60,84). EMA-CO is the preferred initial treatment over the MAC regimen for patients with a high-risk prognostic score (Table 4) (96).

Patients with central nervous system metastasis are given whole-brain irradiation in addition to chemotherapy. In addition intrathecal or high dose (1 gm/M^2) methotrexate must be used. About 50% of patients can be cured with this aggressive treatment (97,98). Liver metastasis from gestational trophoblastic disease is particularly ominous. Three out of nine patients from the Southeastern Regional Trophoblastic Disease Center and none of 6 patients from the Brewer Trophoblastic Disease Center survived (84,99). Grumbine et al. (100) described a technique to control hemorrhage from hepatic metastasis by using silicone balloons to occlude selective hepatic arteries. Chemotherapeutic regimens used in

TABLE 6. *Gestational trophoblastic disease multiagent chemotherapy*

MAC
Methotrexate 15 mg i.v. or i.m., days 1–5
Actinomycin D 0.5 mg i.v., days 1–5
Cyclophosphamide 3 mg/kg i.v., or chlorambucil 10 mg p.o., days 1–5
or
Methotrexate 1.0 mg/kg i.m. days 1, 3, 5, and 7
Folinic acid 0.1 mg/kg i.m. days 2, 4, 6, and 8
Actinomycin D 12 μg/kg i.v. days 1–5
Cyclophosphamide 3 mg/kg i.v. days 1–5
Interval between courses is 10–14 days
EMA-CO
Course 1: EMA
Day 1
Actinomycin D 0.5 mg i.v.
Etoposide 100 mg/M^2 i.v.
Methotrexate 100 mg/M^2
Methotrexate 200 mg/M^2 i.v. 12-hr infusion
Day 2
Actinomycin D 0.5 mg i.v.
Etoposide 100 mg/M^2 i.v.
Folinic acid 15 mg/M^2 i.m. or orally every 12 hr for four doses
Course 2: CO
Day 8
Vincristine 1.0 mg/M^2 i.v.
Cyclophosphamide 600 mg/M^2 i.v.
Course 1 to begin again on day 14

resistant trophoblastic disease include: cis-platinum, vinblastine, and bleomycin (VPB) (101) and cisplatinum, vincristine, methotrexate, and bleomycin (POMB) (102,103).

Reproductive Performance

The treatment of gestational trophoblastic disease in adolescent girls with cytotoxic drugs leads to concern over their future reproductive performance and incidence of congenital malformations, pregnancy complications, and recurrent molar pregnancies. It is known that intensive chemotherapy induces amenorrhea and depletion of ovarian germ cells and sterility (104). Infertility after chemotherapy has been reported with Hodgkin's disease (105,106). Premature ovarian failure with loss of primordial follicles that is age and dose related has been shown in women treated for Hodgkin's disease with nitrogen mustard, vinblastine, procarbazine and prednisolone (105). However, chemotherapy in patients with gestational trophoblastic disease does not appear to affect subsequent pregnancy rates (107–111). Song et al. (108) reviewed 265 cases of choriocarcinoma and invasive mole in young women treated between 1959–1980 at a hospital in Beijing, China. Patients received 6-mercaptopurine, 5-Fluorouracil, an agent similar to actinomycin D, and other agents. Over half the patients had metastatic disease and 80% of patients received at least three courses of chemotherapy. There were 355 pregnancies in the 265 patients. There was no difference in the rates of fetal wastage, malformations, twin pregnancies, and neonatal and infantile deaths than the normal population. Cytogenetic study of the peripheral lymphocytes of 94 of the children revealed no increase of chromosomal aberrations. Long-term follow-up of the mothers also revealed no increase in the rate of recurrence of gestational trophoblastic disease.

In several studies, the incidence of spontaneous abortions has been reported higher in patients prior to and after gestational trophoblastic disease indicating that gestational trophoblastic disease may be a part of a spectrum of abnormal reproductive performance. Patients who develop spontaneous abortions and molar pregnancies may be caused by chromosomal disorders which sometimes led to a halt in development as in a spontaneous abortion and other times to abnormal development as in gestational trophoblastic disease (109,112, 113).

Cytotoxic drugs can be teratogenic when given during pregnancy, but studies of women treated for gestational trophoblastic tumors suggest that they do not have a deleterious effect on later conceptions (114). It has been suggested to delay conception for a year from cessation of chemotherapy to allow elimination of damaged ova from exposure to cytotoxic agents (107). In addition, methotrexate has been shown to be retained in mammalian tissues for up to 8 months (115).

The only remarkable obstetrical complication noted in gestational trophoblastic patients is an increased risk of placenta accreta (placenta which has invaded the uterine musculature.) Van Thiel et al. (116) reviewed 90 pregnancies in 51 women treated for gestational trophoblastic disease and found 4 patients with partial placenta accreta complicating the pregnancies which was higher than the reported incidence in the general population. All four of their patients also had at least one other risk factor for placenta accreta like hysterotomy and curettage. Song et al. (109) discovered eight cases of placenta accreta out of 303 deliveries. The adherent placenta may be due to destruction of the endometrium by trophoblastic disease and curettage.

Chemotherapeutic agents are known carcinogens and have been known to cause other malignancies after curing a cancer. However, there have been no reports of increased incidence of secondary malignancies after being treated for gestational trophoblastic neoplasms. Rustin et al. (117) reviewed 457 long-term survivors treated for choriocarcinoma or invasive mole between 1958 and 1978. All but two patients received methotrexate and 57% received other cytotoxic drugs. After a mean period of 7.8 years since beginning treatment, only two neoplasms developed: acute leukemia in one and breast cancer in the other. This was less than the expected 3.5 cases for this group.

A patient who has had a molar pregnancy is at an increased risk of developing repeat trophoblastic disease in subsequent conceptions. The incidence of repeat gestational trophoblastic disease has been reported to occur in 0.6 to 2.6% of patients (118). Patients who do develop repeat molar pregnancies with subsequent gestations are at an increased risk of having persistent trophoblastic disease with their subsequent molar pregnancies (119,120). Sand et al. (118) reviewed 22 patients with repetitive gestational trophoblastic disease. After two gestational trophoblastic disease episodes, 72% of patients conceived and 44% delivered normal viable infants. However, 28% went on to have a third trophoblastic disease episode.

Evaluation for gestational trophoblastic disease should be performed when irregular bleeding or suggestions of metastatic tumor occurs in the adolescent of reproductive age. β-hCG testing and ultrasound examination are essential techniques for obtaining an early diagnosis, that can be critical for survival.

REFERENCES

1. Huffman JW. Tumors of the uterus, uterine tubes, and broad ligaments. In: *The gynecology of childhood and adolescence*. Philadelphia: W.B. Saunders, 1981;260–76.
2. Koh KS, Blajer S, Vadas G. Adenocarcinoma of the endometrium in a teenager. *CMA J* 1975;112:980–1.
3. Carlson JA. Gynecologic neoplasms. In: Lavery JP, Sanfilippo JS, eds. *Pediatric and adolescent obstetrics and gynecology*. New York: Springer-Verlag, 1985;124–48.
4. Jafari K, Javaheri G, Ruiz G. Endometrial adenocarcinoma and the Stein-Leventhal syndrome. *Obstet Gynecol* 1978;51:97–100.
5. Huang SJ, Amparo EG, Fu YS. Endometrial hyperplasia: histologic clarification and behavior. *Surg Pathol* 1988;1:215–29.
6. Kurman RJ, Kaminski RP, Norris HJ. The behavior of endometrial hyperplasia-A long-term study of "untreated" hyperplasia in 170 patients. *Cancer* 1985;56:403–12.
7. Speroff L, Glass RH, Kase NG. Anovulation. In: *Clinical gynecologic endocrinology and infertility*. 4th ed. Baltimore: Williams and Wilkins, 1989;213–31.
8. Wiscot AL, Neimand KM, Rosenthal AH. Symptomatic myoma in a 13-year-old girl. *Am J Obstet Gynecol* 1969;105:639–41.
9. Augensen K. Uterine myoma in a 15-year-old girl. *Acta Obstet Gynecol Scand* 1981;60:591.
10. Farber M, Stein A, Adashi E. Rokitansky-Kuster-Hauser syndrome and leiomyoma uteri. *Obstet Gynecol* 1977;51:70s–3s.
11. Chumas JC, Mann WJ, Tseng L. Malignant mixed mullerian tumor of the endometrium in a young woman with polycystic ovaries. *Cancer* 1983;52:1478–81.
12. Amr SS, Tavassoli FA, Hassan AA, Issa AA, Madanat FF. Mixed mesodermal tumor of the uterus in a 4-year-old girl. *Int J Gynecol Pathol* 1986;5:371–8.
13. Craig JK. Inversion of the uterus associated with a malignant tumor in a girl of 14 years of age. *J Obstet Gynaecol Br Comm* 1958;65:497–9.
14. Geoffray A, Covanet D, Montagne JP, Leclere J, Flamant F. Ultrasonography and computed tomography for diagnosis and followup of pelvic rhabdomyosarcomas in children. *Pediatr Radiol* 1987;17:132–6.
15. Hays DM, Shimada H, Raney RB, et al. Clinical staging and treatment results in rhabdomyosarcoma of the female genital tract among children and adolescents. *Cancer* 1988;61:1893–903.
16. Young RH, Kleinman GM, Scully RE. Glioma of the uterus. Report of a case with comments on histogenesis. *Am J Surg Pathol* 1981;695–9.
17. Rose PG, O'Toole RV, Keyhani-Rofagha S, Qualman S, Boutselis JG. Malignant peripheral primitive neuroectodermal tumor of the uterus. *J Surg Oncol* 1987;35:165–9.
18. Ehrmann RL, Griffiths CT. Malignant hemangioendothelioma of the uterus. *Gynecol Oncol* 1979;8:376–83.
19. Egwuatu VE. Non-Hodgkin's lymphoma of the uterus in a child. *J Pediatr Surg* 1989;24:220–2.
20. Bittencourt AL, Britto JF, Fonseca LE. Wilms' tumor of the uterus: the first report of the literature. *Cancer* 1981;47:2496–9.
21. Wakely PE, Sprague RI, Kornstein MJ. Extrarenal Wilms' tumor: an analysis of four cases. *Hum Pathol* 1989;20:691–5.
22. Henshaw SK, Kenney AM, Somberg D, Van Vort J. *Teenage pregnancy in the United States. The scope of the problem and state responses*. New York: Alan Guttmacher Institute. 1989:7–43.
23. *Gestational trophoblastic disease: World Health Organization Technical Report Series 692*. Geneva: WHO, 1983.
24. Grimes DA. Epidemiology of gestational trophoblastic disease. *Am J Obstet Gynecol* 1984;150:309–18.
25. Hayashi K, Braken MB, Freeman DH, Hellenbrand K. Hydatidiform mole in the United States (1970–1977): a statistical and theoretical analysis. *Am J Epidemiol* 1982;115:67–77.
26. Stone M, Bagshawe KD. An analysis of the influences of maternal age, gestational age, contraception method, and the mode of primary treatment of patients with hydatidiform moles on the incidence of subsequent chemotherapy. *Br J Obstet Gynaecol* 1979;86:782–92.
27. Teoh ES, Dawood MY, Ratnam SS. Epidemiology of hydatidiform mole in Singapore. *Am J Obstet Gynecol* 1971;110:415–20.
28. Bandy LC, Clarke-Pearson DL, Hammond CB. Malignant potential of gestational trophoblastic disease at the extreme ages of reproductive life. *Obstet Gynecol* 1984;64:395–9.
29. Slocumb JC, Lund CJ. Incidence of trophoblastic disease: increased rate in youngest age group. *Am J Obstet Gynecol* 1969;104:421–3.

30. Curry SL, Hammond CB, Tyrey L, Creasman WT, Parker R. Hydatidiform mole: diagnosis, management and long-term follow-up of 347 patients. *Obstet Gynecol* 1975;45:1–8.
31. Franke HR, Risse KJ, Kenemans P, Vooijs GP, Stolk JG. Epidemiologic features of hydatidiform mole in the Netherlands. *Obstet Gynecol* 1983;62:613–6.
32. Marquez-Monter H, de la Vega GA, Robles M, Bolio-Cicero A. Epidemiology and pathology of hydatidiform mole in the General Hospital of Mexico. *Am J Obstet Gynecol* 1963;85:856–64.
33. Vassilakos P, Riotton G, Kajii T. Hydatidiform mole: two entities. A morphologic and cytogenetic study with some clinical considerations. *Am J Obstet Gynecol* 1977;127:167–70.
34. Szulman AE, Surti U. The syndromes of hydatidiform mole. I. Cytogenetic and morphologic correlations. *Am J Obstet Gynecol* 1978; 131:665–71.
35. Kajii T, Ohama K. Androgenetic origin of hydatidiform mole. *Nature* 1977;268:633–4.
36. Szulman AE, Surti U. The syndromes of hydatidiform mole. II. Morphologic evolution of the complete and partial mole. *Am J Obstet Gynecol* 1978;132:20–7.
37. Jacobs PA, Wilson CM, Sprenkle JA, Rosenshein NB, Migeon BR. Mechanism of origin of complete hydatidiform moles. *Nature* 1980; 286:714–6.
38. Jacobs PA, Hunt PA, Matsuura JS, Wilson CC. Complete and partial hydatidiform mole in Hawaii: cytogenetics, morphology and epidemiology. *Br J Obstet Gynaecol* 1982;89:258–66.
39. Lurain JR, Brewer JI, Torok EE, Halpern B. Natural history of hydatidiform mole after primary evacuation. *Am J Obstet Gynecol* 1983; 145:591–5.
40. Czernobilsky B, Barash A, Lancet M. Partial moles: a clinicopathologic study of 25 cases. *Obstet Gynecol* 1982;59:75–7.
41. Stone M, Bagshawe KD. Hydatidiform mole: two entities. *Lancet* 1976;1:535–6.
42. Szulman AE, Surti U. The clinicopathologic profile of the partial hydatidiform mole. *Obstet Gynecol* 1982;59:597–602.
43. Rice LW, Berkowitz RS, Lage JM, Goldstein DP, Bernstein MR. Persistent gestational trophoblastic tumor after partial hydatidiform mole. *Gynecol Oncol* 1990;36:358–62.
44. Elston CW, Bagshawe KD. The diagnosis of trophoblastic tumours from uterine curettings. *J Clin Pathol* 1972;25:111–8.
45. Mazur MT, Kurman RJ. Choriocarcinoma and placental site trophoblastic tumor. In: Szulman AE, Buchsbaum HJ, eds. *Gestational trophoblastic disease*. New York: Springer-Verlag, 1987;45–68.
46. Bagshawe KD. Risk and prognostic factors in trophoblastic neoplasia. *Cancer* 1976;38: 1373–85.
47. Tsukamoto N, Kashimura Y, Sano M, et al. Choriocarcinoma occurring within the normal placenta with breast metastasis. *Gynecol Oncol* 1981;11:348–63.
48. Guvener S, Kazancigil A, Erez S. Long latent development of trophoblastic disease. *Am J Obstet Gynecol* 1972;114:679–84.
49. Lathrop J, Wachtel TJ, Meissner GF. Uterine choriocarcinoma fourteen years following bilateral tubal ligation. *Obstet Gynecol* 1978; 51:477–82.
50. Aranda JM, Martinez I. Choriocarcinoma in Puerto Rico. *Bol Asoc Med PR* 1968;60:523–35.
51. Teoh ES, Dawood MY, Ratnam SS. Observations on choriocarcinoma in Singapore. *Obstet Gynecol* 1972;40:519–24.
52. Ringertz N. Hydatidiform mole, invasive mole and choriocarcinoma in Sweden 1958–1965. *Acta Obstet Gynecol Scand* 1970;49:195–203.
53. Rolan PA, de Lopez BH. Malignant trophoblastic disease in Paraguay. *J Reprod Med* 1979; 23:94–6.
54. Mazur MT, Lurain JR, Brewer JI. Fatal gestational choriocarcinoma. Clinicopathologic study of patients treated at a trophoblastic disease center. *Cancer* 1982;50:1833–46.
55. Libshitz HI, Baber CE, Hammond CB. The pulmonary metastases of choriocarcinoma. *Obstet Gynecol* 1977;49:412–6.
56. Kumar J, Ilancheran A, Ratnam SS. Pulmonary metastasis in gestational trophoblastic disease: a review of 97 cases. *Br J Obstet Gynecol* 1988;95:70–4.
57. Kelly MP, Rustin GJS, Ivory C, Phillips P, Bagshawe KD. Respiratory failure due to choriocarcinoma: a study of 103 dyspneic patients. *Gynecol Oncol* 1990;38:149–54.
58. Nisula BC, Taliadouros GS. Thyroid function in gestational trophoblastic neoplasia: evidence that the thyrotropic activity of chorionic gonadotropin mediates the thyrotoxicosis of choriocarcinoma. *Am J Obstet Gynecol* 1980; 138:77–85.
59. Miller SM, Lurain JR. Classification and staging of gestational trophoblastic tumor. *Obstet Gynecol North Am* 1988;15:477–90.
60. Hammond CB, Borchert LG, Trey L, Creasman WT, Parker RT. Treatment of metastatic trophoblastic disease: Good and poor prognosis. *Am J Obstet Gynecol* 1973;115: 451–7.
61. Miller DS, Lurain JR. Classification and staging of gestational trophoblastic tumors. *Obstet Gynecol Clin* 1988;15:477–90.
62. Bagshawe KD. Risk and prognostic factors in trophoblastic neoplasia. *Cancer* 1976;38: 1373–85.
63. Bagshawe KD. Treatment of high-risk choriocarcinoma. *J Reprod Med* 1984;29:813–20.
64. Munyer TP, Callen PW, Filly RA, et al. Further observations on the sonographic spectrum of gestational trophoblastic disease. *J Clin Ultrasound* 1981;9:349–58.
65. Hill LM, Buchsbaum, Kanal E. Radiographic techniques in diagnosis and management. In: Szulman AE, Buchsbaum HJ, eds. *Gestational trophoblastic disease*. New York: Springer-Verlag, 1987:101–11.
66. Roberts DK, Wells MM, Horbelt DV. Dysger-

minoma in the differential diagnosis of hydatidiform mole. *Obstet Gynecol* 1986;67:92S–4S.

67. Reid MH, McGahan JP, Oi R. Sonographic evaluation of hydatidiform mole and its look-alikes. *Am J Radiol* 1983;140:307–11.
68. Taylor KJW, Schwartz PE, Kohorn EI. Gestational trophoblastic neoplasia: diagnosis with doppler US. *Radiology* 1987;165:445–8.
69. Goldstein DP, Berkowitz RS, Bernstein MR. Management of molar pregnancy. *J Reprod Med* 1981;26:208–12.
70. Kohorn EI, McGinn RC, Gee BL, et al. Pulmonary embolization of trophoblastic tissue in molar pregnancy. *Obstet Gynecol* 1978;51:16–24.
71. Berkowitz RS, Goldstein DP. Diagnosis and management of the primary hydatidiform mole. *Obstet Gynecol Clin North Am* 1988;15:491–503.
72. McDonald TW, Ruffolo EH. Modern management of gestational trophoblastic disease. *Obstet Gynecol Surv* 1983;38:67–83.
73. Morrow CP, Kletzky OA, DiSaia PJ, Townsend DE, Mishell DR, Nakamura RM. Clinical and laboratory correlates of molar pregnancy and trophoblastic disease. *Am J Obstet Gynecol* 1977;128:424–30.
74. Goldstein DP. The chemotherapy of gestational trophoblastic disease: principles of clinical management. *JAMA* 1972;220:209–13.
75. Stone M, Dent J, Kardana A, Bagshawe KD. Relationship of oral contraception to development of trophoblastic tumor after evacuation of a hydatidiform mole. *Br J Obstet Gynaecol* 1976;83:913–6.
76. Berkowitz RS, Goldstein DP, Marean AR, Bernstein M. Oral contraceptives and postmolar trophoblastic disease. *Obstet Gynecol* 1981;58:474–7.
77. Morrow P, Nakamura R, Schlaerth J, Gaddis O, Eddy G. The influence of oral contraceptives on the postmolar human chorionic gonadotropin curve. *Am J Obstet Gynecol* 1985;151:906–14.
78. Franke HR, Risse EKJ, Kaneman SP, Houx PCW, Stolk JG, Voijs GP. Plasma human chorionic gonadotropin disappearance in hydatidiform mole: a central registry from the Netherlands. *Obstet Gynecol* 1983;62:467–73.
79. Goldstein DP. Prevention of gestational trophoblastic disease by use of actinomycin D in molar pregnancies. *Obstet Gynecol* 1974;43:475–9.
80. Fascoli M, Ratti E, Franceschi S, La Vecchia C, Pecorelli S, Mangioni C. Management of gestational trophoblastic disease: Results of a cooperative study. *Obstet Gynecol* 1982;60:205–9.
81. Kashimura Y, Kashimura M, Sugimori H, et al. Prophylactic chemotherapy of hydatidiform mole. Five to 15 years follow-up. *Cancer* 1986;58:624–9.
82. Ayhan A, Ergeneli MH, Yuce K, Yapar EG, Kisnisci AH. Effects of prophylactic chemotherapy for postmolar trophoblastic disease in patients with complete hydatidiform mole. *Int J Gynecol Obstet* 1990;32:39–41.
83. Kim DS, Moon H, Kim KT, Moon YJ, Hwang YY. Effects of prophylactic chemotherapy for persistent trophoblastic disease in patients with complete hydatidiform mole. *Obstet Gynecol* 1986;67:690–4.
84. Lurain JR, Brewer JI, Torok EE, Halpern B. Gestational trophoblastic disease. Treatment results at the Brewer Trophoblastic Disease Center. *Obstet Gynecol* 1982;60:354–60.
85. Smith EB, Weed JC, Tyrey L, et al. Treatment of nonmetastatic gestational trophoblastic disease: results of methotrexate alone versus methotrexate-folinic acid. *Am J Obstet Gynecol* 1982;144:88–92.
86. Rotmensch J, Rosenshein N, Donehower R, Dillon M, Villar J. Plasma methotrexate levels in patients with gestational trophoblastic neoplasia treated by two methotrexate regimens. *Am J Obstet Gynecol* 1984;148:730–4.
87. Bleyer WA. The clinical pharmacology of methotrexate. New application of an old drug. *Cancer* 1978;41:36–51.
88. Rustin GJS, Bagshawe KD. Gestational trophoblastic tumors. *CRC Crit Rev Oncol Haematol* 1984;3:103–42.
89. Lurain JR. Chemotherapy of gestational trophoblastic disease. In: Deppe G, ed. *Chemotherapy of gynecologic cancer.* 2nd ed. New York: Wiley-Liss, 1990;273–301.
90. Hammond CB, Hertz R, Ross GT, Lipsett MB, Odell WD. Primary chemotherapy for nonmetastatic gestational trophoblastic neoplasms. *Am J Obstet Gynecol* 1967;98:71–8.
91. Hammond CB, Weed JC, Currie JL. The role of operation in the current therapy of gestational trophoblastic disease. *Am J Obstet Gynecol* 1980;136:844–58.
92. Goldstein DP, Berkowitz RS. Nonmetastatic and low-risk metastatic gestational trophoblastic neoplasms. *Semin Oncol* 1982;9:191–7.
93. Wilson RB, Beecham CT, Symmonds RE. Conservative surgical management of chorioadenoma destruens. *Obstet Gynecol* 1965;26:814–20.
94. Maroulis GB, Hammond CB, Johnsrude IS, Weed JC, Parker RT. Arteriography and infusional chemotherapy in localized trophoblastic disease. *Obstet Gynecol* 1975;45:397–406.
95. Lurain JR, Brewer JI. Treatment of high-risk gestational trophoblastic disease with methotrexate, actinomycin D, and cyclophosphamide chemotherapy. *Obstet Gynecol* 1985;65:830–6.
96. DuBeshter B, Berkowitz RS, Goldstein DP, Cramer DW, Bernstein MR. Metastatic gestational trophoblastic disease: Experience at the New England Trophoblastic Disease Center, 1965 to 1985. *Obstet Gynecol* 1987;69:390–5.
97. Weed JC, Hammond CB. Cerebral metastatic choriocarcinoma: intensive therapy and prognosis. *Obstet Gynecol* 1980;55:89–94.
98. Athanassiou A, Begent RHJ, Newlands ES, Parker D, Rustin GJS, Bagshawe KD. Central nervous system metastases of choriocarci-

noma: 23 years' experience at Charing Cross Hospital Center. *Cancer* 1983;52:1728–35.

99. Surwit EA, Hammond CB. Treatment of metastatic trophoblastic disease with poor prognosis. *Obstet Gynecol* 1980;55:565–70.
100. Grumbine FC, Rosenshein NB, Brereton HD, Kaufman SL. Management of liver metastases from gestational trophoblastic neoplasia. *Am J Obstet Gynecol* 1980;137:959–61.
101. Gordon AN, Kavanagh JJ, Gershenson DM, Saul PB, Copeland LJ, Stringer CA. Cisplatin, vinblastine, and bleomycin combination therapy in resistant gestational trophoblastic disease. *Cancer* 1986;58:1407–10.
102. Newlands ES, Bagshawe KD. Activity of high-dose cisplatinum in combination with vincristine and methotrexate in drug-resistant gestational choriocarcinoma. *Br J Cancer* 1979; 40:943–5.
103. Newlands ES. New chemotherapeutic agents in the management of gestational trophoblastic disease. *Semin Oncol* 1982;9:239–43.
104. Damewood MD, Grochow LB. Prospects for fertility after chemotherapy or radiation for neoplastic disease. *Fertil Steril* 1986;45:443–60.
105. Chapman RM, Sutcliffe SB, Malpas JS. Cytotoxic induced ovarian failure in women with Hodgkin's disease: hormone function. *JAMA* 1979;242:1877–81.
106. Schilsky RL, Lewis BJ, Sherring RJ, Young RC. Gonadal dysfunction in patients receiving chemotherapy for cancer. *Ann Intern Med* 1980;93:109–14.
107. Walden PAM, Bagshawe KD. Pregnancies after chemotherapy for gestational trophoblastic tumors. *Lancet* 1979;2:1241.
108. Song H, Wu P, Wang Y, Yang X, Dong S. Pregnancy outcomes after successful chemotherapy for choriocarcinoma and invasive mole: Long-term follow-up. *Am J Obstet Gynecol* 1988; 158:538–45.
109. Pastorfide GB, Goldstein DP. Pregnancy after hydatidiform mole. *Obstet Gynecol* 1973; 42:67–70.
110. Van Thiel DH, Ross GT, Lipsett MD. Pregnancies after chemotherapy of trophoblastic neoplasms. *Science* 1970;169:1326–7.
111. Rustin GJS, Booth M, Dent J, Salt S, Rustin F, Bagshawe KD. Pregnancy after cytotoxic chemotherapy for gestational trophoblastic tumours. *Br Med J* 1984;288:103–6.
112. Meizner I, Leiberman JR, Insler V. Risk factors for gestational trophoblastic neoplasia. *Am J Obstet Gynecol* 1986;155:456–7.
113. Messerli ML, Lilienfeld AM, Parmley T, Woodruff JD, Rosenshein NB. Risk factors for gestational trophoblastic neoplasia. *Am J Obstet Gynecol* 1985;153:294–300.
114. Ross GT. Congenital anomalies among children born of mothers receiving chemotherapy for gestational trophoblastic neoplasms. *Cancer* 1976;37:1043–7.
115. Charache S, Condit PT, Humphreys SR. Studies on the folic acid vitamins. IV. The persistence amethopterin in mammalian tissues. *Cancer* 1960;13:236–40.
116. Van Thiel DH, Grodin JM, Ross GT, Lipsett MB. Partial placenta accreta in pregnancies following chemotherapy for gestational trophoblastic neoplasms. *Am J Obstet Gynecol* 1972;112:54–8.
117. Rustin GJS, Rustin F, Dent J, Booth M, Salt S, Bagshawe KD. No increase in second tumors after cytotoxic chemotherapy for gestational trophoblastic tumors. *N Engl J Med* 1983; 308:473–6.
118. Sand PK, Lurain JR, Brewer JI. Repeat gestational trophoblastic disease. *Obstet Gynecol* 1984;63:140–4.
119. Parazzini F, Mangili G, Belloni C, LaVecchia C, Liati P, Marabini R. The problem of identification of prognostic factors for persistent trophoblastic disease. *Gynecol Oncol* 1988;30:57–62.
120. Rice LW, Lage JM, Berkowitz RS, Goldstein DP, Bernstein MR. Repetitive complete and partial hydatidiform mole. *Obstet Gynecol* 1989;74:217–9.

Pediatric and Adolescent Gynecology,
edited by S. E. Carpenter and J. A. Rock.
Raven Press, Ltd., New York © 1992.

26

Benign and Malignant Tumors of the Ovary

*,†Ira R. Horowitz and †Ricardo Sainz de la Cuesta

**Departments of Gynecology and Obstetrics, and Oncology, The Johns Hopkins University School of Medicine; and †Department of Gynecologic Oncology, The Union Memorial Hospital, Baltimore, Maryland 21218*

The evaluation and treatment of a pelvic mass at any age is a traumatic experience. Tumors in childhood and adolescence, although infrequent, are especially devastating to young patients and their families.

Ovarian cancer is the second most common malignancy for women over the age of 35. Druing the first three decades of life, ovarian neoplasms are rare, with less than 5% of ovarian malignancies occurring in children and adolescents.

Ovarian tumors in childhood and adolescent females account for approximately 1% of all tumors for these age groups and 3% of all ovarian neoplasm (1). Sixty-five percent of all ovarian tumors are benign, and the remaining 35% have malignant features (Table 1). A review by Breen and Mayson (3) of 1,002 ovarian neoplasms in patients under 20 years of age revealed that germ cell tumors constituted 67.2% of all ovarian neoplasms.

FUNCTIONAL CYSTS

Functional cysts are the most frequent cysts present in the human ovary. They can

TABLE 1. *Ovarian tumors in patients under 20 years of age*

	Tintera, 1990 (2)		Norris-Jensen, 1972 (73)		Junaid, 1981 (74)	
	n	%	n	%	n	%
Germ cell	28	59.6	205	58	51	30.2 (67.1)
Mature teratoma	11		71		38	
Malignant teratoma	2		28		4	
Dysgerminoma	2		48		7	
Endodermal sinus tumor	8		32		2	
Mixed or Choriocarcinoma	5		26		0	
Epithelial	18	38.3	67	19	8	4.7 (10.5)
Cystadenoma and adenofibroma	14		59		4	
Borderline	3		5		1	
Cystadenocarcinoma	1		3		3	
Sex cord stromal	1	2.1	62	18	13	7.7 (17.1)
Fibrothecoma	0		23		4	
Androblastoma	1		14		2	
Grannulosa cell tumor	0		12		6	
Nonspecific	0		13		1	
Miscellaneous	0	0	19	5	97	57.4 (5.3)
Lymphoma	0		2		93	
Other	0		17		4	
Total	47	100	353	100	169	100 (100)

Numbers in parentheses represent percentage relative to 76 nonlymphoma tumors.
Modified from ref. 2.

present as follicular, corpus luteum, and theca lutein cysts. All are benign and usually self-limited.

The diameter of these cysts can range up to 8 cm. These cysts usually occur secondary to an abnormality in gonadotropin production and resolve in 4–8 weeks. The majority of follicular cysts are an incidental finding on physical examination; however, large cysts may rupture and cause a transient peritonitis. Although peritoneal signs and symptoms are present, they usually resolve in 24 hr. It is imperative that other causes of peritonitis such as pelvic infections, appendicitis, ruptured ectopic pregnancy, and hemorrhagic cysts be ruled out prior to following a plan of observation. A laparoscopic evaluation should be performed if the etiology of peritonitis is uncertain.

Corpus Luteum Cysts

Corpus luteum cysts, although less common than follicular cysts, are persistently functioning corpora lutea. Corpora lutea are considered corpus luteum cysts when their diameter is more than 3 cm. Corpus lutea have normal endocrine function and may express a prolonged progesterone secretion. Haldan (4) described a classic triad of persistently functioning corpus luteum cysts, which includes a normal menses followed by spotting, unilateral pelvic pain, and a slightly enlarged tender adnexal mass

TABLE 2. *Clinical features (173 patients)*

	n	%
Age (range, 12–52 yr)		
$>$40 years	17	10
$<$20 years	20	12
Parity		
Nulliparous	66	38
Multiparous	92	53
Unknown	15	9
Prior ovarian cyst operation	9	5
Using intrauterine contraceptive device	19	11
Ovulation induced by clomiphene citrate	2	1.15

From ref. 6.

TABLE 3. *Clinical features (173 patients)*

	n	%
Location		
Right ovary	114	66
Left ovary	56	32
Unknown	3	2
Abdominal pain	173	100
Onset with intercourse	29	17
Right ovary	21	72
Left ovary	8	28
Duration		
Less than 24 hr	94	54
1–7 days	40	23
Over 7 days	14	8
Unknown	25	15
Nausea or vomiting or diarrhea	60	35

From ref. 6.

(5). The spontaneous rupture and hemorrhage of these cysts may result in a hemoperitoneum requiring operative intervention to control bleeding. Patients on anticoagulation therapy, such as coumarin or heparin, are at greater risk of a hemorrhagic corpus luteum and as such are frequently treated with oral contraceptives to suppress ovulation. Hallatt et al. (6) reported the most common symptoms identified in 173 patients who required surgical intervention (Tables 2 and 3).

Treatment

The treatments for functional cysts and corpus luteum cysts are essentially the same. These cysts, if left alone, usually will resolve in 4–8 weeks. Spanos (7) has reported 80% resolution of cysts 4–6 cm in patients taking oral contraceptives to suppress ovulation. Grimes and Hughes (8) estimated the rate of hospitalization as 472–522 per 100,000 women for functional ovarian cysts, aged 15–44, while using multiphasic oral contraceptives between 1979 and 1986 (Fig. 1). Alternative therapies include oral or intramuscular progesterone.

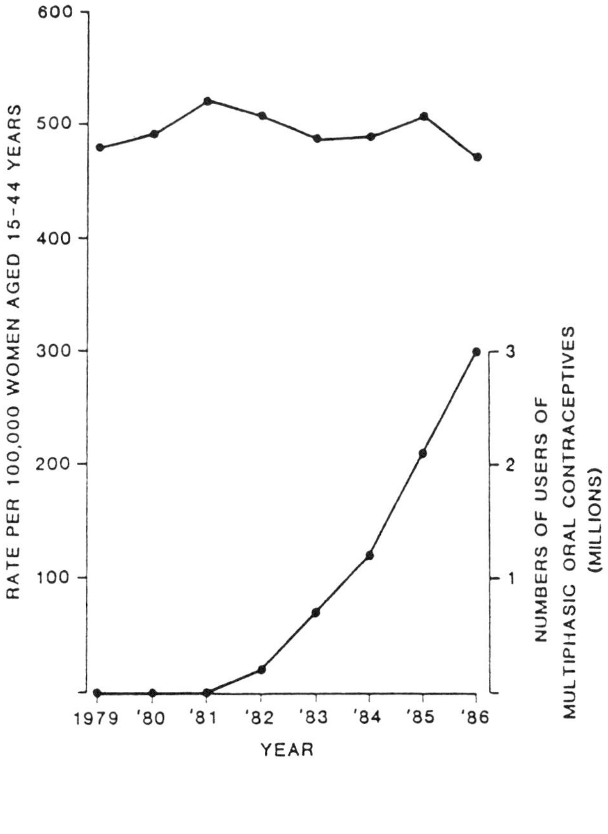

FIG. 1. Rates per 100,000 women of hospitalization for functional ovarian cysts among women aged 15–44 years and use of multiphasic oral contraceptives, United States, 1979–1986. (From ref. 8, with permission.)

Cysts persisting for more than 4–8 weeks require operative intervention. Simple follicular cysts can be drained or excised using operative endoscopy if no evidence suggesting a malignant neoplasm is present. Patients with a ruptured corpus luteal cyst usually present with severe abdominal pain. The differential diagnosis includes a ruptured ectopic pregnancy, endometrioma, adnexal torsion, hemorrhage, a ruptured spleen, or perforated abdominal viscus. A culdocentesis will only assess for the presence of nonclotting blood. A serum pregnancy test for human chorionic gonadotropin (HCG) should be obtained in all patients with this presentation. If the hematocrit continues to drift downward, a laparoscopy is indicated to make a diagnosis, and if bleeding cannot be controlled, an exploratory laparotomy is imperative. Conservative therapy is advocated in the form of a cystectomy and/or cauterization of the bleeding vessels. This is a benign condition and usually does not require an oophorectomy to obtain hemostasis.

Theca Lutein Cysts

Theca lutein cysts are the least common of the functional ovarian cysts and are usually bilateral. Approximately 50% of molar pregnancies and 10% of choriocarcinomas have theca lutein cysts present (5). Multiple gestations, diabetes, and Rh sensitization can result in increased stimulation in the presence of thecal luteum cysts. Clomiphene citrate, GnRH analogs, human menopausal gonadotropins (HMG), and HCG frequently result in overstimulation of the ovaries and the presence of theca lutein cysts. Thecal luteum cysts are frequently large and may be as great as 30 cm in diameter. These multicystic ovaries result in masculinization of the female fetus in approximately 30% of cases.

Treatment

Theca lutein cysts regress spontaneously and do not require operative intervention. If the cysts should persist or result in torsion, an exploratory laparatomy and resection of the involved cyst or adnexa is suggested. In the presence of an intrauterine pregnancy during the first trimester, consultation with a perinatologist should be obtained for possible treatment with progesterone.

Although benign, functional cysts may persist and result in torsion, requiring operative intervention and a possible adnexectomy.

BENIGN TUMORS AND BENIGN NEOPLASMS

Endometriosis

Although most frequent in the third and fourth decade of life, endometriosis can be present in childhood and adolescent females. A thorough discussion of endometriosis can be found in the chapter by Hesla (this volume).

There are several proposed mechanisms for the etiology of endometriosis, which includes retrograde menstruation, coelomic metaplasia, lymphatic and vascular metastasis, immunologic deficiencies, and genetic predisposition. Endometriosis is most frequently found in menstruating women. It can present itself as small implants on the peritoneal surface of the ovaries as well as large endometriomas measuring several centimeters. The classic symptoms include severe dysmenorrhea and infertility. Occasionally patients may present with an adnexal mass, which upon evaluation reveals diffuse endometriosis and a large ovarian endometrioma. This entity is benign and can be treated as described in the chapter by Hesla (this volume).

Mature Cystic Teratomas

Benign ovarian teratomas are the most commonly found ovarian tumor, accounting for approximately 11% of all ovarian neoplasms (9,10). The median age of occurrence is 30 years of age, with a range of 2–88 years of age (9).

Macroscopic

The mature cystic teratoma (dermoid cyst) develops from totipotential cells and is composed of well differentiated ectodermal, endodermal and mesodermal elements. This teratoma is bilateral in 7.9–15% of patients. In gross appearance, the tumor can be round, oval, or globular with a smooth surface and measure less than 1 cm to greater than 30 cm in diameter. Cross-section reveals bone, hair, nerve tissue, sebaceous material, and fully developed teeth representing the three germ cell layers. Skin, hair, and sebaceous material are present in the majority of cystic teratomas excised.

Microscopic

Microscopic layers of the cyst are composed of ovarian stroma forming an outer wall and a cavity lined with squamous epithelium containing abundant sebaceous and sweat glands (apocrine and eccrine glands). The various germ cell layers can be readily identified.

Treatment

These tumors are benign; however, their large size predisposes them to undergo torsion and/or rupture, which can result in acute peritonitis. Malignant transformation occurs in 1–3% of benign teratomas. Squamous cell carcinoma rising from the ectodermal layers accounts for 80% of the malignant transformations (11). Adenocarcinomas and melanomas are extremely rare (11–13).

An abdominal x-ray frequently reveals a soft tissue mass with a calcification resembling a tooth. Additional studies, such as CAT scans or MRI, can identify both the calcification and the fat content of dermoid cysts. The treatment of choice for benign cystic teratomas is ovarian cystectomy. Technology is available to perform this procedure with operative endoscopy in the patients with small lesions. Large lesions without normal ovarian stroma identified should be removed through an exploratory laparotomy; oophorectomy or cystectomy can be performed to avoid rupture and spill of the mucin contents. Recurrence followed conservative treatment is less than 1% (14). The contralateral ovary should always be evaluated to rule out the possibility of bilateral lesions. The presence of mature unilateral cystic teratomas does not necessitate a wedge resection or bivalving the contralateral ovary.

Functional Teratomas

The presence of thyroid tissue in a benign cystic teratoma occurs in 5–20% of benign teratomas (15–18). A diagnosis of stroma ovarii is made only when the majority of the solid component is composed of thyroid tissue. Thyrotoxicosis has been associated with struma ovarii (19–21). The diagnosis of struma ovarii is made upon excision of the pelvic mass and microscopic evaluation. Most of these lesions are benign, and excision of the thyroid tissue is usually adequate.

Carcinoid tumors can be present in benign cystic teratomas. Although an ovarian carcinoid secondary to gastrointestinal metastasis may be present, these lesions are usually bilateral as compared to unilateral carcinoids present in mature cystic teratomas. Unlike metastatic carcinoids of the ovaries, ovarian carcinoids frequently present with the classic carcinoid syndrome of flushes, diarrhea, cardiac valvular lesion, or bronchial constriction (22).

Treatment

Treatment consists of excision of the ovarian lesion.

SEX CORD TUMORS

Thecomas

Thecomas are rare before puberty and uncommon before the age of 30. These tumors are frequently associated with estrogen production and present in the perimenopausal and menopausal years.

Fibromas

Fibromas account for 4% of all ovarian tumors (5,23). Less than 10% of fibromas are encountered in patients under the age of 30. These tumors comprise approximately 0.5–2% of all ovarian tumors found in infancy and childhood (24–26). Forty percent of patients with fibromas greater than 10 cm present with intraperitoneal ascites (27). Patients with ovarian fibromas may present with Mieg's triad, which includes ascites, pleural effusion, and a fibrous ovarian tumor.

Microscopic

Microscopically fibromas are composed of intersecting bundles of spindle cells that produce collagen. Mitotic figures of one to three per high power field can be present and still be considered a benign neoplasm.

Treatment

In the young adolescent female, resecting the fibroma is recommended.

Gonadoblastomas

Originally described by Scully (28), these tumors consist of a germ cell and sex cord stromal element. These gonads act as a source for germ cell tumors, including dysgerminoma and extraembryonal cell tumors. The patients with gonadoblastomas frequently have a Y chromosome in their karyotype. Patients with gonadal dysgenesis and Y chromosomes are at markedly increased risk for the development of a gonadoblastoma and/or malignant germ cell tumor. This is an uncommon tumor, occurring predominantly in young patients under the age of 30 (29). The patients are usually phenotypic females in a ratio of 4:1 (15–18). Their presentation includes primary amenorrhea, virilization, and/or developmental abnormalities. Thirty-eight percent of the lesions are bilateral.

Microscopic

Microscopically, tubules with unencapsulated germ cells and calcified bodies are present. Coexistence with other germ cell components is common (15–18).

Macroscopic

Gonadoblastomas can present in size as a microscopic tumor removed in patients with gonadal dysgenesis to 8 cm masses (12,13).

Treatment

Treatment for patients with gonadoblastomas includes exploratory laparotomy and bilateral excision of gonads. Regardless of whether or not the lesions are bilateral, the gonads in these patients should be removed. The prognosis is excellent in patients who have gonadectomies. Frequently, a germ cell tumor, such as a dysgerminoma, will be present. These patients, as well as those with an endodermal sinus tumor, or immature teratoma, should be treated as outlined in the following sections on germ cell tumors.

MALIGNANT OVARIAN NEOPLASMS

The most common malignant ovarian neoplasms in patients under 20 years of age are germ cell carcinomas. Seventy percent of ovarian tumors in this age group are of germ cell origin, with approximately 23% being malignant germ cell tumors. Sixty-six percent of ovarian malignancies in patients under 20 years of age are of germ cell origin (24,30).

Epithelial tumors of the ovary occur in women older than 40 years of age. Epithelial tumors in patients under age 30 tend to be of a low malignant potential (25).

Clinical Features

Signs and Symptoms

It is difficult to identify abnormal adnexal pathology in the premenarcheal female. Complaints of urinary frequency, dysuria, rectal discomfort, and abdominal fullness with a decrease in appetite are nonspecific and require further evaluation. Although large pelvic masses can be palpated upon abdominal examination, the majority of small lesions require radiologic evaluation and/or an examination under anesthesia. In the menarcheal patient, the above symptoms as well as menstrual irregularities may be present. As with adults, ascites, abdominal distention, and pleural effusion are indications of advanced disease. The presence of a pelvic mass is the most common finding in more than 90% of cases.

Physical Examination

In the menarcheal female, a thorough physical examination should be performed with particular note of sexual development including Tanner stages. Germ cell tumors that produce hormones may result in precocious sexual development. A pelvic examination, including a rectal examination, should be performed to identify any adnexal or pelvic pathology.

In the premenarcheal female, it is frequently difficult to perform such an examination, and various imaging techniques should be initiated.

Radiology

Ultrasound, CAT scans, and MRI have all been used to evaluate the pelvic area for ovarian pathology. Ultrasound is the imaging technique of choice secondary to the low cost, minimal complexity, and discomfort to the patient. Imaging techniques afford us an opportunity to identify cystic, solid, and complex components of the adnexal mass. Those masses with complex components have a high probability of being malignant.

CAT scans and MRI technique are superior in evaluating metastatic lesions to the liver, lung, brain, kidney, and lymph nodes compared to ultrasound. When evaluating for pulmonary metastases, a chest x-ray is usually sufficient to identify large lesions. Further evaluation may require a CAT scan.

TUMOR MARKERS

Monoclonal Antibodies

Monoclonal antibodies that react with antigens associated with various malignancies are extremely useful in the differential diagnosis and subsequent follow-up of ovarian cancers. Germ cell tumors secrete marker substances that aid in the diagnosis and subsequent evaluation of successful treatment protocols (Fig. 2).

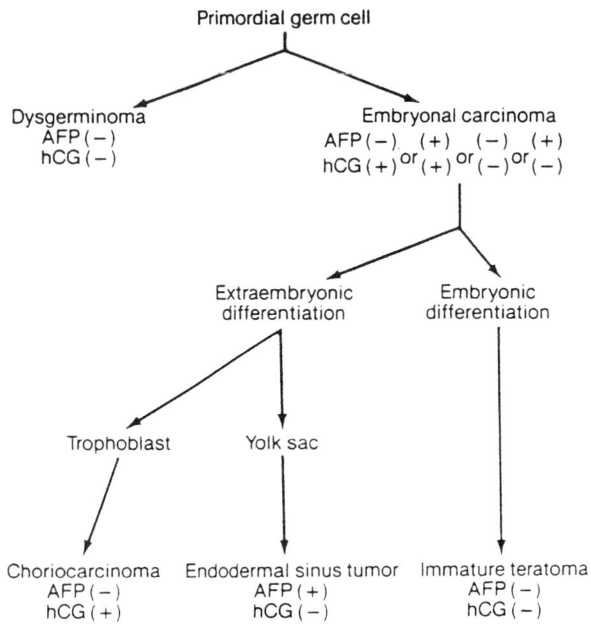

FIG. 2. Relationship between examples of pure malignant germ cell tumors and their secreted marker substances. AFP, alpha-fetoprotein; hCG, human chorionic gonadotropin. (From ref. 31, with permission.)

CA-125

CA-125 was the first widely available monoclonal antibody against epithelial ovarian cancer (32). The specificity of CA-125 is poor, and it may be elevated with a multitude of intraperitoneal processes such as Crohn's disease, pelvic inflammatory disease, endometriosis, pregnancy, and a host of abdominal malignancies. Although this limits its value, the CA-125 level of premenopausal females can be followed after the diagnosis of a malignancy to assist in determining the level of treatment response. Changes in antigen level correlate with treatment response in approximately 90% of patients (33).

Alpha-Fetoprotein

Alpha-fetoprotein (AFP) is an oncofetal antigen, a glycoprotein normally expressed by the fetus and reexpressed by endodermal sinus tumors, mixed germ cell tumors, and immature teratomas. It is a reliable marker with a high sensitivity, which permits diagnosis and treatment evaluation of patients with pure endodermal sinus tumors or tumors with endodermal sinus components. Fewer than 10% of epithelial ovarian carcinomas produce AFP (34).

Human Chorionic Gonadotropin

HCG is produced by trophoblastic cells. It is produced by normal human placental tissue as well as hydatidiform moles, placental site trophoblastic tumors, choriocarcinoma, and embryonal ovarian carcinomas with trophoblastic differentiation. Embryonal carcinomas can produce AFP as previously mentioned.

Carcinoembryonic Antigen

Carcinoembryonic antigen (CEA) has been produced by epithelial and germ cell tumors. CEA may be markedly elevated in colon carcinoma patients and with mucinous carcinomas. In selected situations, it can be an additional marker that assesses clinical response to treatment protocols.

SURGICAL STAGING

Ovarian carcinomas are surgically staged. Surgical staging is classified according to the International Federation of Gynecologists and Obstetricians (FIGO) for primary carcinoma of the ovary (Table 4). A thorough physical examination must be performed. In the premenarcheal female, this may necessitate a twilight or general anesthetic. Prior to surgical intervention, a complete chemistry profile including liver function tests and electrolytes as well as a hemogram should be obtained. Cystoscopic, colonoscopic, and barium enema examinations are performed in those patients where bladder or colon infiltration is suspected. If gross or occult blood is present in the patient's stool, a thorough evaluation of the colon should be performed including a barium enema and/or colonoscopy. A radiologic evaluation with one of the imaging techniques previously described should be obtained prior to surgery.

Intravenous pyelography (IVP) is performed to outline the course of the ureters, their displacement by the pelvic mass, and the presence of a pelvic kidney, abnormal collecting system, or hydronephrosis. Many gynecologic oncologists have replaced this study with a CAT scan using contrast. Although the CAT scan can iden-

TABLE 4. *FIGO staging for carcinoma of the ovary*[a]

Stage	Findings
I	Growth limited to the ovaries
IA	Growth limited to one ovary; no ascites present containing malignant cells. No tumor on the external surface; capsule intact
IB	Growth limited to both ovaries; no ascites present containing malignant cells. No tumor on the external surfaces; capsules intact
IC[b]	Tumor classified as either stage IA or IB but with tumor on the surface of one or both ovaries; or with ruptured capsule(s); or with ascites containing malignant cells present or with positive peritoneal washings
II	Growth involving one or both ovaries, with pelvic extension
IIA	Extension and/or metastases to the uterus and/or tubes
IIB	Extension to other pelvic tissues
IIC[b]	Tumor either stage IIA or IIB but with tumor on the surface of one or both ovaries; or with capsule(s) ruptured; or with ascites containing malignant cells present or with positive peritoneal washings
III	Tumor involving one or both ovaries with peritoneal implants outside the pelvis and/or positive retroperitoneal or inguinal nodes. Superficial liver metastasis equals stage III. Tumor is limited to the true pelvis but with histologically proven malignant extension to small bowel or omentum
IIIA	Tumor grossly limited to the true pelvis with negative nodes but with histologically confirmed microscopic seeding of abdominal peritoneal surfaces
IIIB	Tumor of one or both ovaries with histologically confirmed implants of abdominal peritoneal surfaces none exceeding 2 cm in diameter; nodes are negative
IIIC	Abdominal implants greater than 2 cm in diameter and/or positive retroperitoneal or inguinal nodes
IV	Growth involving one or both ovaries, with distant metastases. If pleural effusion is present, there must be positive cytologic findings to allot a case to stage IV. Parenchymal liver metastasis equals stage IV.

[a]Staging of ovarian carcinoma is based on findings at clinical examination and by surgical exploration. The histologic findings are to be considered in the staging, as are the cytologic findings as far as effusions are concerned. It is desirable that a biopsy be taken from suspicious areas outside of the pelvis.

[b]*Notes about the staging:* To evaluate the impact on prognosis of the different criteria for allotting cases to stage IC or IIC, it would be of value to know whether the rupture of the capsule was spontaneous or caused by the surgeon and if the source of malignant cells detected was peritoneal washings or ascites.

From ref. 35.

tify abnormal collecting systems, hydronephrosis and pelvic kidneys, it does not enable the surgeon to follow the course of the ureter through the pelvis with ease.

Evaluation of neoplasms in childhood and adolescence should include CA-125, AFP, beta HCG, and CEA tumor marker levels.

SURGERY

The temptation to enter the abdomen through a transverse incision is to be avoided. A vertical incision that may be extended in a cephalad direction will enable a thorough evaluation and tumor debulking in the upper abdomen. Upon entering the peritoneal cavity, all ascitic fluid should be aspirated and sent to cytopathology for evaluation. If ascites is not present, abdominal washings from all quadrants should be obtained and sent to cytologic evaluation. A survey of the upper abdomen, including the diaphragm, liver, spleen, colon, pelvic and periaortic lymph nodes, kidneys, adrenals, and small bowel should be performed to ascertain the spread of tumor. If a large pelvic mass is present, it should be resected and sent to pathology for frozen-section evaluation prior to examining the upper abdomen. This practice decreases the risk of rupturing the mass. For small lesions, after the abdomen is explored, the ovarian mass should be resected and sent to pathology for immediate frozen section histologic evaluation. If the ovarian tumor returns with a benign diagnosis, a thorough evaluation should be made of the contralateral ovary prior to completing the surgical procedure. Suspicious areas in the peritoneal cavity should be biopsied and sent to pathology for histologic evaluation.

Surgical extirpation and staging of malignant ovarian neoplasms may be less aggressive in the female patient in childhood and adolescence, when compared to women who have completed childbearing. Early lesions that appear to be confined to a single ovary without excrescences are treated with a unilateral adnexectomy. The patients with bulky disease should undergo a resection of all visible tumor, infracolic omentectomy, pelvic and periaortic lymph node sampling, total abdominal hysterectomy, and bilateral salpingooophorectomy.

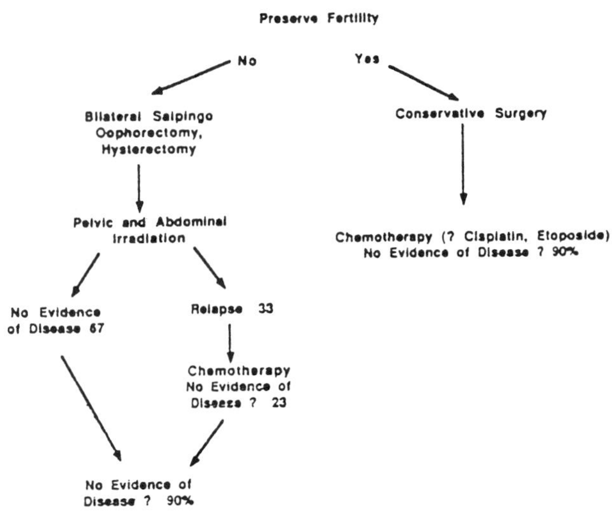

FIG. 3. Theoretical outcome and proposed management for stage IB, II, and III disease. (From ref. 36, with permission.)

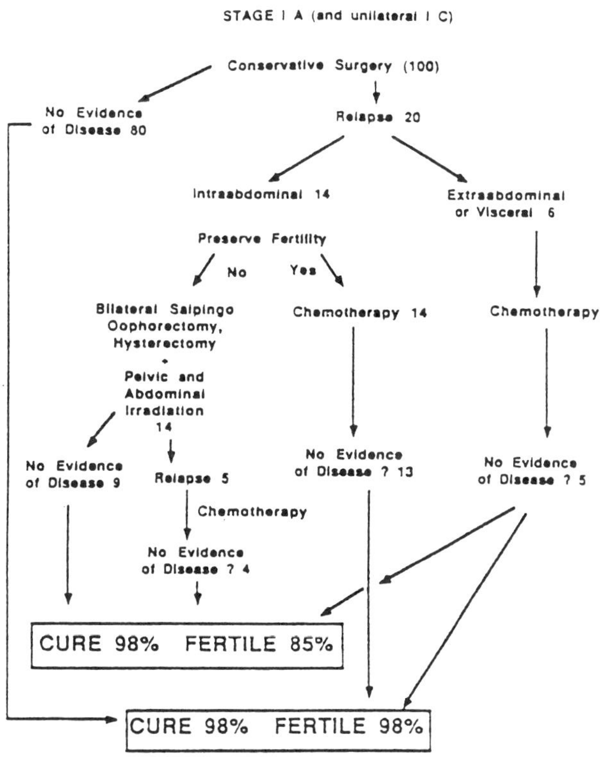

FIG. 4. Theoretical outcome after initial conservative surgery with salvage therapy for relapse. (From ref. 36, with permission.)

Dysgerminomas are frequently bilateral, and a wedge resection of the contralateral ovary should be performed. The exception to the above recommendations are patients with advanced dysgerminomas, who can be treated conservatively to preserve fertility even in the presence of metastatic disease. A unilateral adnexectomy with chemotherapy has enabled conservative surgery and acceptable response rates (Figs. 3 and 4).

GERM CELL TUMORS

Germ cell tumors are the most common ovarian neoplasm in childhood and adolescent patient. Germ cell tumors arise from a primitive germ cell that can develop into two different tumors: dysgerminomas and embryonal carcinomas. The latter is further classified into extraembryonic and embryonic tumors (Fig. 5).

Dysgerminoma

Dysgerminoma is the most common malignant germ cell neoplasm occurring in pure form (30,37). It accounts for approximately 1–2% of primary ovarian neoplasms and 2–5% of ovarian malignancies (38–41). Ninety percent of patients with dysgerminomas are found in patients younger than 30 years of age (42). Fortunately, the prognosis of these patients is excellent if identified promptly and appropriately treated.

Survival rates are in the range of 75–90% (43,44). Unlike epithelial germ cell and stromal tumors, bilateral involvement is present in 10–15% of the patients.

Macroscopic

Macroscopically, dysgerminoma are solid tumors, round, lobulated, or oval with a

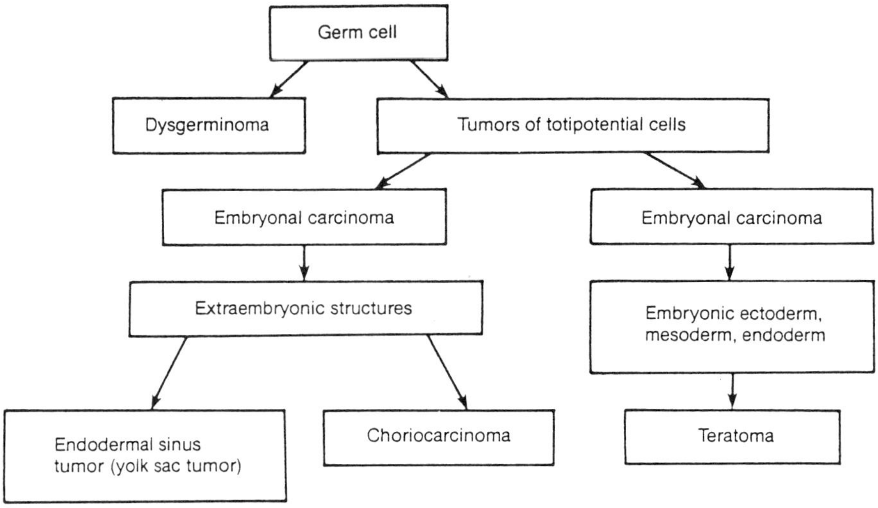

FIG. 5. Histogenesis of germ cell tumors. (From ref. 5, with permission.)

smooth grey-white fibrous capsule. Cystic areas may be present in mixed germ cell tumors coexisting with immature teratomas, choriocarcinoma, and endodermal sinus tumors.

Microscopic

Microscopically, there are aggregates of large uniform cells with varying amounts of connective tissue, stroma, and lymphocytic infiltrate. Moderate pleomorphorism and more than 10 mitoses per high-power field may be present (45). These tumors have a propensity for lymphatic spread to the periaortic region (44,46,47).

Treatment

Until recently, the primary treatment protocol entailed surgical debulking followed by total abdominal radiation. This approach was based on the highly sensitive nature of the tumor to radiation therapy. The standard therapy advanced by Piver in 1979 for dysgerminomas treated the entire abdomen with 2,000 rads by a moving strip technique with a ^{50}Cobalt unit or open fields employing a 25 mev photon beam. A pelvic boost of 1,500–2,000 rads is then administered. In patients with periaortic involvement, an additional 1,000–1,500 rads was administered, followed by mediastinal and superclavicular radiation over 3 weeks following a 4-week hiatus status postinitial treatment. Until recently, chemotherapy was utilized when the bulk of the residual disease precluded radiotherapy.

In recent years, chemotherapy has been used as the primary treatment modality for patients with ovarian dysgerminomas (48,49). Dysgerminomas are thought to be equally sensitive to chemotherapy and radiation therapy. This has permitted the preservation of potential fertility and epiphyseal plate growth in premenarcheal patients. The chemotherapy regimens utilized to treat dysgerminomas and germ cell tumors are outlined in Table 5. Bleomycin, etoposide, and cisplatin are most frequently administered as a result of the ability of chemotherapeutic agents to preserve future fertility.

It is imperative that patients receiving bleomycin have pulmonary function tests prior to each course of therapy. A decrease of 25% in diffusing lung capacity or forced

TABLE 5. *Combination chemotherapy for germ cell tumors of the ovary*

Regimen drugs	Dose and schedule
VAC[a]	
Vincristine	1–1.5 mg/m^2 on day 1 every 4 weeks
Actinomycin-D	0.5 mg/day × 5 days every 4 weeks
Cytoxan	150 mg/m^2/day × 5 days every 4 weeks
VBP[a]	
Vinblastine	20 mg/m^2 days 1 and 2 every 3 weeks
Bleomycin	15 units/m^2/week × 5; then on day 1 of course 4
Cisplatin	100 mg/m^2 on day 1 every 3 weeks
BEP[b]	
Bleomycin	10–15 mg on day 1, 2, 3 every 4 weeks
Etoposide	100 mg/m^2 on day 1, 2, 3 every 4 weeks
Cisplatin	100 mg/m^2 on day 1 every 4 weeks
EP[a]	
Etoposide	100 mg/m^2/day × 5 days every 3 weeks
Cisplatin	20 mg/m^2/day × 5 days, or 100 mg/m^2/day × 1 day every 3 weeks

[a]Data from refs. 12 and 13.
[b]Data from ref. 50.
All doses given intravenously.

expiratory volume (FEV_1) indicates the need for discontinuation of this treatment protocol. These drugs and their toxicity are identified in Table 5. The ideal number of chemotherapeutic courses has not been determined.

In patients with no residual disease, the recommendation is four to six courses. A second-look laparotomy is controversial because these are rapidly growing tumors, and recurrences can be documented within 4–6 months radiographically. Since this tumor recurs in a short time period following completion of therapy, it is advisable to defer pregnancy for approximately 1 year following chemotherapy. Dysgerminoma has an overall 5-year survival of 85% (36).

Endodermal Sinus Tumor

Endodermal sinus tumors were first described by Teilum in 1946. He described the extraembryonal germ cell origin of a tumor that resembled the endodermal sinus of Duval in the yolk sac of the rat placenta and named it "endodermal sinus tumor." This tumor is the second most common germ cell tumor, including mixed forms (51,52). The median age of presentation is 19 years, with a range of 7–37 years (53). Although usually bilateral, 5% of these lesions coexist with a benign cystic teratoma. Only 10% of patients presenting with endodermal sinus tumors are asymptomatic. The majority of patients present with complaints of abdominal and/or pelvic pain (54). As noted in Fig. 2, endodermal sinus tumors produce AFP. Occasionally, low levels of alpha-1-antitrypsin (AAT) may be present. The levels of AFP correlate with the amount of disease and can be used as a tumor marker to track treatment response.

Macroscopic

This tumor is usually large measuring more than 10 cm and is an encapsulated globular firm mass. A cystic appearance may be secondary to tumor necrosis and/or hemorrhage.

Microscopic

Microscopically, a variety of histologic patterns coexist, including microcytic, endodermal sinus, solid, alveolar-glandular, polyvesicle vitelline, myxomatous, papillary, macrocytic, heptoid, or intestinal (55).

The microcystic pattern is the most frequently encountered. Schiller-Duval bodies are spaces lined by a single layer of fine endothelium which protrudes a glomerular-like tuft with blood vessels in the center. The Schiller-Duval body is present in 68% of the tumors (53). Other components include hyaline bodies and a myxoid stroma.

Treatment

Optimal treatment consists of surgery followed by an aggressive combination of chemotherapy agents. These tumors are aggressive and highly malignant, with 33% occurring in the premenarcheal female. The rapid growth of endodermal sinus tumors and intraabdominal spread necessitates immediate surgery and chemotherapy. VAC, VBP, and BEP have all been used successfully to treat this lesion (56–59) (Table 5). We conclude the best treatment today for an endodermal sinus tumor is a cisplatin base combination. Bleomycin, etoposide, and cisplatin is the recommended first line of therapy since it does not have the neurotoxicity present with vincristine. If a marker is not present, the patient should be treated for four courses. If, however, a marker is present at least one or two courses of therapy should be administered after the marker falls within normal range. The value of a second-look laparotomy has not been established.

Embryonal Carcinoma

The median age of patients presenting with embryonal carcinoma is 14 years of age (51). These lesions are large, unilateral masses measuring more than 10–15 cm (12,13). Embryonal carcinomas can differentiate into embryonic tumors, teratomas, polyembryomas, endodermal sinus tumors, and choriocarcinomas. As a result of the totipotential nature of these tumors, they can present with elevated levels of HCG and AFP (51).

Macroscopic

Macroscopic presentation is usually a large solid tumor with occasional cystic areas secondary to hemorrhage and necrosis.

Microscopic

Microscopically, the tumor consists of pleomorphic epithelial like cells with marked nuclear hypochromism and eosinophilic cytoplasm. Giant cells or multinucleated cells may be present and can resemble syncytiotrophblasts.

Treatment

These are aggressive tumors and should receive prompt treatment. Surgical exploration, tumor debulking, and unilateral adnexectomy should be performed prior to administering chemotherapy. As with all germ cell tumors, it appears that the cisplatin regimen may be superior (60).

Polyembryoma

Polyembryoma is an extremely rare tumor that tends to occur predominantly in premenarcheal patients.

Macroscopic

Macroscopically, this tumor is usually solid with necrotic and hemorrhagic areas.

Microscopic

Microscopically, it is composed of numerous embryoid bodies. The tumor can exhibit signs of early embryonic differentiation including formation of an amniotic cavity, embryonic disk, atypical yolk sac, and extraembryonic mesenchyme (55).

Treatment

This is a highly aggressive tumor and should be treated with one of the regimens outlined in Table 5.

Choriocarcinoma

Nongestational choriocarcinoma is extremely rare. The majority of patients presenting with pure nongestational choriocarcinoma of the ovary are usually less than 20 years of age, with 50% exhibiting signs of isosexual precocity (24).

Macroscopic

Macroscopically, an enlarged adnexal mass is usually unilateral in presentation with a positive pregnancy test.

Microscopic

Microscopically, syncytial trophoblast cells are present.

Treatment

These patients can be treated with bleomycin and etoposide and cisplatin or vinblastin, bleomycin, and cisplatin as outlined in Table 5. Alternative therapy would include methotrexate, actinomycin D, and cyclophosphamide triple therapy protocols used to treat gestational trophoblastic neoplasia. Prior to instituting chemotherapy, tumor debulking should be performed with radicality depending on the patient's desire for future fertilty. As with gestational trophoblastic disease, BHCG titers can be followed to determine the effectiveness and response to therapy.

Immature Teratomas

Immature teratomas usually present in the first three decades of life, with a median age of 21 years (61). These lesions are unilateral, although they may coexist with benign cystic teratomas in the contralateral ovary. Immature teratomas are rare and account for 30% of the deaths due to ovarian cancer in the first two decades of life (24). The diagnosis and presentation of these tumors is similar to that of a benign cystic teratoma. A soft-tissue mass may be present upon physical examination, or an abdominal x-ray will reveal calcification. These tumors rarely produce steroids, and tumor markers are negative unless a mixed germ cell tumor is present.

Treatment

Surgical therapy remains the mainstay of treatment in these lesions. In the young patient desiring future fertility, a unilateral salpingooophorectomy should be performed if no evidence of metastatic disease is present. For those who have completed childbearing, a total abdominal hysterectomy and a bilateral salpingooophorectomy is required. Tumors that do not appear to be confined to the ovary should undergo staging as previously described. VAC, PVB, BEP, and EP are effective chemotherapeutic regimens in treating this lesion. Patients with IAG_1 lesions do not require chemotherapy. The remaining patients should receive at least four to six courses of the above noted therapy. Second-look laparotomy is strongly suggested for those patients who have advanced stage tumors. Patients receiving adjuvant therapy, i.e., Stage 1-A Grade 2 and 3 do not require second-look laparotomy.

SEX CORD STROMAL TUMORS IN CHILDHOOD AND ADOLESCENCE

Sex cord stromal tumors account for 5–8% of ovarian malignancies (12,13). Fewer than 10% of all ovarian tumors are of stromal origin; these include tumors containing granulosa, theca, Sertoli, Leydig, and collagen-producing stromal cells or their embryonic precursors. This section concentrates on two malignant tumors: juvenile granulosa cell tumors and Sertoli-Leydig cell tumors. Granulosa cell tumors of childhood constitute less than 7% of all ovarian tumors in the first two decades of life. The majority are of the juvenile type (62–66). Approximately 80% of these patients present with isosexual precocity secondary to a hyperestrogenic state produced by the tumor (64). The majority of granulosa tumors occurring in the first two decades of life are of the juvenile type. Their clinical presentation is usually that of precocious puberty and an abdominal mass. Inhibin levels may be elevated in patients with juvenile granulosa cell tumors (67,68).

Macroscopic

These tumors can vary in size, although the majority are large and can measure more than 10 cm. These tumors frequently rupture and result in bloody ascites.

Microscopic

Microscopically, the cells have large luteinized cytoplasm occurring in a macrofollicular pattern. Call-Exner bodies are present in adult granulosa tumors but not in juvenile tumors.

These tumors are considered to be of low-grade malignancy. If the lesion is unilateral without any evidence of spread beyond the capsule, a unilateral salpingooophorectomy is appropriate therapy. With extensive or residual disease, combination chemotherapy should be incorporated in the treatment protocol. Zambetti (69) reported a 66% response rate in the treatment of granulosa cell tumors with cisplatin, etoposide, and bleomycin. The adult granulosa cell tumors have been treated with vincristine, adriamycin, and cytoxin (VAC), and cisplatin, adriamycin, and cytoxin (PAC) (12,13).

SERTOLI-LEYDIG CELL TUMORS

Sertoli-Leydig (arrhenoblastoma) cell tumors account for less than 0.2% of all ovarian neoplasms. They are derived from sex cord and stroma of the embryonic gland that differentiates in the male direction (24). A typical Sertoli-Leydig cell produces androgens and thereby causes virilization of the female patient (69a). Sertoli-Leydig cell tumors are usually of low-grade malignant potential, although fully differentiated tumors can occur.

Clinical presentation includes signs of virilization such as acne, hirsutism, clitoromegaly, male pattern baldness, breast atrophy, and voice changes. Serum testosterone and androstenedione are usually elevated with dehydroepiandrosterone sulfate (DHEAS) being normal or elevated (24).

Macroscopic

Macroscopically, these lesions are usually large and are complex in nature, containing both cystic and solid components. Tumors can be 10–20 cm and weigh 25 lb (12,13).

Microscopic

Microscopically, Sertoli-Leydig cell tumors include the Sertoli tumor with tubules lined with columnar cells and the Leydig cell with their lipid content and Reinke crystals (12,13,70).

Treatment

In light of the benign nature of this lesion and the predominance of low grade lesions, a unilateral salpingooophorectomy with evaluation of the contralateral ovary and of the peritoneal cavity is sufficient treatment. For those patients who have completed childbearing, a total abdominal hysterectomy and bilateral salpingooophorectomy should be performed. Radiation and chemotherapy have been used in patients with persistent disease (69,71).

EPITHELIAL TUMORS OF THE OVARY

The incidence of epithelial ovarian tumors in young women varies from 4% to 13% (72). Tumors presenting in the first three decades of life are usually of low malignant potential (25). In light of the relative infrequency of these lesions in patients in the first two decades of life, we will not provide further discussion.

SUMMARY

An ovarian tumor can be a catastrophic event to the patient and her family. During the past few decades, treatment has evolved into a conservative approach with increased emphasis on preserving fertility and contralateral ovarian function. A multitude of chemotherapeutic regimens have been reviewed in this chapter and have proven to be efficacious.

Dysgerminomas, which have been traditionally treated with radiation, are now treated with chemotherapeutic agents, enabling us to decrease early and later radiation toxicity as well as preserve ovarian function and fertility. As research in this area advances and new drugs are identified, the ability to provide therapeutic protocols that result in complete responses and 5-year survivals above 90% will be enhanced.

REFERENCES

1. Acosta A, Kaplan AL, Kaufman RH. Gynecologic cancer in children. *Am J Obstet Gynecol* 1972;20:607–25.
2. Tintera H, Mitarnum W. Ovarian neoplasms in childhood and adolescents in Songklanagarind Hospital, February 1983–March 1989. *J Med Assoc Thai* YEAR 73:375–80.
3. Breen JL, Mayson WS. Ovarian tumors in children and adolescents. *Clin Obstet Gynecol* 1977;20:607–25.
4. Haldan (1915).
5. Droegemueller W. Benign gynecologic lesions. In: Droegemueller W, Herbst AL, Mishell DR Jr, Stenchever MA, eds. *Comprehensive Gynecology*. St. Louis: CV Mosby, 1987;440–92.
6. Hallatt JG, Steele CH, Snyder M. Ruptured corpus luteum with hemoperitoneum: a study of 173 surgical cases. *Am J Obstet Gynecol* 1984;149:6.
7. Spanos WJ. Preoperative hormonal therapy and cystic adnexal masses. *Am J Obstet Gynecol* 1973;116:551.
8. Grimes DA, Hughes JM. Use of multiphasic oral contraceptive and hospitalizations of owmen with functional ovarian cysts in the United States. *Obstet Gynecol* 1989;73:1037–9.
9. Surti U, Hoffner L, Chakravariti A, Ferrell RE. Genetics and biology of human ovarian teratoma. I: Cytogenetic analysis and mechanism of origin. *Am J Hum Genet* 1990;47: 635–43.
10. Gargano G, DeLeonardia A, et al. Ovarian bilateral cystic teratomas: Diagnosis and therapy in a young woman. *Clin Exp Obstet Gynecol* 1990;17(1).
11. Woodruff JD, Protos P, Pterson WF. Ovarian teratomas: Relationship of histologic and oncogenic factors to prognosis. *Am J Obstet Gynecol* 1968;102:702.
12. Berek JS. Epithelial ovarian cancer. In: Berek JS, Hacker NF, eds. *Practical gynecologic oncology*. Baltimore: Williams & Wilkins, 1989; 327–64.
13. Berek JS. Nonepithelial ovarian and tubal cancer. In: Berek JS, Hacker NF, eds. *Practical gynecologic oncology*. Baltimore: Williams & Wilkins, 1989;365–90.
14. Engel T, Greeley DU, Swenney WJ III. Recurrent dermoid cysts of the ovary: report of 2 cases. *Obstet Gynecol* 1965;26:757.
15. Scully RE. Sex cord tumor with annular tubules: a distinctive ovarian tumor of Peutz-Jeghers syndrome. *Cancer* 1970;25:1107.
16. Scully RE. Gonadoblastoma. *Cancer* 1970; 25:1340.
17. Scully RE. Recent progress in ovarian cancer. *Hum Pathol* 1970;1:73.
18. Scully RE. Germ cell tumors of the ovary. In: Sturgis SH, Taymore ML, eds. *Progress in gynecology, vol. 5*. New York: Grown & Stratton, 1970;329–48.
19. Grosfeld (1970).
20. Smith FG. Pathology and physiology of stroma ovarii. *Arch Surg* 1946;53:603.
21. Sailers S. Stroma ovarii. *Am J Clin Pathol* 1943;13:271.
22. Oates JA. The carcinoid syndrome. In: Thorn GW, Adams RD, Braunwald E, Isselbucher KJ, Petersdorf RG, eds. *Harrison's principles of internal medicine*. 8th ed. New York: McGraw Hill, 1977;634–42.

23. Bosch-Banyeras JM, Lucaya X, Bernet M, et al. Calcified ovarian fibroma in prepubertal girls. *Eur J Pediatr* 1989;48:749–50.
24. Scully RE. Tumors of the ovary and maldeveloped gonads. In: *Atlas of tumor pathology*. Fascicle 16, Washington, DC: Armed Forces Institute of Pathology, 1979.
25. Towne BH, Mahour GH, Woolley MM, Issacs H Jr. Ovarian cysts and tumors in infancy and childhood. *J Pediatr Surg* 1975;10:311–20.
26. Charache H. Ovarian tumors in childhood: report of six new cases and a review of the literature. *AMA Arch Surg* 1959;79:573–80.
27. Samanth KK, Black W. Benign ovarina stromal tumors associated with free peritoneal fluid. *Am J Obstet Gynecol* 1970;197;538.
28. Scully (1953).
29. Huffman JW. Ovarian tumors in children and adolescents. In: Huffman JW, Dewhurst CJ, Capraro VJ, eds. *The gynecology of childhood and adolescence*. Philadelphia: WB Saunders, 1981;277–349.
30. Berek JS, Hacker NF, Lagasse LD. Ovarian and fallopian tube cancer. In: Haskell CM, ed. *Cancer treatment*. 2nd ed. Philadelphia: WB Saunders, 1983:409–29.
31. Griffiths CT, Parker L. Cancer of the ovary. In: Knapp RC, Berkowitz RS, eds. *Gynecologic oncology*. New York: MacMillan, 1986:364.
32. Bost RC Jr, Feeney M, Lazarus H, et al. Reactivity of a monocolonal antibody with human ovarian carcinoma. *J Clin Invest* 1981;68:1331.
33. Davis HM, Zurawiski VRJ, Bost RC Jr, Ulung TL. Characterization of the CA-125 antigen associated with human epithelial ovarian carcinomas. *Cancer Res* 1986;46:6143.
34. Casper S, Van Nagell S Jr, Powell DF, et al. Immunohistochemical localization of tumor markers in epithelial ovarian cancer. *Am J Obstet Gynecol* 1984;149:154.
35. American College of Obstetricians and Gynecologists. *Technical Bulletin* 1991;155:3.
36. Thomas GM, Dembo AJ, Hacker NF, DePetrillo AD. Current therapy for dysgerminoma of the ovary. *Obstet Gynecol* 1987;70:268–75.
37. DePaolo G, Lattuada A, Kenda R, et al. Germ cell tumors of the ovary: the experience of the National Cancer Institute of Milan. I: Dysgerminoma. *Int J Radiol Oncol Biol Phys* 1987;13:853–60.
38. Boyes DA, Pankratz E, Galliford BW, White GW, Fairey RN. Experience with dysgerminomas at Cancer Control Agency of British Columbia. *Gynecol Oncol* 1978;6:123–9.
39. Kreport G, Smith JP, Rutledge F, de Lchosi. The treatment for dysterminoma of the ovary. *Cancer* 1978;41:986–90.
40. Mueller CW, Topkins P, Lapp WA. Dysgerminoma of the ovary: An analysis of 427 cases. *Am J Obstet Gynecol* 1950;60:153.
41. Santesson L. Clinical and pathological survey of ovarian tumors treated at the Radium Hemmet S. Dysgerminoma. *Acta Radiol (Stockh)* 1947;28:643.
42. Mitchell MF, Gershenson DM, Soeters RP, et al. The long term effects of radiation in therapy on patients with ovarian dysgerminoma. *Cancer* 1991;67:1084–90.
43. Gordon A, Lipton D, Woodruff JD. Dysgerminoma: a review of 58 cases from the Emil Novak Ovarian Tumor Registry. *Obstet Gynecol* 1981;58:497–504.
44. Asadourian A, Taylor HB. Dysgerminoma: an analysis of 105 cases. *Obstet Gynecol* 1969;33:370–9.
45. Bjorkholm E, Lundell M, et al. Dysgerminoma: the radium hemmet series 1927–1984. *Cancer* 1990;65:38–44.
46. Santoni P, Cionini L, et al. Dysgerminomas of the ovary: a report on 29 patients. *Clin Radiol* 1987;38:203–6.
47. DePaolo G, Pilotti S, Kenda R, et al. Natural history of dysgerminoma. *Am J Obstet Gynecol* 1982;143:799–807.
48. Aalders VR, Sleifer JG. Treatment of malignant germ cell tumors of the ovary with cisplatin, vinblastine and bleomycin (PVB). *Canad Treat Rep* 1984;68:719.
49. Gershenson DM, Wharton JT, et al. Chemotherapeutic complete remission in patients with metastatic ovarian dysgerminoma. *Cancer* 1986;58:2594.
51. Kurman RJ, Norris HJ. Endodermal sinus tumor of the ovary. *Cancer* 1976;38:2404.
52. Kurman RJ, Norris HJ. Malignant mixed germ cell tumors of the ovary. *Hum Pathol* 1977;8:551.
53. Gershenson DM, del Junco G, Herson J, Rutledge FN. Endodermal sinus tumor of the ovary: the MD Anderson experience. *Obstet Gynecol* 1983;61:194–202.
54. Cangir A, Smith J, VanEys J. Improved prognosis in children with ovarian cancers following modified VAC (vincristine sulfate, dactinomycin, and cyclophosphamide) chemotherapy. *Cancer* 1978;42:1234.
55. Talerman A. Germ cell tumors of the ovary. In: Kurman RJ, ed. *Blaustienin's pathology of the female genital tract*. New York: Springer-Verlag, 1987;659–721.
56. Gershenson DM, Morris M, Cangir A, et al. Treatment of malignant germ cell tumors of the ovary with belomycin, etoposide and cisplatin. *J Clin Oncol* 1990;8:715–20.
57. Hicks MC, Maxwell SL, Krim W. Management of advanced endodermal sinus tumor of the ovary with preservation of reproductive function. *Henry Ford Hosp Med J* 1990;38:76–8.
58. Curtin JP, Rubin SC, et al. Second-look laparotomy in endodermal sinus tumor: a report of two patients with normal levels of AFP and residual tumor at re-exploration. *Obstet Gynecol* 1989;73:893.
59. Athaniker N, Saikia TK, et al. Aggressive chemotherapy in endodermal sinus tumor. *J Surg Oncol* 1989;40:17–20.

60. Gershenson DM, Wharton JT. Malignant germ cell tumors of the ovary. In: Albert DS, Surwit EA, eds. *Ovarian cancer.* Boston: Martinus Nijhoff, 1985;227–69.
61. Kouios JP, Hoffman JF, Steinhoff MM. Immature teratoma of the ovary. *Gynecol Oncol* 1989;34:46–9.
62. Roofat F, Ulys H, Rylance G. Juvenile granulosa cell tumor. *Pediatr Pathol* 1990;10:617–23.
63. Fox H. Sex-cord stromal tumors of the ovary. *J Pathol* 1985;145:127–48.
64. Young RH, Dickerson GR, Scully RE. Juvenile granulosa cell tumor of the ovary: a clinicopathological analysis of 125 cases. *Am J Surg Pathol* 1984;8:575–96.
65. Young RH, Scully RE. Ovarian sex-cord stromal tumors: recent progress. *Int J Gynecol Pathol* 1982;101–23.
66. Lack EE, Perez AR, Murthy AS, et al. Granulosa theca cell tumors in premenarchal girls: a clinical and pathological study of ten cases. *Cancer* 1981;48:1846–54.
67. Nishida M, Shoji J, Masapumi H, Hayoshi I, Kim T, Tenaka H. Juvenile granulosa cell tumor in association with a high serum inhibin level. *Gynecol Oncol* 1991;VOL:PAGES.
68. Lappohn RE, Burger HG, Bouma J, et al. Inhibin as a marker for granulosa cell tumors. *N Engl J Med* 1989;321:790–3.
69. Zambetti M, Esrobedo A, Pilotti S, DePaolo G. Cisplatinum/vinblastine/bleomycin combination chemotherapy in advanced or recurrent granulosa cell tumors of the ovary. *Gynecol Oncol* 1990;36:317–20.
69a. Slayton RE. Management of germ cell and stromal tumors of the ovary. *Semin Oncol* 1984;11:299.
70. Woodruff JD. Pathology. In: Berek JS, Hacker NF, eds. *Practical gynecologic oncology.* Baltimore: Williams & Wilkins, 1989;109–66.
71. Slayton RE, Hreshchyshyn MM, Silverberg SC, et al. Treatment of malignant ovarian germ cell tumors: response to vincristine, dactinomycin and cyclophosphamide. *Cancer* 1978; 42:390.
72. Smith JP, Day TG. Review of ovarian cancer at the University of Texas Systems Cancer Center, MD Anderson Hospital and Tumor Institute. *Am J Obstet Gynecol* 1979;135:984–93.
73. Norris HJ, Jensen RD. Relative frequency of ovarian neoplasms in children and adolescents. *Cancer* 1972;30:713.
74. Junaid TA. Ovarian neoplasms in children and adolescents in Ibadan, Nigeria. *Cancer* 1981; 47:610–4.
75. Abell MR, Johnson VJ, Holtz F. Ovarian neoplasms in childhood and adolescence. I: Tumors of germ cell origin. *Am J Obstet Gynecol* 1965;92:1059.
76. Abell MR. Ovarian neoplasms in childhood and adolescence. *J Arkansas Med Soc* 1967;63:279.
77. Barber HR, Graber EA. Gynecological tumors in childhood and adolescence. *Obstet Gynecol Surv* 1973;28:357.
78. Blackwell WJ, Dockerty MB, Masson JC, Mussey RD. Dermoid cysts of the ovary: clinical and pathological significance. *Am J Obstet Gynecol* 1946;51:151.
79. Bonazzi C, Columbo N, Lissoni A, et al. Alpha-fetal protein in the management of germ cell tumors of the ovary. *J Nucl Med Allied Sci* 1989;33(suppl 1):53–8.
80. Breen JL, Neubecker RD. Malignant teratoma of the ovary: an analysis of 17 cases. *Obstet Gynecol* 1963;21:669.
81. Breen JL, Mayson WS, Gregoli CA. Ovarian malignancies in children. In: Sciarra JJ, Bushsloaum HJ, eds. *Obstetrics and gynecology,* vol 4. Philadelphia: Harper & Row, 1980:1–12.
82. Brody S. Clinical aspects of dysgerminomas of the ovary. *Acta Radiol (Stockh)* 1961;56:209.
83. Carter J, Stkinson K, Coppleson M. A comparative study of proliferating (borderline) and invasive epithelial ovarian tumors in your women. *Aust NZ J Obstet Gynaecol* 1989; 29:245.
84. Cheung TH, Wong WSF, Shio W, Chay A. A new combination chemotherapy for the treatment of endodermal sinus tumor. *Aust NZ Obstet Gynecol* 1989;3:346.
85. Christman JE, Ballon SC. Ovarian fibrosarcoma associated with Maffucci's syndrome. *Gynecol Oncol* 1990;37:290–1.
86. Creasman WT, Fetter BF, Hammond CB, Parker RT. Germ cell malignancies of the ovary. *Obstet Gynecol* 1979;53:226.
87. Forney JP. Pregnancy following removal and chemotherapy of ovarian endodermal sinus tumor. *Obstet Gynecol* 1978;52:360–4.
88. Gershenson DM, del Junco G, Copeland LJ, Rutledge FN. Mixed germ cell tumors of the ovary. *Obstet Gynecol* 1984;64:200.
89. Lucraft HH. A review of thirty-three cases of ovarian dysgerminoma emphasizing the role of radiotherapy. *Clin Radiol* 1979;30:585–9.
90. Herbst AL. Neoplastic diseases of the ovary. In: Droegemueller W, Herbst AL, Mischell DR Jr, Stenchever MA, eds. *Comprehensive gynecology.* St. Louis: CV Mosby, 1987:833–87.
91. Herson J, Rutledge FN. Endodermal sinus tumor of the ovary: The MD Anderson experience. *Obstet Gynecol* 1983:61:194–202.
92. James P, Lapolla MN, Fiorica JV, et al. Successful therapy of metastatic embryonal carcinoma coexisting with gonadoblastoma in a patient with 46, XY pure gonadal dysgenesis (Swyers syndrome). *Gynecol Oncol* 1990; 37:417–21.
93. Javaheri G, Lifsche ZA, Valle J. Pregnancy following removal of and long-term chemotherapy for ovarian malignant teratoma. *Obstet Gynecol* 1983;61:85–95.
94. Jimerson GK, Woodruff JD. Ovarian extraembryonal teratoma. *Am J Obstet Gynecol* 1977; 127:73–9.
95. Jolles CJ, Karayianis S, Smotkin D, Delia JE. Advanced ovarian dysgerminoma with cure of

tumor persistent in meninges. *Gynecol Oncol* 1989;33:389–91.
96. Kawai M, Kano T, Furuhashi Y, Mizunok, et al. Prognostic factors in yolk sac tumors of the ovary: a clinicopathologic analysis of 29 cases. *Cancer* 1991;67:184–91.
97. Muram D, Gale CL, Thompson E. Functional ovarian cysts in patients cured of ovarian neoplasms. *Obstet Gynecol* 1990;75:680.
98. Norris HJ, Zirkin HG, Berson WL. Immature (malignant) teratoma of the ovary. *Cancer* 1976;37:2359–72.
99. Peterson WF, Prevost EC, Edmunds FT, Huntley JN Jr, Morris FK. Benign cystic teratomas of the ovary: a clinico-statistical study of 1007 cases with a review of the literature. *Am J Obstet Gynecol* 1955;70:368.
100. Piver MS, Lorain JL. Childhood ovarian cancers: new advances and treatment. *NY State J Med* 1979;79:1196.
101. Savage MO, Lowe DG. Gonadal neoplasia and abnormal sexual differentiation. *Clin Endocrinol* 1990;32:519–33.
102. Schellhas HF, Trujillo JM, Rutledge FN, Cork A. Germ cell tumors associated with XY gonadal dysgenesis. *Am J Obstet Gynecol* 1971; 109:1197.
103. Scully RE. Gonadoblastoma: a gonadal tumor related to dysgerminoma (seminoma) and capable of sex hormone production. *Cancer* 1983;6:455.
104. Scully RE. World Health Organization classification and nomenclature of ovarian cancer. *Natl Cancer Inst Monogr* 1975;42:5–7.
105. Scully RE. Ovarian tumors. *Am J Pathol* 1977;87:686–720.
106. Serov SF, Scully RE, Robin LH. *Histological typing of ovarian tumors. International Histological Classification of Tumors 1973 (Monograph 9)*. Geneva: World Health Organization (WHO), 1973.
107. Slayton RE, Park RC, et al. Vincristine, dactinomycin, and cyclophosphamide in the treatment of malignant germ cell tumors of the ovary. *Cancer* 1985;56:243–8.
108. Susnerwala SS, Pande SC, et al. Dysgerminoma of the ovary: review of 27 cases. *J Surg Oncol* 1991;46:43–7.
109. Swanson SA, Norris HJ, Kelsten ML, Wheeler JE. DNA content of juvenile granulosa tumors determined by flow cytometry. *Int J Gynecol Pathol* 1990;9:101–9.
110. Ueda G, Abe Y, Yoshioa M, Fujiwara T. Embryonal carcinoma of the ovary: a six year survey. *Int J Gynecol Obstet* 1990;31:287–92.
111. Williams SD, Blessing JA, Moore DH, Homesley HD, Adcock L. Cisplatin, vinblastine, and bleomycin in advanced and recurrent ovarian germ cell tumors: a trial of the Gynecologic Oncology Group. *Ann Intern Med* 1989;111:22–7.
112. Young RH, Scully RE. Ovarian Sertoli-Leydig cell tumors: a clinical pathological analysis of 207 cases. *Am J Surg Pathol* 1985;9:543–69.
113. Young RC, Faks Z, Huskins WJ. Cancer of the ovary. In: DeVita VT Jr, Hellman S, Rosenberg SA, eds. *Cancer: principles and practice of oncology*. 3rd ed. Philadelphia, JB Lippincott; 1989;1162–96.
114. Zalouche KC, Norris JH. Granulosa tumors of the ovary in children: A clinical and pathologic study of 32 cases. *Am J Surg Pathol* 1982; 6:503–12.

Pediatric and Adolescent Gynecology,
edited by S. E. Carpenter and J. A. Rock.
Raven Press, Ltd., New York © 1992.

27

Disorders of the Breast

Eric A. Wiebke* and John E. Niederhuber**

**Department of Surgery, Indiana University Medical Center, Indianapolis, Indiana 46202-5124;*
***Department of Surgery, Stanford University Medical Center, Stanford, California 94305*

Pediatric breast disorders represent a varied set of abnormalities best grouped into distinct categories for an ordered method of evaluation and a rational approach to treatment. For example, pediatric disorders of the breast may involve the breast gland, or the nipple-areolar complex; and disorders of the gland can be congenital, acquired, developmental, neoplastic, or infectious. A nipple discharge is a frequent problem in the pediatric age group, and such discharges can be endocrine or nonendocrine. Pediatric breast disorders in males, most often gynecomastia and galactorrhea, provide a distinct set of diagnostic and therapeutic issues and are best considered as a separate category.

A summary of this algorithm and the various groups to be discussed is presented in Table 1. As might be expected, a proportionally large number of breast disorders are classed as congenital or developmental. Therefore, a brief discussion of breast embryology and normal development is presented to serve as an introduction to the congenital and developmental problems seen in the pediatric patient population.

BREAST EMBRYOLOGY AND DEVELOPMENT

Embryology

At 4 weeks gestation, two mammary ridges develop on the ventral body wall of the embryo (Fig. 1). These are symmetrical thickenings of ectoderm that extend from the inguinal to axillary regions. At 6 weeks gestation, all but the thoracic component has disappeared, and a downgrowth of epidermis into the underlying mesenchyme occurs. This represents the primary mammary bud. By 16 weeks, the primary bud

TABLE 1. *Pediatric and adolescent breast disorders*

Congenital
- Polythelia
- Polymastia
- Amastia
- Nipple inversion

Acquired
- Amastia
  - Iatrogenic injury
  - Irradiation
  - Breast bud excision
- Hypoplasia
  - Burns and skin contracture

Developmental
- Neonatal hypertrophy (see "Nipple discharge")
- Premature thelarche
- Precocious puberty
  - Central
  - Peripheral
  - Idiopathic
- Asymmetry (gigantomastia)
- Tuberous breast abnormality

Nipple discharge
- Galactorrhea
  - Adolescents and children
  - Neonatal hypertrophy
- Nonmilky discharge

Masses
- Infections
  - Mastitis
  - Abscess
- Cystic disease
  - Simple
  - Juvenile papillomatosis
  - Fibrocystic disease
- Neoplasms
  - Fibroadenomas
  - Phylloides tumors
  - Carcinoma

Disorders in males
- Gynecomastia
  - Physiologic
  - Hypogonadism
  - Testicular/adrenal neoplasms
- Galactorrhea

has grown and branched into multiple secondary buds, which represent early lactiferous ducts. During the last trimester of development, maternal hormones induce a canalization of the primordial ducts; and through the last 8 weeks of gestation, final differentiation occurs with a large increase in breast mass (1–3).

The nipple-areolar complex develops during the late fetal period. A mammary pit can be seen by the 12th week of gestation

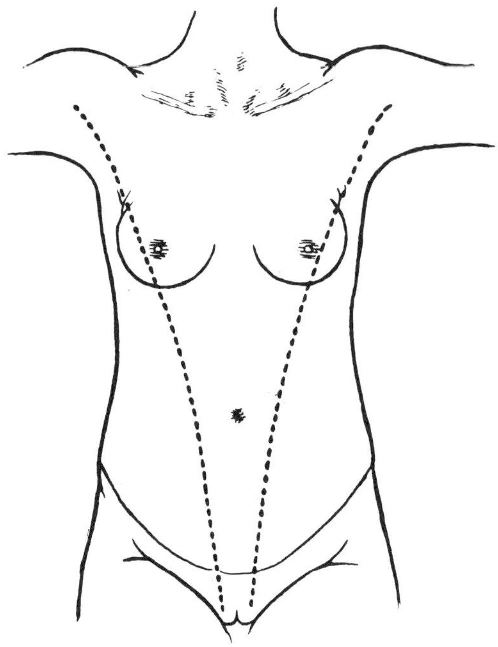

FIG. 1. The "milk line" corresponding to the embryologic mammary ridge. Accessory nipples, the most common congenital anomaly, and accessory breast tissue occur along these lines.

from continued epidermal downgrowth, and mesenchymal proliferation beneath the developing mammary gland produces a thickening corresponding to the future areola. By 20–24 weeks, a pigmented areola is recognizable, but a nipple is not present—developing later during the perinatal period. At birth, the nipple is often inverted; and further nipple development continues during infancy (1–3).

At birth, there is no difference between the breasts of males and females. During childhood, the breasts are relatively dormant structures, remaining so until puberty (1,4).

Congenital Anomalies

The most common congenital anomaly in both males and females is the accessory nipple (polythelia). Accessory nipples are often mistaken for moles, often located in the inframammary area. They may be excised, but treatment is not necessary in most instances. Less commonly, accessory breast tissue is found, usually in the axilla (polymastia). Polythelia and polymastia occur in 2–6% of women (5). The etiology appears to be failure of appropriate involution of the mammary ridge. In contrast, complete involution of the mammary ridge results in amastia. Amastia is a rare abnormality and usually unilateral. Ninety percent of cases of amastia are associated with underlying chest wall deformities, and Poland's Syndrome is a classic example of this association (absence of pectoralis muscle, chest wall deformity, and amastia) (1,6). Figure 2 reveals a young woman with Poland's Syndrome and marked mammary hypoplasia.

Nipple inversion is common and usually not a significant problem. The nipples are generally inverted at birth but become

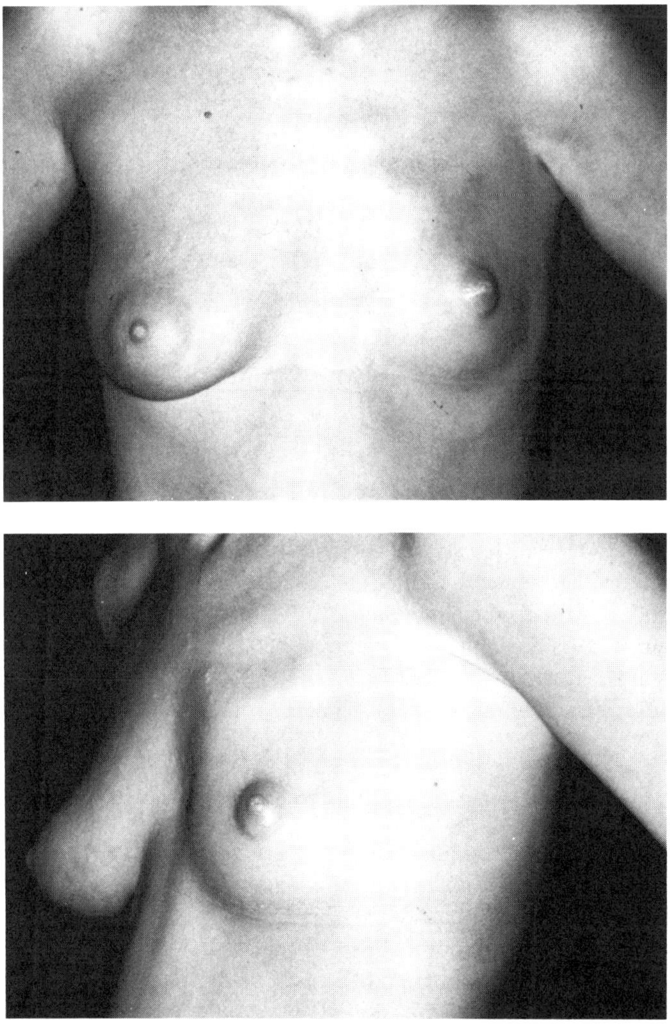

FIG. 2. Two views of significant breast asymmetry in a young woman with Poland's Syndrome. Note small breast, poorly developed nipple-areolar complex, and lack of pectoral contour on affected side. (Courtesy of Craig Vander Kolk, M.D., Johns Hopkins Hospital.)

everted within a few days to weeks postpartum. Nipples that remain inverted in females make nursing difficult, but this is the exception. They pose no other significant problem in males or nulliparous females other than cosmetic. Rarely, nipple inversion can predispose to infection and breast abscess formation. Nipple inversion can be a difficult anomaly to treat successfully and, in general, surgery is avoided. A significant percentage of patients who undergo surgical correction will have recurrence of the inversion, a poor cosmetic result, or significant damage to the ducts, making nursing difficult or impossible.

Acquired Abnormalities

Injuries to the breast bud occurring during infancy and childhood result in failure of normal breast development. Biopsy of the hypertrophied breast bud in the neonate and of the preadolescent breast mound are devastating injuries, each requiring reconstructive surgery during late adolescence. Iatrogenic injury often occurs in the neonate or premature infant because of the lack of pigmentation of the areola to serve as a landmark. Chest wall irradiation and trauma (burns, tube thoracostomy) can also affect normal breast development. Burns often result in skin contractures, with an intact breast bud underneath. Contracture release with skin grafts or flaps during early breast growth will allow for near normal breast development (7).

Development

The onset of breast development (thelarche) occurs early in puberty, usually between the ages 9 and 12 years (1,8). Adrenarche (the development of secondary sexual characteristics), the growth spurt, and menarche follow. Early puberty is marked by increased secretion of gonadotropin-releasing hormone by the hypothalamus. This results in increased secretion of the gonadotropins by the pituitary and of sex steroids by the ovaries. Estradiol secretion correlates best with breast development, but the gonadotropins and somatomedin appear to be required (9–11). Histologically, growth of the glandular elements, the stromal and fatty elements of the breast occurs. Glandular tissue accounts for less than 20% of normal breast mass when fully developed (9).

TABLE 2. *Tanner stages of breast development during puberty*

Stage	Findings
1	Preadolescent; nipple elevation only
2	Breast bud stage; elevation of breast and nipple as small mound, with enlargement of areola diameter
3	Further enlargement of breast and areola; increased pigmentation of areola
4	Further areola enlargement and pigmentation; nipple and areola now form secondary mound above level of breast
5	Mature stage; smooth contour; projection of nipple only with recession of areola to level of breast

Gross breast development has been characterized in the classic publication by Tanner (8). In his studies, normal development is divided into the five Tanner Stages summarized in Table 2. These morphologic descriptions have proven useful in describing normal and abnormal adolescent development.

Developmental Abnormalities

Up to 70% of normal newborns develop neonatal hypertrophy and nipple discharge, so-called "witches milk." Small breast enlargement in both newborn males and females (gynecomastia) is felt to occur secondary to the influence of maternal estrogens. Estrogen withdrawal at birth stimulates the pituitary to produce prolactin. This results in nipple discharge. This is usually a self-limited process and requires no intervention. On occasion, continued manipulation of an infant's breast bud in an effort to decompress it of milk by an unsuspecting parent results in continued production of prolactin by the pituitary and, therefore, continued breast enlargement and discharge in the child. Cessation of breast manipulation results in a prompt return to normal.

Developmental abnormalities that occur later in childhood and at puberty include premature thelarche and precocious puberty, breast asymmetry, idiopathic or virginal hypertrophy (gigantomastia), and tuberous breast abnormality, and hypoplasia.

Premature thelarche is defined as isolated early breast development, usually before age 7–8 years, and most commonly is a benign condition. Premature thelarche must be differentiated, however, from true precocious puberty, a pathological disorder resulting in many other developmental abnormalities due to premature estrogen production (12). Table 3 lists some of the characteristics that help to differentiate these two entities.

Differentiation of these two entities is very important, but sometimes difficult. Premature thelarche requires no treatment and only close follow-up. Studies have shown that thelarche before age two usually regresses completely and, after age 2, persists more frequently, but usually represents the first stage of an early, normal puberty (4,13). Similar findings have been described in other reports (14).

True precocious puberty left untreated results in pubic hair growth, behavioral changes, short stature due to early epiphyseal closure, and accelerated bone maturation, in addition to the early breast development. True precocious puberty is often idiopathic. A variety of other conditions, however, can cause precocious puberty including central nervous system lesions, hypothyroidism (central precocious puberty), ovarian tumors, and adrenal lesions (peripheral precocious puberty) (15). A defined structural or endocrinological abnormality can often be successfully treated. For example, thyroid replacement therapy completely reverses the developmental changes associated with hypothyroidism (16,17). Idiopathic precocious puberty must be treated early with hormonal manipulation, most commonly with long acting gonadotropin releasing hormone analogues (18–20).

Breast development during puberty can be asymmetrical and is usually of no consequence. With time, breast development equilibrates resulting in symmetrical

TABLE 3. *Differentiating premature thelarche and precocious puberty*

Premature thelarche	Precocious puberty
Breast development <3 years of age only (to Tanner Stage 3)	Breast development, menarche, pubic hair development <8 years of age
LHRH stimulator: FSH-predominant (LH:FSH <1.0)	LHRH stimulator: LH-predominant (LH:FSH <1.0)
No growth spurt	Growth spurt
Normal bone development for age	Advanced bone age
Routine lab tests normal	Routine labs test normal
	Other tests
	Hypothyroidism
	Ultrasound of ovaries for tumor
	Head CT for pituitary hypothalamus tumor
	Elevated urinary steroids
	Body odor
	Vaginal discharge
	Acne

breasts. A small amount of asymmetry in fully developed breasts is normal. An underlying mass, such as fibroadenoma, accounts for size differences in most cases (21–24). Asymmetry not related to a mass that persists can be corrected surgically if the young woman finds the difference cosmetically unacceptable. Sizes can be normalized by either reduction or augmentation mammoplasty. Rarely, one or both breasts continue to enlarge in an uncontrolled fashion resulting in massive virginal hypertrophy or gigantomastia (Fig. 3A). The cause of gigantomastia is not clear, but may be related to increased sensitivity of the breast to hormones or to an abnormal estrogen-androgen ratio at the time of thelarche (25–27). Plastic reconstruction represents the only effective treatment and consists of either reduction mammoplasty or subcutaneous mastectomy and nipple-areola complex conservation with prosthetic reconstruction (Fig. 3B). Recurrence after reduction mammoplasty is not uncommon, leading some authors to recommend subcutaneous mastectomy as the initial treatment (26).

The tuberous breast abnormality is a

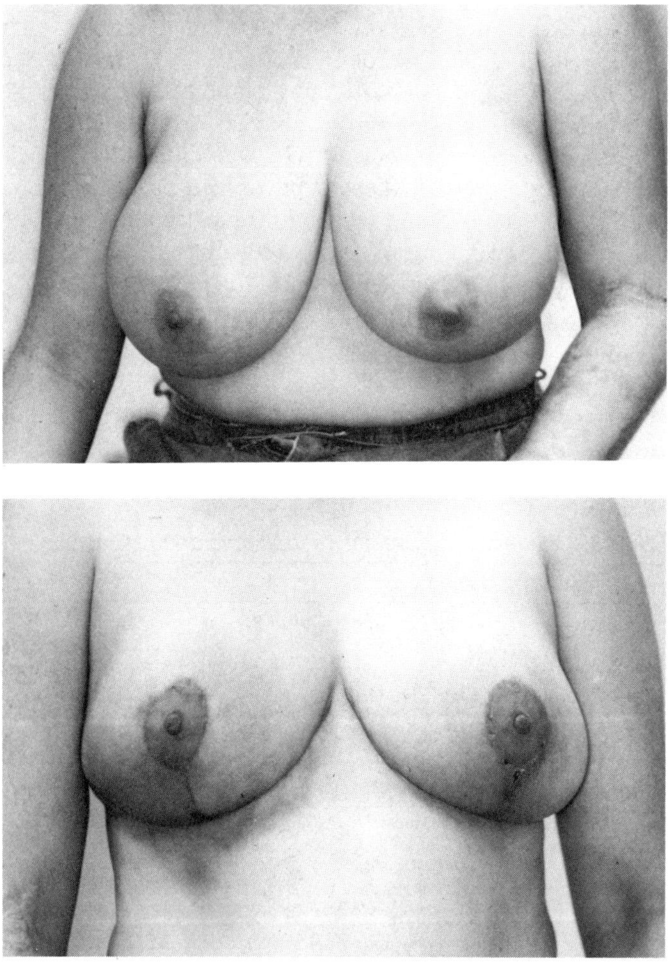

FIG. 3. A: Gigantomastia in a teenage girl. **B:** Postoperative appearance after bilateral reduction mammoplasty. (Courtesy of Sheri Slezak, M.D., University of Maryland Hospital.)

very rare condition described by Rees and Aston in 1976 (28). They describe an abnormality characterized by an apparent over-enlargement of the nipple-areola complex in addition to underdevelopment of breast tissue. The nipple and areola appear to be on a thickened stalk. Plastic reconstruction with breast augmentation is the treatment of choice.

Primary breast hypoplasia may be idiopathic (due to injury or surgery), or it may be constitutional. Bilateral constitutional atrophy (secondary hypoplasia) may occur after aggression dieting, in the setting of certain eating disorders (anorexia nervosa) and in the post partum period.

Figure 4 is an example of a young woman with bilateral idiopathic hypoplasia treated by augmentation mammoplasty. The breast tissue present functions normally, and lactation and nursing are unaffected. Menstruation is normal. Considerable psychological distress may result from small breasts, and surgical augmentation may be very beneficial.

Hypoplasia secondary to delayed pu-

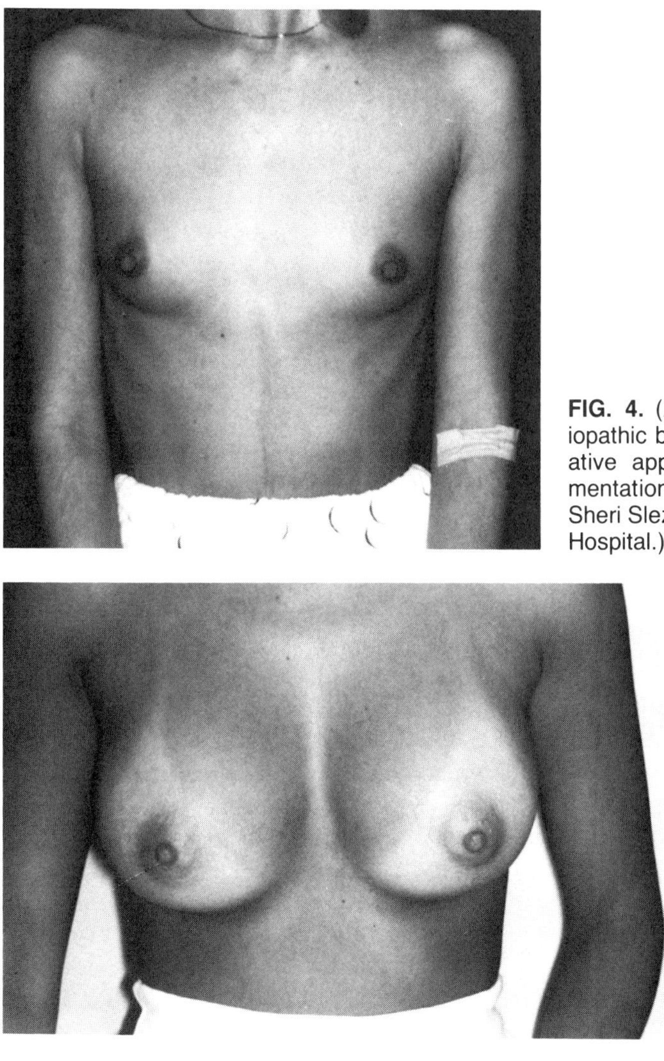

FIG. 4. (**A**); A 30-year-old woman with idiopathic breast hypoplasia. (**B**); Postoperative appearance after successful augmentation mammoplasty. (Courtesy of Sheri Slezak, M.D., University of Maryland Hospital.)

berty is rare. Delayed puberty is defined as puberty beginning after age 15. These conditions are divided into chromosomal defects, such as Turner's syndrome or hormonal defects, such as end-organ unresponsiveness. Turner's syndrome is characterized by classic phenotypic features (webbed or short neck, short stature). The majority of affected females also have hypoplastic nipples and breasts associated with amenorrhea. The diagnosis is made on chromosomal analysis. Estrogen replacement effectively treats amenorrhea and may improve status of breast development if started early in the patient's teenage years (29).

Unilateral hypoplasia can occur after injury or surgery in childhood, or in the setting of severe chest wall anomalies. These topics have been discussed previously in this chapter.

NIPPLE DISCHARGE

Nipple discharge in females can be divided into endocrine and nonendocrine etiologies. Endocrine causes result in a milky discharge (galactorrhea). The majority of nonendocrine discharges, which may be purulent, bloody, or serous, are related to infections and benign conditions such as fibrocystic disease.

Galactorrhea

Galactorrhea is a term used to describe inappropriate lactation. Inappropriate lactation is lactation that (a) is not related to pregnancy or that (b) continues postpartum in the absence of breast feeding. Galactorrhea in newborns has already been discussed and seems to be related to maternal estrogen stimulation and withdrawal. In children and adolescents, however, other conditions are prevalent. Rohn and Daughaday (30,31) have classified the causes into six groups: neurogenic, hypothalamic, pituitary, hormonal/endocrine, drug-induced, and idiopathic.

Neurogenic causes are extremely uncommon and include chest wall disorders (traumatic, malignant, and infectious) resulting in local irritation or stimulation, chronic nipple manipulation, and psychiatric disorders. Presumably, with these etiologies, the hypothalamic-pituitary axis is stimulated. Hypothalamic causes are even more rare. Pituitary causes, however, are commonly reported and have received tremendous attention in the literature as interesting and treatable cases, especially in adults. The most common causative tumor of the pituitary is the prolactinoma. The incidence of these tumors in children and adolescents is not well known but is presumably extremely low. Pituitary adenomas represent 1–10% of all intracranial tumors in the pediatric age group (30,32). In one report of 25 children and adolescents with these tumors, failure of sexual maturation and galactorrhea were the most common presenting symptoms (32). Visual problems and headaches were notably rare in contrast to adults. They were successfully treated by transsphenoidal resection. Currently, prolactinomas are quite effectively treated with bromocriptine. Galactorrhea may also be caused by endocrine disorders or hormonal manipulation.

Nipple discharge may result from estrogen withdrawal, such as that which occurs upon cessation of oral contraceptives, but this represents a tiny proportion of oral contraceptive users (25,30). Polycystic ovarian disease and tumors of the adrenal gland, or gonadal tumors, only rarely cause galactorrhea in children and adolescents (30). Hypothyroidism is a rare cause of galactorrhea in neonates and children, as documented by occasional case reports (33,34). Once hypothyroidism is documented as the likely cause of galactorrhea, return to the euthyroid state by the administration of exogenous thyroid hormone results in cessation of nipple discharge in most cases.

Finally, certain medications may cause galactorrhea; but, again, this has generally been described in adults and not children. Galactorrhea has been ascribed to the use of neuroleptics, estrogens, opiates, and many other agents (25). A common denominator seems to be the antidopaminergic effects of many of these substances, as dopamine inhibits prolactin secretion. Withdrawal of the medication results in cessation of discharge.

The work-up of galactorrhea in children and adolescents must be complete, since a pathologic etiology is common. This, again, contrasts with adult women where the majority of galactorrhea occurs with normal menstruation and is, therefore, not likely to be pathologic. Amenorrhea and galactorrhea, on the other hand, require aggressive work-up. The history must include drug use including oral contraceptives, a menstrual and pregnancy history, a history of nipple manipulation, description of sexual maturation, headaches, visual disturbances, and findings suggestive of hypothyroidism. Pertinent physical findings would include goiter, visual field cuts, breast masses and quality of discharge, chest wall abnormalities, and extent of sexual maturation. Thyroid function and prolactin levels should be determined. If hyperprolactinemia is discovered, the sella should be evaluated by computed tomography or magnetic resonance imaging.

Treatment is directed by the results of the above evaluation. Offending drugs should be stopped, hypothyroidism should be treated, and behavioral changes in the setting of nipple manipulation should be introduced. Prolactin secreting pituitary adenomas are currently treated with bromocriptine, which acts as a dopaminergic agonist. Rarely is surgery indicated. If the evaluation is unrevealing, these female patients should be followed closely for the development of prolactinoma, especially if sexual maturation is delayed.

Other Nipple Discharges

In contrast to galactorrhea, nonmilky nipple discharges often require surgical intervention. Infections can cause purulent discharge and can usually be treated with antibiotics. If the discharge fails to clear with antibiotics, or is chronic, drainage and duct excision may be required (35). Serous discharge can be related to fibrocystic disease and is usually self-limited. Bloody or blood-stained discharge should make one suspicious of malignancy, but this is extremely rare in children and adolescents. Intraductal papillomata and duct ectasia are the usual cause of bleeding in children or adolescents, and should be excised.

MASSES

Table 4 lists the common causes of breast masses. The differential diagnoses include infections (mastitis and abscess), benign cystic diseases, and neoplasms (fibroadenoma, phylloides tumors, and cancer). Neoplasms of the breast usually require biopsy to establish the diagnosis. The differential diagnosis includes the normal breast bud, which should not be excised.

Infections

Infections of the breast or areolar area may present as masses. In newborns, mastitis may present as a mass with overlying erythema. This is often caused by parental manipulation in the setting of hypertrophy or galactorrhea. Treatment ranges from cessation of manipulation and warm packs

TABLE 4. *Breast masses in children and adolescents*

Inflammatory
Mastitis
Abscess
Cystic abnormalities
Simple cyst
Papillomatosis
"Fibrocystic disease"
Neoplastic
Fibroadenomas
Juvenile or giant
Adult
Phylloides tumors
Carcinoma

to intravenous antibiotics. Surgical drainage is rarely necessary. Mastitis and abscess occur more commonly in females after thelarche. Often the etiology is unknown. Self-manipulation and breast feeding are associated with some cases, but the majority are idiopathic. Mastitis may initially be treated with antibiotics that cover oral anaerobes and the staphylococci. Breast feeding may continue during cases of mastitis that develop while nursing. Mastitis that progresses to frank abscess or that does not resolve on antibiotics should be surgically drained. Adipose loculations and septations in the breast make drainage difficult with local anesthesia, and most cases need to be performed under general anesthesia.

Cystic Diseases

Simple Cysts

Cystic disease of the breast occurs after the onset of breast development. Benign simple cysts are relatively common. They present as painless soft masses that are not fixed to surrounding breast tissue. They are usually single and unilateral. Needle aspiration of the cyst results in complete disappearance of the mass. The fluid may be serous or brown in color. The aspirate should be sent for cytological examination, though the yield of this test is very low even in adults. If a mass remains or recurs after aspiration, a biopsy should be considered.

Juvenile Papillomatosis

Juvenile papillomatosis is a lesion of adolescents and young women first described in 1980 (36). It has received attention because certain histological findings in juvenile papillomatosis may be considered premalignant in older women. Indeed, there may be an increased risk of breast cancer developing in the patient with juvenile papillomatosis, as well as in her female relatives. Juvenile papillomatosis is uncommon. The presentation is of a painless mobile mass, initially felt to be a fibroadenoma. After excision, exam reveals multiple cysts; histologic changes are varied and include papillomatosis, cysts, marked epithelial proliferation, and epithelial necrosis.

A report of 180 cases of juvenile papillomatosis revealed a mean age of 23 years; 96% were unilateral (37). Fifty patients (28%) reported the presence of breast cancer in one or more relatives. Additionally, seven patients (4%) had concurrent breast cancer, and two developed breast cancer years later. Given the possible cancer association, treatment consists of wide excision and careful long term follow-up.

"Fibrocystic Disease"

Fibrocystic disease of the breasts, often a multifocal and bilateral problem, presents with breast masses and pain (35). Excisional biopsy may be needed when symptoms are severe or there is a question of malignancy. In general, fibrocystic disease is a problem of older women and not an issue for adolescent females.

Neoplasms

Fibroadenomas

The most common masses of the breast in adolescents and young adults are fibroadenomas. These tumors are benign and have no malignant potential. They present as a single rubbery, round, mobile, and painless mass. Two types have been described: adult and juvenile. Adult fibroadenomas are usually small. Observation is appropriate with surgical excision reserved for growing lesions or when there is diagnostic uncertainty. The juvenile type are more rare, generally much larger (>5 cm), and occur in a slightly younger age group (5). These should not be observed. Early surgical excision is recommended to avoid significant asymmetry and deformity (22). There may be a relation between juvenile fibroadenoma and phylloides tumors.

Phylloides Tumors

Phylloides tumors (cystosarcoma phylloides) are unusual tumors consisting of two important histologic features. Phylloides tumors have both stromal hypercellularity and benign glandular elements, in contrast to fibroadenomas (38,39). Grossly, they may be large, but they usually remain well circumscribed. Generally considered benign lesions, many reports describe aggressive local recurrence after resection and even occasional metastases (40–45). These masses present as large, painless, rapidly growing lesions. The median age at time of diagnosis is 45 years, and very few present in women under age 25 (39,46). The tumors feel multilobular and are not fixed. Most physicians would recommend, for a benign lesion, wide excision with 2 cm margin.

For histologically malignant lesions, however, or lesions that are so large that the cosmetic result would be poor, recommendation would be that mastectomy be performed. This therapy appears too aggressive for the adolescent patient, and current strategies are for local excision of the mass only and close follow-up, regardless of the histology (41,42,47). In a report of nine adolescents with this disorder, eight were treated by excision alone with no recurrences (41). A review of the literature revealed 44 adolescents who had this tumor resected with only three recurrences (41). Recurrent disease can be treated by local reexcision, often repeatedly (40–43,46).

Carcinoma

Cancer of the breast in children is rare, representing <1% of childhood cancers and <0.1% of all breast cancers (48,49). In 1966, McDivitt and Stewart (50) reported on seven children, aged 3–15, with breast cancer, representing the largest series published. All were females presenting with a painless, slow-growing mass adjacent to the nipple. Four were treated by excisional biopsy, one of whom ultimately required mastectomy for recurrence. No axillary nodal disease was present in any patient, and all were alive 3–15 years after operation without metastases. Histology of the tumors revealed a morphology distinct from adult breast cancer. These tumors showed a prominent secretory pattern, and such juvenile breast cancers have subsequently been termed secretory breast cancer. Secretory breast cancer has also been described in adults. In general, further reports confirm the less aggressive nature of these malignancies (48,51,52).

A subsequent review of eighteen reported cases of secretory breast cancer in children included three boys (48). A review of operative therapy revealed no consistent approach to this problem. There were eight excisional biopsies, two quadrantectomies, and eight mastectomies (four simple, one modified radical, and three radical). Two excisional biopsy patients experienced local recurrence. Seven patients had axillary node sampling or dissection, and three had metastatic nodal deposits. No distant metastases or deaths due to secretory breast cancer in children have been reported through 1985.

Breast cancers of the nonsecretory histology are even more rare in children and adolescents. Descriptions in the literature consist of case reports only (53–57). Inflammatory breast cancer and infiltrating ductal cancer have been described (53,56,57).

Recommended therapy for breast cancer in childhood remains poorly defined. Some authors claim that secretory breast cancer, because of its benign course, should be treated by excisional biopsy only (50). Others feel that the 25% local recurrence rate following excision justifies simple mastectomy as initial therapy (48). Karl et al. (48) also urges that adjuvant therapy not be used for secretory breast cancer with axillary nodal metastases. Other authors find these recommendations untenable and recommend that children have aggressive therapy as used in adults (52,53). In reality, nothing in the literature is convincing enough to support that childhood breast cancer, regardless of histology, should be managed any differently than adult breast cancer. Even the secretory type can recur locally and metastasize to axillary nodes.

Currently, women with breast cancer primaries of smaller size (<5 cm) and favorable location (outer quadrants) are candidates for conservative excisional therapy (partial mastectomy), axillary sampling or dissection, and radiation of the breast. Table 5 shows the current TNM staging of breast cancer. Numerous studies have shown similar survival rates between adult patients undergoing modified radical mastectomy and those undergoing partial mastectomy with axillary dissection plus radiation for Stage 1 and Stage 2 breast cancer (58,59). There is also a trend toward breast preservation for tumors with less favorable locations.

Children with breast cancer should probably be treated in a manner similar to identically staged adults. Such therapy consists of partial mastectomy, when feasible, with axillary sampling. While the role of radiation therapy in children with breast cancer is unknown, it must be considered. Cases should be carefully staged, and treatment strongly influenced by the histopathology. Likewise, there is no described experience of treating childhood breast cancer with axillary metastases with adjuvant therapy. In premenopausal women, additional chemotherapy is given, often consisting of cytoxin, 5-fluorouracil, and adriamycin. Such use of adjuvant therapy should be carefully considered for children and adolescents with non-secretory cancers. Therapy will need to be tailored to each child depending on age, sex, histology of tumor, markers of risk, and evidence of nodal metastases. Successful results from conservative therapy, if undertaken, will depend on close follow-up for extended periods of time. The rarity of such tumors in the adolescent female precludes prospective trials designed to evaluate different therapies.

TABLE 5. *TNM staging system*

	Findings		
Stage	T	N	M
I	T_1	N_0	M_0
II	T_1 or T_2	N_1	M_0
	T_2	N_0	M_0
III	T_1 or T_2	N_2	M_0
	T_3	Any N	M_0
	T_4	Any N	M_0
IV	Any T	Any N	M_1

T: 1, <2 cm in size; 2, 2–5 cm in size; 3, >5 cm in size; 4, any size tumor extending into chest wall or through skin. N: 0, no involved axillary nodes; 1, mobile ipsilateral nodes involved with tumor; 2, fixed ipsilateral nodes involved with tumor; 3, involved supraclavicular nodes or arm edema. M: 0, no evidence distant metastases; 1, distant metastases, including skin beyond breast.

MALE BREAST DISORDERS

Gynecomastia

Breast development in boys occurs in response to normal hormonal changes at two ages. During the neonatal period, as previously described, maternal estrogens often cause physiologic gynecomastia in boys. The process is usually self-limited, and no intervention is needed. During puberty, an imbalance between estrogen and androgen levels and tissue sensitivities results in gynecomastia in many boys. Upward of 70% of young males aged 14 developed gynecomastia in one study (60). Another report revealed that 39% of Boy Scouts aged 11–14 developed gynecomastia (61). Physiologic gynecomastia usually resolves spontaneously in less than two years (5,60).

Pathologic causes of gynecomastia include hypogonadism, Klinefelter's syndrome, and testicular and adrenal neoplasms. Drugs such as digoxin, tetrahydrocannabinol (THC), and neuroleptics can cause gynecomastia in boys. These are all rare. It is estimated that 66% of patients with Klinefelter's syndrome develop gynecomastia during puberty, but it is not clear that this is very different than the incidence in the normal population; nor is the natural history described (60).

Treatment of gynecomastia in boys consists of stopping offending drugs if indicated. Observation and reassurance is the cornerstone of managing this embarrassing problem in the adolescent male. Persistent breast enlargement justifies excision of all breast tissue through a circumareolar incision under a general anesthetic. Figure 5 is an example of gynecomastia in a 16-year-old boy requiring surgery.

Galactorrhea

Nipple discharge in boys is abnormal. A pituitary tumor should be sought once drug-induced galactorrhea has been excluded. A prolactinoma is the most common cause of galactorrhea young males (30). A prolactin level and evaluation of the sella turcica are needed. Breast self-manipulation is a rare cause. Three adolescent boys whose self-manipulation to reduce gynecomastia resulted in galactorrhea were described in one report (62). Hypothyroidism causing galactorrhea has not been reported in adolescent males.

Treatment of prolactinoma has been discussed. If prolactin levels are normal and no other cause of galactorrhea can be

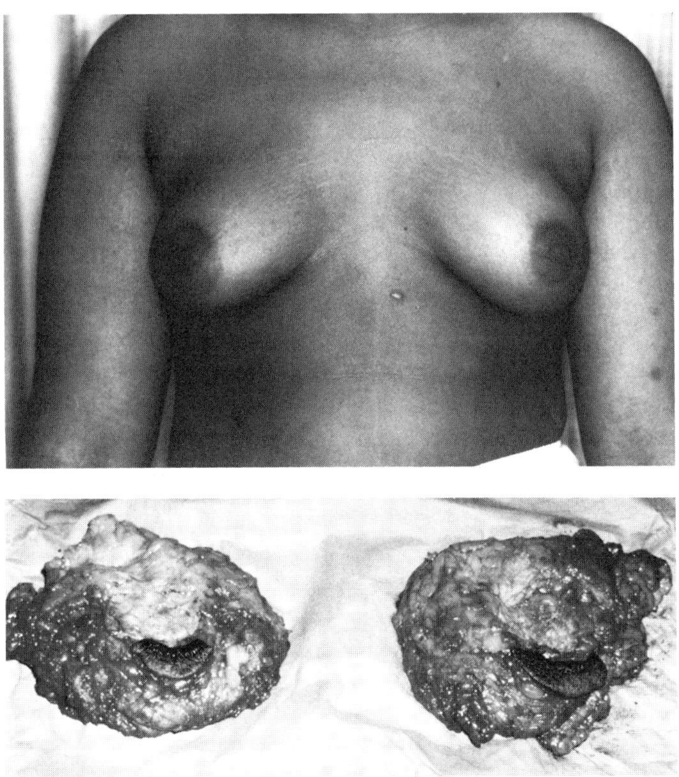

FIG. 5. A: Gynecomastia in teenage boy. Observation is the only necessary treatment in 90% of cases. Tamoxifen may be used when breasts are <6 cm and adverse psychologic effects are severe. **B:** Subcutaneous mastectomy effectively treats gynecomastia present for many years or when breasts are >6 cm in size. Medical therapy is not likely to be effective in these situations.

found, very close follow-up is necessary. A pathologic cause may declare itself. If prolactin levels are high and evaluation of the sella turcica unrevealing, then the child should have yearly CT or MRI evaluation of the sella turcica until the end of puberty, even if the galactorrhea resolves (30).

REFERENCES

1. Osborne MP. Breast development and anatomy. In: Harris JR, Hellman S, Henderson IC, Kinne DW, eds. *Breast diseases*. Philadelphia: JB Lippincott, 1987:1–14.
2. Moore KL. *The developing human. Clinically oriented embryology*. Philadelphia: WB Saunders, 1973:354–6.
3. Snell RS. *Clinical embryology for medical students*. 3rd ed. Boston: Little, Brown, 1983; 340–1.
4. Freni-Titulaer LW, Cordero JF, Haddock L, Lebron G, Martinez R, Mills JL. Premature thelarche in Puerto Rico. *Am J Dis Child* 1986; 140:1263–7.
5. Greydanus DE, Parks DS, Farrell EG. Breast disorders in children and adolescents. *Pediatr Clin North Am* 1989;36:601–38.
6. Ravitch MM. Poland's syndrome—a study of an eponym. *Plast Reconstr Surg* 1977;59:508–12.
7. McCauley RL, Beraja V, Rutan RL, et al. Longitudinal assessment of breast development in adolescent female patients with burns involving the nipple-areolar complex. *Plast Reconstr Surg* 1989;83:676–80.
8. Marshall WA, Tanner JM. Variations in pattern of pubertal changes in girls. *Arch Dis Child* 1969;44:291–303.
9. Drife JO. Breast development in puberty. *Ann NY Acad Sci* 1986;464:58–65.
10. Rosenfield RI, Furlanetto R, Bock D. Relationship of somatomedin-C concentrations to pubertal changes. *J Pediatr* 1983;103:723–8.
11. Sizonenko PC. Endocrinology in preadolescents and adolescents. I. Hormonal changes during normal puberty. *Am J Dis Child* 1978; 132:704–12.
12. Pescovitz OH, Hench KD, Barnes KM, Loriaux DL, Cutler GB. Premature thelarche and central precocious puberty: the relationship between clinical presentation and the gonadotropin response to luteinizing hormone-releasing hormone. *J Clin Endocrin Metab* 1988;67:474–9.
13. Pasquino AM, Tebaldi L, Cioschi L, et al. Premature thelarche: a follow up study of 40 girls. *Arch Dis Child*. 1985;60:1180–92.
14. Mills JL, Stolley PD, Davies J, Moshang T. Premature thelarche. Natural history and etiologic investigation. *Am J Dis Child* 1981;135:743–5.
15. Cutler GB. Precocious puberty. In: JW Hurst, ed. *Medicine for the practicing physician*. Boston: Butterworth, 1988;526–530.
16. Hemady ZS, Siler-Khodr TM, Najjar S. Precocious puberty in juvenile hypothyroidism. *J Pediatr* 1978;92:55–9.
17. Costin G, Kershnar AK, Kogut MD, Turkington RW. Prolactin activity in juvenile hypothyroidism and precocious puberty. *Pediatrics* 1972; 50:881–9.
18. Mansfield MJ, Beardsworth DE, Loughlin JS, et al. Long-term treatment of central precocious puberty with a long-acting analogue of luteinizing hormone-releasing hormone. *N Engl J Med* 1983;309:1286–90.
19. Pescovitz OH, Comite F, Hench K, et al. The NIH experience with precocious puberty: diagnostic subgroups and response to short-term luteinizing hormone releasing hormone analogue therapy. *J Pediatr* 1986;108:47–54.
20. Comite F, Cassorla F, Barnes KM, et al. Luteinizing hormone releasing hormone analogue therapy for central precocious puberty. *JAMA* 1986;255:2613–6.
21. Bryant WM, Archer RR. Unilateral breast enlargement in the adolescent. *Am Surg* 1972; 38:560–2.
22. Davis C, Patel V. Surgical problems in the management of giant fibroadenoma of the breast. *Am J Obstet Gynecol* 1985;152:1010–5.
23. Bauer BS, Jones KM, Talbot CW. Mammary masses in the adolescent female. *Surg Gynecol Obstet* 1987;165:63–5.
24. Stone AM, Shenker IR, McCarthy K. Adolescent breast masses. *Am J Surg* 1977;134:275–7.
25. Frantz AG, Wilson JD. Endocrine disorders of the breast. In: Wilson JD, Foster DW, eds. *Textbook of endocrinology*. 7th ed. Philadelphia: WB Saunders, 1985:402–21.
26. Samuelov R, Siplovich L. Juvenile gigantomastia. *J Pediatr Surg* 1988;23:1014–5.
27. Marynick SP, Nisula BC, Pita JC, Loriaux DL. Persistent pubertal macromastia. *Clin Endocrinol* 1980;50:128–30.
28. Rees TD, Aston SJ. The tuberous breast. *Clin Plast Surg* 1976;3:339–45.
29. Hall JG, Gilchrist DM. Turner syndrome and its variants. *Pediatr Clin North Am* 1990; 37:1421–40.
30. Rohn RD. Galactorrhea in the adolescent. *J Adol Health Care* 1984;5:37–49.
31. Daughaday WH. The adenohypophysis. In: Williams RH, ed. *Textbook of endocrinology* 6th ed. Philadelphia: WB Saunders, 1981:73–116.
32. Richmond IL, Wilson CB. Pituitary adenomas in childhood and adolescence. *J Neurosurg* 1978;49:163–8.
33. Van Wyck JJ, Grumbach MM. Syndrome of precocious menstruation and galactorrhea in juvenile hypothyroidism: an example of hormonal overlap in pituitary feedback. *J Pediatr* 1960; 57:416–35.
34. Macaron C. Galactorrhea and neonatal hypothyroidism. *J Pediatr* 1982;101:576–7.
35. Love SM, Schnitt SJ, Connolly JL, Shirley RL. Benign breast disorders. In: Harris JR, Hellman S, Henderson IC, Kinne DW, eds. *Breast diseases*. Philadelphia: JB Lippincott, 1987;15–53.

36. Rosen PP, Cantrell B, Mullen DL, DePalo A. Juvenile papillomatosis (Swiss cheese disease) of the breast. *Am J Surg Pathol* 1980;4:3–12.
37. Rosen PP, Holmes G, Lesser ML, Kinne DW, Beattie EJ. Juvenile papillomatosis and breast cancer. *Cancer* 1985;55:1345–52.
38. Vorherr H, Vorherr UF, Key CR. Cystosarcoma phyllodes: epidemiology, pathohistology, pathobiology, diagnosis, therapy, and survival. *Arch Gynecol* 1985;236:173–81.
39. Rosai J. Breast. In: *Ackerman's surgical pathology*. 7th ed. St. Louis: C.V. Mosby, 1989: 1246–9.
40. Chua CL, Thomas A. Cystosarcoma phyllodes tumors. *Surg Gynecol Obstet* 1988;166:303–6.
41. Briggs RM, Walters M, Rosenthal D. Cystosarcoma phylloides in adolescent female patients. *Am J Surg* 1983;146:712–4.
42. Stromberg BV, Golladay ES. Cystosarcoma phylloides in the adolescent female. *J Pediatr Surg* 1978;13:423–5.
43. Hart J, Layfield LJ, Trumbull WE, Brayton D, Barker WF, Giuliano A. Practical aspects in the diagnosis of management of cystosarcoma phyllodes. *Arch Surg* 1988;123:1079–83.
44. Hoover HL, Trestioreanu A, Ketcham AS. Metastatic cystosarcoma phylloides in an adolescent girl: an unusually malignant tumor. *Ann Surg* 1975;181:279–82.
45. Gibbs BF, Roe RD, Thomas DF. Malignant cystosarcoma phylloides in a pre-pubertal female. *Ann Surg* 1968;167:229–31.
46. Salvadori B, Cusumano F, del Bo R, et al. Surgical treatment of phyllodes tumors of the breast. *Cancer* 1989;63:2532–6.
47. Mollitt DL, Golladay ES, Gloster ES, Jimenez JF. Cystosarcoma phylloides in the adolescent female. *J Pediatr Surg* 1987;22:907–10.
48. Karl SR, Ballantine TVN, Zaino R. Juvenile secretory carcinoma of the breast. *J Pediatr Surg* 1985;20:368–71.
49. Ferguson TB, McCarty KS, Filston HC. Juvenile secretory carcinoma and juvenile papillomatosis: diagnosis and treatment. *J Pediatr Surg* 1987;22:637–9.
50. McDivitt RW, Stewart FW. Breast carcinoma in children. *JAMA* 1966;195:144–6.
51. Oberman HA, Stephens PJ. Carcinoma of the breast in childhood. *Cancer* 1972;30:470–4.
52. Heydenrych JJ, Villet WT, Von Der Heyden U. Carcinoma of the breast in children. *S Afr Med J* 1980;57:1005–8.
53. Close MB, Maximov NG. Carcinoma of breast in young girls. *Arch Surg* 1965;91:386–9.
54. Byrne MP, Fahey MM, Gooselaw JG. Breast cancer with axillary metastasis in an eight and one-half-year-old girl. *Cancer* 1973;31:726–8.
55. Hartman AW, Magrish P. Carcinoma of breast in children. Case report: six-year-old boy with adenocarcinoma. *Ann Surg* 1955;141:792–8.
56. Ramirez G, Ansfield FJ. Carcinoma of the breast in children. *Arch Surg* 1968;96:222–5.
57. Nichini FM, Goldman L, Lapayowker MS, Levy WM, Maier W, Rosemond GP. Inflammatory carcinoma of the breast in a 12-year-old girl. *Arch Surg* 1972;105:505–8.
58. Kinne DW. Primary treatment of breast cancer surgery. In: Harris JR, Hellman S, Henderson IC, Kinne DW, eds. *Breast diseases*. Philadelphia: JB Lippincott, 1987:259–84.
59. Harris JR, Hellman S. Primary treatment of breast cancer. Conservative surgery and radiotherapy. In: Harris JR, Hellman S, Henderson IC, Kinne DW, eds. *Breast disease*. Philadelphia: JB Lippincott, 1987:299–324.
60. Knorr D, Bidlingmaier F. Gynaecomastia in male adolescents. *Clin Endocrinol Metab* 1975; 4:157–71.
61. Nydick M, Bustos J, Dale JH. Gynecomastia in adolescent boys. *JAMA* 1961;178:449–54.
62. Rohn RD. Benign galactorrhea in adolescent males. *J Adol Health Care* 1982;3:141.

Pediatric and Adolescent Gynecology,
edited by S. E. Carpenter and J. A. Rock.
Raven Press, Ltd., New York © 1992.

28
Child Sexual Abuse

Lawrence S. Wissow

Department of Pediatrics, The Johns Hopkins Hospital, Baltimore, Maryland 21205

Estimates of the incidence of child sexual abuse vary enormously by the study methods employed (1a). In 1982, sexual abuse made up about 7% of all suspected reports of maltreatment made in the United States (1). Most authorities agree, however, that the true incidence greatly exceeds reported or disclosed cases. Sexual abuse may be more likely than other forms of abuse to remain hidden for years after its onset (2). Visible scars are rare, the victims often feel stigmatized (or suffer memory repression), and adults often react with anger and disbelief when children make disclosures. In population surveys, 5–20% of women report having had unwanted sexual experiences during childhood, and upwards of 50% give affirmative responses to more detailed probes about the occurrence of sexual maltreatment (3).

Although the figures may be biased to some extent by disclosure and referral patterns, studies have found that for many, if not the majority, of child victims, sexual abuse begins in the first few years of life (4,5). This early onset is one of the factors that contributes to delays in disclosure: young children are easily misled into believing that the activities are "special" and must be kept secret. Child sexual abuse is characterized by dynamics to which young, dependent children are particularly vulnerable. The perpetrator assures them that should they disclose, that dire consequences will ensue to themselves, other family members, or the perpetrator.

The legal definition of child sexual abuse includes both sexual contact (either intrusion into body orifices, fondling, or requiring the child to fondle or fellate the perpetrator) and noncontact acts (such as exhibitionism, involvement in child pornography, and deliberate exposure of children to sexually explicit materials). Sexual abuse of children generally begins with acts that may be confusing or frightening for children but that do not involve physical harm. Contacts may slowly increase in intensity and intrusiveness, often over a period of years. Thus, physical findings in a child who has disclosed may be minimal if the disclosure is relatively early in the course of the abuse, or if the perpetrator has avoided or not yet begun intrusive activities.

APPROACH TO THE PHYSICAL EXAMINATION

Parents and children are often very anxious about examinations conducted in the course of evaluations for suspected maltreatment. After an initial disclosure, while the family is still in a state of crisis and unable to offer adequate support, the child may have undergone an initial exam in an emergency room, possibly conducted by a physician who was pressed for time or not comfortable with being involved in that type of case. If no previous exam has taken place, both parent and child may be worried that what has been arranged is the child's first "internal" exam, with the parent unable to conceal from the child his or her own distaste for such procedures. Thus, at the time the examination is scheduled, it is important to ask about such experiences and concerns and to outline what will be taking place. Families are usually greatly reassured to learn that the upcoming examination will not involve any instrumentation besides the use of a bright light and possibly some magnifying apparatus.

When the child's condition permits, it is preferable to speak to the child and parent before asking the child to disrobe. It is important to remember that the examination of a potentially abused child must be therapeutic as well as diagnostic. Both the child and the parent may feel or actually be victimized, or they may be feeling an acute lack of control and personal security, even if only from being required to follow through with evaluations because of the suspicion of abuse. Even more than with other medical encounters, it is vital that the clinician show respect for the family's concerns, privacy, and modesty.

In general, children suspected of being victims of maltreatment have or will be questioned closely by professionals who specialize in conducting forensically correct interviews. Such encounters must follow careful procedures to document questions and responses, avoid any appearance of leading the child or suggesting answers, and provide reassurance about the availability of support during the investigation. The interviews accompanying medical evaluations usually focus only on symptoms that may yield clues to infection or trauma. It is reasonable, however, for the clinician to tell the child that he or she would be happy to hear about what has happened if the child is comfortable telling the story. If the child says "no," the clinician can use information from the parents, police, or social service agencies to guide the evaluation. If the child is willing to provide some details, they should be noted carefully in the medical record. The clinician should try to make his or her questions and replies as open-ended and nonspecific as possible. Questions that ask whether a specific person performed a specific act (for example, "Did Mr. Smith ever put his penis in your mouth?") should be avoided at all costs. Better questions are, "Did anyone else do anything?" and "Did he do anything else?" It can also be important to reassure the child that the clinician is asking these questions to guide the exam and better help the child. Often, if the child has been questioned before, the child will think that the clinician is repeating the questions because he or she does not believe the previous statements.

The examination of a possibly abused child should extend from head to toe, regardless of the type of abuse suspected. Perhaps the most important reason for this is to help the child become accustomed to the clinician's touch, and to allow the clinician to demonstrate that he or she can be trusted to talk about the steps in the exam and respond to the child's signs of distress or discomfort. This period of adjustment is critical for the parent as well as for the child, since the parent's discomfort will be quickly transmitted to the child even if the child herself is not apprehensive. A second reason for conducting a thorough exam is that various forms of child abuse often occur together: signs of physical abuse or neglect may also be present. Finally, manifestations of sexual abuse are not confined to the genitalia and rectum. As discussed below, there may be injuries to the mouth or breasts, or physical findings suggestive of disseminated sexually transmitted diseases.

Depending upon the type of case and the extent of preparation for the visit, children may sometimes refuse all or part of the examination. Unless some serious injury or infection is suspected, it is preferable to defer the exam until another date (often after the child has had the opportunity to meet with a counselor or therapist) rather than use force or undue emotional pressure to obtain compliance. There is always some risk that the child's refusal represents an attempt to manipulate the parents or clinician, but this is far outweighed by the possibility that insisting will be revictimization of a child whose bodily integrity has already been violated. Refusals can often be avoided by careful preparation of the family prior to the visit, exploring the parent's reservations as well as the child's, and taking the exam slowly, giving the child ample opportunity to know what is happening and to take control to the extent possible.

Documentation plays a critical role in examinations of suspected abuse. Information in medical records may be admissible in court even though it could otherwise be kept out of discussion by rules about hearsay; for example, a child's identification of a perpetrator, made because the nature of the assault is important for the planning of diagnosis and treatment, may be admissible in court even if the child ultimately cannot testify herself or himself. As with other medical-legal cases, records will likely be scrutinized both by attorneys and by other clinicians, sometimes with the goal of discounting the findings or clouding their interpretation. It is thus crucial that clinicians clearly describe procedures and findings, and then separately discuss their conclusions. It is best to avoid words that may have specific legal meanings or emotional value (and that frequently lack any real medical significance) such as "intact" to describe a hymen or "marital" to describe the introitus. "Penetration," to a physician, may indicate insertion of an object into the anal canal or vagina; to an attorney, it may be legally defined as simple placement of a penis between the labia or buttocks; a child may report the sensation of "having something stuck inside me" after vulvar coitus or pressure on the perirectal skin. It is essential that the clinician give a description of the physical findings that can serve as primary data for other professionals to interpret independently along with the clinician.

EXTRAGENITAL LESIONS SUGGESTIVE OF SEXUAL ABUSE

Bites inflicted in the context of sexual abuse or assault may injure the breasts, stomach, or genitals themselves (6). Bite marks may also be found on the arms, nose, or earlobes; they may be inflicted in order to damage or hurt the victim, as well as for sexual gratification. Bites can provide important evidence in cases of suspected abuse because they may give some clue as to the identity of the abuser. Human bites cause a combination of crush injury with superficial laceration. Soon after the bite, only an elliptical or oval set of indentations may be visible in the skin, perhaps with a reddened area in the center from the force of sucking or folding the skin. Later, the outline of the bite may be visible as bruises that correspond to the locations of the teeth. Although the skin does not provide good medium for making a perfect casting of the bite, it is often possible to assess the distance between the maxillary canine teeth: intercanine distances of greater than 3 cm most likely represent adult dentition (7). Fresh bites can also be swabbed for salivary residue and processed in the same manner as other forensic specimens.

The mouth should also be examined in cases of suspected sexual abuse or assault. Ulcers or exudates may be signs of sexually transmitted diseases. The frenula attaching the gums to the upper and lower lip or tongue may be lacerated from the application of gags or from forceful feedings. Erythema, petechiae, and bruising of the palate may occur after fellatio (8).

TECHNIQUES OF GENITAL EXAMINATION

Because of the scrutiny likely to follow any examination for suspected abuse, clinicians need to document not only their findings but how their examination was conducted. Recent work by McCann et al. (9,10) has demonstrated that differences in technique alter the types of observations that can be made about the prepubertal genitalia and the apparent size of the structures observed.

Three approaches are commonly used to examine prepubertal female genitalia. (a) The most common is the so-called supine separation technique. A child is asked to lie on her back, either on a parent's lap or examining table, with the hips fully abducted and the heels touching. The examiner applies lateral and slightly downward traction on the labia majora with the fingertips, exposing the hymen and vagina. (b) The supine traction variant of this technique is conducted in the same position, but instead the labia are held gently and pulled laterally, slightly forward, and slightly up. These supine positions are probably the most comfortable for the child, and they offer the best view of the labia, vestibule, and posterior fourchette. The separation technique, however, is least efficient in spreading out the hymen, and allowing its configuration and any opening to be seen. (c) A third possibility for an examination is the knee-chest position. The child is asked to kneel on an examining table with her back swayed, chest flat on the table, and knees slightly apart. The examiner then stands behind her, and gently spreads and pulls back the tissues adjacent to the introitus. Although it may be harder to prepare the child for this approach, it offers the greatest possibility of seeing up into the vagina and looking for foreign bodies or injury without the use of a speculum.

Regardless of the position used, good lighting and usually some magnification are important to the examination. Colposcopes are widely recommended for use in examinations for suspected maltreatment, but their benefits have also been debated (11). Major advantages of colposcopes are their excellent illumination, ability to take photographs, and distance that they afford between the examiner and child. Disadvantages include cost, lack of availability, and visualization of detail that, given the present state of knowledge, may be more suitable to research than clinical activities.

Time and patience are perhaps the most essential tools for examining small children's genitalia. Relaxation has a major impact on both how much visualization can be obtained and on the appearance of the structures visualized. The effort to avoid any direct instrumentation, even with only a moistened swab, means that traction often must be applied, relaxed, or reapplied to free up moist, adherent tissues, and then observations made in another position. This is only possible if the child is cooperative and the parent supportive.

EXAMINATION OF THE VULVA

The labia minora extend from the clitoris anteriorly to the area known as the posterior fourchette. The tissue that normally joins them posteriorly, known as the frenulum, is often stretched tightly when lateral traction is placed on the labia majora. Before puberty, the skin of the frenulum is very thin and superficial midline lacerations may often occur during examination. Vulvar irritation from either mechanical or infectious causes can also lead to increased friability. One study that was able to compare both probably abused with probably unabused girls found an increased prevalence of friability among both those with a history of sexual abuse and those who had been referred for vaginitis, vulvitis, and dysuria (12). Some unabused girls also have a midline, avascular appearing area in the posterior fourchette (10). These areas may be more pronounced with greater degrees of traction, and then seem to disappear as traction is relaxed. Of ongoing concern is how such areas might be distinguished from scars that could be attributed to prior trauma.

Friability in the posterior fourchette is often seen in conjunction with adhesions of the labia minora. Small adhesions are usually posterior, extending anteriorly from the fourchette. Because labial adhesions are thought to be caused by prior trauma or irritation, it would seem logical to expect them to be more common among children who have been sexually abused. Observations recorded in the literature, however, yield a confusing picture. Berkowitz et al. (13) reported finding labial adhesions in 10 of 375 girls younger than 5 years old referred for evaluation of possible sexual abuse (about 3%). This figure was higher than the "less than 1%" prevalence described in textbooks. In a comparative study that included older prepubertal girls, Emans et al. (12) found labial adhesions in nine of 127 "normals" (7%), four of 59 with vaginal problems (7%), and 21 of 118 with a history of sexual abuse (18%). When the results were analyzed separately by race, however, white girls had no difference in the prevalence of adhesions among the three study groups. There was a trend for abused black and Hispanic girls to have more adhesions, but the number of cases available for analysis was small. Finally, in the study of McCann et al. (10) of girls aged 1–10 years who had been screened to exclude likely cases of abuse, the prevalence of labial adhesions was nearly 40% among 90 girls examined in the supine position and 14% among 86 girls examined in the knee-chest position. These widely varying prevalence rates suggest major differences in the populations studied and the criteria used to make observations. Until more uniform data are developed, the association of adhesions with abuse is likely to remain a matter of conjecture.

A variety of conditions can cause changes in the vulvar tissue that can be mistaken for possible maltreatment (14). Perhaps the most problematic are the skin conditions such as lichen sclerosis and related disorders that can cause subepidermal bleeding, blisters, and superficial lacerations after minor trauma. Genital warts are a second very problematic finding. As discussed in the chapter by Tjaden and Rock (this volume), neither the natural history nor means of transmission of human papilloma virus (HPV) infection are well defined. Warts in toddlers and younger children may possibly be associated with perinatal infection, whereas it is more difficult to postulate nonsexual HPV infection in older children. When the concern for maltreatment arises because of a particular physical finding, and not because of a child's disclosure, it is important to carefully gather other medical information and to probe tactfully for evidence of behavioral or family problems before reaching a clinical conclusion. Once a concern for abuse is raised, it is very difficult to retract.

EXAMINATION OF THE HYMEN

Examination of the hymen has been the most intense focus of studies hoping to demonstrate findings diagnostic of sexual abuse in prepubertal girls. The normal hymen varies a great deal in appearance, although congenital absence apparently does not occur except in the case of major genitourinary malformations (15). Pokorny (16) has proposed the following classification:

- The fimbriated hymen has "redundant, gathered skirts" of tissues with a scalloped rim that attaches to all 360° of the rim of the hymenal ring.
- The circumferential hymen is composed of a "smooth, unfolded skirt" of tissue that also attaches to the full circumference of the hymenal ring.
- The posterior rim hymen appears as a crescent of tissue that runs generally from about 2 or 3 o'clock on the hymenal ring along the posterior edge to a symmetrical location on the opposite side. Partial openings in hymens are usually either central or anterior, probably reflecting how the urogenital sinus and the Müllerian structures join during embryogenesis. Anterior/posterior septae are also sometimes seen.
- The hymen may sometimes be imperforate. In that case, its appearance will differ from that of a large labial adhesion in that the urethra will not be covered. The fact that the membrane appears thin instead of thick helps to differentiate an imperforate hymen from agenesis of the vagina. Having the child cough should make the truly imperforate hymen bulge.

Before making a final determination of configuration, however, the clinician should check for relaxation and consider making observations in another examining position. In the study of McCann et al. (10), hymens that had appeared to be fimbriated using the supine separation method took on a smoother, crescentic appearance when traction was applied or the child was examined in the knee-chest position.

Early attempts to diagnose sexual abuse attempted to determine sizes of the hymenal opening that might be indicative of prior trauma. The landmark study in this area was reported by Cantwell (17), a comparison of findings among over 250 girls 12 and younger who had been admitted to a crisis care facility for treatment of various kinds of abuse. In this population, a hymenal opening of greater than 4 mm was strongly associated with a history of sexual abuse. A subsequent study by Emans et al. (12), however, offered some important methodologic improvements and questioned the utility of Cantwell's 4 mm cut-off point. Table 1 gives dimensions of the hymenal opening (measured supine) among children 3–6 years old, comparing asymptomatic children with those who gave a history of sexual abuse and those who had genital complaints. Although the asymptomatic children had, on the average, smaller openings, only four of the 55 children in the abused group had openings outside the range found in the asymptomatic girls. Based on these and other data, the authors concluded that the horizontal diameter of the hymenal opening was not a good indicator of previous vaginal or vulvar trauma, although girls with openings greater than 6 mm might be in a group at increased risk if they did not currently have some other vaginal complaint.

The study of McCann et al. (10) of apparently not abused girls provided further evidence against the 4 mm cut-off point, although it was not a comparison of abused

TABLE 1. *Horizontal diameter of the hymenal opening in girls 3–6 years of age*

Group	n	Mean (mm)	Range (mm)
History of sexual abuse	55	4.0	1–10
Asymptomatic	34	2.9	1–6
Vaginal complaints	19	4.1	2–10

Adapted from ref. 12.

and nonabused children. The study also demonstrated the extent of difference in hymenal opening diameter that could be attributed to a child's age and to examination techniques. Table 2 shows mean horizontal diameters for three age groups of children and three examination techniques. Average diameter increases with age, and is generally larger in the supine traction and knee-chest positions, although this difference is most important in young children. An important caveat in comparing these figures to Emans' is that McCann and colleagues did not average in the opening size of zero for those girls whose hymens appeared redundant and without an opening. This represented about 20% of the girls examined with the supine separation technique and 8% of those examined with supine traction or in the knee-chest position. This would tend to make McCann's average measurements larger than those made by other investigators who might have included all cases. The ranges reported by McCann, however, are similar to those reported by Emans and support the idea that diameters substantially larger than 4 mm may be normal findings. It is also important to note that vertical diameters tend to be larger than horizontal, and that studies comparing which dimension is most affected by injury, or which might ultimately provide the most sensitive or specific indicator of maltreatment, have yet to be reported. There are also some data to suggest that after injury and stretching the hymenal diameter may decrease over time (18). How rapidly and to what extent this may occur are not known, however.

Despite questions about its utility, measurement of the hymenal diameter continue to be an expected part of examining a prepubertal girl for suspected sexual abuse. Once variation in relaxation and examination technique are accounted for, colposcopes offer the most precise method of measurement. The very narrow depth of field allows the examiner to focus on the hymen, take a photograph, and subsequently photograph a ruler or other measuring device at exactly the same focal length and magnification. If the two images are printed at the same size, the ruler can be used to measure distances on the photograph. This procedure is complicated and subject to some error if the plane of the hymenal opening is not parallel to the plane of the colposcope lens, but it is far superior to holding a measuring device on the perineum and squinting down the vaginal canal toward the hymenal ring. Some clinicians use a probe of known diameter and hold it in or near the hymenal orifice. This can be successful if the child does not become

TABLE 2. *Horizontal diameter of hymenal opening in nonabused girls: variation by age and examining position*[a]

Age group	Examination method	n	Mean diameter (mm)	Range
2–4 years	Separation	21	3.9	1.0–5.5
	Knee-chest	29	4.6	2.5–7.5
	Traction	24	5.2	2.0–8.0
5–7 years	Separation	39	4.2	1.0–8.0
	Knee-chest	41	5.6	2.5–8.5
	Traction	43	5.6	1.0–9.0
8 years to Tanner Stage II	Separation	19	5.7	3.0–8.5
	Knee-chest	21	7.3	4.0–11.0
	Traction	20	6.9	2.5–10.5

[a]The children examined were volunteers who had been screened to determine risk factors or history that might be suggestive of maltreatment. See text for descriptions of examination methods and cautions about comparing figures with other published data.

Adapted from ref. 10.

frightened or if the probe does not touch sensitive tissues.

Several other characteristics of hymens may serve to demonstrate that an individual has a higher likelihood of having been sexually abused. These are well illustrated in the color atlas of prepubertal genital and rectal findings developed by the California Medical Association (19). Perhaps the most significant is a cleft or tear in the hymen posteriorly, especially at about the 6 o'clock position. Anecdotal reports (20,21) suggest that this is the area most likely to be damaged in violent sexual assault or attempted penile penetration (Fig. 1). In the study by Emans et al. (12), the presence of a cleft or healed tear in the hymen did not distinguish among abused, asymptomatic, and symptomatic girls. Only three girls, however, had a tear at 6 o'clock, and these were all individuals who had given a history of pain and penetration. Bumps on the hymen in the 3 o'clock to 9 o'clock region, adhesions of the hymen to the vaginal wall, attenuation of the hymen (narrowing of the rim), and increased vascularity of the hymen or surrounding tissue have all been found among children with a history of abuse, but Emans and colleagues found them in roughly equal or greater proportion among children with other vaginal complaints. These are all observations based on a relatively small number of studies and patients. Other studies reported to be in progress will certainly add to what is known.

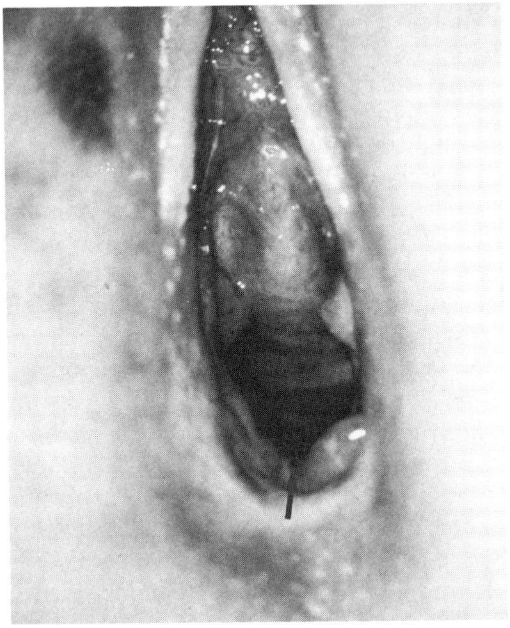

FIG. 1. Colposcopic photograph of a prepubertal girl's genitalia. The hymen is attenuated, and there is a cleft or interruption at about 6 o'clock. (Courtesy of Dr. T. Doran, Sinai Hospital of Baltimore.) (© 1990, The Williams and Wilkins Co., Baltimore)

INTRAVAGINAL FINDINGS

Especially by examining a child in the knee-chest position, it is often possible to see through the opening of the hymen and into the vagina. Anterior/posterior ridges (columns) run lengthwise, with transverse rugae branching out from them laterally. The length of the vagina varies a great deal with age and among individuals. From birth to about 7 years of age it is about 4–5 cm long (22). Just before puberty it is about 6–7 cm deep along its anterior wall and about 8–11 cm deep posteriorly (23). Penetration with an object larger than a single adult finger is said, after only a few episodes, to cause the vagina to lengthen and its folds to flatten.

The possibility of sexual abuse is often raised when a vaginal foreign body is found. Young children sometimes do put small objects in convenient orifices, and this is probably not a sign of molestation or abnormal psychosexual development unless it happens repeatedly or seems to be associated with an excessive amount of self-stimulatory behavior. What is unusual is for children to insert objects that would mimic coitus, or to do anything to themselves that one might anticipate to be painful. Such episodes suggest inflicted injury or, if self-inflicted, exposure to explicit sexual material. If a foreign body is suspected under these circumstances, an evaluation under anesthesia may be preferable to instrumentation or even irrigation in the office setting. Noninvasive approaches such as ultrasound might be considered first.

PERIRECTAL LESIONS

The prevalence of rectal injury in child abuse may well be underestimated, if only because knowledge of normal variations and the manifestations of trauma is even more scanty than for the genitalia. Serious injury to the rectum seems to be relatively uncommon in prepubertal sexual abuse, possibly because many child sexual abusers go to great lengths not to inflict trauma that will be detected. In addition, the anus is very expansive: Many stools are larger than the adult penis and can be accommodated without injury; therefore, penile penetration of the rectum may go undetected. Healing also appears to be quite rapid, so that minor injuries may be virtually undetectable by 2–3 weeks after a sexual encounter. More serious injuries may take place when the assailant is another child (and not capable of preventing detectable abuse), in the setting of violent sexual assault (rape), or among adolescents who are abused by adults practicing rectal sexual practices with violence or without lubrication such as in the insertion of hands ("fisting") or foreign bodies. It seems likely that as more sexual abuse victims come forward that the true prevalence of anal injuries will be found to be relatively high.

The types of injuries found in children or adults correspond to various aspects of the anatomy of the perirectal area (8,23). When the buttocks are first parted, the hyperpigmented skin of the anal verge can be seen surrounding the anterior-posteriorly oriented slit of the anus itself. The anal verge is roughly circular, and its skin is loosely applied over a thin layer of involuntary muscle and an easily disrupted network of small blood vessels (the inferior hemorrhoidal plexus). The muscle layer normally keeps the skin folded into multiple shallow furrows that fan out from the anus more or less symmetrically in all directions. Penetration with a single finger or other small object, especially if it is relatively well lubricated, may leave no visible mark on the anal verge except possibly for a shallow abrasion, possibly from a fingernail (24). Larger objects, however, especially if no lubricant is used, will tend to draw the anal verge skin inward with them. The fragile blood vessels under the skin may break, causing either localized or circumferential bruising (25). The skin itself may tear, causing a shallow fissure that may bleed. More extensive tears extending beyond the skin of the anal verge, either onto the adjacent skin of the buttocks or down into the rectal mucosa, are clearly unusual and suggest some nonphysiologic (abusive) trauma. On the other hand, shallow fissures are indistinguishable from the injuries that can be caused by the passage of a large, hard stool, or from the friability and maceration encountered with wearing diapers or poor hygiene.

Anecdotal reports suggest that unless there is chronic abuse most minor lesions of the anal verge resolve within a period of weeks. Areas of blue discoloration or hematomas resolve in a period of days, sometimes leaving small skin tags that may persist for an additional 2–3 weeks (24). These can be confused with midline skin tags in or near the anal verge, which are often a normal finding. In those cases, the tag will be noted to have been present since birth. Some observers (25) feel that increased prominence of the venous markings under the skin of the anal verge, or more pronounced filling and emptying of these vessels, may be a sign of prior trauma. Hemorrhoids may also be found and potentially are signs of prior trauma since otherwise they are rare in childhood. Other causes of hemorrhoids include perirectal infections and inflammatory bowel disease. Shallow fissuring in the past may leave fine scars that appear to be triangular, with the point of the triangle facing the anal opening, when the skin folds of the anal verge are spread during an examination. Although some authorities have felt that scars created by objects passing out of the rectum look different from those created by objects going in, others (23) feel that these two scenarios generally leave the same markings. The latter base their opinion on the fact that the configuration of the scar appears to be determined by the action of the underlying musculature rather than the mechanics of the injury. McCann et al. (26), in their study of children who were thought *not* to be victims of abuse, reported finding shinier, triangular-shaped "smooth" areas in the perirectal skin anteriorly and posteriorly (at the 6 and 12 o'clock positions), which they attributed to the distribution of the underlying musculature.

Chronic abuse does appear to alter the skin of the anal verge. It becomes thickened from repeated abrasion and flattened as the underlying muscle becomes stretched. In extreme cases, the perianal area may take on a "funnel-shaped" appearance, so that the apparent opening of the anus is within the perianal skin, above its normal location at the point that the rectal mucosa begins. Although this finding is said to be rare in children, one group of physicians has reported seeing it in six of 224 prepubertal children examined for suspicion of sexual abuse (27).

The anal canal is the passage that links the lower rectum to the exterior of the body at the anus. It ranges from about 1 cm long in children to 3 cm in adults. The external part of the canal is made up of skin similar to that of the anal verge: delicate and very sensitive to pain, because it is innervated by the somatic sensory system. The internal portion is lined with a mucous membrane that is relatively insensitive to pain, because it derives its innervation from the autonomic system. The internal and external portions meet near the so-called dentate line, which gets its name from the appearance of the puckered, longitudinal folds (known as Morgagni's, anal, or rectal columns) of the internal portion. The dentate line is at the level at which the anal canal passes through the levator ani musculature. At the ends of the anal columns are blind folds known as anal valves. The "crypt" within each valve contains glands that serve to lubricate the area and that can be involved with perirectal infections and ultimately in the development of perianal abcesses (28).

Both trauma and infection (with chlamydia, gonorrhea, or herpes virus, for example) may produce erythema and edema of the anal mucosa (proctitis). Symptoms include a burning sensation and pain on defecation. If the irritation is caused by a single episode of trauma and is not associated with infection, it will resolve spontaneously. The anal mucosa may also be lacerated (with or without involving the deeper muscle layers), causing pain and bleeding. Laceration may be caused by insertion of the penis, other body parts, or an object of some kind. Care must be taken to assure that the laceration has not perforated the wall of the anal canal or of the rectum. These are very distensible structures and perforation suggests either great force or the introduction of a relatively large or sharp object. Perforations may enter either the peritoneal cavity or the perineal tissues. The former type of perforation usually presents rapidly with signs of peritonitis and free air in the abdomen, but the latter may not be readily apparent until cellulitis develops. Initial evaluation can include checking the hemocrit and vital signs to determine the extent of bleeding, and an upright abdominal film to search for a foreign body or free air in the peritoneal cavity. Children suspected of having serious acute, rectal trauma should be hospitalized for observation, surgical consultation, and possibly proctoscopy.

The anal sphincter is composed of two sets of overlapping musculature, the internal and external sphincters. The internal sphincter, which lies closest to the bowel, is an involuntary muscle innervated by the autonomic nervous system while the external sphincter, which wraps around the internal sphincter and extends the entire length of the anal canal, is striated, voluntary muscle. The external sphincter has no opposing muscles to force it to open; defecation is possible when the muscle relaxes from its usually contracted position.

Acute stretching of the sphincter may cause it to remain open for a period of hours. If the muscle fibers have not actually been ruptured (sometimes visible at the site of a laceration of the anal skin or mucosa) the injury will be followed by spasm. Injury to the anal area that does not stretch the sphincter may also result in spasm as the muscles attempt to "splint" sensitive tissues and reduce discomfort. Past the acute period, unless there has been repeated penetration or tearing, the sphincter will appear normal. Repeated penetration can result in stretching the sphincter so that it easily accommodates wide objects (several centimeters in diameter) and loses some of its strength (manifested as a decreased "grip" on an examiner's fingers). Scarring from an old laceration, or splinting because of an abscess or fissure, may produce increases in tone or asymmetry in the shape of the anus when closed.

One of the standard findings in routine physical examinations of children and adults is the so-called anal wink, a reflex tightening of the external sphincter in response to stimulation of the perirectal skin. The reflex is also sometimes triggered by simply spreading the buttocks. It can be abolished by lesions of the sacral segments of the spinal cord or of the pelvic nerves, and individuals can learn to inhibit it if they have experienced frequent stimulation in the perirectal area or in order to be cooperative with the examiner. Physicians who perform digital rectal examinations in adults, for example, know that with coaching and relaxation a patient can relax the sphincter to allow entry of a finger or an instrument. Children who have had repeated rectal examinations, or frequent enemas or other instrumentation, may also learn to inhibit contraction of the sphincter. It follows that failure to observe a strong wink, or the ability to relax the sphincter during observation or digital examination, is a nonspecific finding that may have many interpretations.

Some children tighten the anus when the buttocks are spread, and others relax it slightly, often allowing a small amount of flatus to escape. Both of these reactions are probably normal (23). If traction is applied to the perirectal skin to "test" the sphincter, the mucocutaneous junction of the anal canal can often easily be seen in normal individuals because it is actually just at or below the bottom edge of the sphincter muscles. McCann et al. (26) in their study of children thought not to be abused provide the only data regarding how far the anus should normally open when the buttocks are spread. In that study, more than half the children would gradually relax the sphincter if gentle traction was maintained for a sufficient time (average about 60 sec). The degree of relaxation frequently fluctuated during the exam. McCann's team observed rectal openings, when the examinations were conducted in the knee chest position, of up to 2 cm measured anterior-posteriorly (average 1 cm). Putting McCann's observations together with those of Paul (23), one could develop the following criteria for judging whether a child's rectum might be abnormally dilated:

- large diameter (> 2 cm) in the absence of stool in the rectal ampulla
- asymmetry of the anus when dilated
- apparently fixed opening—no gradual relaxation or fluctuation in diameter observed
- thickening and smoothing of the skin of the anal verge (although smoothing alone, during relaxation, is probably normal, reflecting only relaxation of the underlying muscles)

- decreased "grip" on digital exam (if one believes that digital exams are appropriate in cases of suspected sexual abuse).

If the child is willing or able to talk about what has happened, he or she should be asked in an open ended, nonleading way about discomfort or pain associated with the incident of abuse. Anal penetration is usually painful both initially and on withdrawal. This pain is often sharp, and children sometimes will report that the assailant "put a knife in my rear." This may sometimes actually be the case, but it is important to ask the child if a knife or other sharp object was actually seen. The discrepancy between this type of account and a finding of only minor or no lasting trauma often serve erroneously to discredit the child's statement. Clinicians can help by explaining the probable source of the child's perception. There is usually a dull aching sensation after anal penetration, or continued sharp pain if there has been more extensive trauma. Even with minimal trauma, there may be pain on defecation for 2 or 3 weeks, sometimes accompanied by a change in bowel habits.

If it is not appropriate to ask about the incident of abuse, or if one has not yet been disclosed, it is still important to enquire about other rectal symptoms such as burning or pain on defecation, passing blood, or problems with large, hard stools or chronic constipation. These questions can be asked as they would be normally, by asking about the frequency of defecation and medications or enemas that may have been administered. Changes in bowel habits are also of potential significance, as are episodes of encopresis after toilet training or apparent leakage of stool.

The perirectal exam must be more than a "quick look." Relaxation and good lighting are vital. The child should initially be assured that the exam will be totally external and not painful. He or she may be comfortable in a variety of positions including supine, bent over prone (standing or on a special proctoscopy table) or on the side. The knee-chest position also offers good visibility but may be the most embarrassing.

When the child is relaxed the buttocks can be spread gently and the configuration and reaction of the anus observed. As discussed above, either a reflex tightening or gentle relaxation is probably normal. If there is any doubt about the competency of the sphincter, the perirectal skin can be stimulated to provoke a wink, but a negative response in a relaxed child may not have great meaning. The anus itself should be a relatively uniform anterior-posterior slit, surrounded by a symmetrical area of hyperpigmented skin. The buttocks themselves should be examined for bruises and scars.

The perirectal skin should be examined for redness, scars, hemorrhoids, skin tags, fissures, ulcers, or warts. Irritation may be secondary to poor hygiene or pinworm infection. The folds of the anal verge can be gently spread tangentially to look for shallow fissures or scars that may not be immediately visible. Inspection and gentle palpation of the skin around the anal verge, especially anteriorly, may reveal bulging or tenderness suggestive of a perirectal abscess or fistula. Finally, traction on either side of the anal verge will allow inspection of the most distal portion of the anal canal, possibly revealing other hemorrhoids either external or internal (if they have prolapsed).

For most children with a normal examination, or with no findings suggestive of chronic abuse, no further inspection may be performed. A digital examination is not likely to yield any further information, except, perhaps, if there is reason to suspect a vaginal foreign body that might be felt through the anterior wall of the rectum. If there is reason to suspect serious acute or complicated chronic injury (perforation, fistula, foreign body), a specialist should be consulted for an examination with an appropriate instrument, probably under anesthesia.

When chronic abuse is suspected, but no acute injury is present, a digital exam may be the easiest way to determine the extent of stretching and decrease in strength, or alternatively the extent of scarring. The digital exam is best performed with a gloved, lubricated finger (29). Gentle pressure should be exerted with the ball of the finger, not the tip. Older children can be asked to bear down as if they were going to the bathroom. They should be warned that they may feel as if they are about to defecate but that this is not the case. As the sphincter relaxes, the finger can be rotated forward so that the tip enters first. If relaxation fails to occur, or there is tightening, waiting for a moment with the finger in place and reassuring the child may help. Once the finger is inserted, it can be rotated gently to assess first the uniformity of the superficial portion of the external sphincter and then the deep portion of the sphincter and the wall of the rectum.

FORENSIC PROCEDURES IN CASES OF SEXUAL ABUSE OR ASSAULT

When abuse or assault has taken place within 48 to 72 hours, it may be possible to detect materials from the abuser on the victim's body or clothing. This may provide important evidence to demonstrate that abuse has taken place and may sometimes help to identify the abuser. Procedures must be carefully followed to adequately collect and preserve available evidence.

Clothing

If the victim is still wearing the clothing worn at the time of the assault, he or she should stand on a large, clean cloth or paper sheet and remove all clothing. The clothing should be wrapped in the sheet, taking care not to spill any small objects that may have fallen onto it, and the bundle labelled and safely stored until it can be handed over to a police laboratory.

Examination for Traces of Semen

Finding traces of semen on a victim's body or clothing can be strong evidence that sexual contact of some kind took place. A first goal is to demonstrate that semen is present, and a second is to isolate genetic markers in the semen that may be linked with a particular perpetrator.

Examination for Semen on Skin

Victims may have semen from the abuser on their skin, often at sites adjacent to target areas for sexual contact. Ultraviolet (UV) light, which causes semen to fluoresce, can be used to aid detection. After a thorough explanation of the procedure, the room can be partially darkened. A few moments are required for the examiner's eyes to adapt to the dark. The UV light can be used to examine the thighs, buttocks, lower abdomen, chest, and lower face. Secretions may also be found in the hair, especially if the victim has tried to spit out ejaculate. If positive areas are found they can be swabbed with saline-moistened swabs that should be air-dried and put into empty, sterile blood collecting tubes or a clean paper envelope. If sealed tubes are used, the swabs must be totally dry to avoid overgrowth of contaminants. Alternatively, if preferred by the local forensic laboratory, the swabs can be immediately frozen instead of being dried. This may help preserve the activity of prostatic enzymes that can be used to identify the material as semen.

Semen is usually identified by looking microscopically for sperm and biochemically for enzymes and other proteins in the ejaculate. Both processes should be applied in all cases: as will be discussed below, the factors that influence retrieval of sperm and other seminal components act in a very variable manner. It is not unusual for sperm to be found in the absence of enzymes or vice versa. (Some abusers and rapists may be impotent, so that even finding no evidence of semen does not rule out genital contact.)

Sperm

Although, normal male ejaculate can contain hundreds of millions of sperm, much smaller numbers are recovered from the vagina, even immediately after intercourse. In addition, the concentration of sperm in any individual's ejaculate may be decreased by elevated testicular temperature, chronic alcohol intake or procedures such as vasectomy.

Sperm recovered from the vagina shortly after sexual contact may still be observed to be moving when examined in wet preparations. The outer limit for finding motile sperm in adult vaginal secretions is often given as eight hours (30), although studies report a great deal of variation. Twelve hours appears to be the longest survival generally reported (31). Nonmotile sperm can be found for much longer periods, with reports ranging from 14 to 26 hours (30,32,33). These figures are all for sperm that, while nonmotile, are morphologically intact. Sperm without tails may be identified for considerably longer (33), but it may be harder to differentiate them from yeasts, debris, or other similar-size objects. Identification of intact sperm is more convincing forensic evidence (34).

Sperm may be found in other body sites besides the vagina. They can survive in the cervix for up to several days after sexual contact, or for a period of hours on the perineal skin. Survival in the anus and rectum is much shorter than the cervix or vagina: Whole sperm can usually be found for only a few hours, although pieces, if they can be properly identified, may be present for up to 2 days (33). In females, small numbers of sperm found in the anus or perirectal area may be contaminants from the vagina (34). Sperm may also be recovered from the oral cavity and surrounding skin. If the index of suspicion for oral sex is high, separate swabs should be taken from the perioral skin, the gums, the tongue, and the pharynx. The gums may be an especially good source. Their protected location in the mouth allows sperm to be retained there for several hours after contact, sometimes despite of the use of mouthwashes or toothbrushing.

A variety of techniques are described for obtaining specimens to examine for sperm. Some clinicians feel that wet preparations are generally not useful (32) because of the variable motility of sperm. Dried, stained smears may be more sensitive, and the have the advantage of creating a permanent record that other observers may examine. Swabs soaked with material to be examined can be immersed in 1 or 2 ml of saline or distilled water, or a portion of the swab can be cut off and dropped into the fluid so that the rest of the swab can be used for biochemical analysis (33). The fluid and swab are agitated to release sperm and then a drop of fluid can be air-dried on a slide and either stained (with Giemsa or hematoxylin and eosin) or processed as a cytopathology specimen.

Biochemical Markers

Semen contains several enzymes and other proteins that can be used to demonstrate its presence in vaginal fluids. The most commonly used biochemical marker for semen is the enzyme acid phosphatase (ACP) which is produced in the prostate. Small amounts of ACP are present in normal adult vaginal secretions, but at levels that are 100–1,000 times smaller than in semen. ACP is measured in international units (IU), with one IU equal to the amount of enzyme required to metabolize one micromole of substrate in 1 min. Several quantitative methods are available to measure ACP activity.

Given the excess of ACP in semen compared to vaginal secretions, it would seem simple to use analysis of ACP in vaginal fluids to detect recent intercourse. Unfortunately, ACP activity diminishes rapidly in the vagina, although it is relatively stable on dry materials such as cloth if kept cool, dark, and relatively acid (35). In the vagina, activity related to prostatic ACP may not be distinguishable from normal vaginal enzyme after about 72 hr following intercourse.

Establishing cut-off values for inferring the presence of prostatic ACP, and determining the rate with which activity decays so that the time of coitus can be estimated, have been hampered by the fact that various collection and assay methods yield different dilutions of specimens and thus different values for "normal." In addition, normal adult vaginal ACP levels do not have a Gaussian (or "bell-shaped") distribution. The distribution of activity levels is log normal; that is, most women have relatively low levels of activity, but a small proportion of have relatively high levels. Pooling data from several studies, Sensabaugh (36) calculated that the 99% upper confidence limit for normal vaginal ACP activity is about 6.6 times a laboratory's average normal vaginal level using a consistent collection technique. For example, if the average ACP activity in adult females is 25 IU/L, a level of about 165 IU/L represents a 99% confidence upper limit of normal. ACP levels higher than this point would be presumed to be caused by the presence of prostatic enzyme. Sensabaugh also calculated multipliers to obtain 99% confidence intervals for estimated ACP activity for various time periods between coitus and when a sample is taken.

Other Tests Potentially Useful for Identifying Assailant

The following procedures may not be required in many cases and, with the exception of the first, can usually be postponed until after the initial examination. The clinician should consult with a police laboratory official or a designated sexual assault center to decide if collection is necessary.

Combings for Hair Samples

It may be useful to search for abuser's hair that has become adherent to the patient's body. If the patient has pubic hair it can be gently combed onto a piece of clean filter paper that is then carefully folded and placed in a labelled envelope for delivery to the police. If the patient struggled with and scratched the assailant, scrapings from under the fingernails may contain tissue useful in identifying the assailant or corroborating the history of struggle. Collection of blood or saliva from the patient may also be useful in differentiating his or her secretions from those of the assailant.

Identification of specific abusers from hair, blood, or semen samples has, until the present, been a difficult and often frustrating task. Most presently available testing has been based on a search for polymorphisms in blood group markers and serum proteins. Although several markers and proteins can be examined (fewer for semen than for blood or other tissues), patterns of variation cannot uniquely identify individuals. It can often be said that only one person in 100 or 1,000 would have a similar pattern of polymorphisms, but these odds are frequently not small enough to be the sole evidence linking a particular individual with a particular crime (37). This situation has been radically altered by the availability of genetic "fingerprinting" techniques based on detection of polymorphisms in human DNA (38).

"CHAIN OF EVIDENCE" FOR MEDICOLEGAL SPECIMENS

It is vital that a "chain of evidence" be maintained for sexually transmitted disease and other laboratory specimens associated with a case of suspected child abuse of any kind. The "chain" is a written record assuring that the specimen which arrived in the laboratory for analysis was the same specimen taken from the patient. Although a medical facility's standard procedures are usually adequate for social service and juvenile court proceedings, they may be challenged and provide a handy defense for an abuser should a case be heard in a criminal court.

The chain may be carried out in many ways. A slip may accompany each specimen and contain spaces for the name and signature of each person handling the specimen (person collecting, transporting, evaluating) with the corresponding date and time handled. Alternatively, the clinician may describe the specimens collected in the medical record, carry them him or herself to the laboratory, and ask the technician to sign the record stating that the specimens were received and giving any laboratory number that may be assigned to them. Specimens collected for the police laboratory may be placed in a locked cabinet or "black box." When a police representative comes to collect the box, he or she should be asked to co-sign a slip describing the box's contents, and the date and time of transfer.

REFERENCES

1. Russell AB, Trainor CM. *Trends in child abuse and neglect: a national perspective*. Denver: The American Humane Association, 1984:Table A-IV-3.
2. Daro D. *Confronting child abuse: research for effective program design*. New York: The Free Press, 1988.
3. Peters SD, Wyatt GE, Finkelhor D. Prevalence. In: Finkelhor D, ed. *A sourcebook on child sexual abuse*. Beverly Hills: Sage Publications, 1986;15–59.
4. White S, Halpin BM, Strom GA, Santilli G. Behavioral comparisons of young sexually abused, neglected and nonreferred children. *J Clin Psychol* 1988;17:53–61.
5. Dube R, Herbert M. Sexual abuse of children under 12 years of age; a review or 511 cases. *Child Abuse Negl* 1988;12:321–30.
6. Trube-Becker E. Bite-marks on battered children. *Z Rechtsmed* 1977;79:73–8.
7. Committee on Early Childhood, Adoption, and Dependent Care. Oral and dental aspects of child abuse and neglect. *Pediatrics* 1986;78: 537–9.
8. Elam AL, Ray VG. Sexually related trauma: a review. *Ann Emerg Med* 1986;15:576–84.
9. McCann J, Voris J, Simon M, Wells R. Comparison of genital examination techniques in prepubertal girls. *Pediatrics* 1990;85:182–7.
10. McCann J, Wells R, Simon M, Voris J. Genital findings in prepubertal girls selected for nonabuse: a descriptive study. *Pediatrics* 1990; 86:428–39.
11. Ricci LR. Medical forensic photography of the sexually abused child. *Child Abuse Negl* 1988; 12:305–10.
12. Emans SJ, Woods ER, Flagg NT, Freeman A. Genital findings in sexually abused, symptomatic, and asymptomatic girls. *Pediatrics* 1987; 79:778–85.
13. Berkowitz CD, Elvik SL, Logan MK. Labial fusion in prepubescent girls: a marker for sexual abuse? *Am J Obstet Gynecol* 1987;156:16–20.
14. Bays J, Jenny C. Genital and anal conditions confused with child sexual abuse trauma. *Am J Dis Child* 1990;144:1319–22.
15. Jenny C, Kuhns MLD, Arakawa F. Hymens in newborn female infants. *Pediatrics* 1987;80: 399–400.
16. Pokorny SF. Configuration of the prepubertal hymen. *Am J Obstet Gynecol* 1987;157:950–6.
17. Cantwell HB. Vaginal inspection as it relates to child sexual abuse in girls under thirteen. *Child Abuse Negl* 1983;7:171–6.
18. Cantwell HB. Update on vaginal inspection as it relates to child sexual abuse in girls under thirteen. *Child Abuse Negl* 1987;11:545–6.
19. Chadwick DL, Berkowitz CD, Kerns DL, McCann J, Reinhart MA, Strickland SL. *Color atlas of child sexual abuse*. Chicago: Year Book Medical Publishers, 1989.
20. Wynne JM. Injuries to the genitalia in female children. *S Afr Med J* 1980;57:47–50.
21. Herman-Giddens ME, Frothingham TE. Prepubertal female genitalia: examination for evidence of sexual abuse. *Pediatrics* 1987;80: 203–8.
22. Cowell CA. The gynecologic examination of infants, children, and young adolescents. *Pediatr Clin North Am* 1981;28:247–66.
23. Paul DM. "What really did happen to baby Jane?"—the medical aspects of the investigation of alleged sexual abuse of children. *Med Sci Law* 1986;26:85–102.
24. Paul DM. The medical examination in sexual offences against children. *Med Sci Law* 1977; 17:251–8.
25. Hobbs CJ, Wynne JM, Buggery in childhood—a common syndrome of child abuse. *Lancet* 1986;2:792–8.
26. McCann J, Voris J, Simon M, Wells R. Perianal findings in prepubertal children selected for non-

abuse: a descriptive study. *Child Abuse Negl* 1989;13:179–93.

27. Wright C, Fraser EM, Denman M, Duke L. Detection of sexual abuse in children [Letter]. *Lancet* 1987;2:218.
28. Storer EH, Goldberg SM, Nivatvongs S. Colon, rectum, and anus. In: Schwartz SI, ed. *Principles of surgery*. 2nd ed. New York: McGraw-Hill, 1974.
29. Seidel HM, Ball JW, Dains JE, Benedict GW. *Mosby's guide to physical examination*. St. Louis: C.V. Mosby, 1987:471–89.
30. Rupp JC. Sperm survival and prostatic acid phosphatase activity in victims of sexual assault. *J Forensic Sci* 1969;14:177–83.
31. Bach CM. *Medical-legal consultation*. Seattle, Washington: Harborview Medical Center, August, 1980.
32. Dahlke MB, Cooke C, Cunnane M, Chawla J, Lau P. Identification of semen in 500 patients seen because of rape. *Am J Clin Pathol* 1977;68:740–6.
33. Willott GM, Allard JE. Spermatozoa—their persistence after sexual intercourse. *Forensic Sci Int* 1982;19:135–54.
34. Enos WF, Beyer JC. Spermatozoa in the anal canal and rectum and in the oral cavity of female rape victims. *J Forensic Sci* 1978;23:231–3.
35. Findley TP. Quantitation of vaginal acid phosphatase and its relationship to time of coitus. *Am J Clin Pathol* 1977;68:238–42.
36. Sensabaugh GF. The quantitative acid phosphatase test. A statistical analysis of endogenous and postcoital acid phosphatase levels in the vagina. *J Forensic Sci* 1979;24:346–65.
37. Tribe LH. Trial by mathematics: precision and ritual in the legal process. *Harvard Law Rev* 1971;B4:1329.
38. Gill P, Jeffreys AJ, Werrett DJ. Forensic applications of DNA "fingerprints." *Nature* 1985; 318:577–9.
39. Wissow, LS. *Child advocacy for the clinician*. Williams & Wilkins, Baltimore, 1990.

Pediatric and Adolescent Gynecology,
edited by S. E. Carpenter and J. A. Rock.
Raven Press, Ltd., New York © 1992.

29

Gynecologic Care for the Mentally Handicapped Individual

Sue Ellen Koehler Carpenter

Department of Obstetrics and Gynecology, Division of Reproductive Endocrinology, The Johns Hopkins School of Medicine, Baltimore, Maryland 21205

There is a great need to provide quality gynecologic care to mentally handicapped individuals. In general, these individuals now have greater life expectancy than previously. Those with mild to moderate retardation are being encouraged to fulfill their highest potential by living in society at large or in sheltered situations with a high degree of normalization. Severely affected individuals, who might have succumbed at a young age to the medical complications of their disorder, are living through puberty and surviving their parents. Issues of sexuality, contraception, menstrual hygiene, and premenstrual syndrome with severe behavioral disorders can become important. Management of common gynecologic disorders such as vaginal discharge, dysfunctional uterine bleeding, and pelvic pain becomes difficult due to limitations in communication and examination. At Johns Hopkins and other locations, multispecialty clinics have been created to serve these patients (1).

MENSTRUAL HYGIENE

Issues of menstrual hygiene are common. Frequently, behavior modification successfully trains mildly and moderately retarded women. These programs may be less successful for profoundly affected patients unless toilet training has been successful previously (2). Oral contraceptives can be useful for limiting the volume of menstrual flow. Alternatively, menstrual suppression with depo-medroxyprogesterone acetate 150 mg IM every 3 months can be used. Hysterectomy must be reserved for patients with documented failure of training programs, gynecologic disease, severe anemia, or contraindications to hormonal therapy. A case of hepatitis-positive blood being spattered uncontrollably (one could imagine HIV-positive blood as well) and posing a substantial threat to housemates and caregivers has been reported to justify a hysterectomy (3). Dysfunctional uterine bleeding will certainly exacerbate problems of hygiene. Dysfunctional bleeding should be evaluated as it would be in the general population. Obesity and thyroid dysfunction, which occur commonly in Down's syndrome, may predispose those patients to abnormal uterine bleeding. Accurate menstrual records should be kept. Alterations in previously normal cycles may herald other medical conditions.

PREMENSTRUAL SYNDROME

Premenstrual syndrome with exacerbation of autism, temper tantrums, irritability, restlessness, disobedient behavior, and seizure activity has been noted. The value of an accurate menstrual calendar for interpreting these behavioral changes is obvious. Some behavior problems reflect dysmenorrhea, which severely handicapped persons are unable to communicate. This will respond to timely, generous administration of nonsteroidal antiinflammatory drugs. Others may respond to low-dose oral contraceptives or depo-medroxyprogesterone acetate. If GnRH analogs catch on for treatment of PMS in the general population, they are likely to be useful for patients with cyclic severe behavioral disorders (4).

SEXUALITY

Issues surrounding sexual behavior are best dealt with in group educational and individual counseling sessions. Individuals who are integrated into the community often cannot interpret media representations of sexual behavior. They need help understanding the nature of appropriate relationships and learning to take responsibility for their actions. They must be taught to avoid situations that could lead to sexual abuse. Parent groups focus on helping parents learn to accept their children's sexuality and establish realistic goals for the maturing family member. More severely affected persons need limitations placed on unacceptable public displays of sexual behaviors and sexual self-abuse.

CONTRACEPTION

Providing adequate contraception can be difficult. Oral contraceptives and barrier methods demand a level of compliance that may be beyond the scope of an individual's abilities. However, oral contraceptives can be supervised by caregiver. The intrauterine device may be appropriate in a few cases; however, they will be unacceptable to the extent that they increase dysmenorrhea and menstrual flow. Sterilization is the focus of immense legal and societal debate. Depo-medroxyprogesterone has been used secondarily for contraception. The new contraceptive, Norplant, may find a very significant role in this population. Norplant does not carry the contraindications of estrogen-containing oral contraceptives. Its greatest single side effect is breakthrough bleeding, which is minimal in volume and may be acceptable to these patients and their caregivers.

STERILIZATION

The question of involuntary sterilization inevitably arises in a clinic where patients with mental retardation who are deemed incapable of giving informed consent are seen. The history of the procedure in the United States dates from the turn-of-the-century when the eugenics movement advocated involuntary sterilization to avoid genetic transmission of mental retardation. In 1927, the Supreme Court affirmed the constitutionality of eugenic sterilization in an opinion on *Buck vs. Bell* written by Justice Oliver Wendell Holmes: "It is better for all the world if instead of waiting to execute degenerative offspring for crime or let them starve of their imbecility, society can prevent those who are manifestly unfit from continuing their kind . . . three generations of imbeciles are enough" (5).

Today, most readers of the opinion of Justice Holmes would find it very disturbing. However, the decision set the stage for a 15-year period during which 37 states passed eugenic sterilization legislation. In 1942, the Supreme Court, with a completely different membership, heard *Skinner vs. Oklahoma*. Skinner had been convicted three times of shoplifting and other similar offenses. Under the Oklahoma habitual criminal sterilization act, anyone convicted of specific crimes (including larceny) would be sterilized. The law excluded other equally serious offenses. Skinner argued that this differential treatment violated his right to equal protection. The opinion of the Supreme Court held the Oklahoma statute unconstitutional. In the words of Justice Douglas, "We are dealing here with legislation which involves one of the basic civil rights of man. Marriage and procreation are fundamental to the very existence and survival of the human race. The power to sterilize, if exercised, may have subtle, far reaching and devastating effects . . . there is no redemption for the individual whom the law touches . . . He is forever deprived of a basic liberty" (6).

The Skinner decision set the stage for the current debate on involuntary sterilization. The physician is placed in a difficult position when a patient and her family seem to have a reasonable request for sterilization because the individual cannot or does not wish to meet the demands of child rearing. Vining and Freeman (7) have appealed for a moderate approach that is guided by the level of retardation of the patient. In some cases, the level of supervision required for the severely affected patient makes sexual activity and, thus, the fear of pregnancy unreasonable. In the case of mildly retarded individuals who are able to marry and maintain themselves in the community, sterilization should not be an issue. For a middle group, living in a sheltered situation, increased efforts at normalization have led to acceptance of the right to sexual satisfaction, and sterilization may offer the best chance for normalcy. Advocacy for individual rights should include the possibility of obtaining sterilization under circumstances where the procedure allows patients to best fulfill their own potential.

Currently, the physician liability issues with regard to involuntary sterilization depend upon state laws. There are three categories to consider: (a) potential liability when a state statute authorizes involuntary sterilization, (b) liability when a court orders sterilization at the request of the guardian without a specific statute, and (c) liability when there is no statute or court order (8). Approximately 19 states now have legislation enabling sterilization of mentally incompetent persons. The statutes have generally been upheld if they contain enough procedural protection for the patient. The New Jersey court invoked the *parens patriae* doctrine to order sterilization (9). The purpose of the doctrine is to protect the rights of mental incompetents. The judge interpreted sterilization as a procedure to which the patient had a right when it was clearly in her best interest. The court sought to protect that right. In some states where there is no statute, it may be possible to obtain a court order for sterilization when due process and equal protection under the law are emphasized. Other state courts have been unwilling to conclude that there is anything in their common law powers that enables them to mandate sterilization.

The substituted consent of parents alone, without a valid court order, will not suffice. The current attitude of the courts in such cases implies that physicians incur tremendous liability if they perform such procedures.

Rauh (10) has pleaded for a moderate approach to the issue: for a statute that would enable sterilization under specific circumstances. Applications would be reviewed by local courts or hospital review committees (10). Rauh's proposed model statute would include the following:

1. The individual is presumed capable of procreation.
2. The individual is or is likely to be sexually active.
3. Pregnancy would not usually be intended by a competent person facing analogous choices.
4. All alternative contraceptive methods have proved unworkable or been shown inapplicable.
5. The individual's guardian agrees that sterilization is the best course of action in the case.
6. Comprehensive medical, psychological, and social evaluations recommend sterilization for the individual.
7. The individual is represented by independent legal counsel with demonstrated competence in dealing with medical, legal, social, and ethical issues involving sterilization.
8. The individual, regardless of her level of competence, has been informed in full by one able to make her understand and up to her level of competence shows awareness of the method of sterilization, the consequences of sterilization, the likelihood of success, alternative methods of sterilization and birth control, and the consequences of pregnancy and parenthood.

HYSTERECTOMY

Frequently, patients' families present to the clinic with requests for hysterectomy. This must be considered on an individual basis. The least harmful form of care consistent with the patients' best interest should be employed. Families sometimes present with this request even before menstruation begins or when the patient is amenorrheic. Patients often have significant medical risks for surgery, which the family does not consider in their request. The family's specific concerns must be addressed with sensitivity, practical advice, and assurances of support. Questions of menstrual hygiene should be answered with adequate training programs and medication as needed. Contraception should be provided. Information that hysterectomy will not ameliorate PMS or prevent sexual abuse should be presented. Parent support groups and social work intervention may be encouraged. At times, a parent requests hysterectomy as part of a larger, sometimes overwhelming, agenda dealing with the physical, emotional, and financial demand that the maturing dependent places upon the family.

McNeeley and Elkins (11) have reported on their experience with major gynecologic surgery in 15 mentally handicapped women. The indications for hysterectomy were menorrhagia (n = 3), leiomyomata (n = 9), and ovarian neoplasm (n = 3). All decisions for major surgery or sterilization in their clinic are presented to a societally based committee prior to admission (12). Six of the 13 women undergoing major abdominal surgery in this series developed significant complications. All three quadriplegic patients with cerebral palsy developed aspiration pneumonia. Pelvic cellulitis occurred in one case. Urinary tract infection and fecal impaction occurred in two others—one with associated small bowel obstruction. In this report, another 22 minor procedures including dilatation and curettage, and laparoscopic sterilization were performed without incident. Abdominal hysterectomy for sterilization alone is certainly contraindicated by its increased morbidity. Most of the patients in this series presented with advanced gynecologic pathology probably due to the difficulty of providing routine gynecologic examinations in this population.

ROUTINE EXAMINATION

The initial evaluation of patients with mental retardation who present for routine gynecologic care should include a complete medical history, a gynecologic history with a menstrual calendar if available, and a physical examination. A recent social work evaluation and psychological evaluation (with IQ testing) should also be available. A pelvic examination should be performed if possible, and a pap smear obtained in patients with abnormal vaginal bleeding or vaginal discharge, patients over age 30, or patients who are sexually active. When pelvic examination cannot be performed, a pelvic ultrasound may be a useful alternative. However, in some cases, sonogram will not be an adequate alternative to examination under anesthesia. At the University of Michigan, an anesthesiologist is available in the clinic one day each month to provide sedation, which allows otherwise impossible examinations to be performed (13).

Routine complaints such as vaginal discharge require a practical approach. Urinary frequency, crying on urination, or foul smelling urine suggest a urinary tract infection. Anal itching suggests the presence of pinworms. Vulvar irritation can result from or cause excessive masturbatory behavior. Hypoestrogenism may be a cause of discomfort, especially if hygiene is difficult. This responds to a regimen of frequent sitz baths, air drying, and soothing ointment such as Balmex. Hydrocortisone cream 1% may be used as well. Recent antibiotic use or a thick white discharge suggest Candida infection and an empiric trial of an antifungal agent is appropriate. If the discharge is persistent or recurrent, a complete pelvic examination to rule out foreign body and obtain complete cultures for Candida, gonorrhea, chlamydia, strep, and fecal pathogens is required. A saline prep should be examined for trichomonas and gardnerella. Appropriate treatment is then instituted. If cultures are positive for a sexually transmitted disease, an RPR and HIV testing along with an investigation for sexual abuse may be required if consensual sexual activity cannot be confirmed.

In summary, the gynecologic care of mentally retarded adolescents requires special care. It is best provided by individuals with an interest in the field and the ability to consider the patient's unique medical and social circumstances when providing services. A common sense approach to the patient's best interests is needed. The breadth of experience in the academic center clinics may be informative for those who provide community-based care for these special patients.

REFERENCES

1. Elkins TE, Gafford LS, Wilks CS, Muram D, Golden G. A model clinic approach to the reproductive health concerns of the mentally handicapped. *Obstet Gynecol* 1986;68:185–8.
2. Kreutner AK. Sexuality, fertility and the problems of menstruation in mentally retarded adolescents. *Pediatr Clin North Am* 1981;28:275.
3. Elkins TE, McNeeley SG, Punch M, Kope S, Heaton C. Reproductive health concerns in Down syndrome. *J Reprod Med* 1990;35:745–50.
4. Muse KN, Cetel NS, Futterman LA, Yen SSC. The premenstrual syndrome: effects of "medical oophorectomy." *N Engl J Med* 1984;311:1345–9.
5. *Buck v Bell* 274, U.S. 200, U.S. Supreme Court, 1927.
6. *Skinner v Oklahoma* 36, U.S. 535, U.S. Supreme Court, 1942.
7. Vining EPG, Freeman JM. Sterilization and the retarded female: is advocacy depriving individuals of their rights? *Pediatrics* 1978;62:850–3.
8. Letterie GS, Fox WF. *Fertil Steril* 1990;53: 391–8.
9. In *re Grady*, 85 NJ 235, 426 A. 2d. 467, 1981.
10. Rauh JL, Dine MS, Biro FM, Rauh TD. Sterilization for the mentally retarded adolescent. *J Adolesc Health Care* 1989;10:467–72.
11. McNeeley SG, Elkins TE. Gynecologic surgery and surgical morbidity in mentally handicapped women. *Obstet Gynecol* 1989;74:155–8.
12. Elkins TE, Strong C, Wolfe AR, Brown D. An ethics committee in a reproductive health clinic for mentally handicapped persons. *Hastings Cent Rep* 1986;16:20–2.
13. Elkins TE, McNeeley SG, Rosen D. A clinical observation of a program to accomplish pelvic exams in difficult-to-manage patients with mental retardation. *Adolesc Pediatr Gynecol* 1988; 1:195–8.

Subject Index

B